THE NETTER COLLECTION
OF MEDICAL ILLUSTRATIONS

Nervous System

Part II—Spinal Cord and Peripheral Motor and Sensory Systems

3rd Edition

VOLUME 7

A compilation of paintings prepared by **FRANK H. NETTER, MD**

Edited by

Michael J. Aminoff, MD, DSc, FRCP
Distinguished Professor Emeritus
Department of Neurology
School of Medicine
University of California
San Francisco, California

Scott L. Pomeroy, MD, PhD
Bronson Crothers Professor of Neurology
Harvard Medical School
Chair, Department of Neurology
Neurologist-in-Chief
Boston Children's Hospital
Boston, Massachusetts

Kerry H. Levin, MD
Professor of Neurology
Cleveland Clinic Lerner College of Medicine of Case Western
Reserve University
Chairman, Department of Neurology
Director, Neuromuscular Center
Cleveland Clinic
Cleveland, Ohio

Additional Illustrations by

Carlos A.G. Machado, MD

CONTRIBUTING ILLUSTRATORS
John A. Craig, MD
Tiffany S. DaVanzo, MA, CMI
DragonFly Media
Anita Impagliazzo, MA, CMI
Paul Kim, MS
Kristen W. Marzejon, CMI
James A. Perkins, MS, MFA

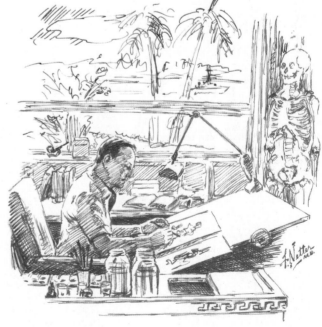

Self portrait by Dr. Netter

ELSEVIER

Elsevier
1600 John F. Kennedy Blvd.
Suite 1600
Philadelphia, Pennsylvania

THE NETTER COLLECTION OF MEDICAL ILLUSTRATIONS: NERVOUS SYSTEM,
PART II: SPINAL CORD AND PERIPHERAL MOTOR AND SENSORY SYSTEMS,
VOLUME 7, THIRD EDITION

ISBN: 978-0-323-88085-5

Notices

Knowledge and best practice in this field are constantly changing. As new research and experience broaden our understanding, changes in research methods, professional practices, or medical treatment may become necessary.

Practitioners and researchers must always rely on their own experience and knowledge in evaluating and using any information, methods, compounds, or experiments described herein. In using such information or methods they should be mindful of their own safety and the safety of others, including parties for whom they have a professional responsibility.

With respect to any drug or pharmaceutical products identified, readers are advised to check the most current information provided (i) on procedures featured or (ii) by the manufacturer of each product to be administered, to verify the recommended dose or formula, the method and duration of administration, and contraindications. It is the responsibility of practitioners, relying on their own experience and knowledge of their patients, to make diagnoses, to determine dosages and the best treatment for each individual patient, and to take all appropriate safety precautions.

To the fullest extent of the law, neither the Publisher nor the authors, contributors, or editors, assume any liability for any injury and/or damage to persons or property as a matter of products liability, negligence or otherwise, or from any use or operation of any methods, products, instructions, or ideas contained in the material herein.

Publisher: Elyse O'Grady
Senior Content Strategist: Marybeth Thiel
Publishing Services Manager: Catherine Jackson
Senior Project Manager/Specialist: Carrie Stetz
Book Design: Patrick Ferguson

Printed in India

Last digit is the print number: 9 8 7 6 5 4 3 2 1

Working together
to grow libraries in
developing countries

www.elsevier.com • www.bookaid.org

"Clarification is the goal. No matter how beautifully it is painted, a medical illustration has little value if it does not make clear a medical point."

—Frank H. Netter, MD

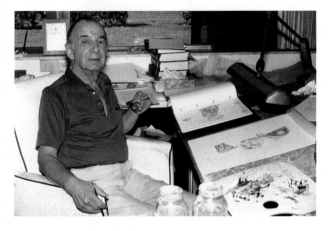

Dr. Frank Netter at work.

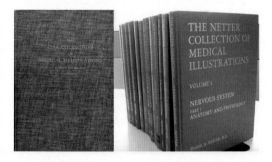

The single-volume "Blue Book" that preceded the multivolume *Netter Collection of Medical Illustrations* series, affectionately known as the "Green Books."

The Netter Collection
OF MEDICAL ILLUSTRATIONS
3rd Edition

Dr. Frank Netter created an illustrated legacy unifying his perspectives as physician, artist, and teacher. Both his greatest challenge and greatest success was charting a middle course between artistic clarity and instructional complexity. That success is captured in *The Netter Collection,* beginning in 1948 when the first comprehensive book of Netter's work was published by CIBA Pharmaceuticals. It met with such success that over the following 40 years the collection was expanded into an 8-volume series—with each title devoted to a single body system. Between 2011 and 2016, these books were updated and rereleased. Now, after another decade of innovation in medical imaging, renewed focus on patient-centered care, conscious efforts to improve inequities in healthcare and medical education, and a growing understanding of many clinical conditions, including multisystem effects of COVID-19, we are happy to make available a third edition of Netter's timeless work enhanced and informed by modern medical knowledge and context.

Inside the classic green covers, students and practitioners will find hundreds of original works of art. This is a collection of the human body in pictures—Dr. Netter called them *pictures,* never paintings. The latest expert medical knowledge is anchored by the sublime style of Frank Netter that has guided physicians' hands and nurtured their imaginations for more than half a century.

Noted artist-physician Carlos Machado, MD, the primary successor responsible for continuing the Netter tradition, has particular appreciation for the Green Book series. "*The Reproductive System* is of special significance for those who, like me, deeply admire Dr. Netter's work. In this volume, he masters the representation of textures of different surfaces, which I like to call 'the rhythm of the brush,' since it is the dimension, the direction of the strokes, and the interval separating them that create the illusion of given textures: organs have their external surfaces, the surfaces of their cavities, and texture of their parenchymas realistically represented. It set the style for the subsequent volumes of *The Netter Collection*—each an amazing combination of painting masterpieces and precise scientific information."

This third edition could not exist without the dedication of all those who edited, authored, or in other ways contributed to the second edition or the original books, nor, of course, without the excellence of Dr. Netter. For this third edition, we also owe our gratitude to the authors, editors, and artists whose relentless efforts were instrumental in adapting these classic works into reliable references for today's clinicians in training and in practice. From all of us with the Netter Publishing Team at Elsevier, thank you.

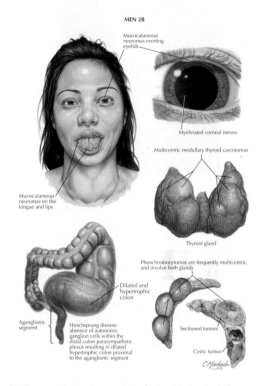

An illustrated plate painted by Carlos Machado, MD.

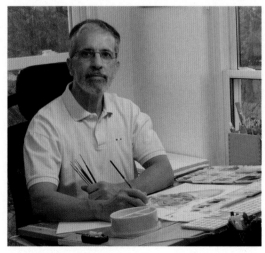

Dr. Carlos Machado at work.

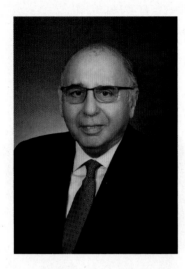

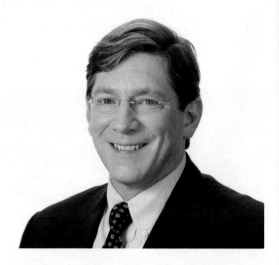

Michael J. Aminoff, MD, DSc, was born and educated in England, graduating from University College London in 1962 and from University College Hospital Medical School as a physician in 1965. He subsequently trained in neurology and clinical neurophysiology at The National Hospital for Neurology and Neurosurgery (Queen Square) in London and also undertook basic research on spinal physiology at its affiliated Institute of Neurology, which led to the award of an MD degree (which, in England, is an advanced medical degree based on research) on completion of his thesis. In 1974 he moved from England to the University of California San Francisco (UCSF) School of Medicine, where he became Professor of Neurology in 1982 and Distinguished Professor of Neurology in 2010 and is now Distinguished Professor Emeritus. He directed the Clinical Neurophysiology Laboratories at UCSF until July 2004 and then served as Executive Vice Chair of the Department of Neurology (2004–2017).

Dr. Aminoff is the author of over 240 original medical and scientific articles, more than 200 book chapters on neurologic topics, and the author or editor of numerous books, many of which have gone into several editions. His published scientific contributions led to the award of a Doctorate in Science (an advanced doctorate in the Faculty of Science) in 2000 by the University of London. He is the one of the two editors-in-chief of the four-volume *Encyclopedia of the Neurological Sciences*

published by Academic Press in 2003 (2nd edition, 2014). He is also one of the series editors of the prestigious multivolume *Handbook of Clinical Neurology* (Elsevier). He was Editor-in Chief of the journal *Muscle and Nerve* from 1998 to 2007 and also serves on numerous other editorial boards of medical and scientific journals. His other interests include medical history, and he has written biographies of Brown-Séquard (Raven Press, 1993; Oxford University Press, 2011), Sir Charles Bell (Oxford University Press, 2016), and Victor Horsley (Cambridge University Press, 2022).

The awards that he has received include the Lifetime Achievement Award of the American Association of Neuromuscular and Electrodiagnostic Medicine in 2006, the A.B. Baker Award of the American Academy of Neurology in 2007 for lifetime achievements and contributions to medical education, and the Robert S. Schwab Award for outstanding contributions to research in peripheral clinical neurophysiology from the American Clinical Neurophysiology Society in 2019. An endowed chair is to be named after him at UCSF, and a lectureship has been named for him within the Division of Neurology at Miami Neuroscience Institute, South Florida.

He served for 8 years as a director of the American Board of Psychiatry and Neurology, serving as chairman of the board in 2011. He is married, lives in San Francisco, and has a daughter who is a pediatrician and two sons who are attorneys.

Scott L. Pomeroy, MD, PhD, was born and educated in Southwest Ohio, graduating from Miami University in 1975 and the MD/PhD program of the University of Cincinnati in 1982. His doctoral research focused on brainstem neurophysiology and pain inhibition. After a pediatric residency at Boston Children's Hospital, he trained in child neurology at St. Louis Children's Hospital and studied nervous system development as a postdoctoral fellow of Dale Purves at Washington University in St. Louis, work for which he won the Child Neurology Society Young Investigator Award in 1989. After returning to Boston Children's Hospital and Harvard Medical School in 1991, he cofounded the neuro-oncology service and conducts basic research to understand how normal development of brain cells becomes derailed to cause childhood brain tumors. He currently is the Chair of the Department of Neurology and Neurologist-in-Chief of Boston Children's Hospital, the Bronson Crothers Professor of Neurology at Harvard Medical School, and Co-director of the Eunice K. Shriver National Institutes of Child Health and Human Development–funded Intellectual and Developmental Disabilities Research Center of Boston Children's Hospital and Harvard Medical School.

Dr. Pomeroy served as an editor of the second edition of this atlas and is one of four editors of the widely read textbook *Bradley and Daroff's Neurology in Clinical Practice* (Elsevier). He served as Associate Editor of *Annals of Neurology* from 2013 to 2021 and has served on the editorial boards of several other journals in the fields of neurology and neuro-oncology. He has contributed more than 200 peer-reviewed papers and book chapters.

Dr. Pomeroy has won numerous awards for his research and clinical care of children with brain tumors, including the Sidney Carter Award of the American Academy of Neurology, the Daniel Drake Medal of the University of Cincinnati College of Medicine, the Compassionate Caregiver Award of the Schwartz Center for Compassionate Healthcare, and the Bernard Sachs Award of the Child Neurology Society. He was elected as a member of the National Academy of Medicine in 2017. Dr. Pomeroy and his wife, Marie, live in Boston and spend much of their time devoted to their children and seven grandchildren, who live in Maryland and Colorado.

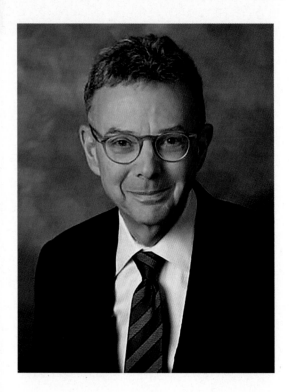

Kerry Levin, MD, graduated from the Johns Hopkins University School of Arts and Sciences in 1973 and the Johns Hopkins University School of Medicine in 1977. After an internal medicine residency at the Case Western Reserve University Hospitals of Cleveland, he completed a neurology residency at the Hospital of the University of Chicago and an EMG/Neuromuscular Fellowship at Mayo Clinic, Rochester, Minnesota.

Dr. Levin has practiced neurology and neuromuscular medicine at Cleveland Clinic since 1984. He has served as Director of the Neurology Residency Program and the Clinical Neurophysiology and Neuromuscular Medicine Fellowship programs. At Cleveland Clinic he has been Chair of the Department of Neurology since 2008 and Director of the Neuromuscular Center since 2006. He has authored and edited numerous publications and texts, including two clinical neurophysiology volumes of the *Handbook of Clinical Neurology* (Elsevier). He formerly served on the editorial board of *Continuum*, a publication of the American Academy of Neurology. Dr. Levin was a director of the American Board of Psychiatry and Neurology for 8 years and served as its chairman in 2017. In 2021 he received the Distinguished Physician Award of the American Association of Neuromuscular and Electrodiagnostic Medicine. He has one daughter and lives with his wife in Cleveland.

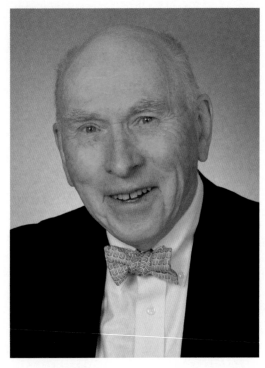

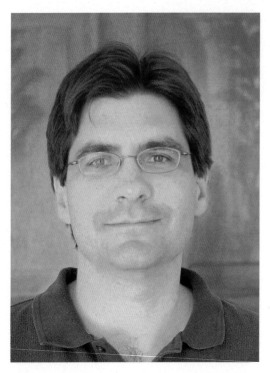

H. Royden Jones Jr, MD, died in June 2013, shortly after the previous edition of this book was published. He had been instrumental in its development, assembling us as an editorial team to see it to fruition, and was particularly proud of it, for he had known Frank Netter personally. He was greatly missed as we worked on this new (third) edition.

Dr. Jones received his medical degree in 1962 from Northwestern University Medical School and trained in neurology and clinical neurophysiology at the Mayo Clinic. He joined the Lahey Clinic in 1972 and was appointed the Jaime Ortiz-Patiño Chair in Neurology in 1996. He was an outstanding physician and teacher who specialized in neuromuscular disorders and a clinical electromyographer who founded the EMG Laboratory at the Lahey Clinic; he also directed the laboratory at Boston Children's Hospital. He was a Director of the American Board of Psychiatry and Neurology (1997–2004) and in 2007 received the Distinguished Physician Award from the American Association of Neuromuscular and Electrodiagnostic Medicine, a well-deserved tribute. Dr. Jones taught each of us and touched our lives in many other ways. He is missed by all who knew him.

Ted M. Burns, MD, died in June 2022. He was one of the editors of the second edition of this book, and his contributions to its structure and content live on in this new edition. A leader in American neurology, he has left a legacy of excellence in clinical care, scholarship, and service to his own institution and many professional societies. Although his chosen area of interest was neuromuscular disorders, his goal was to advance neurologic knowledge and its access to practicing neurologists nationally and internationally. In his honor, the American Brain Foundation and American Academy of Neurology established the annual Ted M. Burns Humanism in Neurology Award in 2020. At the time of his death, Ted was the Vice Chair of Clinical Affairs in the Department of Neurology at the University of Virginia and held an Endowed Chair as the Harrison Distinguished Teaching Professor. He was head of the Neuromuscular Disorders Division and Director of the Electromyography Laboratory. We miss him.

PREFACE

Ten years have passed since the last edition of this volume was published. They have been exciting years in the neurosciences and in clinical neurology. Advances in molecular biology have led to a greater understanding of many disease processes. Disease prediction, prognostication, and treatment are becoming tailored more completely to individual patients, as exemplified by the management of brain tumors. With advances in genomics and other factors, personalized medicine is becoming an increasing reality, something quite unimaginable just a few years ago.

Recent advances, expanding knowledge, and increasing specialization within all branches of clinical medicine have made it difficult for trainees and non-neurologists to grasp the essentials of clinical neurology and for established neurologists to remain abreast of developments in subspecialities other than their own. These factors have prompted the development of this new edition of *The Netter Collection of Medical Illustrations: Nervous System.*

Frank Netter's initial atlas of neurologic structure and function, first published in 1957, provided a very concise introduction to the nervous system for generations of students. He was able to simplify complicated anatomic components and physiologic processes and to illustrate them memorably in paintings that were both arresting and pleasing. The initial single-part publication provided a stimulating introduction to many intriguing and important clinical aspects of neurologic medicine. Although the scope was somewhat limited in its clinical depth, the vivid and intriguing plates that accompanied each topic provided a means of learning about the neurosciences that was both exciting and satisfying. To widen the content of the work, a second volume was published in 1986, and these two parts are generally referred to as the first edition of *Netter's Collection of Medical Illustrations of the Nervous System.*

When we developed the second edition, published in 2013, we expanded the scope of the volumes to bring them up to date and make them more comprehensive, helped by a superb group of medical artists who were able to follow Frank Netter's original style. We discussed many neurologic disorders from both basic science and clinical perspectives, supplementing the system-based approach now used in many medical schools. Encompassing the many advances in genetics, immunology, and imaging that had occurred was challenging, especially because the size of the volume had to be limited if it was to retain its utility.

Such is the pace of medical advance that now—just 10 years later—we have felt the need to prepare this new edition. We hope that today's medical students will find it an exciting introduction to the study of the nervous system in health and disease and will derive as much pleasure from the illustrations as we have been fortunate enough to enjoy.

ACKNOWLEDGMENTS

The editors thank their many neuroscience colleagues who contributed to this text, as well as our many patients through whom we learned the art and science of neurology. We also express our admiration and thanks to our artist colleagues Carlos A.G. Machado, MD, Kristen W. Marzejon, MS, MFA, Tiffany S. DaVanzo, MA, CMI, Paul Kim, MS, and James A. Perkins, MS, MFA, who have so carefully upheld Frank Netter's approach to medical illustration. These dedicated artists have expertly created a number of outstanding new plates for these volumes. Finally, the entire Elsevier editorial team, particularly Marybeth Thiel, Elyse O'Grady, and Carrie Stetz, have been gracious and cooperative in supporting our goals. It has been a distinct pleasure having such professional and dedicated colleagues.

DEDICATION

These two volumes are dedicated to our wives, children, and grandchildren, whose love and support gave us the time to work on this project; to our students, residents, and fellows, who challenged us to be fine teachers; and to our many and dear patients for whom we have been honored to care.

Michael J. Aminoff
Scott L. Pomeroy
Kerry H. Levin

FOREWORD TO THE SECOND EDITION

Combining Dr. Frank Netter's classic medical illustrations with a first-rate, current text is a brilliant idea. The choice of authors could not be better; as a group they are well-regarded clinicians whose experience as teachers, having national and sometimes international reputations, is well illustrated by the clarity of their writing. Very clearly there has been great attention to achieving a supple, readable style. The added images, such as the MRIs and other visual tools, are very well chosen. Their clarity for teaching purposes matches the text in quality, and these are nicely integrated with Netter's classic imagery. The most impressive thing about this effort is the marvelous embedding of Netter's illustrations into the text with preservation of coherence.

The original publication of these illustrations in the first Netter atlas was a regular, albeit unofficial, part of medical school neurologic learning early in my career during the 1960s. Concomitantly, Netter's corollary bimonthly white-covered slim paperback *Clinical Symposia* was always welcome with the new mail...more than one issue was frequently strewn on my desk. These were essentially mini atlases always centered by a striking illustration immediately telling you what the dedicated subject would be. Each new edition was always accompanied by 15 to 20 new and now classic Netter illustrations. It was not clear how Ciba Pharmaceutical wanted to specifically influence us in trade for their marvelous free teaching aids. Now I wish I had saved many of them.

Dr. Netter's style is absolutely distinctive. It has the look of mid-20th-century illustration art, somewhat like Norman Rockwell's. Not unlike a Rockwell, one can recognize a Netter illustration across the room. He is consistent no matter what his subject; his work, including its vivid coloration, is always particularly serious despite its sometimes cartoonish appearance. Netter is distinctive the way all truly great artists' work invariably is, no matter what the level of sophistication. Think of Mondrian. Think of Francis Bacon. Totally different than Netter, they are good examples of great "high" art that are similarly distinctive and consistent. And such consistency, regardless of the subject, is surely part of what makes for genius with subsequent fame and greatness. Accompanied by their new text in two detailed parts covering the brain as well as the spinal cord and its related peripheral motor sensory units, Frank Netter's art has been beautifully resurrected once again. These will surely provide learning with pleasure to yet another generation of medical students during their neurologic studies.

Nicholas A. Vick, MD
Clinical Professor of Neurology
Pritzker School of Medicine
University of Chicago
Chicago, Illinois
Department of Neurology
NorthShore University Health System
Evanston, Illinois

While attending a major medical meeting more than 2 decades after using the first Netter *Nervous System,* published in 1957, I met a representative of the Ciba Pharmaceutical Medical Education division—the corporation that sponsored Dr. Frank Netter's medical artistic career for more than 40 years—and inquired about the possibility of having him create paintings relevant to the peripheral motor and sensory unit and, particularly, the major peripheral nerves. Within a few months, I was surprised to receive a handwritten letter from Dr. Netter, asking for more detailed suggestions. This led to an invitation to meet with him at his Florida beachfront home and to advise him in reference to his current orthopedic disorders project.

Frank was a humble and engaging person entirely dedicated to his goal of illustrating all human anatomy and related clinical disorders. A day in his studio might be dedicated to interviewing physicians to discuss their area of expertise, who would provide him with a full appreciation of the subject before he started on his drawings. Sometimes after lunch he took a break from his ever-present cigars and his studio to play two or three holes of golf before returning to his various challenges. Most other days were dedicated to conceptualization, drawing, or painting sessions. Dr. Netter had an unbridled passion for his work. His artistic abilities were truly amazing—he was under contract to provide 93 new illustrations annually, which amounts to one every 4 days. He worked with vigor every day of the week until his death at age 85.

Unknown to me when we initially met, Frank previously had commenced his work on a new edition of his *Neuroscience Atlas,* having recognized the relatively limited scope of his initial volume. After we worked together for awhile, he showed this project to me, noting that it had remained dormant for a few years; subsequently, he asked me to become its clinical editor. There were to be two parts. *Part I,* dedicated to traditional basic neuroanatomy and neurophysiology, was essentially completed. The clinical portion of his revised atlas, *Part II, Neurologic and Neuromuscular Disorders,* required extensive new artwork and text and was first published in 1986. However, production costs and time restraints limited its clinical breadth and depth. Therefore Frank and I envisioned production of a more complete set of texts within 5 to 10 years to add further to these volumes. Although long overdue, thanks to the foresight of Elsevier, these volumes are now completed. There is no doubt that Dr. Netter would be extremely pleased with these results subsequent to the dedication of so many expert neurologic physicians. The new two-part volume supports his dream of very comprehensive, relevant, and totally up-to-date neuroscience atlases.

H. Royden Jones, MD

INTRODUCTION TO THE FIRST EDITION—PART II

In the introduction to Part I of this volume on the nervous system, I wrote of why, after almost 35 years of widespread acceptance, it was necessary to revise and update the original atlas, Volume 1 of *The Ciba Collection of Medical Illustrations*. I also told there of how, as I progressed with the revision, the amount of material to be included grew to such a magnitude that it was decided to publish it in two parts. Part I, published in 1983, contained a depiction of what may be called the "basic science" of the nervous system; that is, the bony encasements, the gross anatomy, the vasculature of the brain and spinal cord, the autonomic nervous system, the cranial nerves, the nerve plexuses and peripheral nerves, the embryology, and the physiology and functional neuroanatomy of the nervous system. Part II, presented herewith, is devoted to portraying the disorders and diseases of the nervous system. But once again, to my dismay, as I progressed with picturing the pathology and clinical aspects of those multitudinous ailments, the volume of material grew to such an extent that I was hard put to confine it to the limits of one book. Furthermore, the fantastic progress that was being made in the field even as I worked added to the difficulty of space limitation. Accordingly, I tried to place emphasis on those disorders most threatening to mankind because of incidence or severity, with due consideration for timeliness, diagnostic difficulty, and potential for beneficial management.

I believe that, in studying many of the conditions portrayed in this book, the reader will find it most helpful to refer repeatedly to Part I of this volume for an understanding of the basic science aspects underlying the disorder. For example, study of stroke in this book may be enhanced by reference to the arterial supply and functional subdivisions of the brain, as covered in Part I. Likewise, study of the peripheral neuropathies may call for a review of nerve conduction as well as of the course and distribution of the peripheral nerves.

But the nervous system is not an isolated entity. It is intimately involved with the function of every other system of the body as portrayed in other volumes of the *Ciba Collection*. The association is, however, most marked with the musculoskeletal system. Indeed, there is great overlap between the fields of neurology and neurosurgery with the field of orthopedics, both diagnostically and therapeutically. Cerebral palsy and poliomyelitis are, of course, basically neurologic diseases, and they are so presented in this volume. But the aftercare, corrective surgery, and rehabilitation of such patients are usually in the hands of the orthopedists. Accordingly, those aspects of these diseases will be covered in the forthcoming atlases on the musculoskeletal system, on which I am now at work. Intervertebral disc herniation and spinal stenosis likewise fall into both fields of practice, and thus, though presented herein, their management will be amplified in the musculoskeletal volume. The neuromuscular diseases are among many other examples of overlap between the two disciplines.

The trials and tribulations of the production of this atlas were far outweighed by the pleasure and stimulation I received from working on it. This was largely due to those wonderful people, my consultants and collaborators, who helped me, taught me, advised me, and supplied me with the pertinent reference material as a basis for many of my illustrations. They are all listed separately herein and I thank them, each and every one, for the knowledge they imparted to me and for the time they so graciously gave me.

I was especially fortunate to have had the guidance and counsel of that delightful personality, Dr. H. Royden Jones, Jr. ("Roy" to me), of the Lahey Clinic. The many long hours we spent together planning and organizing the material to be included were not only informative and productive but exceedingly pleasurable as well. I was constantly impressed by his broad knowledge, his unique ability to define the essence of each subject we dealt with, and his ability to call upon knowledgeable consultants for special topics, yet maintaining an overall perspective of the project in relation to the total field of medical practice and neurology in particular. Our collaboration thus developed into a lasting friendship that I cherish highly.

I express here also my appreciation for the help and encouragement I received from Dr. William (Bill) Fields, professor and chairman of the Department of Neuro-oncology at the MD Anderson Hospital and Tumor Institute, Houston. He was not only a definitive collaborator for some specific subjects but readily gave me much practical advice and counsel throughout the undertaking. I thank Mr. Philip Flagler, director of Medical Education for the CIBA Company, and Dr. Milton Donin, a relative newcomer to our team, for their continuous efforts in coordinating the varied aspects of the undertaking, to keep it moving along, and to ensure that each person involved understood and felt happy in their contribution to it. My accolades go also to Gina Dingle for her diverse editorial activities, for her untiring and patient attention to frustrating details, for her great organizing accomplishments, and especially for her ever-present personality. Finally, I express once more my appreciation of the CIBA Pharmaceutical Company and its executives for their understanding of the significance of this project and for the free hand they have given me in its creation.

Frank H. Netter, 1986

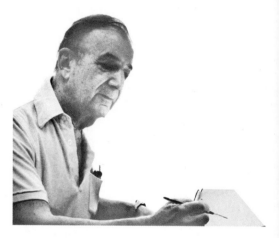

EDITORS-IN-CHIEF

Michael J. Aminoff, MD, DSc, FRCP
Distinguished Professor Emeritus
Department of Neurology
School of Medicine
University of California
San Francisco, California
EDITOR: PART I: SECTIONS 6, 7, 11, 14;
　　PART II: SECTIONS 1, 2, 3, 7, 9
AUTHOR: PART I: PLATE 7.18; PART II: PLATES
　　2.1–2.29

Scott L. Pomeroy, MD, PhD
Bronson Crothers Professor of Neurology
Harvard Medical School
Chair, Department of Neurology
Neurologist-in-Chief
Boston Children's Hospital
Boston, Massachusetts
EDITOR: PART I: SECTIONS 1, 2, 3, 4, 5, 8, 12;
　　PART II: SECTION 8

Kerry H. Levin, MD
Professor of Neurology
Cleveland Clinic Lerner College of Medicine of Case
　　Western Reserve University
Chairman, Department of Neurology
Director, Neuromuscular Center
Cleveland Clinic
Cleveland, Ohio
EDITOR: PART I: SECTIONS 9, 10, 13;
　　PART II: SECTIONS 4, 5, 6, 10, 11, 12

CONTRIBUTORS

Valérie Biousse, MD
Reunette Harris Chair in Ophthalmology
Professor of Ophthalmology and Neurology
Emory Eye Center
Atlanta, Georgia
PLATES 1.8–1.19

Lennox Byer, BA
Resident, Neurology
UCSF Weill Institute for Neurosciences
University of California, San Francisco
San Francisco, California
PLATES 1.1–1.7, 1.20–1.50

Melissa Cook, MD
Fellow, Neuromuscular Neurology
University of Minnesota
Minneapolis, Minnesota
PLATES 9.5–9.6

Basil T. Darras, MD
Associate Neurologist-in-Chief
Department of Neurology
Boston Children's Hospital
Joseph J. Volpe Distinguished Professor of
　　Neurology
Department of Neurology
Harvard Medical School
Boston, Massachusetts
PLATES 9.1–9.2

William S. David, MD, PhD
Associate Professor of Neurology
Harvard Medical School
Massachusetts General Hospital
Boston, Massachusetts
PLATE 10.5–10.11

Feza Deymeer, MD, MS (Epid)
Professor of Neurology, Memorial Şişli Hospital
Istanbul Faculty of Medicine
Istanbul University
Istanbul, Türkiye
PLATE 11.11

Elliot L. Dimberg, MD
Assistant Professor of Neurology
Mayo Clinic College of Medicine and Science
Consultant, Department of Neurology, Mayo Clinic
Jacksonville, Florida
PLATES 12.1–12.6

Anne G. Douglas, MD
Fellow, Neurohospitalist
University of California, San Francisco
San Francisco, California
PLATES 1.1–1.7, 1.20–1.50

P. James B. Dyck, MD
Professor of Neurology
Head of the Peripheral Nerve Pathology Laboratory
　　and Section
Mayo Clinic
Rochester, Minnesota
PLATES 6.3, 6.7–6.25, 6.27–6.29

Alexander Fay, MD, PhD
Assistant Professor of Neurology
School of Medicine
University of California, San Francisco
San Francisco, California
PLATES 9.3–9.4

Nathaniel H. Fleming, MD, MS
Clinical Fellow, Neurology
UCSF Weill Institute for Neurosciences
School of Medicine
University of California, San Francisco
San Francisco, California
PLATES 1.1–1.7, 1.20–1.50

Partha Ghosh, MD
Associate Professor of Neurology
Harvard Medical School
Director, EMG Laboratory
Boston Children's Hospital
Boston, Massachusetts
PLATES 12.8–12.10

Namita Goyal, MD
Professor of Neurology
University of California, Irvine
Irvine, California
PLATES 11.7–11.8, 11.12, 12.7, 12.11–12.21

Peter B. Kang, MD
Professor and Vice Chair of Research, Department of
　　Neurology
Director, Paul & Sheila Wellstone Muscular Dystrophy
　　Center
University of Minnesota Medical School
Minneapolis, Minnesota
PLATES 9.5–9.6

Christopher J. Lamb, MD
Assistant Professor of Neurology
Mayo Clinic
Jacksonville, Florida
PLATES 6.1–6.25, 6.27–6.29, 10.1–10.4, 11.3–11.6

Yuebing Li, MD, PhD
Staff Physician, Neurology
Cleveland Clinic
Cleveland, Ohio
PLATES 11.1–11.2, 11.9–11.10

John Markman, MD
Vice Chair, Neurosurgery
Professor, Neurology
University of Rochester School of Medicine
Rochester, New York
PLATES 8.1–8.23

Tahseen Mozaffar, MD
Professor of Neurology
University of California, Irvine
Irvine, California
PLATES 11.7–11.8, 11.12, 12.7, 12.11–12.21

Nancy J. Newman, MD
LeoDelle Jolley Chair in Ophthalmology
Professor of Ophthalmology and Neurology
Instructor in Neurological Surgery, Director
　　of Neuro-ophthalmology
Emory University School of Medicine
Atlanta, Georgia
PLATES 1.8–1.19

Katharine Nicholson, MD
Assistant in Neurology
Instructor, Harvard Medical School
Massachusetts General Hospital
Boston, Massachusetts
PLATES 10.5–10.11

Fajar Pasha, MD
Human Subject Research Coordinator
Department of Neurosurgery
University of Rochester
Rochester, New York
PLATES 8.1–8.23

Douglas Pet, MD
Assistant Professor, Neurology
UCSF Weill Institute for Neurosciences
School of Medicine
University of California, San Francisco
San Francisco, California
PLATES 1.1–1.7, 1.20–1.50

CONTENTS OF COMPLETE VOLUME 7—NERVOUS SYSTEM: TWO-PART SET

CONTENTS

CRANIAL NERVE AND NEURO-OPHTHALMOLOGIC DISORDERS

DISTRIBUTION OF MOTOR AND SENSORY FIBERS

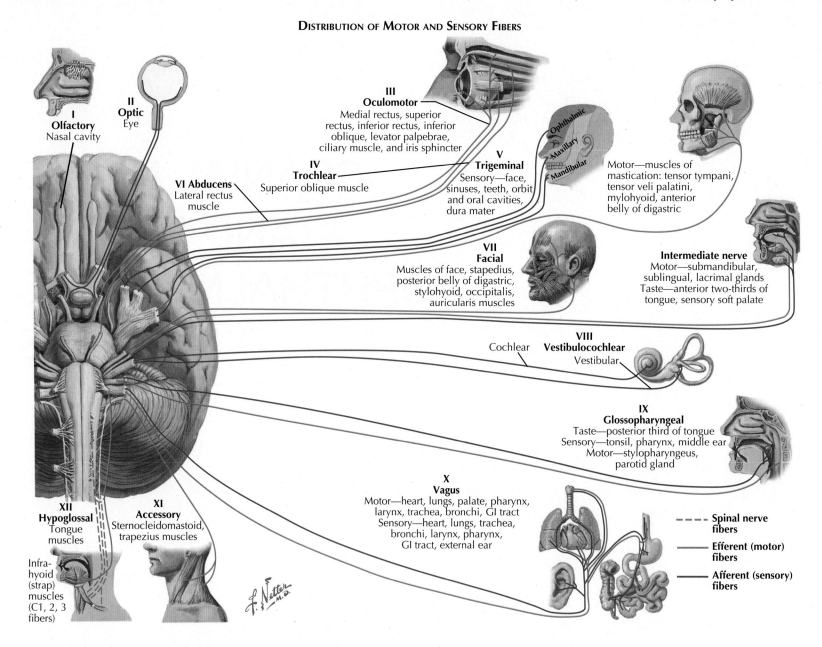

I Olfactory Nasal cavity

II Optic Eye

VI Abducens Lateral rectus muscle

III Oculomotor Medial rectus, superior rectus, inferior rectus, inferior oblique, levator palpebrae, ciliary muscle, and iris sphincter

IV Trochlear Superior oblique muscle

V Trigeminal Sensory—face, sinuses, teeth, orbit and oral cavities, dura mater

Ophthalmic
Maxillary
Mandibular

Motor—muscles of mastication: tensor tympani, tensor veli palatini, mylohyoid, anterior belly of digastric

VII Facial Muscles of face, stapedius, posterior belly of digastric, stylohyoid, occipitalis, auricularis muscles

Intermediate nerve Motor—submandibular, sublingual, lacrimal glands Taste—anterior two-thirds of tongue, sensory soft palate

VIII Vestibulocochlear Cochlear Vestibular

IX Glossopharyngeal Taste—posterior third of tongue Sensory—tonsil, pharynx, middle ear Motor—stylopharyngeus, parotid gland

X Vagus Motor—heart, lungs, palate, pharynx, larynx, trachea, bronchi, GI tract Sensory—heart, lungs, trachea, bronchi, larynx, pharynx, GI tract, external ear

XII Hypoglossal Tongue muscles

Infra-hyoid (strap) muscles (C1, 2, 3 fibers)

XI Accessory Sternocleidomastoid, trapezius muscles

- - - Spinal nerve fibers
—— Efferent (motor) fibers
—— Afferent (sensory) fibers

OVERVIEW OF CRANIAL NERVES

The brainstem is the source of all the cranial nerves (CNs) and provides sensory, motor, and, through the vagus nerve, parasympathetic preganglionic innervation to the face, head, thorax, and most of the abdominal viscera. Distinct motor and sensory nuclei within the brainstem project axons to the various structures of the head to provide (1) general sensory information from the face, ears, and oropharynx and (2) motor innervations for facial movement and expression, mastication, extraocular eye movements, and complex functions such as speech and swallowing. The specialized olfactory, visual, auditory, and gustatory senses are provided by highly specialized receptor cells and end organs, with ultimately wide cortical projections.

Cranial nerve motor nuclei are located medially, whereas the sensory nuclei are generally found more lateral. Three types of motor nuclei are present, innervating voluntary striated muscles (somatic), muscles of facial expressions and mastication (special motor

derived from embryonic branchial arch structures), and autonomic smooth muscles (visceral). Each cranial nerve serves a regional skull area and may provide more than one function to that area and therefore is not restricted to a single nucleus or nerve type. For example, the facial nerve provides voluntary motor innervations to the face, as well as taste sensation to the anterior tongue. The pure motor nerves (except for perhaps some proprioceptive function) are the oculomotor (III), trochlear (IV), abducens (VI), spinal accessory nerve (XI), and hypoglossal (XII). The special sensory nerves are the olfactory (I), optic (II), and vestibulocochlear (VIII). Mixed cranial nerves are the trigeminal (V), facial (VII), glossopharyngeal (IX), and vagus (X). A summary of the origin, course, and distribution of each cranial nerve is outlined on the following pages.

Cranial neuropathies can manifest as a single cranial neuropathy or, less commonly, as multiple cranial neuropathies. Single cranial neuropathies are discussed in their respective sections. For example, idiopathic facial neuropathy (Bell palsy) is reviewed on Plate 1.30. Multiple cranial neuropathies involve any combination of

CNs, although CNs III, V, VI, and VII are the most commonly affected in most clinical series. The manifestations of multiple cranial neuropathies reflect the sites of injury and function of the cranial nerves affected. Causes are numerous and include infectious, neoplastic, autoimmune, traumatic, and vascular processes. Infections associated with multiple cranial neuropathies include Lyme disease, tuberculous meningitis, cryptococcosis, histoplasmosis, botulism, mucormycosis, infections with certain viruses (e.g., herpes simplex virus, varicella-zoster virus), and bacterial meningitis. Guillain-Barré syndrome (GBS) and the Miller Fisher variant of GBS are monophasic, autoimmune polyradiculoneuropathies that can frequently involve multiple CNs. Neoplasms cause multiple cranial neuropathies either by direct compression and local extension, such as with meningiomas, schwannomas, and nasopharyngeal tumors, or by diffuse dissemination and meningeal infiltration, such as with lymphoma and various carcinomas. Myasthenia gravis (MG) can mimic multiple cranial neuropathies, but the site of autoimmune attack in MG is directed at the neuromuscular junction rather than the nerve.

Plate 1.2

Cranial Nerve and Neuro-ophthalmologic Disorders

Name and number: Type of fibers	Origin, course, and distribution	Chief functions
Olfactory (I): *Special sensory*	Olfactory cells in nasal mucosa aggregate into olfactory nerves that penetrate the cribriform plate and join to form the olfactory bulb. The bulb's posteriorly extending tract divides into a medial branch, which fans into the parolfactory and subcallosal areas, and a lateral branch, which ends in the uncus and the parahippocampal gyrus.	*Smell*
Optic (II): *Special sensory*	Axons of the inner retinal *ganglion cell layer* form the retina's *nerve fiber layer* and gather at the optic disk (optic nerve head) before turning 90 degrees and penetrating the scleral canal to exit the globe, now myelinated, as the *optic nerve*. The *optic chiasm* is the intersection of the optic nerve from each eye coming through the optic canal and is located above the pituitary body within the sella turcica. Axons from the temporal retina (nasal field) remain ipsilateral as they pass through the chiasm to the optic tract. In contrast, the nasal retinal fibers decussate, carrying temporal visual field information to the contralateral side. Inferior nasal fibers decussate within the chiasm more anteriorly than superior ones. As the inferior nasal retinal fibers approach the posterior aspect of the chiasm, the fibers shift to occupy the lateral aspect of the contralateral optic tract. The optic tract leads to the lateral geniculate bodies. The lateral geniculate nucleus (LGN) is a thalamic nucleus that serves as the synapse point of the retinal ganglion cells and relays visual information through the optic radiations to the striate occipital cortex.	*Vision*
Oculomotor (III): *Motor* *Visceral motor*	This nerve emerges as a collection of nine rostral midbrain subnuclei located ventral to the aqueduct at the level of the superior colliculus and includes the *accessory autonomic (Edinger-Westphal) nucleus*. Axons from the CN III subnuclei gather into a fascicle that arcs through the red nucleus and emerge at the medial surface of the cerebral peduncle. In the interpeduncular cistern, the nerve passes beneath the posterior cerebral artery, then pierces the dura crossing next to the internal carotid artery en route to the cavernous sinus. From the lateral wall of the cavernous sinus, it enters the orbit through the superior orbital fissure to supply the superior rectus, medial rectus, inferior rectus, and inferior oblique muscles. The fibers subserving pupillary constriction are located superficially and are susceptible to compression but are less prone to microvascular or ischemic changes than the deeper fibers are. These parasympathetic fibers split off the oculomotor nerve in the orbit and synapse in the ciliary ganglion from which postganglionic *short ciliary nerves* supply the pupillary sphincter and ciliary muscles.	*Somatic motor:* Upper lid elevation (levator palpebrae superioris) and extraocular movements upward, medially, and downward *Visceral motor:* Parasympathetically mediated pupillary constriction and accommodation reflex
Trochlear (IV): *Motor*	The CN IV nuclei are located in the midbrain at the level of the inferior colliculi off midline at the anterior edge of the periaqueductal gray. Axons from the trochlear nucleus arc posteriorly around the periaqueductal gray and cross the midline to emerge laterally beneath the inferior colliculus and wrap forward around the medial border of the brachium conjunctivum. CN IV completely decussates, a unique feature among the cranial nerves, and exits the brainstem from its posterior aspect. It passes the ambient cistern and through the lateral wall of the cavernous sinus to then enter the orbit via the superior orbital fissure. The trochlear nerve innervates a single extraocular muscle, the superior oblique.	*Somatic motor:* Superior oblique muscle, extraocular eye movement downward and intorsion
Trigeminal (V): *Somatic sensory and special motor*	The *trigeminal somatic sensory column* is a posterolateral series of nuclei extending from the mid pons to the upper cervical cord; these nuclei receive general sensory input from the eye, orbit, face, forehead, upper and lower jaws, sinuses, teeth, and nasopharynx. Proprioceptive fibers in the extraocular and masticatory muscles end in the *mesencephalic nucleus*. Pain, touch, and temperature fibers end in the *principal (pontine) sensory nucleus* and *spinal nucleus of the trigeminal nerve*. The *trigeminal motor nucleus* in the upper part of the pons is the origin of special branchiomotor fibers to the muscles of mastication. Large sensory and smaller motor roots enter and emerge laterally at the midpons level. As the trigeminal nerve exits the posterior fossa, it expands over the apex of the petrous temporal bone into the *trigeminal (semilunar) ganglion* made of sensory nuclei from the *ophthalmic, maxillary,* and *mandibular* nerves that pass through the superior orbital fissure, foramen rotundum, and foramen ovale, respectively. The *ophthalmic nerve* divides into lacrimal, frontal, and nasociliary branches, which participate in innervating the eye, nose, and scalp. The *maxillary nerve* traverses the pterygopalatine fossa, enters the infraorbital groove (canal), and emerges as the *infraorbital nerve* through infraorbital foramen; supplies meningeal, zygomatic, superior alveolar, inferior palpebral, nasal, and superior labial branches; and is connected with pterygopalatine ganglion through which it supplies orbital, nasal, palatine, and pharyngeal branches. The *mandibular nerve* is joined by the entire motor root of trigeminal nerve in the foramen ovale and gives off meningeal, buccal, auriculotemporal, lingual, and inferior alveolar branches, as well as motor nerves supplying masticatory muscles, the tensors of the soft palate, and the tympanic membrane.	*Somatic sensory (touch, pain, and temperature):* Eyes, face, anterior scalp, sinuses, teeth, and oral and nasal cavities as well as the dura mater *Proprioceptive sensory (deep pressure, position, and movement):* Teeth, temporomandibular joint, hard palate, and muscles of mastication *Special motor:* Branchiomotor fibers to the muscles of mastication, anterior belly of the digastrics, tensor tympani, tensor veli palatini, and mylohyoid
Abducens (VI): *Motor*	The abducens CN VI nucleus is in the floor of the fourth ventricle just lateral to the median eminence of the pons. It is enveloped by looping CN VII fibers (genu) that form the facial colliculus. The CN VI nucleus contains two physiologically distinct groups of neurons: one innervating the ipsilateral lateral rectus muscles and the other projecting across the midline up the contralateral medial longitudinal fasciculus to the ventral nucleus of the contralateral CN III nuclear complex. These internuclear connections produce the simultaneous activation of the contralateral medial rectus muscle and the ipsilateral lateral rectus that ensures conjugate lateral horizontal gaze. The CN VI fasciculus projects anteriorly and caudally to exit the inferior edge of the pons just medial to the corticospinal tracts. The nerve ascends between the pons and the clivus within the pontine cistern. It pierces the dura and then enters the lateral cavernous sinus proximate to the carotid artery and intimate with the sympathetic fibers. It reaches the orbit through the superior-orbital fissure.	*Somatic motor:* Lateral rectus muscle extraocular eye movement, and eye abduction

Nerves and Nuclei Viewed in Phantom From Behind

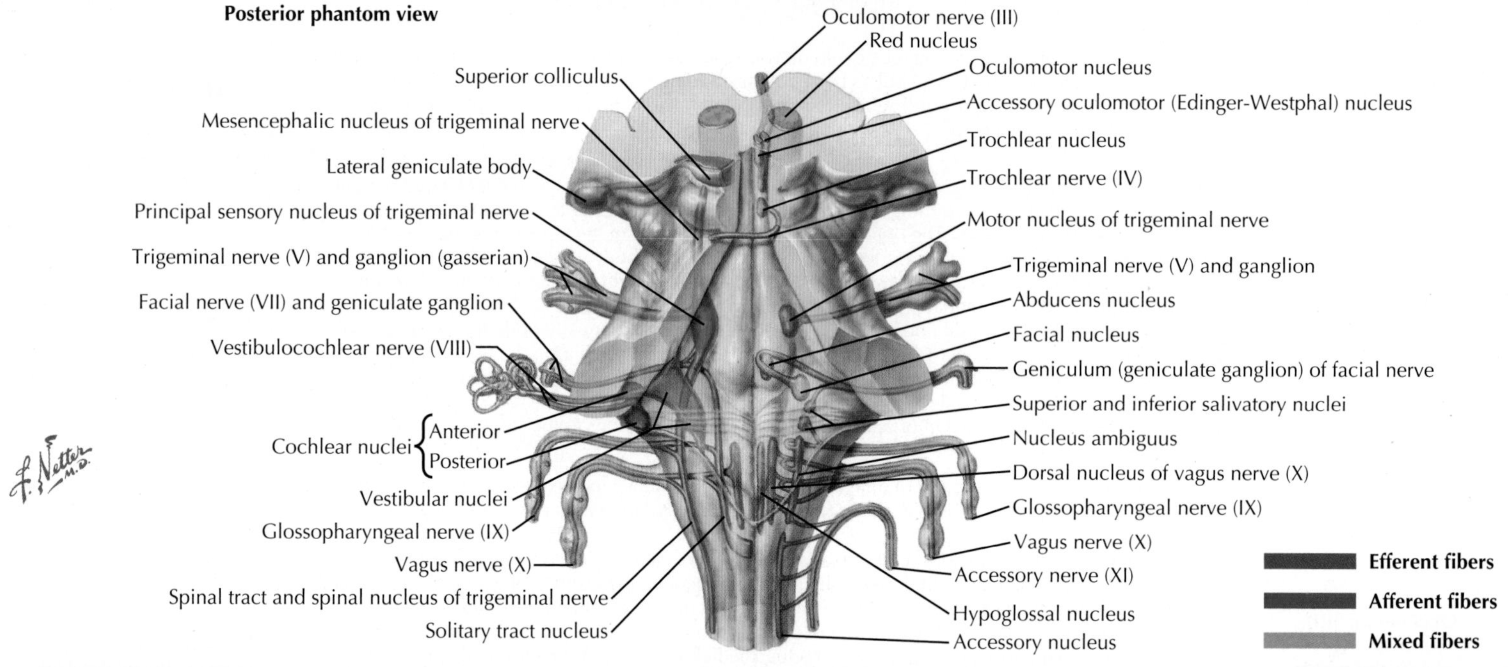
Posterior phantom view
Oculomotor nerve (III)
Red nucleus
Superior colliculus
Oculomotor nucleus
Accessory oculomotor (Edinger-Westphal) nucleus
Mesencephalic nucleus of trigeminal nerve
Trochlear nucleus
Lateral geniculate body
Trochlear nerve (IV)
Principal sensory nucleus of trigeminal nerve
Motor nucleus of trigeminal nerve
Trigeminal nerve (V) and ganglion (gasserian)
Trigeminal nerve (V) and ganglion
Facial nerve (VII) and geniculate ganglion
Abducens nucleus
Facial nucleus
Vestibulocochlear nerve (VIII)
Geniculum (geniculate ganglion) of facial nerve
Superior and inferior salivatory nuclei
Cochlear nuclei
Anterior
Posterior
Nucleus ambiguus
Dorsal nucleus of vagus nerve (X)
Vestibular nuclei
Glossopharyngeal nerve (IX)
Glossopharyngeal nerve (IX)
Vagus nerve (X)
Vagus nerve (X)
Accessory nerve (XI)
Spinal tract and spinal nucleus of trigeminal nerve
Hypoglossal nucleus
Solitary tract nucleus
Accessory nucleus
Efferent fibers
Afferent fibers
Mixed fibers
F. Netter M.D.

Name and number: Type of fibers	Origin, course, and distribution	Chief functions
Facial (VII): ***Special motor*** ***General visceral motor*** ***Somatic sensory*** ***Special sensory***	Branchiomotor fibers arise from the *facial nucleus* in the lower pons and ascend to loop around the abducens nucleus and then descend anterolaterally between the spinal trigeminal complex and CN VII motor nucleus. The nerve emerges as two divisions through the recess between the inferior cerebellar peduncle and the medulla: a larger *motor root* and smaller *nervus intermedius* containing mainly afferent special sensory fibers for taste and secretomotor fibers to the *pterygopalatine ganglion* (lacrimation and mucous membrane secretory function in the mouth and nose). Both divisions of the facial nerve, along with CN VIII, then pass through the internal acoustic meatus. At the level of the geniculate ganglion secretomotor fibers (originating from the *superior lacrimal/salivatory nucleus*), separate and proceed superiorly to the pterygopalatine ganglion. The chorda tympani (carrying secretomotor fibers to the submandibular ganglion and special sensory taste fibers from the anterior two-thirds of tongue and soft palate) separates distal to the geniculate nucleus and joins the lingual nerve to the tongue. The remaining branchiomotor fibers continue their course, proceeding through the bony facial canal and emerging in the face anterior to the mastoid process from the stylomastoid foramen. These fibers enter the parotid gland to divide into diverging branches toward the facial muscles and the platysma (see Plate 1.27).	***Special motor:*** Muscles of facial expression, stapedius, stylohyoid, and posterior belly of the digastric muscle ***General visceral motor:*** Parasympathetic innervations of the submandibular, sublingual, lacrimal, and nasal/oral mucous membrane glands ***Somatic sensor:*** External auditory meatus and skin over mastoid ***Special sensory:*** Taste anterior two-thirds of the tongue
Vestibulocochlear (VIII): ***Special sensory***	The vestibulocochlear nerve emerges through the internal acoustic meatus at the pontomedullary angle posterolateral to the facial nerve. The primary neurons are bipolar cells located in the vestibular and multiple spiral ganglia. Peripheral processes pass from special auditory (cochlea) and vestibular (ampullae, utricle, and saccule) receptors, while the central processes project to two cochlear and four vestibular brainstem nuclei, respectively. The ventral and dorsal cochlear nuclei are located at the level of the inferior cerebellar peduncle in the superior medulla. Most cochlear nuclear fibers decussate through the trapezoid body, after which third- and fourth-order neurons then ascend the lateral lemniscus to the inferior colliculus with projections ultimately to the auditory cortex. The superior, inferior, medial, and lateral vestibular nuclei lie in the anterolateral floor of the fourth ventricle and connect with the cerebellum, the nuclei of CNs III, IV, and VI (through the medial longitudinal fasciculus) and to anterior horn cells controlling muscles of head and neck (vestibulospinal tract).	***Hearing*** ***Equilibrium and balance*** ***Reflexive eye movements***
Glossopharyngeal (IX): ***Special motor*** ***General visceral motor*** ***Special sensory*** ***General visceral sensory*** ***Somatic sensory***	Special branchiomotor fibers arise from cranial end of nucleus ambiguous and supply the stylopharyngeus muscle. Secretomotor fibers arise from inferior salivatory nucleus and proceed as parasympathetic fibers through the tympanic nerve to the otic ganglion; postganglionic fibers (lesser petrosal nerve) innervate the parotid gland. Special sensory taste fibers from the posterior third of the tongue have their cell bodies in the petrosal ganglion and then project centrally to the solitary tract nucleus. "Visceral" sensory fibers from the posterior tongue, fauces, tonsil, tympanic cavity, eustachian tube, and mastoid cells end in a combined dorsal glossopharyngeal vagal nucleus, with ordinary sensory fibers probably ending in the spinal tract and nucleus of trigeminal nerve. Special visceral afferents from pressure receptors in the carotid sinus mediate decreased heart rate and blood pressure through vagus nerve connections. The nerve emerges from the medulla above the vagus nerve and leaves the skull through the jugular foramen. It runs forward between the internal carotid artery and internal jugular vein and curves over the stylopharyngeus muscle, to end in branches for the tonsils, and mucous membrane and glands of pharynx and pharyngeal part of tongue. The tympanic branch forms the main part of the tympanic plexus, which supplies the tympanic cavity and the lesser petrosal nerve carrying secretomotor fibers for the parotid gland.	***Special motor:*** Stylopharyngeus; elevation of pharynx ***General visceral motor:*** Parotid and mucous glands secretion ***Special sensory:*** Taste posterior third of the tongue, and numerous taste buds in vallate papillae ***General visceral sensory:*** Baroreceptors from carotid body; general sensation from posterior tongue, fauces, tonsil, tympanic cavity, eustachian tube, and mastoid cells ***Somatic sensory:*** Outer ear sensation

Plate 1.4

Cranial Nerve and Neuro-ophthalmologic Disorders

NERVES AND NUCLEI IN LATERAL DISSECTION

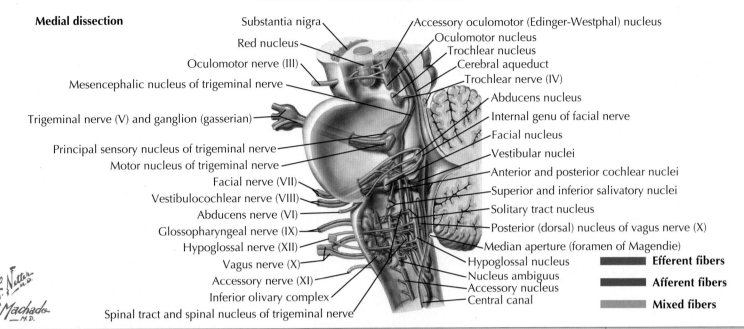

Medial dissection

Substantia nigra
Red nucleus
Oculomotor nerve (III)
Mesencephalic nucleus of trigeminal nerve
Trigeminal nerve (V) and ganglion (gasserian)
Principal sensory nucleus of trigeminal nerve
Motor nucleus of trigeminal nerve
Facial nerve (VII)
Vestibulocochlear nerve (VIII)
Abducens nerve (VI)
Glossopharyngeal nerve (IX)
Hypoglossal nerve (XII)
Vagus nerve (X)
Accessory nerve (XI)
Inferior olivary complex
Spinal tract and spinal nucleus of trigeminal nerve

Accessory oculomotor (Edinger-Westphal) nucleus
Oculomotor nucleus
Trochlear nucleus
Cerebral aqueduct
Trochlear nerve (IV)
Abducens nucleus
Internal genu of facial nerve
Facial nucleus
Vestibular nuclei
Anterior and posterior cochlear nuclei
Superior and inferior salivatory nuclei
Solitary tract nucleus
Posterior (dorsal) nucleus of vagus nerve (X)
Median aperture (foramen of Magendie)
Hypoglossal nucleus
Nucleus ambiguus
Accessory nucleus
Central canal

◼◼◼ **Efferent fibers**
◼◼◼ **Afferent fibers**
◼◼◼ **Mixed fibers**

Name and number: Type of fibers	Origin, course, and distribution	Chief functions
Vagus (X): *Special motor* *General visceral motor* *Somatic sensory* *Visceral sensory* *Special sensory*	The dorsal vagal nucleus is a mixture of visceral efferent and afferent cells forming an elongated column on each side of midline and extending through the length of the medulla, lateral to the hypoglossal nuclei. From here, preganglionic parasympathetic fibers go to parasympathetic ganglia innervating cardiac and unstriated muscles in the thoracic and abdominal viscera. Motor fibers for striated muscles of the larynx and pharynx originate in the midportion of the nucleus ambiguous (ill-defined column of large cells located in the reticular formation). Afferent fibers from visceral receptors have their cell bodies in the inferior vagal (nodose) ganglion and end in the mixed dorsal vagal nucleus. They convey sensation from the pharynx, larynx, trachea, and viscera. However, a few special sensory taste fibers from the epiglottis and the adjacent tongue end in the solitary tract nucleus. General somatic afferents from auricular and meningeal branches with cell bodies in the jugular ganglion end in the spinal tract and nucleus of the trigeminal nerve. The nerve is attached by a series of medullary rootlets located laterally between the olive and inferior cerebellar peduncle. The vagus nerve leaves the skull through the jugular foramen and is soon joined by the cranial part of the accessory nerve to then descend in the neck within the carotid sheath. The vagus nerve continues through the thorax and contributes to cardiac, pulmonary, and esophageal plexuses. It enters the abdomen as the anterior and posterior vagal trunks.	**Special motor:** Intrinsic laryngeal muscles and contribute to pharyngeal constrictors **General visceral motor:** Parasympathetic supply (movement and secretion) to the heart, the great vessels, trachea, bronchi, and alimentary canal and associated glands from pharynx almost to left colic (splenic) flexure **Somatic sensory:** Parts of auricle, external acoustic meatus, and tympanic membrane meninges of posterior cranial fossa **General visceral sensory:** Pharynx, larynx, trachea, and abdominal viscera **Special sensory:** Taste from epiglottis and valleculae
Accessory (XI): *Special motor*	The accessory nerve consists of cranial and spinal roots. Cranial roots arises from cells within the lower end of the nucleus ambiguus and supply intrinsic laryngeal muscles. The spinal roots arise from a group of anterior horn cells in the upper five or six cervical segments (the spinal accessory nucleus) and supply the sternocleidomastoid and trapezius muscles. The cranial root fibers form the internal branch of the accessory nerve and arise as a series of rootlets on the surface of medulla oblongata below, and in line with the glossopharyngeal and vagal nerve rootlets. The spinal rootlets emerge through the lateral white column of the spinal cord and ascend behind the denticulate ligaments and unite to form the external branch of the accessory nerve entering the skull through the foramen magnum behind the vertebral artery. Cranial and spinal roots unite for a short distance, before leaving the skull through the jugular foramen. The internal branch joins the vagus nerve. The external branch runs downward and backward through the sternocleidomastoid muscle, and then it crosses the posterior triangle of neck and ends in the trapezius muscle. It also communicates with branches of spinal nerves C2–C4.	**Special motor** **Internal branch (vagus n.):** Intrinsic muscles of the larynx via the recurrent laryngeal nerve (except cricothyroid-superior laryngeal nerve) and soft palate (except tensor veli palatine-mandibular division of the trigeminal nerve) **External branch:** Sternocleidomastoid and trapezius muscles
Hypoglossal (XII): *Motor*	The hypoglossal nucleus is a medial column of cells situated in the lower floor of the fourth ventricle and extends the length of the medulla anterior to the central canal in the "closed" part of medulla oblongata. Axons from the nucleus course anteriorly and just lateral to the medial lemniscus and cross the most medial portion of the inferior olive to exit the brainstem in the anterolateral sulcus between the pyramidal tract and the prominence of the inferior olive. The fibers emerge as 10–15 rootlets and fuse to form two bundles that unite as they pass through the hypoglossal canal of the occipital bone. The hypoglossal nerve then runs forward between the internal carotid artery and internal jugular vein and inclines upward into tongue. It is joined by a filament from spinal nerve C1, but this soon leaves to form the superior root (descendens hypoglossi) of the ansa cervicalis.	**Somatic motor:** Intrinsic and extrinsic muscles of the tongue

OLFACTORY PATHWAYS

Olfactory bulb cells: schema

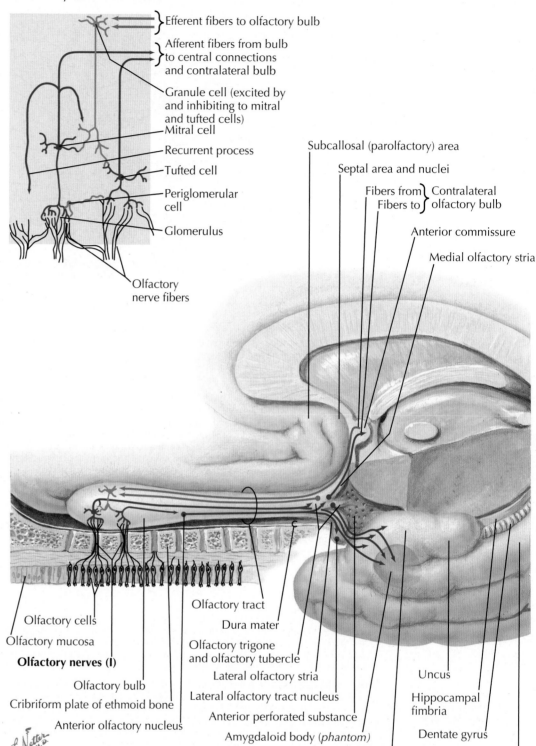

Efferent fibers to olfactory bulb

Afferent fibers from bulb to central connections and contralateral bulb

Granule cell (excited by and inhibiting to mitral and tufted cells)

Mitral cell

Recurrent process

Tufted cell

Periglomerular cell

Glomerulus

Olfactory nerve fibers

Subcallosal (parolfactory) area

Septal area and nuclei

Fibers from } Contralateral
Fibers to } olfactory bulb

Anterior commissure

Medial olfactory stria

Olfactory cells

Olfactory mucosa

Olfactory nerves (I)

Olfactory bulb

Cribriform plate of ethmoid bone

Anterior olfactory nucleus

Olfactory tract

Dura mater

Olfactory trigone and olfactory tubercle

Lateral olfactory stria

Lateral olfactory tract nucleus

Anterior perforated substance

Amygdaloid body (*phantom*)

Piriform lobe

Uncus

Hippocampal fimbria

Dentate gyrus

Parahippocampal gyrus

CRANIAL NERVE I: OLFACTORY NERVE

ANATOMY

The olfactory nerves subserve the special sense of smell. Olfactory nerve fibers are the central processes of bipolar nerve cells located in the olfactory epithelium, which covers most of the superior-posterior nasal septum and the lateral wall of the nasal cavity. The unmyelinated peripheral olfactory fibers aggregate into approximately 20 slender olfactory bundles that make up the olfactory nerve. The nerve traverses the ethmoidal cribriform plate surrounded by finger-like extensions from the dura mater and arachnoid to end in the "glomeruli" of the ipsilateral olfactory bulb. Within the bulb, these fibers synapse with second-order neurons called mitral and tufted cells whose axons constitute the olfactory tract that courses along the frontal lobe base. The olfactory tract then divides into the medial and lateral olfactory striae on either side of the anterior perforated substance and projects directly into the primary olfactory cortex within the temporal lobe. This direct pathway without a central sensory relay site (such as in the thalamic nuclei) is unique among the CNs. Although most of the olfactory tract fibers have ipsilateral central connections, some fibers decussate in the anterior commissure, making the cortical representation of smell bilateral. The human primary olfactory cortex includes the uncus, hippocampal gyrus, amygdaloid complex, and entorhinal cortex.

OLFACTORY NERVE DISORDERS

Anosmia is not always apparent to the patient, and because of the close association of flavor perception and olfaction, it may be reported as altered taste rather than loss of smell. Bilateral anosmia is more common and usually of benign nature, whereas unilateral anosmia should raise suspicion for a more serious disorder, such as an olfactory groove meningioma or frontal basal tumor. The most common causes of anosmia are nasal and paranasal sinus infections with associated inflammation, which are referred to as transport or conductive olfactory disorders. Anosmia is a common clinical feature of viral infection with SARS-CoV-2, the cause of the COVID-19 pandemic. Posttraumatic olfactory dysfunction is the cause for 20% of patients with anosmia and is the result of olfactory nerve shearing as it passes through the cribriform plate. In more substantial damage, the olfactory nerve is torn by fractures involving

the cribriform plate, often causing cerebrospinal fluid rhinorrhea and potential meningeal infection. Posttraumatic anosmia or hyposmia may be either unilateral or bilateral. Tumors of the olfactory groove affect the olfactory bulb and tract, most commonly olfactory groove meningiomas, which are usually histologically benign tumors that gradually cause mostly unilateral, and occasionally bilateral, olfactory dysfunction. Other tumors include sphenoid and frontal osteomas, pituitary tumors, and nasopharyngeal carcinomas. Unless

specifically tested, presentation of these neoplasms with anosmia is unusual because of generally unilateral involvement and slow tumor growth with gradual decline in olfactory function. Once such tumors are large enough (>4 cm in diameter), they cause pressure on the frontal lobes and the optic tracts, with symptoms of headaches, visual disturbances, personality changes, and memory impairment. On rare occasion, very large olfactory groove tumors cause ipsilateral optic atrophy by exerting direct pressure on the optic nerve with

Plate 1.6

Cranial Nerve and Neuro-ophthalmologic Disorders

OLFACTORY RECEPTORS

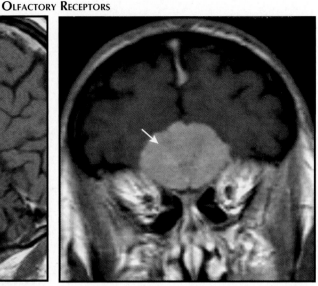

Subfrontal meningioma. T1-weighted, gadolinium-enhanced sagittal and coronal magnetic resonance images show a large enhancing skull-based mass displacing and compressing the olfactory apparatus.

CRANIAL NERVE I: OLFACTORY NERVE (Continued)

contralateral papilledema from increased intracranial pressure. The finding of ipsilateral optic atrophy, contralateral papilledema, and ipsilateral anosmia is known as Foster Kennedy syndrome. Esthesioneuroblastomas arise from the upper nasal cavity and manifest with nasal obstruction and epistaxis. Rarely, they involve the orbit and cause diplopia, visual loss, proptosis, and periorbital swelling. Anosmia is an early sign of neurodegenerative processes, particularly Parkinson disease, Alzheimer disease, and Lewy body dementia. It frequently precedes other neurologic signs, such as motor findings or cognitive changes. Olfactory discrimination is affected by many medications thought to disrupt the physiologic turnover of receptor cells, including opiates, anticonvulsants, and various immunosuppressive agents. Congenital or hereditary anosmia is rare. Kallmann syndrome consists of congenital hypoplasia, or absence of the olfactory bulbs, and hypogonadotropic hypogonadism.

OLFACTORY RECEPTORS

Receptors responsible for the sense of smell are found in the patch of olfactory epithelium that is located on the superior-posterior nasal septum and the lateral wall of the nasal cavity. In addition to the receptor cells, this epithelium contains olfactory (Bowman's) glands and sustentacular cells; both contribute to the mucous secretion that coats the epithelial surface and makes odorants soluble. The sustentacular cells also act as supporting cells for the slender olfactory receptors.

Olfactory receptor cells may be considered specialized, primitive-type, bipolar neurons. Their nuclei are located at the base of the epithelial layer. Basal stem cells located along the basement membrane differentiate into olfactory receptors or supporting cells, replenishing the olfactory epithelium about every 2 weeks. From the nuclear region of the olfactory receptor cell, a thin dendritic process extends toward the surface of the epithelium. At its apical end, this process widens into an olfactory rod, or vesicle, from which 10 to 15 motile cilia project into the mucous layer covering the epithelium. Desmosomes at the base of the olfactory vesicle provide a tight seal between the membranes of olfactory and

Distribution of olfactory epithelium (blue area)

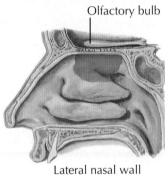

Olfactory bulb

Lateral nasal wall

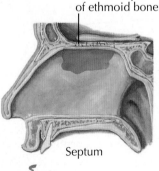

Cribriform plate of ethmoid bone

Septum

Section through olfactory mucosa

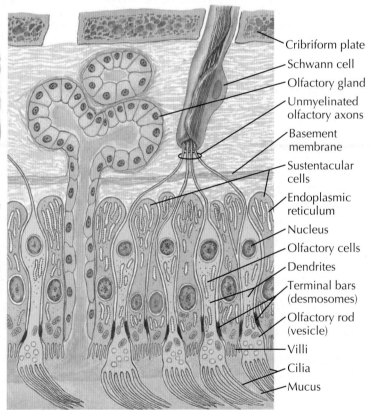

Cribriform plate
Schwann cell
Olfactory gland
Unmyelinated olfactory axons
Basement membrane
Sustentacular cells
Endoplasmic reticulum
Nucleus
Olfactory cells
Dendrites
Terminal bars (desmosomes)
Olfactory rod (vesicle)
Villi
Cilia
Mucus

sustentacular cells, thus preventing external substances from entering the intercellular spaces. At its base, the olfactory receptor cell narrows and gives rise to a fine (0.2–0.3 μm), unmyelinated axon. Large numbers of these axons converge to run together within a single Schwann cell sheath. The fibers then penetrate the cribriform plate to collectively form the olfactory nerve. In humans, this nerve contains approximately 100 million axons.

ODORANT TRANSDUCTION

The cell membranes of the olfactory receptor cells can convert chemical odorants into an electric signal by activation of a G-protein–coupled protein receptor cascade that activates the enzyme adenylate cyclase, which produces cyclic adenosine monophosphate (cAMP) as a second messenger. cAMP then changes the structure of the cell membrane channel proteins to an open state. The channel is permeable to cations that flow from the

OLFACTORY BULB AND NERVE

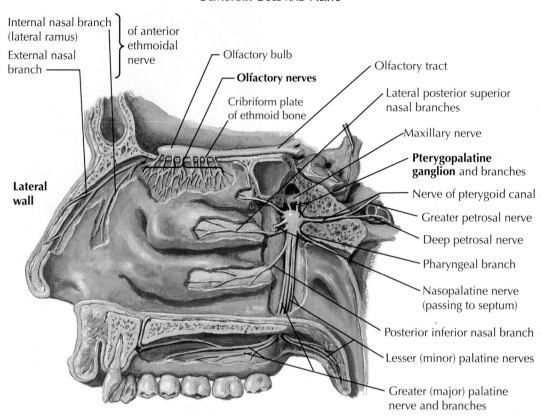

Internal nasal branch (lateral ramus) } of anterior ethmoidal nerve
External nasal branch

Olfactory bulb

Olfactory nerves

Cribriform plate of ethmoid bone

Olfactory tract

Lateral posterior superior nasal branches

Maxillary nerve

Pterygopalatine ganglion and branches

Nerve of pterygoid canal

Greater petrosal nerve

Deep petrosal nerve

Pharyngeal branch

Nasopalatine nerve (passing to septum)

Posterior inferior nasal branch

Lesser (minor) palatine nerves

Greater (major) palatine nerve and branches

Lateral wall

CRANIAL NERVE I: OLFACTORY NERVE (Continued)

nasal mucosa into the cell. The negative resting membrane potential (−70 mV) is shifted to a more positive value. Once a certain threshold is reached, the analog sensor potential is converted to a digital action potential, which is conducted via the axon of the olfactory cell to the brain.

SENSE OF SMELL

As with taste fibers, which may respond to a variety of taste stimuli, individual olfactory nerve fibers respond to several different odors. Humans differentiate the odors of thousands of chemicals; nevertheless, it has not been possible to identify a set of primary odor qualities analogous to the four primary tastes.

OLFACTORY PATHWAY

Olfactory Bulb

About 100 million olfactory afferent fibers enter the olfactory bulb, a flattened, oval mass lying near the lateral margin of the cribriform plate of the ethmoid bone. The incoming olfactory fibers coalesce in the outermost layer of the olfactory bulb to form presynaptic nests, or glomeruli. Each glomerulus is composed of about 25,000 receptor cell axon terminals. The terminals synapse and excite the dendrites of mitral and tufted cells, which are the second-order neurons in the olfactory bulb. Each mitral cell sends its dendrites to only a single glomerulus, whereas each tufted cell sends dendrites to several glomeruli. Olfactory afferents within the glomeruli also activate periglomerular cells, which then inhibit mitral and tufted cells. Further inhibition arises at the dendrodendritic contacts between mitral and tufted cells and the processes of granule cells, which lie deeper still within the olfactory bulb. These contacts are an example of two-way synaptic feedback connections: the granule cells are excited by mitral and tufted cells and, in turn, inhibit them. Integration of olfactory information occurs when excitation is spread throughout the multiple-branched granule cell processes, and also when granule cells are excited by the centrifugal efferent fibers that reach the olfactory bulb from higher centers. Another factor in this highly complex integrative process is the recurrent collaterals of mitral cells that appear to

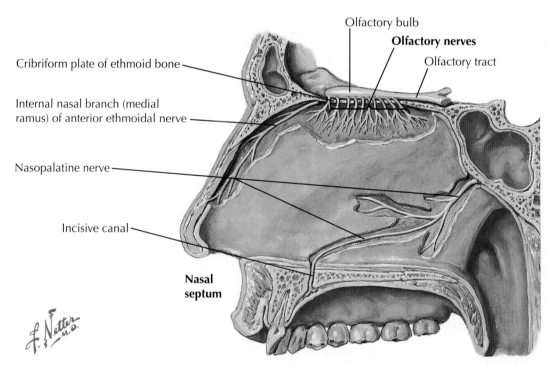

Cribriform plate of ethmoid bone

Internal nasal branch (medial ramus) of anterior ethmoidal nerve

Nasopalatine nerve

Incisive canal

Olfactory bulb

Olfactory nerves

Olfactory tract

Nasal septum

excite mitral, tufted, and granule cells. There is a dramatic transformation in the response to odors between the glomeruli and the mitral cells. The glomeruli respond to different substances based on their physiochemical properties, whereas mitral cells respond to groups of substances that evoke subjective sensations.

Olfactory Tract and Central Connections

The axons of mitral and tufted cells form the olfactory tract, through which they project to the olfactory trigone and into the lateral and medial olfactory striae, establishing a complex pattern of central connections. Some mitral and tufted cell axons terminate in the anterior olfactory nucleus (a continuation of the granule cell layer throughout the olfactory tract) and olfactory tubercle, the sites of origin of the efferent fibers projecting to both the ipsilateral and contralateral olfactory bulbs. Other axons from the lateral stria reach the piriform lobe of the temporal cortex and terminate in the amygdala (amygdaloid body), the septal nuclei, and the hypothalamus.

Plate 1.8   Cranial Nerve and Neuro-ophthalmologic Disorders

EYE

Horizontal section

Zonular fibers (suspensory ligament of lens)

Perichoroidal space   Hyaloid canal

Choroid

Sclera

Fascial sheath
of eyeball
(Tenon's capsule)

Episcleral space

Fovea centralis
in macula (lutea)

Meningeal sheath
of optic nerve

Subara-
chnoid
space

Central retinal
artery and vein

Optic nerve (II)

Lamina cribrosa of sclera

Tendon of medial
rectus muscle

Ciliary part of retina

Ciliary body
and ciliary muscle

Bulbar conjunctiva

Scleral spur

Scleral venous
sinus (canal of
Schlemm)

Iris

Lens

Capsule
of lens

Cornea

Anterior
chamber

Posterior
chamber

Iridocorneal
angle

Ciliary processes

Ora serrata

Tendon of lateral
rectus muscle

Vitreous body

Section through retina

Inner limiting membrane

Axons at surface of retina passing via optic nerve,
chiasm, and tract to lateral geniculate body

Ganglion cell

Müller cell (supporting glial cell)

Amacrine cell

Bipolar cell

Horizontal cell

Rod

Cone

Pigment cells of choroid

CRANIAL NERVE II: OPTIC NERVE

HUMAN EYE

The human eye is a highly developed sense organ containing numerous accessory structures that modify visual stimuli before they reach the photoreceptors. The *extraocular muscles* move the eyeball, thus causing the image of the object viewed to fall on the *fovea*, the retinal area of highest visual acuity. The shape of the eyeball, its surfaces, and the refractive properties of the *tear film, cornea, lens,* and *aqueous* and *vitreous humor* assist in focusing the image on the retina. To allow viewing of near and far objects, this focus can be adjusted by the action of the *ciliary muscle,* which changes the shape of the lens. The intensity of the light reaching the retina is controlled by the muscles of the *iris,* which vary the size of the *pupillary aperture.* Incident light must traverse most of the retinal layers before it reaches the *photoreceptor cells* lying in the outer part of the retina. Beyond the photoreceptors is a layer of *pigment cells,* which eliminates back reflections by absorbing any light passing through the photoreceptor layer.

RETINA

The retina has several distinct layers. *Rods* and *cones* form synaptic connections with bipolar and horizontal cells. *Bipolar cells* are relay neurons that transmit visual

signals from the inner to the outer plexiform layer of the retina; *horizontal cells* are interneurons activated by rods and cones and send their axons laterally to act on neighboring bipolar cells. As a result of the actions of horizontal cells, bipolar cells have concentric receptive fields; that is, their membrane potentials are shifted in one direction by light reaching the center of their receptive field, and in the opposite direction by light reaching the surrounding area. Neither bipolar nor

horizontal cells generate action potentials; all information is transferred by changes in membrane potential, which spread passively through the cell bodies and axons.

The processes of bipolar cells that reach the outer plexiform layer form synapses with ganglion cells and amacrine cells. *Ganglion cells* are output neurons whose axons comprise the optic nerves and optic tracts; *amacrine cells* are interneurons. Unlike other retinal

CRANIAL NERVE II AND VISUAL PATHWAYS

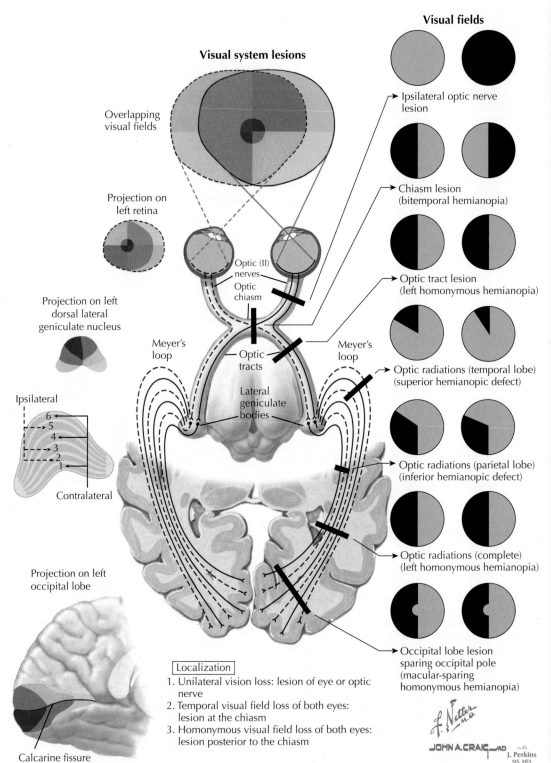

Visual fields

Visual system lesions

Overlapping visual fields

Projection on left retina

Projection on left dorsal lateral geniculate nucleus

Meyer's loop

Meyer's loop

Ipsilateral

Contralateral

Projection on left occipital lobe

Optic (II) nerves

Optic chiasm

Optic tracts

Lateral geniculate bodies

Calcarine fissure

Ipsilateral optic nerve lesion

Chiasm lesion (bitemporal hemianopia)

Optic tract lesion (left homonymous hemianopia)

Optic radiations (temporal lobe) (superior hemianopic defect)

Optic radiations (parietal lobe) (inferior hemianopic defect)

Optic radiations (complete) (left homonymous hemianopia)

Occipital lobe lesion sparing occipital pole (macular-sparing homonymous hemianopia)

Localization
1. Unilateral vision loss: lesion of eye or optic nerve
2. Temporal visual field loss of both eyes: lesion at the chiasm
3. Homonymous visual field loss of both eyes: lesion posterior to the chiasm

JOHN A. CRAIG—AD   with J. Perkins MS, MFA

CRANIAL NERVE II: OPTIC NERVE (Continued)

neurons, both amacrine and ganglion cells generate action potentials.

The *photoreceptor cells* are called rods and cones because of the shapes of their outer segments. *Rods* function as receptors in a highly sensitive, monochromatic visual system, whereas *cones* serve as receptors in the color vision system, which is less sensitive but more acute. Both receptors, however, are activated in a similar manner—they are hyperpolarized by photons of light falling directly upon them. For example, the detection of light in the rod begins with the absorption of photons by the visual pigment, *rhodopsin.* Rhodopsin is a combination of the protein opsin and the *cis* isomer of retinene, a compound derived from vitamin A. It is located within the membranous lamellae of the rod's outer segment, a highly modified cilium associated with a typical basal body. Upon the absorption of a photon, rhodopsin is converted to *lumirhodopsin,* which is unstable and changes spontaneously to *metarhodopsin,* which is then degraded by a chemical reaction known as bleaching. Rhodopsin lost by this bleaching process is restored to its active form by enzymatic reactions that require metabolic energy and vitamin A. After a brief time lag, the absorption of a photon leads to changes in the ionic permeability of the

membrane of the outer segment. The change in the receptor membrane triggered in the rod by light absorption is not the typical increase in ion permeability most sensory receptors undergo when activated; rather, there is a decrease in the permeability of the outer segment membrane to sodium ions (Na^+). In the absence of light, this permeability is relatively high, and there is a steady inward flow of Na^+ (the current flow resulting from this ionic movement, known as the "dark current,"

keeps the entire rod in a depolarized state). When light absorption provokes a decrease in Na^+ permeability, the dark current is cut off and the rod becomes more hyperpolarized. This hyperpolarization influences the synaptic action of the rod on horizontal and bipolar cells. Polarization changes in one rod may also spread to neighboring receptors via electrical synapses. Any photon that is successfully absorbed by photopigment produces the same electrochemical result, regardless of

Plate 1.10

Cranial Nerve and Neuro-ophthalmologic Disorders

OPTIC NERVE APPEARANCE

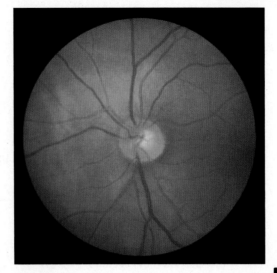

Normal optic nerve

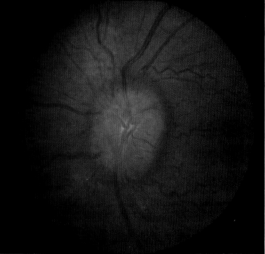

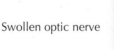
Swollen optic nerve

CRANIAL NERVE II: OPTIC NERVE (Continued)

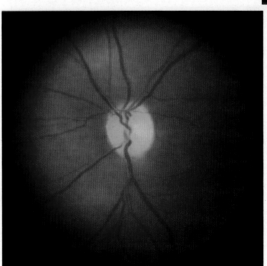

Pale optic nerve

the wavelength of that photon. However, the probability that a photon will be absorbed by photopigment varies considerably with the wavelength of the incident light, and rhodopsin has a maximal absorbency for light with a wavelength of 500 nm. Cones may contain one of three different photopigments, with a maximum absorbency at 445 nm (blue), 535 nm (green), and 570 nm (red). Cone pigments all contain *cis* retinene but have different forms of opsin, which modify the light absorption pattern. By analyzing the relative activity produced by the three types of cones, the central nervous system (CNS) can determine the wavelength of the incident light, and a sensation of color vision results.

RETINOGENICULOSTRIATE VISUAL PATHWAY

In mammals, most retinal ganglion cells send excitatory or inhibitory impulses via the *optic nerves* and *tracts* to the *dorsal lateral geniculate nucleus* of the lateral geniculate body of the thalamus, from where retinal information is relayed to the primary visual cortex via the *geniculostriate projection,* or *optic radiations.* In humans, this cortical area covers both walls of the posterior calcarine fissure and adjacent parts of the occipital pole (Brodmann's area 17). The transmission of information from retina to visual cortex is topographically organized. Stimuli in the right half of the visual field activate neurons in the left half of each retina. Ganglion cells from these areas project to the left lateral geniculate body, which then projects to the left visual cortex. Input from both eyes is relayed by neurons in different layers of the lateral geniculate body. Similarly, stimuli in the left half of the visual field are relayed to the right visual cortex.

The upper and lower visual fields are also topographically mapped onto the lateral geniculate body and visual cortex. The upper field is represented in the lateral parts of the lateral geniculate nuclei and the inferior portions of the visual cortex, and the lower visual field is represented in the corresponding medial and superior regions. The *macula* (central visual field) is represented in the central parts of the lateral geniculate nuclei and the posterior visual cortex, and the *peripheral retina* in

RETINAL PROJECTIONS TO THALAMUS, MIDBRAIN, AND BRAINSTEM

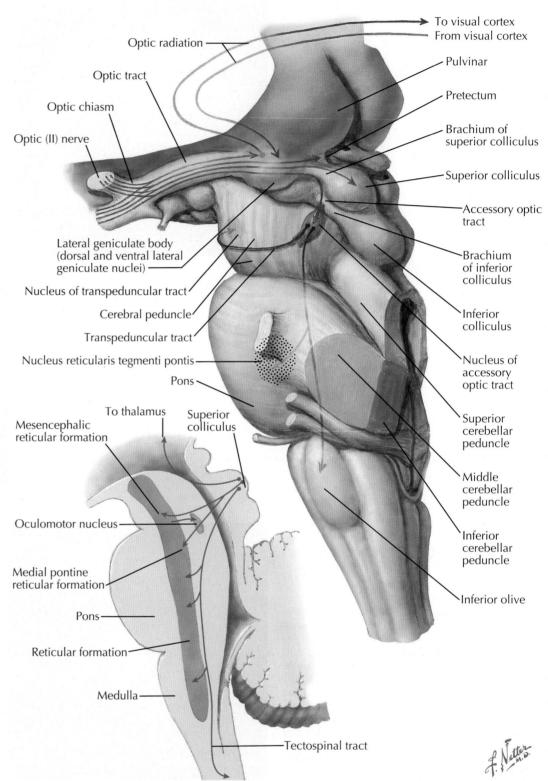

CRANIAL NERVE II: OPTIC NERVE (Continued)

the peripheral parts of the lateral geniculate nuclei and the anterior visual cortex. The fovea, the central spot of the macula, is represented by a proportionally larger cortical area than the periphery of the retina.

NEUROLOGIC DEFICITS OF THE RETINA AND OPTIC NERVE

Neurologic deficits in the visual system can be localized by determining the type and extent of the resultant visual field deficit. Retinal and optic nerve damage produces vision loss in the affected eye. Most retinal lesions will be visible on ophthalmoscopy of the ocular fundus. Optic nerve lesions will produce central scotomas and visual field defects that might respect the horizontal meridian. If the optic nerve is affected in its anterior portion (i.e., where it is visualized on ocular funduscopy), one may see swelling of the optic nerve head during the acute phase of injury. If the retrobulbar portion of the optic nerve is the site of injury, then the optic nerve head (so-called optic disc) will look normal acutely. After several weeks, injury to the optic nerve anywhere along its course will manifest as relative pallor of the optic nerve head. Unilateral or asymmetric bilateral optic nerve damage will cause a relative afferent pupillary defect

(less transmission of light along the more damaged optic nerve to the brain centers controlling pupillary constriction).

CHIASMAL AND POSTCHIASMAL NEUROLOGIC DEFICITS

Lesions at the optic chiasm will result in bitemporal hemianopsia, caused by damage to the fibers from the nasal segment of both retinas. Interruption of the optic

tract (that portion of the visual pathways between the chiasm and lateral geniculate body) results in a contralateral homonymous hemianopsia. Similarly, lesions of the optic radiations or striate cortex will cause partial or complete contralateral homonymous hemianopic defects.

VISUAL SYSTEM: RETINAL PROJECTIONS

The main retinal projection is to the *dorsal lateral geniculate nucleus,* which then projects to the visual

Plate 1.12   Cranial Nerve and Neuro-ophthalmologic Disorders

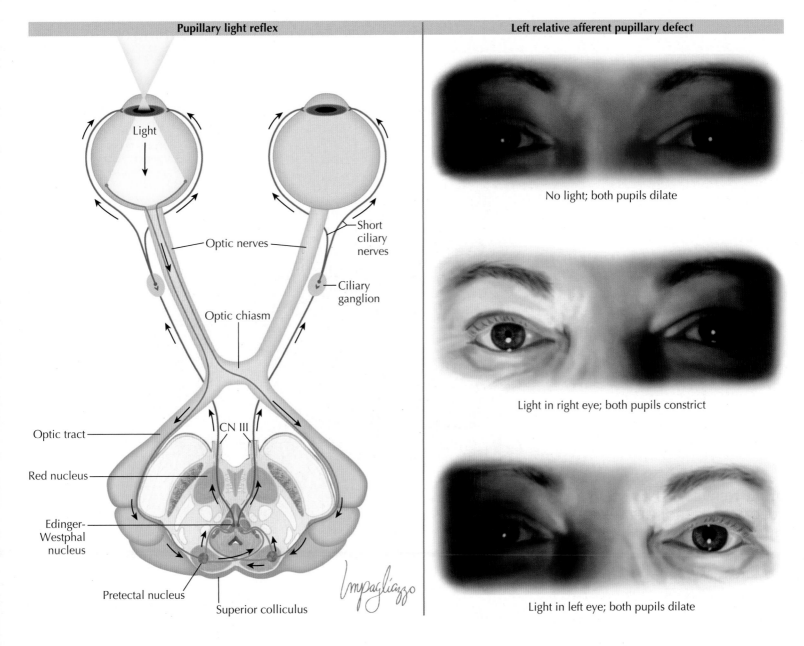

Pupillary light reflex

Light

Optic nerves

Short ciliary nerves

Ciliary ganglion

Optic chiasm

Optic tract

CN III

Red nucleus

Edinger-Westphal nucleus

Pretectal nucleus

Superior colliculus

Impagliazzo

Left relative afferent pupillary defect

No light; both pupils dilate

Light in right eye; both pupils constrict

Light in left eye; both pupils dilate

CRANIAL NERVE II: OPTIC NERVE
(Continued)

cortex. The retinogeniculostriate system thus formed is the basis for essentially the entire visual consciousness in humans.

Other optic nerve fibers terminate within the *superior colliculus.* This multilayered structure plays an important role in orienting the reactions that shift the head and eyes to bring an object of interest into the center of the visual field. In addition to direct optic nerve input, the superior colliculus receives indirect visual input via the visual cortex. As is the case throughout the visual system, this input is topographically organized so that each point within the colliculus corresponds to a particular region within the visual field. Collicular neurons tend to respond best to interesting or moving stimuli, and the discharge of neurons in the deeper layers of the colliculus is closely related to the orienting movements of the eyes evoked by such stimuli.

The deeper collicular layers are the source of several efferent projections. One group of fibers crosses the midline and runs caudally, sending terminals to the brainstem reticular formation and then continuing to cervical and thoracic levels as the *tectospinal tract;* these fibers are probably involved in the orienting movements of the head and body. A second group of fibers projects to the posterior thalamus (pulvinar), which then projects to the cortical association areas. Fiber projections responsible for eye movements relay in the mesencephalic reticular formation below the superior colliculus (vertical eye movements) and in the paramedian pontine reticular formation (horizontal eye movements).

PUPILLARY LIGHT REFLEX AND THE
ACCOMMODATION REFLEX

The *pretectum,* like the superior colliculus, receives visual information from optic nerve fibers not destined to synapse in the lateral geniculate bodies. This area is involved in the pupillary light reflex (which regulates the size of the pupil) and the accommodation reflex (which con-

trols the degree of curvature of the lens). The former is a subcortical reflex and relays in the accessory oculomotor (Edinger-Westphal) nucleus, whereas the latter involves pathways through the cerebral cortex. In the pupillary light reflex, afferent pupillary fibers leave the optic tract before the lateral geniculate bodies, travel in the brachium of the superior colliculus, and synapse in the pretectal nuclei (explaining why lesions of the geniculate bodies, the optic radiations, and the visual cortex do not affect pupillary reactivity, and why lesions of the brachium of the superior colliculus can cause a relative afferent pupillary defect without causing a visual field defect). Both pretectal nuclei receive input from both eyes, and each sends axons to both Edinger-Westphal nuclei. Parasympathetic fibers for pupillary constriction leave the Edinger-Westphal nucleus and travel as part of the ipsilateral third cranial nerve to the ipsilateral ciliary ganglion within the orbit. The postganglionic parasympathetic fibers innervate the pupillary constrictor muscle and the ciliary muscle for accommodation.

OCULOMOTOR (III), TROCHLEAR (IV), AND ABDUCENS NERVES (VI)

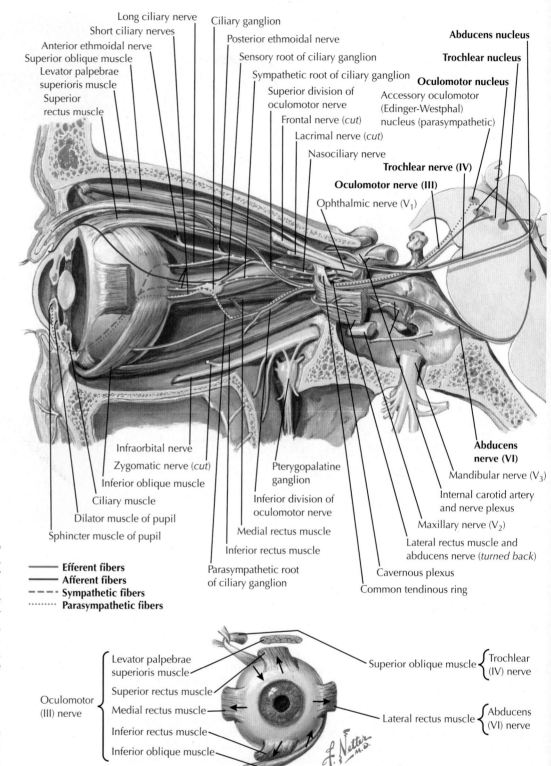

Long ciliary nerve
Short ciliary nerves
Anterior ethmoidal nerve
Superior oblique muscle
Levator palpebrae superioris muscle
Superior rectus muscle

Ciliary ganglion
Posterior ethmoidal nerve
Sensory root of ciliary ganglion
Sympathetic root of ciliary ganglion
Superior division of oculomotor nerve
Frontal nerve (cut)
Lacrimal nerve (cut)
Nasociliary nerve

Abducens nucleus
Trochlear nucleus
Oculomotor nucleus
Accessory oculomotor (Edinger-Westphal) nucleus (parasympathetic)
Trochlear nerve (IV)
Oculomotor nerve (III)
Ophthalmic nerve (V₁)

Infraorbital nerve
Zygomatic nerve (cut)
Inferior oblique muscle
Ciliary muscle
Dilator muscle of pupil
Sphincter muscle of pupil

Pterygopalatine ganglion
Inferior division of oculomotor nerve
Medial rectus muscle
Inferior rectus muscle

Abducens nerve (VI)
Mandibular nerve (V₃)
Internal carotid artery and nerve plexus
Maxillary nerve (V₂)
Lateral rectus muscle and abducens nerve (turned back)

Parasympathetic root of ciliary ganglion

Cavernous plexus
Common tendinous ring

—— Efferent fibers
—— Afferent fibers
--- Sympathetic fibers
····· Parasympathetic fibers

Levator palpebrae superioris muscle
Oculomotor (III) nerve
Superior rectus muscle
Medial rectus muscle
Inferior rectus muscle
Inferior oblique muscle

Superior oblique muscle { Trochlear (IV) nerve
Lateral rectus muscle { Abducens (VI) nerve

CRANIAL NERVES III, IV, AND VI (OCULOMOTOR, TROCHLEAR, AND ABDUCENS)

OCULOMOTOR NERVE

The oculomotor nerve carries somatic motor fibers to the levator palpebrae superioris muscle; the medial, superior, and inferior recti muscles; and the inferior oblique muscle. It also conveys important parasympathetic fibers to intraocular structures, such as the sphincter pupillae and ciliary muscles, and is joined by sympathetic fibers from the internal carotid plexus, which are distributed with its branches. Some oculomotor proprioceptive fibers may reach the midbrain through the oculomotor nerve; most of them join the ophthalmic branch of the trigeminal nerve via its communications with the oculomotor nerve.

Oculomotor Nuclei

The somatic and parasympathetic efferent fibers in the oculomotor nerve are the axons of cells located in the complex oculomotor nuclei situated anterolateral to the upper end of the cerebral aqueduct. The nuclei are composed of groups of large and small multipolar cells. The main groups of large cells are arranged in two columns of *posterolateral, intermediate,* and *anteromedial nuclei,* one on each side of the midline, which control the rectus and oblique extraocular muscles. A single *median nucleus,* composed of similar cells and partly overlying the caudal and posterior aspects of the bilateral columns, controls the levator muscles of the upper eyelids. Cranial to the median nucleus, and also partially overlying the posterior aspects of the main bilateral columns, are two narrow, wing-shaped nuclei,

which are interconnected across the midline at their cranial ends—the *accessory (autonomic) nuclei* (Edinger-Westphal). They are the source of parasympathetic preganglionic fibers for the ciliary ganglion. The multiple subnuclei of the oculomotor nucleus each project ipsilaterally via the oculomotor nerve to the individual muscles that they innervate except for the superior rectus subnucleus, which projects contralaterally via the contralateral oculomotor nerve to the contralateral superior rectus muscle.

Oculomotor Nerve

The axons from the bilateral oculomotor nuclear cells form minute bundles, which run through the mesencephalic tegmentum, traversing the red nuclei to emerge from the mesencephalic oculomotor sulcus as the oculomotor nerve rootlets.

Each *oculomotor nerve* runs forward between the posterior cerebral and superior cerebellar arteries and lateral to the posterior communicating artery in the interpeduncular subarachnoid cistern. It pierces the

Plate 1.14   Cranial Nerve and Neuro-ophthalmologic Disorders

CRANIAL NERVES III, IV, AND VI (OCULOMOTOR, TROCHLEAR, AND ABDUCENS) (Continued)

NERVES OF ORBIT AND CAVERNOUS SINUS

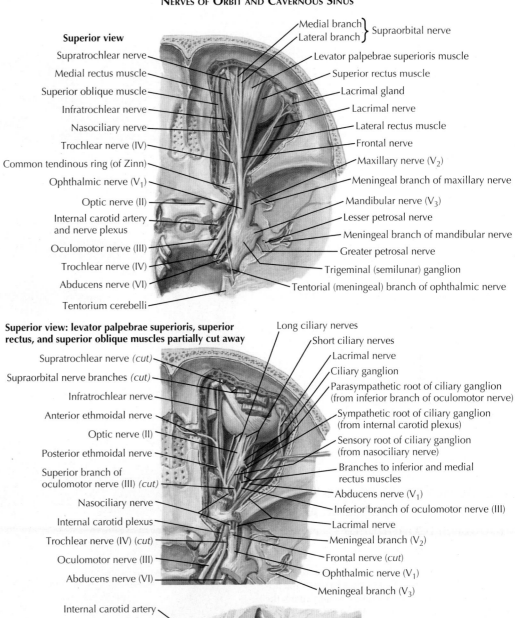

Superior view

Supratrochlear nerve
Medial rectus muscle
Superior oblique muscle
Infratrochlear nerve
Nasociliary nerve
Trochlear nerve (IV)
Common tendinous ring (of Zinn)
Ophthalmic nerve (V₁)
Optic nerve (II)
Internal carotid artery and nerve plexus
Oculomotor nerve (III)
Trochlear nerve (IV)
Abducens nerve (VI)
Tentorium cerebelli

Medial branch } Supraorbital nerve
Lateral branch }
Levator palpebrae superioris muscle
Superior rectus muscle
Lacrimal gland
Lacrimal nerve
Lateral rectus muscle
Frontal nerve
Maxillary nerve (V₂)
Meningeal branch of maxillary nerve
Mandibular nerve (V₃)
Lesser petrosal nerve
Meningeal branch of mandibular nerve
Greater petrosal nerve
Trigeminal (semilunar) ganglion
Tentorial (meningeal) branch of ophthalmic nerve

Superior view: levator palpebrae superioris, superior rectus, and superior oblique muscles partially cut away

Supratrochlear nerve (cut)
Supraorbital nerve branches (cut)
Infratrochlear nerve
Anterior ethmoidal nerve
Optic nerve (II)
Posterior ethmoidal nerve
Superior branch of oculomotor nerve (III) (cut)
Nasociliary nerve
Internal carotid plexus
Trochlear nerve (IV) (cut)
Oculomotor nerve (III)
Abducens nerve (VI)

Long ciliary nerves
Short ciliary nerves
Lacrimal nerve
Ciliary ganglion
Parasympathetic root of ciliary ganglion (from inferior branch of oculomotor nerve)
Sympathetic root of ciliary ganglion (from internal carotid plexus)
Sensory root of ciliary ganglion (from nasociliary nerve)
Branches to inferior and medial rectus muscles
Abducens nerve (V₁)
Inferior branch of oculomotor nerve (III)
Lacrimal nerve
Meningeal branch (V₂)
Frontal nerve (cut)
Ophthalmic nerve (V₁)
Meningeal branch (V₃)

Internal carotid artery
Oculomotor (III) nerve
Trochlear (IV) nerve
Internal carotid artery
Abducens (VI) nerve
Ophthalmic nerve
Cavernous sinus
Maxillary nerve

Optic chiasm
Diaphragma sellae
Pituitary gland

f. Netter M.D.

arachnoid and dura mater in the angle between the free and attached margins of the tentorium cerebelli to enter first the roof of the cavernous sinus and then its lateral wall. Continuing forward above the trochlear nerve, the oculomotor nerve divides into superior and inferior rami as it enters the orbit through the superior orbital fissure.

The smaller *superior division* supplies the superior rectus muscle and the main superficial (voluntary, or striated, muscular) lamina of the levator palpebrae superioris. The deep lamina is a tenuous layer of involuntary, or unstriated, fibers known as the superior tarsal muscle; a similar but even more tenuous inferior tarsal muscle is present in the lower eyelid, and both these tarsal muscles are innervated by sympathetic fibers. The larger *inferior division* supplies the medial and inferior recti and the inferior oblique muscles.

CILIARY GANGLION

The ciliary ganglion is tiny and lies in the posterior part of the orbit between the optic nerve and the lateral rectus muscle. Only the first of its three roots is constant because the sensory and/or sympathetic roots may bypass the ganglion.

Motor Root

The ciliary ganglion is the relay station for preganglionic *parasympathetic fibers,* which originate in the accessory

(autonomic) oculomotor nucleus and reach the ganglion through a short offshoot from the oculomotor branch to the inferior oblique muscle. The postganglionic fibers form the 12 to 20 delicate *short ciliary nerves* that penetrate the sclera around the optic nerve and continue forward in the perichoroidal space to supply the ciliaris and sphincter pupillae muscles and the intraocular vessels.

The *sensory and sympathetic roots* of the ciliary ganglion are derived from the nasociliary nerve and the internal carotid vascular nerve plexus, but they do not always join the ganglion. Instead, their fibers may reach

the eye by joining the ciliary nerves directly, whereas the *sympathetic fibers* (already postganglionic after relaying in the superior cervical trunk ganglia) may follow the ophthalmic artery and its branches to their destinations. The *sensory fibers* convey impulses from the cornea, iris, and choroid and the intraocular muscles.

TROCHLEAR NERVE

The trochlear nerve is slender, and its nucleus of origin is in the midbrain just caudal to the oculomotor nuclei.

DAMAGE TO CRANIAL NERVE III

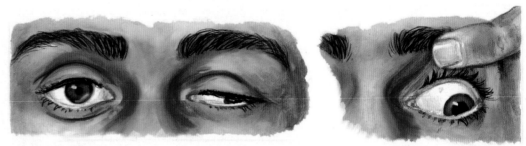

Oculomotor palsy. Affected eye exhibits ptosis and a dilated pupil. The eye is abducted and depressed due to the pull of the two extraocular muscles that are functioning.

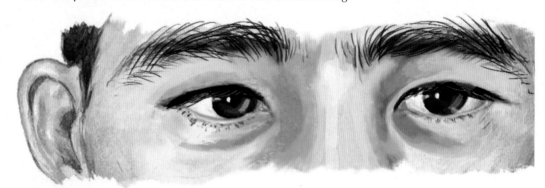

Abducens palsy. Affected eye is adducted due to the loss of abduction by the lateral rectus muscle.

CRANIAL NERVES III, IV, AND VI (OCULOMOTOR, TROCHLEAR, AND ABDUCENS) (Continued)

The trochlear fibers curve posterolaterally and slightly caudally around the cerebral aqueduct to reach the upper part of the superior medullary velum; here the nerve fibers from opposite sides decussate before emerging on either side of the frenulum veli, below the inferior colliculi. No other cranial nerves emerge from the dorsal aspect of the brainstem.

Each trochlear nerve winds forward around the midbrain below the free edge of the tentorium cerebelli, passes between the superior cerebellar and posterior cerebral arteries and above the trigeminal nerve, and pierces the inferior surface of the tentorium near its attachment to the posterior clinoid process to run forward in the lateral wall of the cavernous sinus between the oculomotor and ophthalmic nerves. The nerve enters the orbit through its superior fissure, immediately lateral to the common annular tendon, and passes medially between the orbital roof and the levator palpebrae superioris to supply the *superior oblique muscle.* Proprioceptive fibers are transferred through a communication with the ophthalmic nerve to the trigeminal nerve. The trochlear nerve usually receives sympathetic filaments from the internal carotid nerve plexus.

ABDUCENS NERVE

The abducens nerve arises from the abducens nucleus, which is in the pons, subjacent to the facial colliculus in the upper half of the floor of the fourth ventricle.

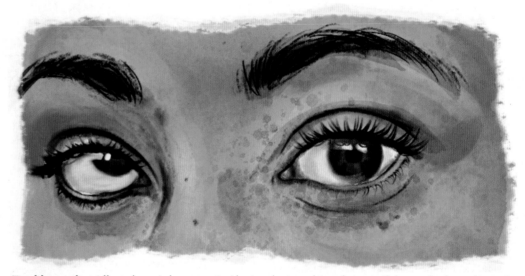

Trochlear palsy. Affected eye is hypertropic (deviated upwards) and extorted due to the loss of superior oblique function.

The nucleus is encircled by fibers of the homolateral facial nerve. The abducens nerve fibers pass forward to emerge near the midline through the groove between the pons and the pyramid of the medulla oblongata. Each abducens nerve then inclines upward in front of the pons, usually behind the inferior cerebellar artery. Near the apex of the petrous part of the temporal bone, the nerve bends sharply forward above the superior petrosal sinus to enter the cavernous sinus, where it lies adjacent to the internal carotid artery. There the abducens may transfer proprioceptive fibers to the ophthalmic branch of the trigeminal nerve and receive sympathetic filaments from the internal carotid nerve plexus. The abducens nerve enters the orbit through the superior orbital fissure, within the common annular tendon, and ends by supplying the *lateral rectus muscle.*

The abducens has a relatively long intracranial route in the posterior cranial fossa and cavernous sinus. Consequently, it is vulnerable to increases in intracranial pressure and to pathologic or traumatic lesions affecting nearby parts of the brain, skull, or sinus.

Plate 1.16

Cranial Nerve and Neuro-ophthalmologic Disorders

CONTROL OF EYE MOVEMENTS

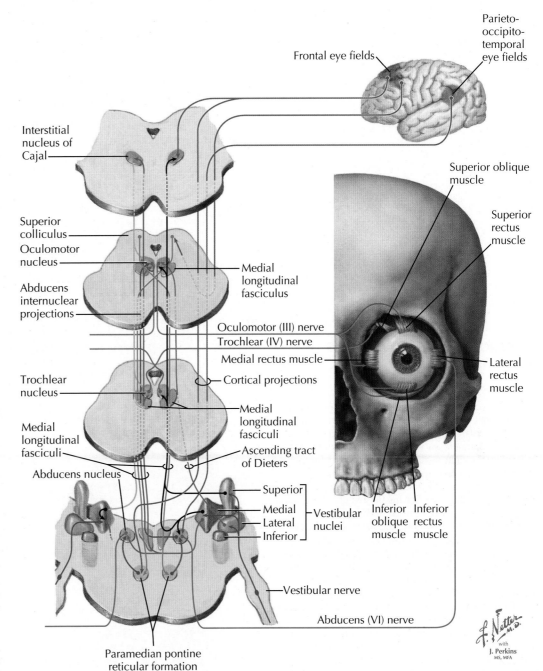

Excitatory endings →→→→→→→→→

Inhibitory endings ⟶

Frontal eye fields

Parieto-occipito-temporal eye fields

Interstitial nucleus of Cajal

Superior colliculus

Oculomotor nucleus

Abducens internuclear projections

Trochlear nucleus

Medial longitudinal fasciculi

Abducens nucleus

Superior oblique muscle

Superior rectus muscle

Medial longitudinal fasciculus

Oculomotor (III) nerve

Trochlear (IV) nerve

Medial rectus muscle

Lateral rectus muscle

Cortical projections

Medial longitudinal fasciculi

Ascending tract of Dieters

Superior

Medial

Lateral

Inferior

Vestibular nuclei

Inferior oblique muscle

Inferior rectus muscle

Vestibular nerve

Abducens (VI) nerve

Paramedian pontine reticular formation

CONTROL OF EYE MOVEMENTS

The extraocular muscles responsible for eye movements are controlled by motor neurons located in various nuclei. Thus the lateral rectus is controlled by the abducens nucleus, the superior oblique by the trochlear nucleus, and the superior, inferior, and medial recti and the inferior oblique muscles by the oculomotor nucleus. Both smooth (pursuit) and rapid (saccadic) eye movements depend on patterns of activity produced in these muscles by direct projections from the vestibular nuclei and the reticular formation, and by indirect activation from the superior colliculus and the cerebral cortex.

The *medial* and *lateral rectus muscles* move the eyeball horizontally, causing the cornea to look medially or laterally. The actions of the superior and inferior rectus muscles and those of the oblique muscles are more complicated. The *superior* and *inferior rectus muscles* move the eyeball upward and downward, respectively. Because they are disposed at an angle of about 20 degrees to the sagittal plane (due to the long axis of each orbit being directed slightly outward), they also impart a minor degree of rotation to the eyeball (intorsion for the superior rectus and extorsion for the inferior rectus). When the eyeball is abducted, the superior and inferior rectus muscles purely elevate and depress the eyeball. The *inferior oblique muscle* rotates the eyeball outward (excyclotorsion) and elevates the eyeball when it is adducted. However, an exact idea of the actions of the extrinsic eye muscles cannot be obtained by considering each muscle separately because, under normal circumstances, none of the six extraocular muscles acts alone. Consequently, all eye movements are the result of highly integrated and delicately controlled agonist and antagonist activities. The actions of individual muscles have been determined from studies of congenital

defects or from functional disturbances caused by disease or injury to the nerve supply.

VESTIBULAR PROJECTIONS IMPORTANT FOR VISUAL FIXATION

The vestibular projection is important for the maintenance of visual fixation during head movements. To effect smooth movement, tracking, and proper visualization, the contraction of one eye muscle must be

accompanied by the relaxation of its antagonist. The action of turning the head excites *vestibular afferent fibers* from semicircular canal receptors. Fibers from an individual semicircular canal excite two specific groups of relay neurons in the *vestibular nuclei*. One group excites the extraocular motor neurons that cause the eyes to move in the direction opposite to the head movement, and the other group inhibits motor neurons that activate movement of the eyes in the same direction as the head. For example, turning the head to the

CONTROL OF EYE MOVEMENTS: PATHOLOGY

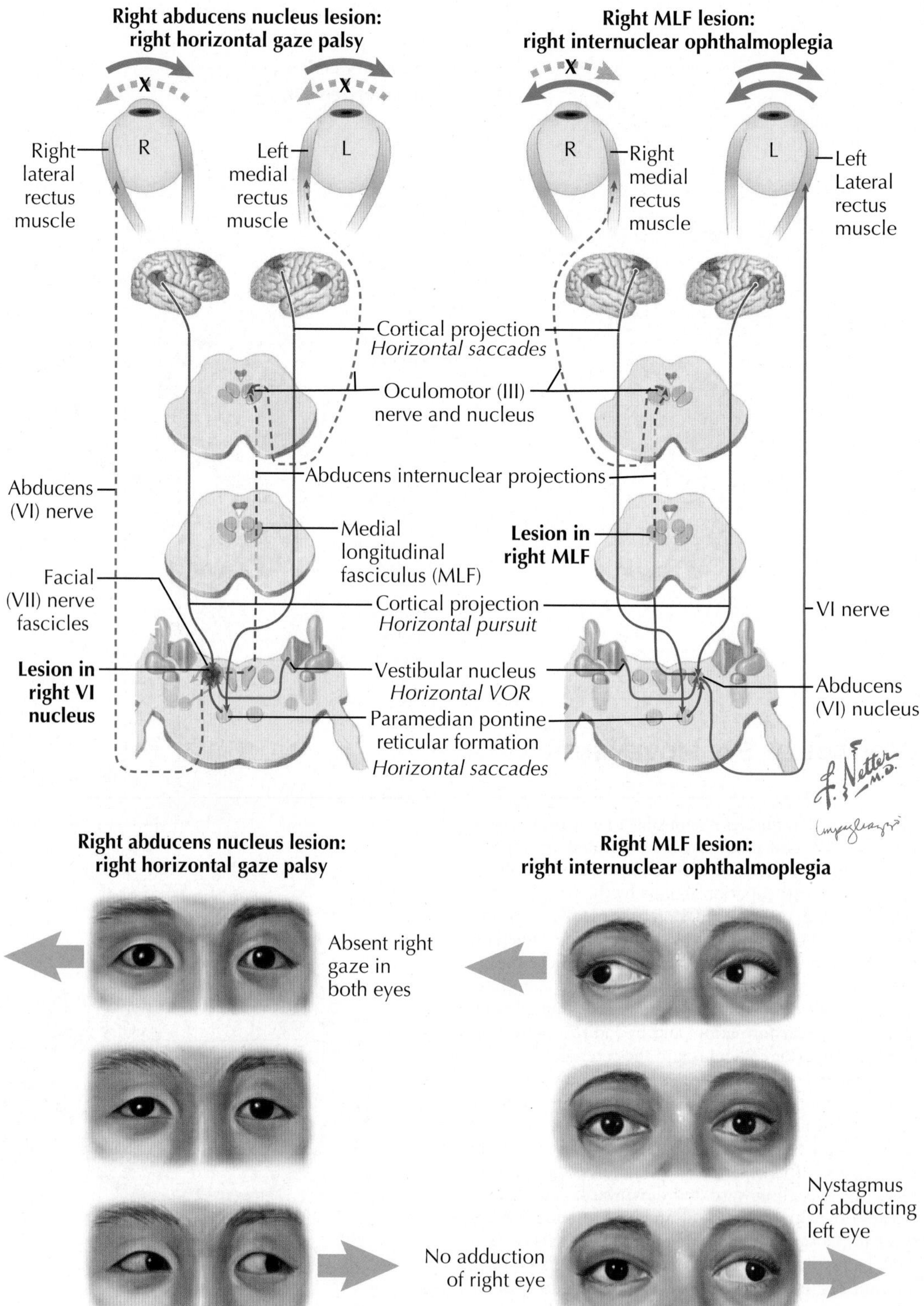

Right abducens nucleus lesion:
right horizontal gaze palsy

Right MLF lesion:
right internuclear ophthalmoplegia

Right lateral rectus muscle

Left medial rectus muscle

Right medial rectus muscle

Left Lateral rectus muscle

Cortical projection
Horizontal saccades

Oculomotor (III) nerve and nucleus

Abducens internuclear projections

Abducens (VI) nerve

Medial longitudinal fasciculus (MLF)

Lesion in right MLF

Facial (VII) nerve fascicles

Cortical projection
Horizontal pursuit

Lesion in right VI nucleus

Vestibular nucleus
Horizontal VOR

Paramedian pontine reticular formation
Horizontal saccades

VI nerve

Abducens (VI) nucleus

CONTROL OF EYE MOVEMENTS
(Continued)

right will excite fibers from the right horizontal semicircular canal, which, in turn, will activate neurons in the right medial and lateral vestibular nuclei. Some of these vestibular neurons will then excite motor neurons controlling the right medial and left lateral rectus muscles. Other vestibular neurons will inhibit motor neurons controlling the right lateral rectus and internuclear neurons controlling the left medial rectus. The result will be a compensatory movement of both eyes to the left. The vestibulocerebellum modulates the vestibulo–extraocular reflex in such a way that the resulting eye movement precisely compensates for the head movement and thus keeps the gaze fixed on the same point.

The connections of the right vestibular nuclei to the *abducens, trochlear,* and *oculomotor nuclei* can be divided into two sections. The first section comprises vestibular projections to motor neurons supplying the superior and inferior rectus and superior and inferior oblique muscles. These motor neurons all receive excitatory input from the contralateral medial nucleus and inhibitory input from the ipsilateral superior nucleus. The innervation of medial and lateral rectus motor neurons, which mediate horizontal eye movements, is organized differently. The medial vestibular nucleus sends excitatory fibers to the contralateral abducens nucleus and inhibitory fibers to the ipsilateral abducens nucleus. These fibers excite or inhibit the lateral rectus motor neurons and another group of neurons within the abducens nucleus, the internuclear neurons, which project to the opposite oculomotor nucleus to excite the medial rectus motor neurons. The latter neurons are also excited by fibers that originate in the lateral vestibular nucleus and pass upward in the ascending tract of Deiters.

Right abducens nucleus lesion:
right horizontal gaze palsy

Right MLF lesion:
right internuclear ophthalmoplegia

Absent right gaze in both eyes

No adduction of right eye

Nystagmus of abducting left eye

In addition to the pathways described above, each ocular motor nucleus also receives input for saccadic and pursuit eye movements that do not involve the vestibular nuclei. These pathways ultimately converge on the final common pathways for horizontal and vertical ocular motor control also used in the vestibulo-ocular system, but initially via different anatomic pathways. For example, saccadic eye movements (fast conjugate eye movements to a fixed target, either voluntary or reflex in origin) are initiated in the frontal and parietal lobes. The horizontal saccade pathway is a crossed pathway. Pathways from the frontal and parietal eye fields descend via the superior colliculus into the brainstem and cross at the level of the midbrain–pontine junction to synapse on the contralateral paramedian pontine reticular formation. The paramedian pontine reticular formation projects to the ipsilateral abducens nucleus, from which abducens neurons project to the ipsilateral

Plate 1.18

Cranial Nerve and Neuro-ophthalmologic Disorders

CONTROL OF EYE MOVEMENTS: PATHOLOGY (CONTINUED)

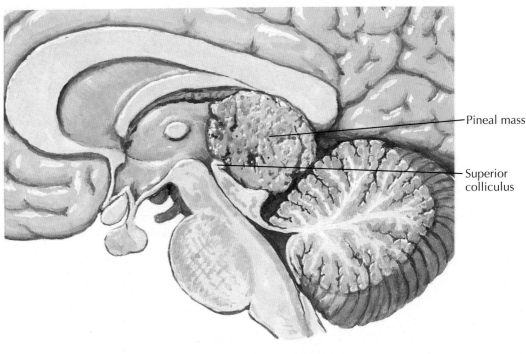

Pineal mass

Superior colliculus

CONTROL OF EYE MOVEMENTS (Continued)

lateral rectus muscle, whereas abducens interneurons project cross the midline to ascend in the contralateral medial longitudinal fasciculus and synapse on the medial rectus subnucleus of the contralateral oculomotor nucleus. The pathways for vertical saccades involve the rostral interstitial nucleus of the medial longitudinal fasciculus, the interstitial nucleus of Cajal, the posterior commissure, and the nucleus of the posterior commissure.

In contrast to the saccadic pathways, the pathways for horizontal smooth pursuit (conjugate maintenance of fixation of the eyes while following a moving target) descend ipsilaterally from cortical centers of eye movement control to synapse directly on the abducens nucleus, and from there to the ipsilateral abducens nerve and lateral rectus and the contralateral oculomotor nerve and medial rectus. This internuclear connection between the abducens nucleus and the contralateral oculomotor nucleus via the medial longitudinal fasciculus is the final common pathway responsible for conjugate horizontal gaze, whether initiated reflexively via the vestibulo-ocular system or voluntarily via the saccadic or pursuit systems.

NEUROLOGIC DEFICITS

Eye movement disorders from brainstem involvement of the pathways subserving horizontal and vertical gaze are usually exquisitely localizing. For example, a lesion in the right abducens nucleus will cause a complete loss of gaze of either eye toward the right (usually with an associated ipsilateral lower motor neuron facial palsy because the fascicles of the facial nerve wrap around the abducens nucleus before exiting the brainstem),

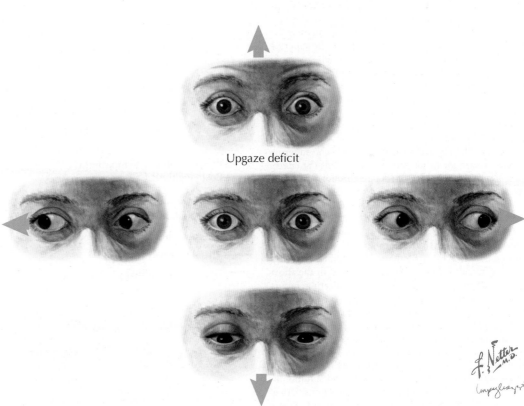

Upgaze deficit

Posterior midbrain syndrome (with upgaze palsy and lid retraction) secondary to a pineal mass

whereas a lesion of just the right paramedian pontine reticular formation will cause an absence of voluntary and reflex saccades to the right, with relative preservation of the vestibulo-ocular reflex and pursuit eye movements. A lesion of the right medial longitudinal fasciculus will disrupt only the abducens interneuron projections, and therefore the patient will have all eye movements intact except for poor adduction of the right eye (poor movement of the right eye toward the nose), a so-called internuclear ophthalmoplegia.

Vertical gaze may be selectively abnormal, with lesions in the midbrain and pretectal area, especially from compression from above, such as typically seen with pineal tumors. If the posterior commissure is primarily involved, these patients may have selective absence of upward eye movements with preservation of all other eye movements. Associated clinical abnormalities include upper lid retraction and nonreactive pupils to light with intact pupillary constriction when viewing a near target (all part of the so-called dorsal midbrain syndrome).

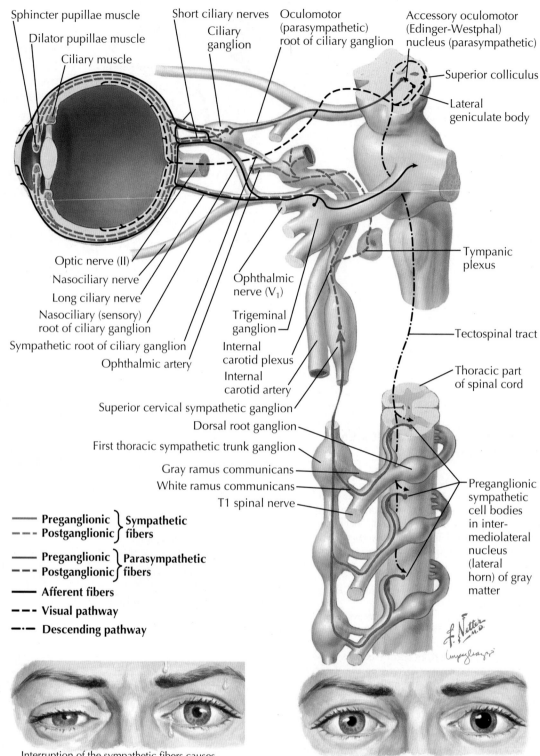

CILIARY GANGLION

Sphincter pupillae muscle
Dilator pupillae muscle
Ciliary muscle
Short ciliary nerves
Ciliary ganglion
Oculomotor (parasympathetic) root of ciliary ganglion
Accessory oculomotor (Edinger-Westphal) nucleus (parasympathetic)
Superior colliculus
Lateral geniculate body
Optic nerve (II)
Nasociliary nerve
Long ciliary nerve
Nasociliary (sensory) root of ciliary ganglion
Sympathetic root of ciliary ganglion
Ophthalmic artery
Ophthalmic nerve (V₁)
Trigeminal ganglion
Internal carotid plexus
Internal carotid artery
Superior cervical sympathetic ganglion
Dorsal root ganglion
First thoracic sympathetic trunk ganglion
Gray ramus communicans
White ramus communicans
T1 spinal nerve
Tympanic plexus
Tectospinal tract
Thoracic part of spinal cord
Preganglionic sympathetic cell bodies in intermediolateral nucleus (lateral horn) of gray matter

—— Preganglionic } Sympathetic
--- Postganglionic } fibers

—— Preganglionic } Parasympathetic
--- Postganglionic } fibers

━━ Afferent fibers
--- Visual pathway
-·- Descending pathway

Interruption of the sympathetic fibers causes ipsilateral ptosis, anhidrosis, and miosis without abnormal ocular motility (Horner syndrome)

Left dilated pupil with no other sign caused by left ciliary ganglion lesion

AUTONOMIC INNERVATION OF THE EYE

SYMPATHETIC FIBERS

The sympathetic *preganglionic fibers* for the eye emerge in the ipsilateral first and second, and occasionally in the third, thoracic spinal nerves. They pass through white or mixed rami communicantes to the sympathetic trunks in which the fibers ascend to the superior cervical ganglion, where they relay, although a proportion may form synapses higher up in the internal carotid ganglia. The *postganglionic fibers* run either in the internal carotid plexus and reach the eye in filaments that enter the orbit through its superior fissure, or else they run alongside the ophthalmic artery in its periarterial plexus.

Some of the filaments passing through the superior orbital fissure form the *sympathetic root of the ciliary ganglion;* their contained fibers pass through it without relaying to become incorporated in the 8 to 10 *short ciliary nerves.* Other filaments join the ophthalmic nerve or its nasociliary branch and reach the eye in the two to three *long ciliary nerves* that supply the radial musculature in the iris (dilator pupillae). Both long and short ciliary nerves also contain afferent fibers from the cornea, iris, and choroid. Fibers conveyed in the short ciliary nerves pass through a communicating ramus from the ciliary ganglion to the nasociliary nerve; this ramus is called the *sensory root of the ciliary ganglion.* The parent cells of these sensory fibers are in the trigeminal (semilunar) ganglion, and their central processes end in the *sensory trigeminal nuclei* in the brainstem. The sensory trigeminal nuclei have multiple interconnections with other somatic and autonomic centers and thus influence many reflex reactions. Other sympathetic fibers from the internal carotid plexus reach the eye through the ophthalmic periarterial plexus and along its subsidiary plexuses around the central retinal, ciliary, scleral, and conjunctival arteries.

PARASYMPATHETIC FIBERS

The parasympathetic preganglionic fibers for the eye are the axons of cells in the accessory, or autonomic (Edinger-Westphal) oculomotor nucleus. They run in the third cranial nerve and exit in the *motor root of the ciliary ganglion,* where they relay. The axons of these ganglionic cells are postganglionic parasympathetic fibers, which reach the eye in the *short ciliary nerves* and are distributed to the constrictor fibers of the iris (sphincter pupillae), to the ciliary muscle, and to the blood vessels in the coating of the eyeball.

NEUROLOGIC DISORDERS

Disruption of the sympathetic innervation to the eye at any level along the sympathetic pathways will result in a Horner syndrome, in which the pupil on the involved side is smaller and dilates poorly, especially notable in the dark, and the upper lid droops slightly (ptosis). Depending on where the sympathetic chain is disrupted, there may also be loss of sweating on the ipsilateral face. A lesion of the ciliary ganglion will cause disruption of the parasympathetic fibers to the pupillary constrictor muscle, and there will be isolated enlargement of the ipsilateral pupil, especially notable in lighted conditions, but no findings such as ptosis or extraocular muscle weakness to suggest a lesion along the course of the oculomotor nerve.

Plate 1.20

Cranial Nerve and Neuro-ophthalmologic Disorders

TRIGEMINAL NERVE (V)

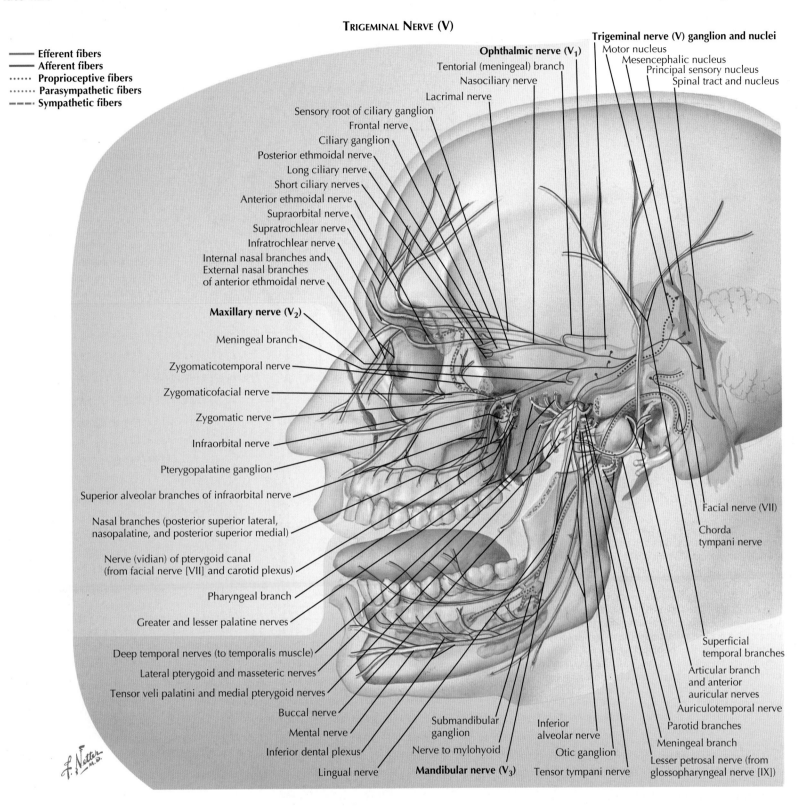

Efferent fibers
Afferent fibers
Proprioceptive fibers
Parasympathetic fibers
Sympathetic fibers

Ophthalmic nerve (V₁)
Tentorial (meningeal) branch
Nasociliary nerve
Lacrimal nerve
Sensory root of ciliary ganglion
Frontal nerve
Ciliary ganglion
Posterior ethmoidal nerve
Long ciliary nerve
Short ciliary nerves
Anterior ethmoidal nerve
Supraorbital nerve
Supratrochlear nerve
Infratrochlear nerve
Internal nasal branches and
External nasal branches
of anterior ethmoidal nerve

Trigeminal nerve (V) ganglion and nuclei
Motor nucleus
Mesencephalic nucleus
Principal sensory nucleus
Spinal tract and nucleus

Maxillary nerve (V₂)
Meningeal branch
Zygomaticotemporal nerve
Zygomaticofacial nerve
Zygomatic nerve
Infraorbital nerve
Pterygopalatine ganglion
Superior alveolar branches of infraorbital nerve
Nasal branches (posterior superior lateral,
nasopalatine, and posterior superior medial)
Nerve (vidian) of pterygoid canal
(from facial nerve [VII] and carotid plexus)
Pharyngeal branch
Greater and lesser palatine nerves
Deep temporal nerves (to temporalis muscle)
Lateral pterygoid and masseteric nerves
Tensor veli palatini and medial pterygoid nerves
Buccal nerve
Mental nerve
Inferior dental plexus
Lingual nerve

Submandibular ganglion
Nerve to mylohyoid
Mandibular nerve (V₃)

Inferior alveolar nerve
Otic ganglion
Tensor tympani nerve

Facial nerve (VII)
Chorda tympani nerve
Superficial temporal branches
Articular branch and anterior auricular nerves
Auriculotemporal nerve
Parotid branches
Meningeal branch
Lesser petrosal nerve (from glossopharyngeal nerve [IX])

CRANIAL NERVE V: TRIGEMINAL NERVE

ANATOMY

The trigeminal nerve is the largest cranial nerve and gives rise to three major branches: the ophthalmic, maxillary, and mandibular nerves. It is a mixed nerve that provides motor innervation to the muscles of mastication and sensory innervation to the cornea, face, anterior scalp, nasal cavity, oral cavity, and dura mater.

The trigeminal nerve emerges from the anterolateral aspect of the upper pons, containing sensory and motor roots that travel over the superior border of the petrous temporal bone near its apex. The large, lateral sensory root conveys touch, pain, and temperature sensation from most of the face and scalp, including the external acoustic meatus, nasopharynx, teeth, temporomandibular joint, and most of the meninges in the anterior and middle cranial fossae. It carries proprioceptive impulses from masticatory and, likely, from extraocular and facial muscles. The sensory root expands into the semilunar-shaped trigeminal ganglion (gasserian ganglion) and contains pseudounipolar cells with peripheral processes conveying sensory impulses from the face and head structures through the three major trigeminal divisions. The smaller, medial motor root supplies muscles derived from the first branchial arch: the masticatory muscles, the mylohyoid, the anterior

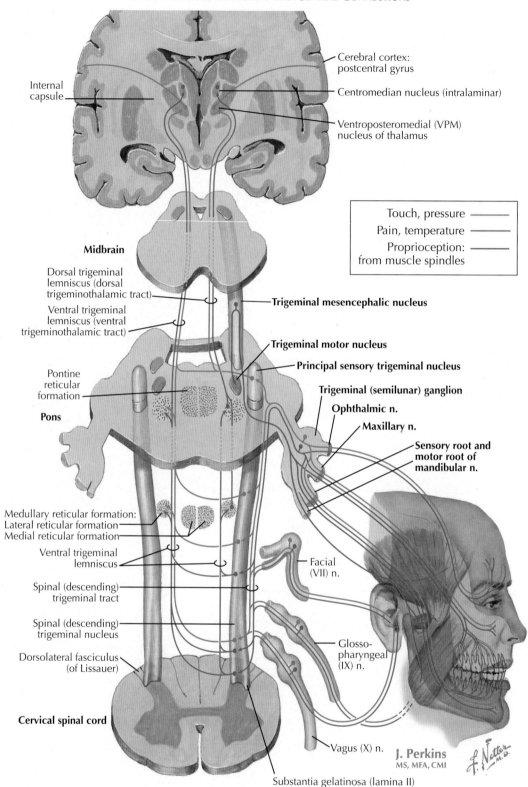

TRIGEMINAL NUCLEI: AFFERENT AND CENTRAL CONNECTIONS

Internal capsule

Cerebral cortex: postcentral gyrus

Centromedian nucleus (intralaminar)

Ventroposteromedial (VPM) nucleus of thalamus

Touch, pressure ⎯⎯⎯
Pain, temperature ⎯⎯⎯
Proprioception: ⎯⎯⎯
from muscle spindles

Midbrain

Dorsal trigeminal lemniscus (dorsal trigeminothalamic tract)

Ventral trigeminal lemniscus (ventral trigeminothalamic tract)

Trigeminal mesencephalic nucleus

Trigeminal motor nucleus

Principal sensory trigeminal nucleus

Trigeminal (semilunar) ganglion

Ophthalmic n.

Maxillary n.

Sensory root and motor root of mandibular n.

Pontine reticular formation

Pons

Medullary reticular formation:
Lateral reticular formation
Medial reticular formation

Ventral trigeminal lemniscus

Facial (VII) n.

Spinal (descending) trigeminal tract

Spinal (descending) trigeminal nucleus

Glosso-pharyngeal (IX) n.

Dorsolateral fasciculus (of Lissauer)

Cervical spinal cord

Vagus (X) n.

J. Perkins
MS, MFA, CMI

Substantia gelatinosa (lamina II)

CRANIAL NERVE V: TRIGEMINAL NERVE (Continued)

belly of the digastric, the tensor veli palatini, and tensor tympani. Numerous parasympathetic and sympathetic fibers join branches of the trigeminal nerve through interconnections with the oculomotor (III), trochlear (IV), facial (VII), and glossopharyngeal (IX) nerves.

Trigeminal nerve processes coalesce to form the sensory root, which enters the brainstem and ends in one of three major nuclear complexes: the spinal (inferior) trigeminal nucleus, the principal sensory (pontine) nucleus, or the mesencephalic nucleus. The spinal tract of the trigeminal nucleus travels from the pons, through the medulla, and into the spinal cord, where it is contiguous with Lissauer's tract. The spinal tract gives off fibers to the medially located nucleus of the spinal tract, which receives pain, temperature, and soft touch input from the face and mucous membranes. From the spinal nucleus, the ascending fibers travel ipsilaterally in the trigeminothalamic tract to the Ventroposteromedial (VPM) and intralaminar nuclei of the thalamus. Projections ascend to the proximal sensory cortex for pain and temperature perception.

The principal sensory nucleus, which is in the lateral pons, receives tactile and proprioceptive sensation. It gives off fibers that travel in the trigeminal lemniscus and the uncrossed dorsal trigeminothalamic tract, both of which terminate in the VPM nucleus of the thalamus. It is represented bilaterally in the cortex.

Moving superiorly, the mesencephalic nucleus contains cell bodies that carry proprioceptive input from masticatory and extraocular muscle spindles. It is the only place in the CNS where cell bodies of primary sensory afferents are found in the CNS and not in sensory ganglia. The trigeminal mesencephalic nucleus

extends from the main sensory nucleus to the superior colliculus of the mesencephalon.

Trigeminal motor fibers originate in the trigeminal motor nucleus. Accompanied by afferent sensory roots, the motor roots of the trigeminal nerve leave the pons and pass through Meckel's cave to form the trigeminal ganglion. This ganglion then divides into the three nerve trunks: the ophthalmic, maxillary, and mandibular nerves. The small motor root passes under the ganglion to join the mandibular nerve.

The ophthalmic nerve (V_1) collects pain, temperature, touch, and proprioceptive information from the upper third of the face, top of the nose, scalp regions, and adjacent sinuses. It is joined by filaments from the internal carotid sympathetic plexus and communicates with the oculomotor, trochlear, and abducens nerves as it runs forward in the lateral wall of the cavernous sinus. Near its origin, it gives off a small recurrent tentorial (meningeal) branch to the tentorium cerebelli and then divides into the lacrimal, frontal, and nasociliary

Plate 1.22

Cranial Nerve and Neuro-ophthalmologic Disorders

TRIGEMINAL NUCLEI: CENTRAL AND PERIPHERAL CONNECTIONS

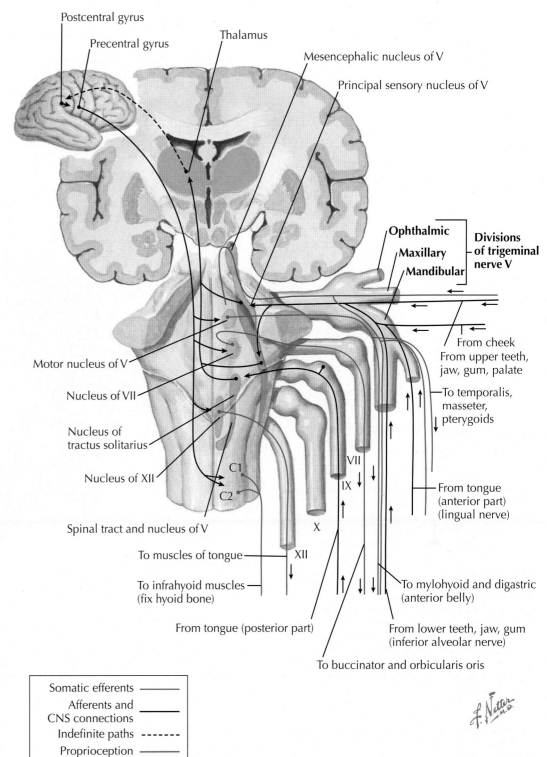

Postcentral gyrus
Precentral gyrus
Thalamus
Mesencephalic nucleus of V
Principal sensory nucleus of V

Ophthalmic
Maxillary
Mandibular
Divisions of trigeminal nerve V

From cheek
From upper teeth, jaw, gum, palate

Motor nucleus of V

To temporalis, masseter, pterygoids

Nucleus of VII

Nucleus of tractus solitarius

Nucleus of XII

C1
C2

VII
IX
X
XII

From tongue (anterior part) (lingual nerve)

Spinal tract and nucleus of V

To muscles of tongue

To infrahyoid muscles (fix hyoid bone)

From tongue (posterior part)

To mylohyoid and digastric (anterior belly)

From lower teeth, jaw, gum (inferior alveolar nerve)

To buccinator and orbicularis oris

Somatic efferents ——————
Afferents and CNS connections ——————
Indefinite paths - - - - - - -
Proprioception ——————

CRANIAL NERVE V: TRIGEMINAL NERVE (Continued)

branches, which enter the orbit through the superior orbital fissure.

Larger than the ophthalmic nerve, the maxillary nerve (V₂) is also sensory. It supplies the side of the forehead, medial cheek, side of the nose, upper lip, palate, upper teeth, nasopharynx, anterior and medial cranial fossae, meninges, and the skin overlying the maxilla. As with the other branches of the trigeminal nerve, it serves as a vehicle for the distribution of autonomic fibers to the skull structures. The maxillary nerve gives off a small meningeal branch to the meninges of the middle cranial fossa before passing through the lower part of the lateral wall of the cavernous sinus. It then leaves the skull through the foramen rotundum and enters the pterygopalatine fossa, where it communicates with the pterygopalatine ganglion and then branches into different directions. In the pterygopalatine fossa, the maxillary nerve superiorly gives off the zygomatic nerve (with the zygomaticotemporal and zygomaticofacial branches), and, inferiorly, the superior posterior alveolar nerves. The superior middle and superior anterior alveolar nerves arise from the infraorbital part of the nerve that descends in the wall of the maxillary sinus between the bone and the mucous membrane. Dental and gingival rami unite to form the superior dental plexus of the upper teeth and gums. The maxillary nerve ultimately moves anterolaterally across the upper part of the posterior surface of the maxilla to traverse the inferior orbital fissure on the way to the orbit. It then passes through the infraorbital groove as the infraorbital nerve, with the external and internal nasal, inferior palpebral, and superior labial branches, which supply the nasal alae, lower lid, upper lip skin, and mucous membranes, respectively.

The mandibular nerve (V₃) is the largest branch of the trigeminal nerve and consists of a large sensory root and a small trigeminal motor root. The sensory portion innervates the side of the head, anterior wall of the external auditory meatus, external wall of the tympanic membrane, the temporomandibular joint, lower lip and jaw, inferior teeth and surrounding gums, mucous membranes of the mouth, anterior two-thirds of the tongue, and the chin. The sensory and motor components leave the skull through the foramen ovale and

unite to form a short nerve that lies between the lateral pterygoid and tensor veli palatini muscles, anterior to the middle meningeal artery. The small otic ganglion closely adheres to the medial side of the nerve. Just below the foramen, the mandibular nerve gives off a meningeal branch (nervus spinosus) to supply the meninges of the middle and anterior cranial fossae and calvaria, and the mucous membrane of the mastoid air cells. Motor nerve fibers supplying the medial pterygoid, tensor veli palatini, and tensor tympani muscles

OPHTHALMIC (V₁) AND MAXILLARY (V₂) NERVES

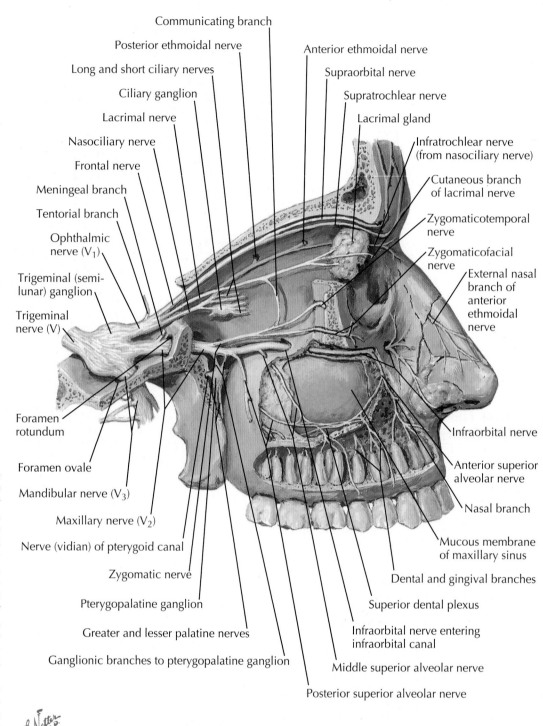

Communicating branch
Posterior ethmoidal nerve
Long and short ciliary nerves
Ciliary ganglion
Lacrimal nerve
Nasociliary nerve
Frontal nerve
Meningeal branch
Tentorial branch
Ophthalmic nerve (V₁)
Trigeminal (semilunar) ganglion
Trigeminal nerve (V)
Foramen rotundum
Foramen ovale
Mandibular nerve (V₃)
Maxillary nerve (V₂)
Nerve (vidian) of pterygoid canal
Zygomatic nerve
Pterygopalatine ganglion
Greater and lesser palatine nerves
Ganglionic branches to pterygopalatine ganglion

Anterior ethmoidal nerve
Supraorbital nerve
Supratrochlear nerve
Lacrimal gland
Infratrochlear nerve (from nasociliary nerve)
Cutaneous branch of lacrimal nerve
Zygomaticotemporal nerve
Zygomaticofacial nerve
External nasal branch of anterior ethmoidal nerve
Infraorbital nerve
Anterior superior alveolar nerve
Nasal branch
Mucous membrane of maxillary sinus
Dental and gingival branches
Superior dental plexus
Infraorbital nerve entering infraorbital canal
Middle superior alveolar nerve
Posterior superior alveolar nerve

CRANIAL NERVE V: TRIGEMINAL NERVE (Continued)

emerge from the medial aspect of the mandibular nerve and travel through the otic ganglion without relay. The main mandibular nerve divides into a small anterior and a larger posterior division. The anterior division contains primarily motor fibers through the nerve to the lateral pterygoid and two or three deep temporal nerves that innervate the temporalis muscle. The anterior portion has one sensory branch, the buccal nerve, which innervates the areas of skin overlying the buccinator muscle and the mucous membranes beneath. The posterior part of the mandibular nerve is primarily sensory and divides into the auriculotemporal, lingual, and inferior alveolar nerves. Its few motor fibers are distributed in the mylohyoid branch of the inferior alveolar nerve, supplying both the mylohyoid muscle and the anterior belly of the digastric.

At its origin, the auriculotemporal nerve divides into anterior and posterior roots that encircle the middle meningeal artery before rejoining to form a single nerve. It ends in the superficial temporal branches that supply the skin and fascia of the temple, as well as adjacent areas of the scalp. The auriculotemporal nerve also gives branches to the temporomandibular joint, the external acoustic meatus, and the tympanic membrane. An anterior auricular branch innervates the skin of the tragus and part of the helix. Additionally, the auriculotemporal nerve supplies filaments containing secretomotor and vasomotor fibers to the parotid gland, which traverse the otic ganglion.

Sensation to the anterior two-thirds of the tongue and floor of the mouth is carried by the lingual nerve. It is joined near its origin by the chorda tympani, a branch of the facial nerve, which conveys taste from the

part of the tongue anterior to the V-shaped sulcus terminalis. The lingual nerve supplies the mucous membrane of the anterior two-thirds of the tongue, lower part of the oropharyngeal isthmus (isthmus of the fauces), and the floor of the mouth, including the lingual surfaces of the lower gums. The branches communicate with the terminal branches of the glossopharyngeal and hypoglossal nerves. The inferior alveolar nerve descends behind the lingual nerve. It gives off its only motor branch, the mylohyoid nerve, before

entering the mandibular foramen. The mylohyoid nerve supplies the mylohyoid muscle and the anterior belly of the digastric. The other branches of the inferior alveolar nerve are the mental nerve and inferior dental and gingival rami, which arise from the nerve as it passes through the mandibular canal. The latter are delicate nerves that unite to form the inferior dental plexus supplying the lower teeth and gums. They may be joined by branches of the buccal and lingual nerves or by filaments from nerves supplying the muscles

Plate 1.24

Cranial Nerve and Neuro-ophthalmologic Disorders

MANDIBULAR NERVE (V₃)

Lateral view

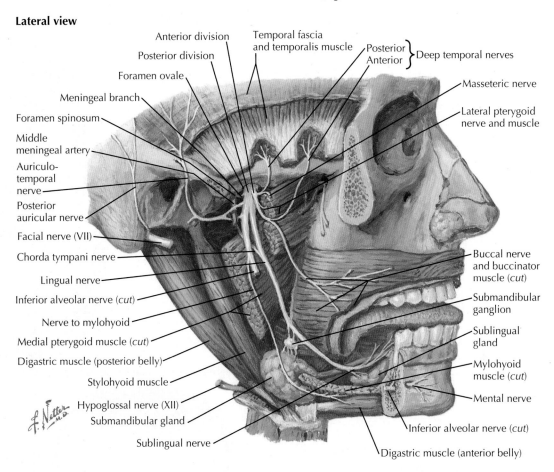

Medial view

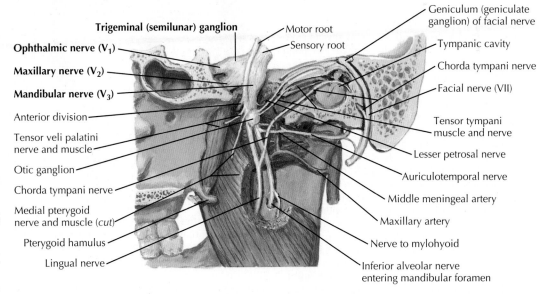

CRANIAL NERVE V: TRIGEMINAL NERVE (Continued)

attached to the mandible. These branches may carry sensory fibers, which explains why blocking the inferior alveolar nerve alone does not always anesthetize the lower teeth.

TRIGEMINAL NERVE DISORDERS

Patients with trigeminal neuropathy frequently report facial numbness. Furthermore, impairment of general sensation from the tongue and palate carried by the trigeminal nerve can, at times, also result in mild taste disturbances, even though the special sensory fibers providing primary taste sensation, supplied by the facial and glossopharyngeal nerves, are not involved. The examination of touch, pain, and temperature in the three divisions of the trigeminal nerve, as well as the blink reflex, is routinely checked. Although the muscles of mastication are frequently difficult to assess, jaw deviation toward the paretic anterior pterygoid muscle on forward protrusion may help indicate trigeminal motor weakness or isolated V₃ division involvement.

Differential diagnosis for trigeminal neuropathy includes trauma, infection, and rarely iatrogenic injuries from maxillofacial procedures with sensory loss depending on the involved site. Herpes zoster is a common viral cause of a trigeminal neuropathy and occurs when latent varicella-zoster virus within the trigeminal ganglion becomes reactivated. A vesicular rash and neuralgic pain along the involved division are characteristic and can lead to a chronic postherpetic neuralgia that may persist for months to years. Herpes zoster ophthalmicus occurs when the ophthalmic division is involved. If not promptly addressed,

the most serious potential complication of this condition is corneal scarring with subsequent visual loss. Rarely, ipsilateral carotid and middle cerebral artery granulomatous angiitis with infarctions may occur as the virus travels retrograde from the ganglion along the trigeminal nerve. Worldwide, leprosy is a leading cause of trigeminal neuropathy. As it affects the coolest areas of the skin, sensory loss confined to the pinna of the ear or tip of the nose raises leprosy as a diagnostic consideration.

Trigeminal ganglionopathy in association with connective tissue disease is likely caused by circulating autoantibodies to ganglion cell bodies. This is particularly seen in scleroderma or Sjögren syndrome. Numbness begins around the mouth and spreads slowly over months to involve all trigeminal divisions. Frequently, the ophthalmic division is less involved or spared. In Sjögren syndrome, trigeminal ganglionopathy is typically part of a more widespread sensory ganglionopathy.

TRIGEMINAL NERVE DISORDERS

Varicella-zoster with probable keratitis

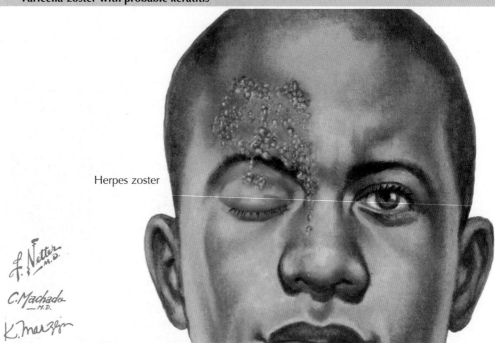

Herpes zoster

Progressive systemic sclerosis (scleroderma)

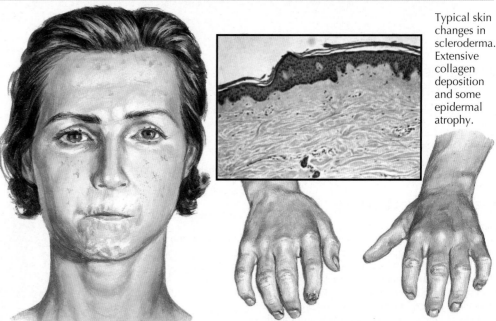

Typical skin changes in scleroderma. Extensive collagen deposition and some epidermal atrophy.

Characteristics. Thickening, tightening, and rigidity of facial skin, with small, constricted mouth and narrow lips, in atrophic phase of scleroderma.

Sclerodactyly. Fingers partially fixed in semiflexed position; terminal phalanges atrophied; fingertips pointed and ulcerated.

CRANIAL NERVE V: TRIGEMINAL NERVE (Continued)

Metastatic neoplasm or tumors involving the face, such as squamous cell carcinoma, microcystic adnexal carcinomas, and keratoacanthoma, may invade cutaneous nerve branches, especially at their exit point from the skull (mental and infraorbital neuropathies), and exhibit focal sensory loss. The numb chin syndrome (or isolated mental neuropathy) consists of unilateral numbness of the chin and adjacent lower lip and may be an ominous sign of primary or metastatic cancer involving the mandible, skull base, or leptomeninges. The most common etiologies are metastatic breast cancer and lymphoproliferative malignancies.

Trigeminal neuralgia, also known as tic douloureux, is an often severe and disabling lancinating or electric facial pain syndrome occurring in the trigeminal nerve distribution (typically maxillary or mandibular) without associated neurologic deficits. It characteristically affects middle-aged people, women more than men, and involves the right side more often than the left. It is rare to have bilateral attacks of trigeminal neuralgia except in the setting of multiple sclerosis. The attacks are mostly unilateral and brief, lasting for seconds to several minutes, and rarely occur during sleep. Paroxysms of pain are frequently provoked by nonnociceptive triggers, including talking, chewing, shaving, drinking hot or cold liquids, or any form of sensory facial stimulation. Between paroxysms, a constant, dull ache can persist, often leading patients to believe the problem is of dental origin. The frequency of attacks fluctuates markedly, disabling a patient for weeks and then remitting for months to years. The etiology is thought to involve loss of myelin insulation within the posterior root of the trigeminal nerve. It may be idiopathic or due to compression at the entry zone of the trigeminal nerve root by an ectatic artery (often a branch of the superior cerebellar artery), multiple sclerosis plaque, infarction, vascular malformation, cerebellopontine (CP) angle tumor, or rarely, posterior communicating or distal anterior inferior cerebellar artery (AICA) aneurysm. Given the potential for underlying structural abnormalities, high-resolution magnetic resonance imaging of the brain with gadolinium and magnetic resonance angiography are indicated for all patients with trigeminal neuralgia. Bilateral symptoms, trigeminal sensory findings, and loss of corneal reflexes are strong indicators of secondary trigeminal neuropathy and should raise concern. Anticonvulsants are the primary medical therapy for trigeminal neuralgia, with most patients responding to carbamazepine and, more recently, oxcarbazepine. Baclofen, an antispasmodic, is advocated by some as an adjuvant treatment to carbamazepine if higher doses alone are inadequate or cause side effects. Tricyclic antidepressants and other anticonvulsants, such as phenytoin, gabapentin, lamotrigine, topiramate, and pregabalin, also may be useful as adjuvant drugs or monotherapy. Several surgical approaches are available for patients who do not respond to medical therapy. Trigeminal neuralgia can recur after any procedure at a lifetime rate of about 20%.

Plate 1.26

Cranial Nerve and Neuro-ophthalmologic Disorders

PONS: LEVEL OF THE GENU OF THE FACIAL NERVE

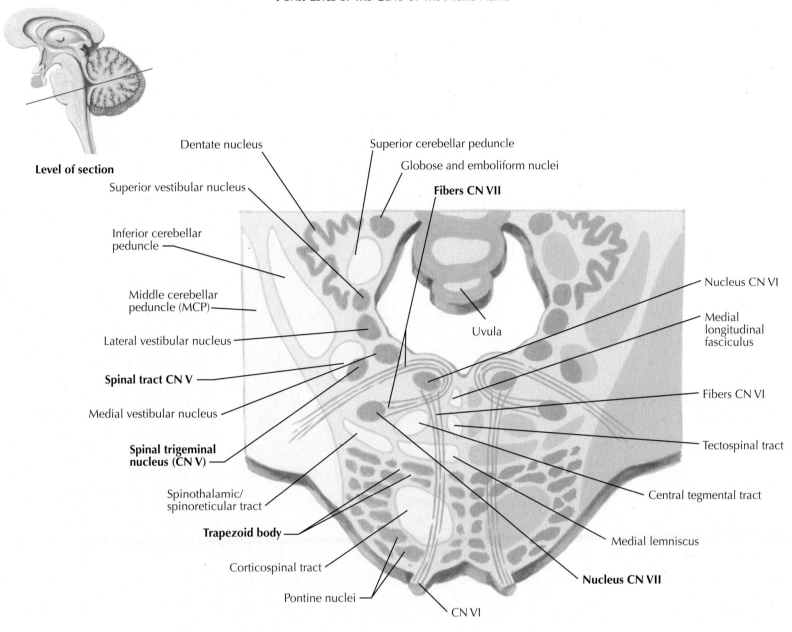

Level of section

Dentate nucleus

Superior cerebellar peduncle

Globose and emboliform nuclei

Fibers CN VII

Superior vestibular nucleus

Inferior cerebellar peduncle

Middle cerebellar peduncle (MCP)

Uvula

Lateral vestibular nucleus

Nucleus CN VI

Medial longitudinal fasciculus

Spinal tract CN V

Medial vestibular nucleus

Fibers CN VI

Spinal trigeminal nucleus (CN V)

Tectospinal tract

Spinothalamic/ spinoreticular tract

Central tegmental tract

Trapezoid body

Medial lemniscus

Corticospinal tract

Nucleus CN VII

Pontine nuclei

CN VI

CRANIAL NERVE VII: FACIAL NERVE

ANATOMY

The facial nerve is a mixed nerve containing special motor, special sensory, general sensory, and parasympathetic fibers. The facial nerve is composed of two roots: (1) a larger motor root, which supplies the facial mimetic musculature, the stapedius, the stylohyoid, and the posterior belly of the digastric; and (2) a smaller sensory root called the nervus intermedius, which carries sensation and parasympathetic fibers.

MOTOR DIVISION

Fibers arise from the motor facial nucleus, located in the reticular formation of the lowest part of the pons. The nucleus is posterior to the superior olive, medial to the nucleus of the spinal tract of the trigeminal nerve, and anterolateral to the nucleus of the abducens nerve. The supranuclear control of facial movements occurs through the corticonuclear fibers originating in the precentral gyrus. These fibers course through the corona radiata, genu of the internal capsule, and the medial portion of the cerebral peduncle to the pons. The posterior portion of the facial nucleus controls the upper facial musculature and receives bilateral supranuclear input, whereas the anterior facial nucleus controls the lower facial muscles and receives predominantly

FACIAL NERVE (VII)

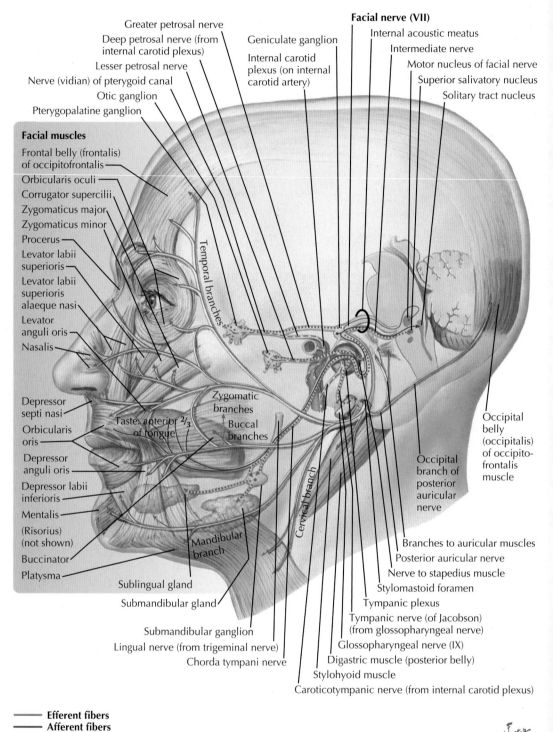

Greater petrosal nerve
Deep petrosal nerve (from internal carotid plexus)
Lesser petrosal nerve
Nerve (vidian) of pterygoid canal
Otic ganglion
Pterygopalatine ganglion

Geniculate ganglion
Internal carotid plexus (on internal carotid artery)

Facial nerve (VII)
Internal acoustic meatus
Intermediate nerve
Motor nucleus of facial nerve
Superior salivatory nucleus
Solitary tract nucleus

Facial muscles
Frontal belly (frontalis) of occipitofrontalis
Orbicularis oculi
Corrugator supercilii
Zygomaticus major
Zygomaticus minor
Procerus
Levator labii superioris
Levator labii superioris alaeque nasi
Levator anguli oris
Nasalis
Depressor septi nasi
Orbicularis oris
Depressor anguli oris
Depressor labii inferioris
Mentalis
(Risorius) (not shown)
Buccinator
Platysma

Temporal branches

Taste, anterior ⅔ of tongue
Zygomatic branches
Buccal branches

Mandibular branch

Sublingual gland
Submandibular gland
Submandibular ganglion
Lingual nerve (from trigeminal nerve)
Chorda tympani nerve

Cervical branch

Occipital branch of posterior auricular nerve

Occipital belly (occipitalis) of occipitofrontalis muscle

Branches to auricular muscles
Posterior auricular nerve
Nerve to stapedius muscle
Stylomastoid foramen
Tympanic plexus
Tympanic nerve (of Jacobson) (from glossopharyngeal nerve)
Glossopharyngeal nerve (IX)
Digastric muscle (posterior belly)
Stylohyoid muscle
Caroticotympanic nerve (from internal carotid plexus)

—— Efferent fibers
—— Afferent fibers
········· Parasympathetic fibers
– – – Sympathetic fibers

CRANIAL NERVE VII: FACIAL NERVE (Continued)

contralateral input. Supranuclear lesions, such as with stroke, therefore produce a pattern of contralateral predominantly lower facial weakness. The efferent fibers of the motor nucleus form a motor root and course around the abducens nucleus superiorly and exit the brainstem laterally in the CP angle (see Plate 1.26). The motor root travels with the nervus intermedius and CN VIII in the CP angle and enters the internal auditory meatus of the temporal bone. Within the temporal bone, there are four portions of the facial nerve. (1) In the meatal (canal) segment, the motor division is on the superoanterior surface of CN VIII, and the nervus intermedius is in between them. (2) In the labyrinthine segment, the motor root and nervus intermedius enter the facial canal in the petrous bone. The labyrinthine segment passes above the labyrinth and reaches the geniculate ganglion, which contains the sensory fiber nuclei of the nervus intermedius. Here, the greater superficial petrosal nerve arises from the geniculate ganglion. This nerve is composed of preganglionic parasympathetic efferents that innervate the nasal, lacrimal, and palatal glands via the pterygopalatine ganglion. The greater superficial petrosal nerve also carries sensory fibers from the external auditory meatus, lateral pinna, and mastoid. (3) The horizontal (tympanic) segment contains the facial nerve as it runs horizontally backward below and medial to the horizontal semicircular canal. (4) In the mastoid (vertical) segment the facial nerve bends inferiorly. The nerve to the stapedius muscle branches off in this segment. The chorda tympani also branches off here and joins the lingual nerve. The chorda tympani contains efferent preganglionic parasympathetic fibers from the superior salivatory nucleus and innervates the submandibular and sublingual glands via the submandibular ganglion. The chorda tympani also contains afferent taste fibers from the anterior two-thirds of the tongue that then

continue to the nucleus of the solitary tract. After the chorda tympani branches off, CN VII exits the facial canal through the stylomastoid foramen and immediately gives off the posterior auricular nerve (to the posterior, transverse, and oblique auricular muscles

and to the occipitalis) and digastric and stylohyoid branches. The facial nerve continues on to pierce the parotid gland and divide into temporofacial and cervicofacial branches, which further divide into temporofrontal, zygomatic, buccal, marginal mandibular, and

Plate 1.28   Cranial Nerve and Neuro-ophthalmologic Disorders

MUSCLES OF FACIAL EXPRESSION: LATERAL VIEW

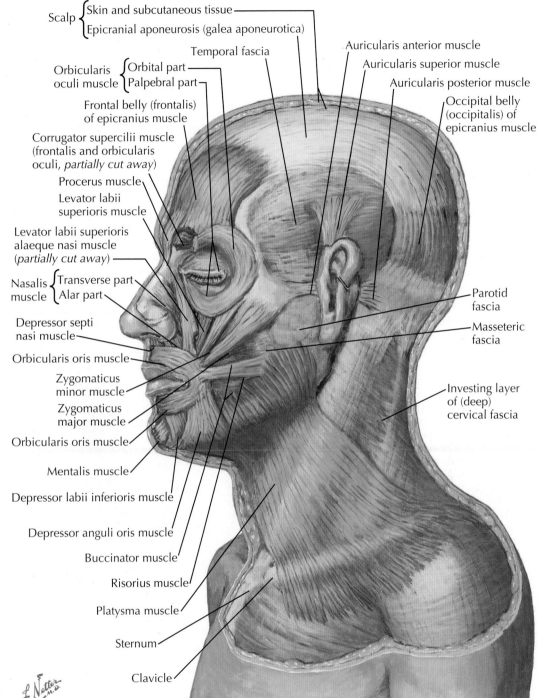

Scalp { Skin and subcutaneous tissue
Epicranial aponeurosis (galea aponeurotica)

Temporal fascia

Auricularis anterior muscle

Auricularis superior muscle

Auricularis posterior muscle

Orbicularis oculi muscle { Orbital part
Palpebral part

Occipital belly (occipitalis) of epicranius muscle

Frontal belly (frontalis) of epicranius muscle

Corrugator supercilii muscle (frontalis and orbicularis oculi, *partially cut away*)

Procerus muscle

Levator labii superioris muscle

Levator labii superioris alaeque nasi muscle (*partially cut away*)

Nasalis muscle { Transverse part
Alar part

Parotid fascia

Depressor septi nasi muscle

Masseteric fascia

Orbicularis oris muscle

Zygomaticus minor muscle

Investing layer of (deep) cervical fascia

Zygomaticus major muscle

Orbicularis oris muscle

Mentalis muscle

Depressor labii inferioris muscle

Depressor anguli oris muscle

Buccinator muscle

Risorius muscle

Platysma muscle

Sternum

Clavicle

CRANIAL NERVE VII: FACIAL NERVE (Continued)

cervical branches that supply the muscles of facial expression.

SENSORY AND PARASYMPATHETIC DIVISION (NERVUS INTERMEDIUS)

The nervus intermedius is the parasympathetic and sensory division of the facial nerve. It carries the preganglionic parasympathetic fibers that ultimately supply the submandibular ganglion via the chorda tympani (and then postganglionic fibers travel to the submandibular and sublingual glands) and supply the pterygopalatine ganglion via the greater petrosal nerve (postganglionic fibers travel to the lacrimal, nasal, and palatal glands). The nervus intermedius also receives sensory fibers originating from nuclei in the geniculate ganglion. This ganglion receives afferents from the mucosa of the pharynx, nose, palate, and skin of the external auditory meatus, lateral pinna, and mastoid, and it carries taste sensation from the anterior two-thirds of the tongue. The superior salivatory nucleus of the pontine tegmentum gives rise to the parasympathetic fibers; the associated lacrimal nucleus contains the fibers controlling lacrimation. The gustatory afferents end in the nucleus of the tractus solitarius in the medulla. Fibers conveying general sensations from the external auditory meatus, lateral pinna, and mastoid likely come through interconnections between the chorda tympani and the auricular branch of the vagus and terminate in the spinal nucleus of the trigeminal nerve. The afferents from the meninges and their arteries in the middle cranial fossa likely reach the facial nerve through the greater petrosal branch.

FACIAL NERVE DISORDERS

Facial weakness is caused by both central and peripheral lesions, and differentiating between the two frequently requires close examination. Peripheral facial weakness involves both the upper and lower part of the face to the same degree, whereas upper motor neuron lesions typically manifest with a gradient of weakness, with relative preservation of movement in the brow and forehead (e.g., frontalis muscles). Supranuclear lesions, such as in suprabulbar palsies, may result in an absence of voluntary facial movements but retention of reflexive movements (e.g., smiling) in response to emotional stimuli.

CENTRAL VERSUS PERIPHERAL FACIAL PARALYSIS

Hyperacusis

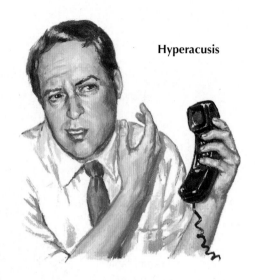

This may be an early or initial symptom of a peripheral VII nerve palsy: patient holds phone away from ear because of hyperacusis, an uncomfortable sensitivity to sound. Loss of taste also may occur on affected side.

CRANIAL NERVE VII: FACIAL NERVE (Continued)

Intrapontine lesions that affect the facial motor nucleus or its exiting fibers often produce weakness that involves both the upper and lower part of the face. An intrapontine lesion may be suspected because symptoms will often be referable to neighboring brainstem structures; for instance, a paramedian pontine reticular formation lesion causing facial weakness would be expected to cause also an ipsilateral conjugate gaze palsy, an associated sixth cranial nerve tract lesion with limited ipsilateral lateral rectus palsy, and/or contralateral hemiparesis of the arm and leg.

The facial nerve can be damaged at any level along its course (see Plate 1.30). Facial musculature paralysis is the hallmark of seventh cranial nerve lesions. The presence or absence of symptoms related to the various other components of the facial nerve is important for further localization. The patient with a *peripheral facial nerve* palsy after its exit from the stylomastoid foramen, with the exception of an early very distal branch lesion within the parotid gland, has weakness of the entire ipsilateral side of their face, with asymmetric smile, inability to close the eye (orbicularis oculi), or wrinkle the forehead (frontalis). *Intracranial, extramedullary lesions* affecting the seventh nerve typically occur within the CP angle and/or internal auditory meatus, most commonly caused by large acoustic neuromas, and often involve the vestibulocochlear nerve. In these cases, diminished hearing, at times initially presenting with tinnitus, usually precede the onset of peripheral facial paresis. Rarely, very large tumors may also involve the ipsilateral trigeminal cranial nerve with accompanying unilateral facial anesthesia and loss of corneal reflex. A *proximal pregeniculate, intracanalicular facial nerve* lesion in the facial canal characteristically also causes diminished lacrimation from greater petrosal nerve involvement, as well as hyperacusis (i.e., increased sensitivity to sound) due to associated stapedius muscle paresis. These lesions also lead to

Left peripheral VII facial weakness

Attempt to close eye results in eyeball rolling superiorly exposing sclera (Bell phenomenon) but no closure of the lid per se

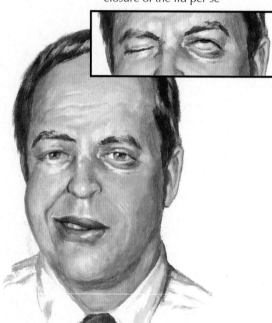

Patient unable to wrinkle forehead; eyelid droops very slightly; cannot show teeth at all on affected side in attempt to smile; and lower lip droops slightly

Left central facial weakness

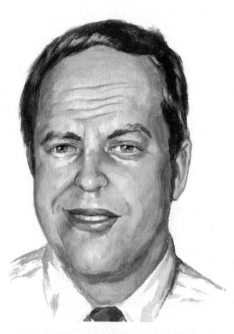

Incomplete smile with very subtle flattening of affected nasolabial fold; relative preservation of brow and forehead movement

diminished salivation, absent or altered taste for the anterior two-thirds of the tongue, and affected somatic sensation for the external auditory canal and mastoid area. Lesions *between the geniculate ganglion and the stapedius nerve* spare lacrimation, because the greater petrosal nerve has already exited. Damage *between the branch points of the stapedius nerve and the chorda tympani* results in hyperacusis and impaired salivation and taste, but not change in lacrimation. Lesions distal to the chorda tympani branch point result in pure

Plate 1.30

Cranial Nerve and Neuro-ophthalmologic Disorders

FACIAL PALSY

Sites of facial (VII) nerve injury

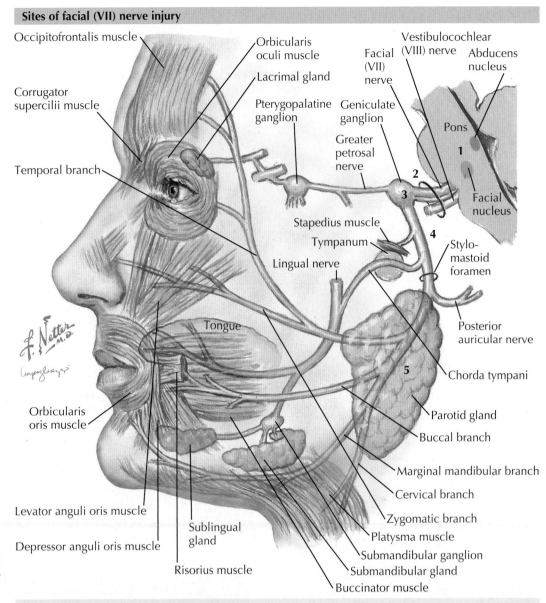

Occipitofrontalis muscle
Corrugator supercilii muscle
Temporal branch
Orbicularis oculi muscle
Lacrimal gland
Pterygopalatine ganglion
Vestibulocochlear (VIII) nerve
Facial (VII) nerve
Abducens nucleus
Geniculate ganglion
Pons
Greater petrosal nerve
Facial nucleus
Stapedius muscle
Tympanum
Lingual nerve
Stylo-mastoid foramen
Tongue
Posterior auricular nerve
Chorda tympani
Orbicularis oris muscle
Parotid gland
Buccal branch
Marginal mandibular branch
Cervical branch
Levator anguli oris muscle
Zygomatic branch
Depressor anguli oris muscle
Sublingual gland
Platysma muscle
Submandibular ganglion
Risorius muscle
Submandibular gland
Buccinator muscle

CRANIAL NERVE VII: FACIAL NERVE (Continued)

ipsilateral facial weakness. Distal lesions that affect individual motor branches result in weakness that may be restricted to individual facial muscles.

"IDIOPATHIC" FACIAL PALSY (BELL PALSY)

Bell palsy is a common cause of unilateral facial weakness. Onset of weakness is acute to subacute, evolving over hours to a few days. The lesion burden is usually proximal, with loss of total motor function on one side of the face, hyperacusis, disturbed taste, and decreased lacrimation. A preceding dull ache behind the ipsilateral ear is a common initial symptom. Nerve edema with subsequent compression and ischemia within the facial canal has been noted pathologically. The cause is believed to be reactivation of latent herpes simplex or varicella-zoster virus. A short course of corticosteroids, if given early in the course, reduces the duration of paralysis and risk of permanent impairment. The long-term prognosis is generally good, but severe cases may result in permanent partial facial paresis; in these cases, a structural etiology such as neoplasm should be investigated. Upon recovery from Bell palsy, facial synkinesis, caused by aberrant regeneration of nerve, may manifest as ipsilateral eye closure occurring with smiling or ipsilateral lip and chin muscle activation during blinking. Excessive lacrimation when eating results from aberrant regeneration of salivatory fibers to the lacrimal glands ("crocodile tears").

OTHER ETIOLOGIES OF FACIAL NEUROPATHY

Lyme disease is a relatively common infectious cause of an acute unilateral or bilateral facial neuropathy. Symptoms typically include systemic symptoms (e.g., arthralgia, fever, rash), as well as other neurologic symptoms (e.g., headache, radiculitis, meningitis, encephalopathy). Herpes zoster infection within the external auditory canal (Ramsay-Hunt syndrome), may cause facial paralysis that may precede the appearance of typical herpetic vesicles in the auditory canal. Extension of otitis media may rarely inflame and damage the facial nerve where it travels through the petrous bone. Leprosy may lead to bilateral facial nerve lesions. Unilateral or bilateral facial neuropathy is a common neurologic manifestation of sarcoidosis. Bilateral facial weakness is common in Guillain-Barré syndrome (acute inflammatory demyelinating polyradiculopathy).

Sites of lesions and their manifestations

1. Intrapontine lesions: Peripheral motor facial paralysis associated with eye movement abnormalities (ipsilateral abducens or horizontal gaze palsies) and contralateral motor paralysis.

2. Intracranial and/or internal auditory meatus: All symptoms of 3, 4, and 5, plus deafness due to involvement of eighth cranial nerve.

3. Geniculate ganglion: All symptoms of 4 and 5 with diminished lacrimation, plus pain behind ear. Herpes of tympanum and of external auditory meatus may occur.

4. Facial canal: All symptoms of 5, plus loss of taste in anterior tongue and decreased salivation on affected side due to chorda tympani involvement. Hyperacusis due to effect on nerve branch to stapedius muscle.

5. Below stylomastoid foramen (parotid gland tumor, trauma): Facial paralysis (mouth draws to opposite side) on affected side with patient unable to close eye or wrinkle forehead; food collects between teeth and cheek due to paralysis of buccinator muscle.

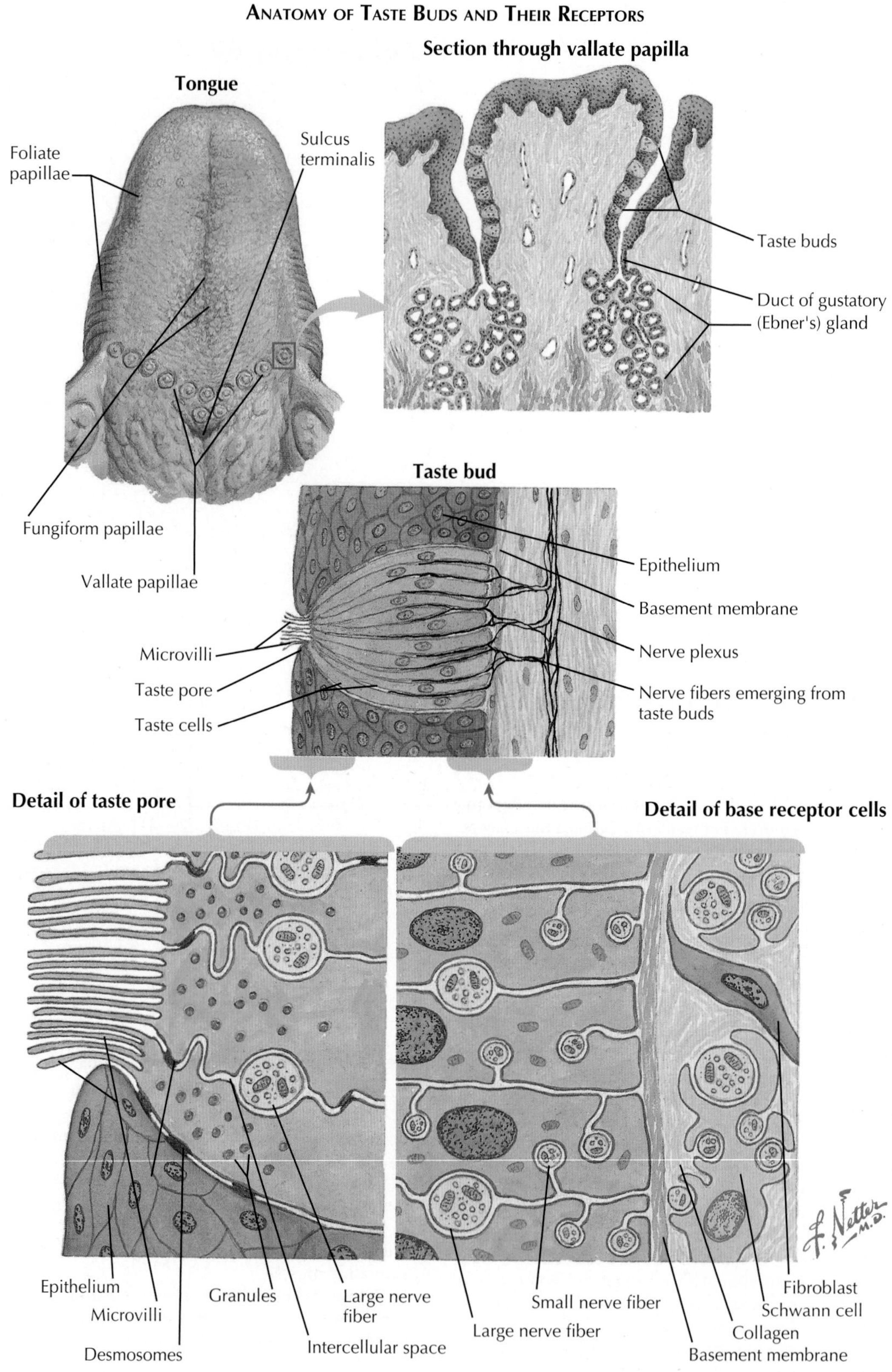

ANATOMY OF TASTE BUDS AND THEIR RECEPTORS

Section through vallate papilla

Tongue

Foliate papillae

Sulcus terminalis

Taste buds

Duct of gustatory (Ebner's) gland

Fungiform papillae

Vallate papillae

Taste bud

Microvilli

Taste pore

Taste cells

Epithelium

Basement membrane

Nerve plexus

Nerve fibers emerging from taste buds

Detail of taste pore

Detail of base receptor cells

Epithelium

Microvilli

Desmosomes

Granules

Large nerve fiber

Intercellular space

Small nerve fiber

Large nerve fiber

Fibroblast

Schwann cell

Collagen

Basement membrane

TASTE RECEPTORS AND PATHWAYS

TASTE RECEPTORS

Taste buds contain the receptors responsible for taste sensation. They are located on the upper surface of the tongue, soft palate, epiglottis, and upper esophagus. The greatest concentration of taste buds is found on the raised protuberances of the tongue called the papillae. The vallate papillae are located at the back of the tongue in front of the sulcus terminalis and are innervated by the glossopharyngeal nerve. The fungiform papillae are located at the apex of the tongue and are innervated by the facial nerve. Foliate papillae are found on the lateral margins of the tongue and are innervated by the facial and glossopharyngeal nerve.

Each taste bud consists of up to 100 polarized neuroepithelial cells that form "islands" of columnar pseudostratified taste cells embedded in the epithelium. Each bud has a central taste pore through which microvilli extend from the cells. Just below their apical ends, taste cells are joined by desmosomes, which seal off the intracellular spaces from the taste pore. Three types of taste cells (types I, II, and III) and basal cells make up the taste bud. Taste buds are constantly being renewed.

Taste buds are innervated by both large and small fibers, which emerge from a subepithelial nerve plexus and enter the bud at its base. The larger fibers run in clefts between taste cells, whereas the smaller fibers (possibly terminal branches derived from large fibers) tend to run in invaginations found in the basal parts of taste cells.

The *sensation of taste* can be divided into five primary qualities: sweet (sucrose), sour (hydrochloric acid), salty (sodium chloride), bitter (quinine), and umami (l-glutamate and other l-amino acids). Sweet foods signal the presence of carbohydrates, which supply energy. Sour foods signal dietary acids and are frequently aversive. Salty taste sensation helps to regulate body water balance and blood pressure. Bitter taste is aversive and guards against poison consumption. Umami reflects the protein content of food. The tip of the tongue is sensitive to all five stimuli but especially to sweet and salty substances, the sides of the tongue to sour substances, and the base of the tongue to bitter substances.

Water-soluble compounds evoke taste sensations by binding to the apical parts (microvilli) of the taste cells. Type I cells are the most abundant and function primarily by terminating synaptic transmission and regulating neurotransmitters. Sweet, bitter, and umami ligands bind to taste-specific receptors on type II cells, resulting in increased cytoplasmic calcium, cell membrane depolarization, adenosine triphosphate release, and further downstream signaling. Type III cells, which mediate sour taste sensation, form synaptic junctions with gustatory afferent nerve fibers and release both serotonin and norepinephrine. Salty taste is

Plate 1.32

Cranial Nerve and Neuro-ophthalmologic Disorders

TONGUE

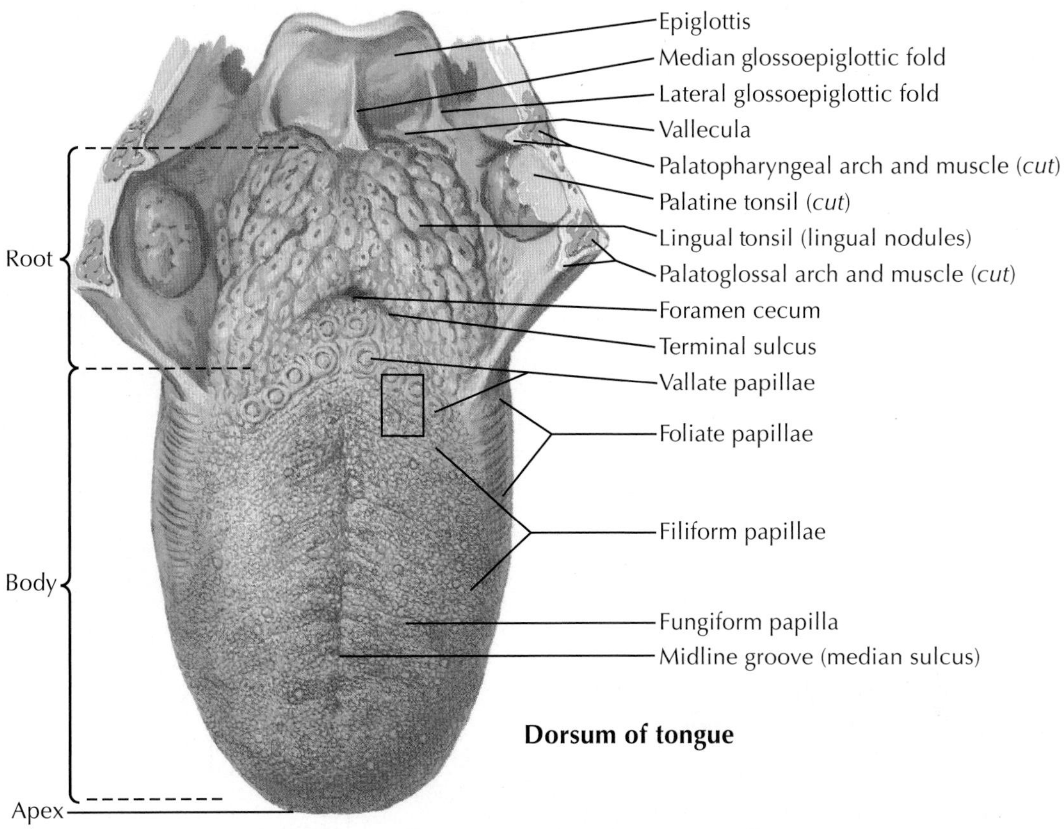

Epiglottis
Median glossoepiglottic fold
Lateral glossoepiglottic fold
Vallecula
Palatopharyngeal arch and muscle (*cut*)
Palatine tonsil (*cut*)
Lingual tonsil (lingual nodules)
Palatoglossal arch and muscle (*cut*)
Foramen cecum
Terminal sulcus
Vallate papillae
Foliate papillae
Filiform papillae
Fungiform papilla
Midline groove (median sulcus)

Root

Body

Apex

Dorsum of tongue

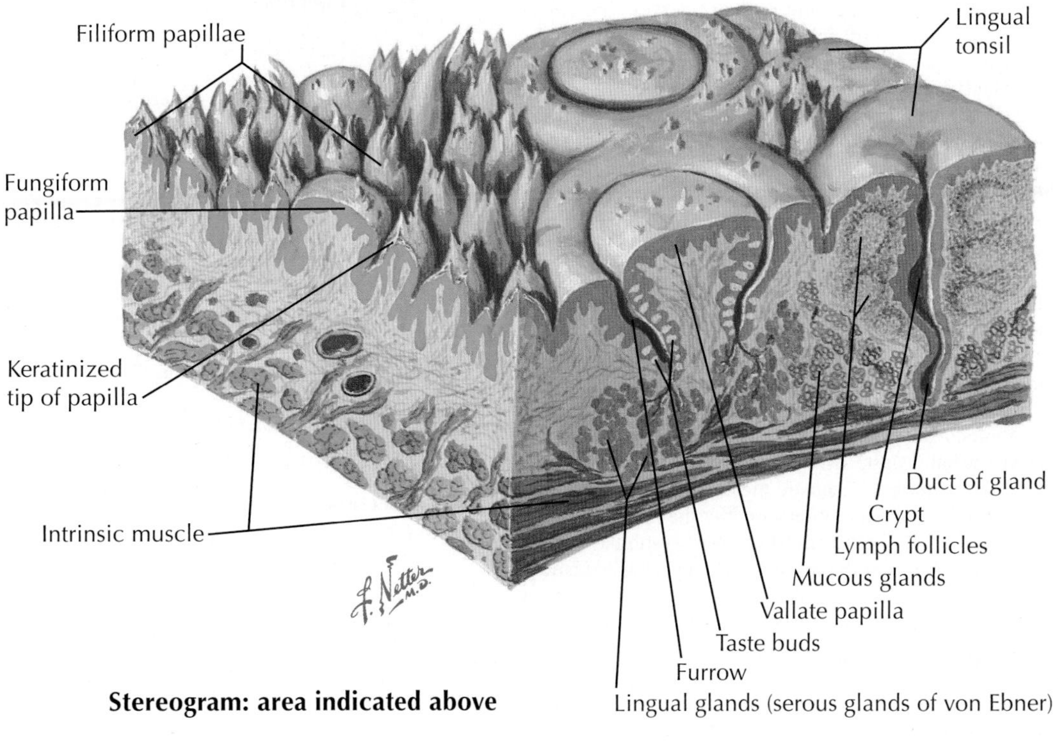

Filiform papillae
Lingual tonsil
Fungiform papilla
Keratinized tip of papilla
Intrinsic muscle
Duct of gland
Crypt
Lymph follicles
Mucous glands
Vallate papilla
Taste buds
Furrow
Lingual glands (serous glands of von Ebner)

Stereogram: area indicated above

TASTE RECEPTORS AND PATHWAYS (Continued)

detected by direct permeation of sodium through membrane ion channels. The cell type underlying salty taste has not been identified, although type I cells have been implicated.

A single-taste cell may respond to more than one of the five primary taste stimuli but not equally to each sensation. Similarly, each afferent gustatory nerve fiber communicates with several taste cells and can carry signals representing multiple taste qualities. The patterns of responses to the five taste stimuli by single fibers are not entirely random because experimental studies of large groups of fibers have revealed a tendency for certain fiber groups to respond specifically to certain sets of stimuli. For instance, a considerable number of fibers have been observed to respond well to both salt and acid stimuli, whereas fibers responding strongly to both salt and sweet stimuli are rare. Even within a given responding group, the relative sensitivity to different stimuli varies widely.

TASTE PATHWAYS

The chemosensitive cells found in the taste buds of the tongue, epiglottis, and larynx are innervated by three groups of sensory neurons.

Sensory Neurons

Based on their location in the oral cavity, taste cells synapse with sensory axons that run in the facial, glossopharyngeal, or vagus nerves and corresponding ganglia. The chorda tympani and greater petrosal branches of the facial nerve carry taste sensation via the geniculate ganglion. The lingual branch of the glossopharyngeal nerve carries taste sensation via the petrosal (inferior) ganglion. The superior laryngeal branch of the vagus nerve passes through the nodose (inferior) ganglion. All three afferent pathways terminate in the medullary nucleus of the tract of solitarius.

Central Connections

From the nucleus of the tract of solitarius, the majority of second-order neurons project ipsilaterally (some

may cross over in the medial lemniscus) up the solitariothalamic bundle to the VPM nucleus of the thalamus. Third-order neurons from the VPM nucleus pass through the posterior limb of the internal capsule to the taste region of the sensory cortex, located just below the facial region. Higher-order taste connections to the hypothalamus and amygdala appear to be primarily involved in reflex and motivational

responses to taste stimuli, and thus mediate consumption behaviors.

Brainstem connections between the taste nuclei and the autonomic nuclei (superior and inferior salivatory nuclei) mediate salivation reflexes that accompany taste responses to food stimuli. "Gustatory sweating," facial and forehead perspiration in response to eating spicy foods, is a normal response, although it can be pathologic if profuse.

VESTIBULOCOCHLEAR NERVE (VIII)

Geniculum (geniculate ganglion) of facial nerve
Facial canal
Tympanic cavity
Chorda tympani nerve
Greater petrosal nerve
Head of malleus
Incus

—— **Afferent fibers**

Cochlear (spiral) ganglion
Vestibular nerve
Cochlear nerve*
Motor root of facial nerve and intermediate nerve
Vestibulocochlear nerve (VIII)
Medulla oblongata (cross section)

Vestibular nuclei (diagrammatic) { Medial, Superior, Inferior, Lateral }

Internal acoustic meatus

Ventral / Dorsal } Cochlear nuclei

Ampulla of lateral semicircular canal
Ampulla of superior semicircular canal
Utricle
Ampulla of posterior semicircular canal
Saccule
Superior division / Inferior division } of vestibular nerve

Inferior cerebellar peduncle (to cerebellum)

Vestibular ganglion

*Note: The cochlear nerve also contains efferent fibers to the sensory epithelium (Plate 1.38). These fibers are derived from the vestibular nerve while in the internal auditory meatus.

Nucleus solitarius
Tractus solitarius
Medial vestibular nucleus
Inferior vestibular nucleus
Reticular formation
Hypoglossal nucleus CN XII
Inferior cerebellar peduncle
Dorsal motor nucleus of CN X
CN X
Spinal tract CN V
Spinal nucleus CN V
Spinothalamic/spinoreticular tract
Inferior olivary nucleus
Pyramid
Medial longitudinal fasciculus
Tectospinal tract
Medial lemniscus

Level of section

f. Netter M.D.
JOHN A. CRAIG—MD

CRANIAL NERVE VIII: VESTIBULOCOCHLEAR NERVE

The vestibulocochlear nerve consists of two separate divisions, the vestibular and cochlear nerves. The vestibular labyrinth of the internal ear, including the semicircular canals (ducts) and the otolith organ (utricle and saccule), subserves equilibration, posture, and muscle tone. Linear acceleration is monitored by the maculae of the utricle and saccule, and angular acceleration is monitored by the cristae in the ampullae of the semicircular canals. The cochlea of the internal ear transmits auditory impulses from the spiral organ. The roots of the vestibular and cochlear nerves are attached to the brainstem posterior to the facial (VII) nerve, in the triangular area bounded by the pons, cerebellar flocculus, and medulla oblongata. The vestibular and cochlear nerves enter the brainstem separately and have different central connections. Sympathetic and parasympathetic fibers likely accompany both parts of the vestibulocochlear nerve. The vestibular and cochlear nerves usually unite over a variable distance as they traverse the internal acoustic meatus below the motor root of the facial nerve interposed by the nervus intermedius, before again splitting into vestibular and cochlear portions at the fundus of the internal acoustic meatus.

VESTIBULAR NERVE

At the fundus of the internal acoustic meatus, the vestibular part of the vestibulocochlear nerve expands to form the vestibular ganglion before dividing into superior and inferior divisions. Both divisions contain peripheral processes of the vestibular bipolar cells, which penetrate tiny foramina in the superior and inferior vestibular areas of the fundus of the internal meatus. The peripheral processes spread to contact hair cell receptors embedded in the neuroepithelium lining the ampullae of the semicircular canals (ducts) and the maculae of the saccule and utricle. The longer central processes of the bipolar cells transmit impulses from these vestibular hair cells to the brainstem. As these

afferent fibers pass posteriorly, the central processes divide into ascending and descending branches, which end predominantly in the superior (cranial), inferior (caudal), medial, and lateral vestibular nuclei located in the medulla oblongata and lower pons. Other branches proceed directly through the ipsilateral inferior cerebellar

peduncle to the flocculonodular cerebellar lobe. Fibers from the superior vestibular nucleus enter the ipsilateral medial longitudinal fasciculus and ascend to end on cells of CNs III, IV, and VI. Fibers from the inferior, medial, and lateral vestibular nuclei all terminate on the contralateral medial longitudinal fasciculus,

Plate 1.34   Cranial Nerve and Neuro-ophthalmologic Disorders

PATHWAY OF SOUND RECEPTION

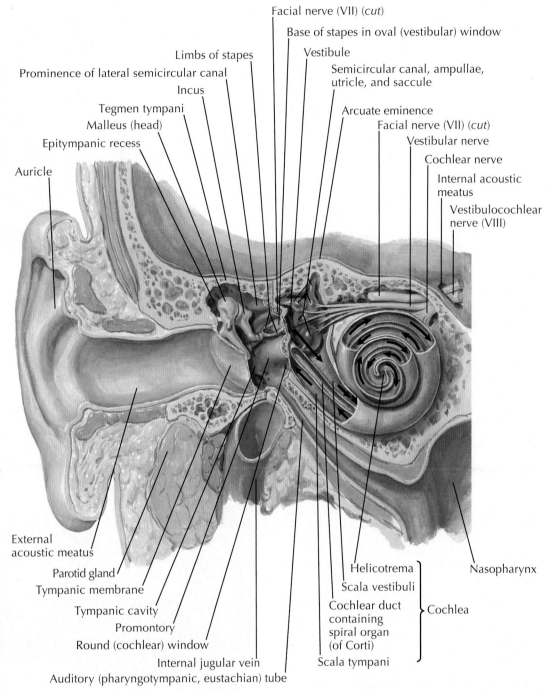

Frontal section

Facial nerve (VII) (*cut*)
Base of stapes in oval (vestibular) window
Limbs of stapes
Vestibule
Prominence of lateral semicircular canal
Semicircular canal, ampullae, utricle, and saccule
Incus
Arcuate eminence
Tegmen tympani
Facial nerve (VII) (*cut*)
Malleus (head)
Vestibular nerve
Epitympanic recess
Cochlear nerve
Auricle
Internal acoustic meatus
Vestibulocochlear nerve (VIII)

External acoustic meatus
Parotid gland
Tympanic membrane
Tympanic cavity
Promontory
Round (cochlear) window
Internal jugular vein
Auditory (pharyngotympanic, eustachian) tube
Helicotrema
Nasopharynx
Scala vestibuli
Cochlear duct containing spiral organ (of Corti)
} Cochlea
Scala tympani

Note: Arrows indicate course of sound waves.

CRANIAL NERVE VIII: VESTIBULOCOCHLEAR NERVE (Continued)

in addition to connecting with the autonomic nuclei, reticular formation, and the intermediolateral column of the cord. These connections play a crucial role in regulating posture and coordinating head, body, and eye movements. Separate vestibular-cerebellum pathways, mainly mediated by the fastigial nuclei, also influence posture and movement coordination. Connections with the autonomic centers and the intermediolateral column likely account for the nausea and vomiting seen, at times, with overstimulation of the vestibular system.

COCHLEAR NERVE

The fibers in the cochlear part of the vestibulocochlear nerve traverse many small, spirally arranged foramina in the fundus of the internal acoustic meatus and enter the modiolus, the central pillar of the cochlea. The fibers run in tiny longitudinal and spiral canals into the conic central modiolus, with numerous enlargements of the spiral cochlear ganglia that contain bipolar nerve cells. The short peripheral processes of these bipolar cells end in special acoustic hair cells in the spiral organ of Corti in the cochlear duct. The hair cells located at the apex of the cochlea are stimulated by low-frequency tones, and those located at the base are stimulated by high-frequency tones. The relatively long afferent central processes of the bipolar cells of the cochlear nerve reach the brainstem lateral to the vestibular part and end in the ventral and dorsal cochlear nuclei located on the lateral aspect of the inferior cerebellar peduncle in the superior medulla. The dorsal nuclei receive high-frequency fibers, and the ventral nuclei receive the low-frequency hair cells. Most cochlear nuclear fibers decussate through the trapezoid body before climbing in the lateral lemniscus to the inferior colliculus, whereas others synapse with neurons in the superior olivary nucleus. Third-order neurons from the inferior colliculus synapse in the medial geniculate body, which is the thalamic auditory relay nucleus. The fourth-order neurons proceed as the auditory radiations and course laterally

through the sublenticular portion of the internal capsule to the primary auditory cortex in the transverse temporal gyri of Heschl (see Plate 1.37).

DISORDERS OF THE VESTIBULOCOCHLEAR NERVE AND SYSTEM

Vestibular

Ménière disease is an idiopathic process characterized by bouts of episodic vertigo, fluctuating but eventually progressive sensorineural hearing loss, tinnitus, and a sensation of aural fullness. Vestibular symptoms classically predominate early, although some patients present primarily with auditory symptoms with only mild and infrequent vertigo. Ménière disease is felt to be secondary to an imbalance of the inner ear's endolymph associated with a pathologic lesion called endolymphatic hydrops. In contrast with the hearing loss and aural fullness seen in Ménière disease, vestibular neuritis is characterized by relatively acute onset of sustained

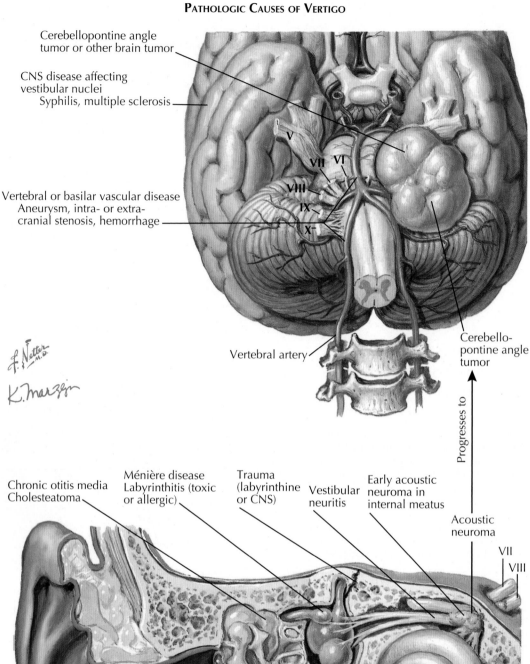

PATHOLOGIC CAUSES OF VERTIGO

Cerebellopontine angle tumor or other brain tumor

CNS disease affecting vestibular nuclei
Syphilis, multiple sclerosis

V

VII VI

VIII

IX

X

Vertebral or basilar vascular disease
Aneurysm, intra- or extra-cranial stenosis, hemorrhage

Cerebello-pontine angle tumor

Vertebral artery

Progresses to

Chronic otitis media Cholesteatoma

Ménière disease
Labyrinthitis (toxic or allergic)

Trauma (labyrinthine or CNS)

Vestibular neuritis

Early acoustic neuroma in internal meatus

Acoustic neuroma

VII

VIII

Acute otitis media

CRANIAL NERVE VIII: VESTIBULOCOCHLEAR NERVE (Continued)

vertigo without hearing loss. *Benign paroxysmal positional vertigo* (BPPV) is caused by errant otolith debris in the semicircular canals that leads to overstimulation with head movement. Bedside maneuvers and vestibular rehabilitation help reposition errant otolith debris and reestablish equal tonic vestibular input (e.g., canalith repositioning or Epley maneuver).

Vestibular schwannoma (also known by the misnomer "acoustic neuroma") is a benign Schwann cell tumor of the vestibular nerve that accounts for 8% of intracranial tumors. Vestibular schwannomas also involve the adjacent cochlear division by compression against the walls of the internal auditory canal. Progressive hearing loss from stretching or compression of the cochlear nerve is the most common symptom, occurring in approximately 95% of patients. High-pitched unilateral tinnitus is often present. Vestibular symptoms are usually limited only to mild gait unsteadiness, presumably due to gradual adaptation of the contralateral vestibular system. Large tumors can lead to facial or trigeminal nerve involvement and, at times, pontine compression.

The eighth cranial nerve is vulnerable to fractures involving the petrous part of the temporal bone and by tumors affecting the brainstem or cerebellum. Vertigo may be caused by central or peripheral pathology, but the distinction is not always readily clear, and thus, diagnostic circumspection is often warranted because posterior circulation strokes may manifest with the complaint of vertigo. Brainstem involvement from stroke or other central processes may often be distinguished from a peripheral etiology by symptoms or signs indicating damage to other brainstem structures, such as dysmetria, diplopia, dysphagia, dysarthria, sensory loss, or weakness.

Cochlear

Conductive hearing loss refers to disrupted sound wave transmission to the cochlea from external ear canal, tympanic membrane, or ossicular dysfunction.

Sensorineural hearing loss relates to impairment of the cochlea (sensory), cochlear nerve or nuclei (neural), or any part of the brain auditory pathway (central).

Auditory nerve dysfunction often results in subjective tinnitus in addition to sensorineural hearing loss. Tinnitus, the sensation of ringing in the ears without significant stimulus, is more frequently noted with peripheral than central lesions. Pulsatile tinnitus is often associated with vascular abnormalities such as venous sinus stenosis, dural arteriovenous fistula, arteriovenous malformations, high-grade carotid stenosis, intracranial aneurysm, blood vessel–rich skull base

Plate 1.36

Cranial Nerve and Neuro-ophthalmologic Disorders

CANALITH REPOSITIONING (EPLEY MANEUVER)

Right ear
Superior
Posterior
Lateral
Utricle
Particles

Head rotated 45 degrees toward right ear, patient moves from seated to supine position.

①

Utricle
Lateral
Particles
②
Superior
Posterior

Vertigo is provoked.
Position sustained 30 seconds or until vertigo subsides.

Utricle
Posterior
Particles
Superior
Lateral
③

Head is rotated to left, still extended at 45 degrees. Left ear is down.

Posterior
Particles
Lateral
Utricle
Superior
④

Head and body are rotated farther so head is down.

Superior
Particles
Lateral
Utricle
Posterior
⑤

With left shoulder down, patient is brought to a seated position.

Fairman
CMI

CRANIAL NERVE VIII: VESTIBULOCOCHLEAR NERVE (Continued)

tumors, and vascular loops. Pulsatile tinnitus is also a feature of idiopathic intracranial hypertension. Bilateral hearing deficits reflect general processes such as ototoxicity (aminoglycosides, salicylates, or loop diuretics), noise exposure, and age-related hearing loss (presbycusis), whereas unilateral hearing loss should raise concern of neoplastic, vascular, neurologic, or inflammatory etiologies. Fluctuating symptoms are seen in Ménière disease, whereas progressive loss may indicate tumor (e.g., vestibular schwannoma). Ménière disease typically results in low roaring tinnitus, whereas high-pitched tinnitus may suggest tumor or presbycusis. Sudden hearing loss occurs with viral neuritis or vascular or compressive processes that occlude the cochlear blood supply from the internal auditory artery (labyrinthine artery), a terminal branch of the AICA or the basilar artery. Strokes from occlusion of the AICA itself are relatively rare, but they are often accompanied by ipsilateral hearing loss and tinnitus, vestibular symptoms, gait ataxia, conjugate gaze palsy, ipsilateral facial paralysis and sensory loss, and contralateral body loss of pain and temperature sensation. Combined symptoms of tinnitus and vertigo may also indicate inner ear pathology of the cochlea, vestibular labyrinth, auditory nerve, or a combination of structures.

CANALITH REPOSITIONING MANEUVERS

First-line therapy for BPPV includes canalith repositioning maneuvers such as the Epley maneuver. The maneuver uses gravity to pull the canalith debris out of the affected semicircular canal and into the utricle, where it lodges in the otolithic membrane of the macula (see Plate 1.39). The maneuver requires sequential movement of the head into four positions, staying in each position for approximately 30 seconds. The Epley maneuver is most useful for posterior canal BPPV. The patient begins in the upright sitting position with the head turned 45 degrees toward the affected side (in the figure, the right ear is affected). The patient then lies down with the affected ear facing the ground and the head in 30 degrees of neck extension (Dix-Hallpike maneuver). Vertigo and nystagmus are elicited, and the position is maintained until the nystagmus ceases. Then the head is rolled 180 degrees until the affected ear is facing up. The patient rolls onto their side until their nose points toward the floor. The patient then rapidly returns to the seated position and remains there for 30 more seconds. The maneuver is repeated until no nystagmus is elicited.

AFFERENT AUDITORY PATHWAYS

Auditory afferent fibers enter the brainstem in the vestibulocochlear nerve and then branch to the dorsal and ventral cochlear nuclei located in the medulla. Neurons in these nuclei have similar properties: each is excited by a relatively narrow range of sound frequencies and may be inhibited by tones outside that range. A tonotopic distribution arises in each nucleus, as neurons sensitive to different frequencies are arranged in an orderly manner.

The fibers of the ventral cochlear nucleus then project to the superior olive located in the medulla. The fibers then project by way of the lateral lemniscus nuclei and other relays to the inferior colliculus. The dorsal cochlear nucleus projects directly to the inferior colliculus via the lateral lemniscus. Fibers from both the ventral and dorsal cochlear nucleus project from the inferior colliculus to the medial geniculate nucleus of the thalamus. Within the colliculi, signals from both ears interact on their way toward the cerebral cortex. From the medial geniculate nucleus, the auditory signals travel to the primary auditory cortex, which is in the temporal lobe and is Brodmann's area 41. Despite the extensive intermixing among afferent fibers, the bulk of the neural activity reaching the auditory cortex originates in the contralateral ear. Tonotopic ordering is preserved throughout the ascending pathway so that individual cortical regions are sensitive to specific frequencies. The width of the band of frequencies to which an individual neuron responds is approximately the same in area 41 as at the level of the cochlear nuclei.

In the analysis of acoustic information, relatively little is known about the function of the various stages along the auditory pathway. Neurons within the superior olivary complex are specifically adapted for analyzing the location of a sound in space. The lateral superior olive (LSO) receives excitatory input from the ipsilateral cochlea via the medial nucleus of the trapezoid body. There is an ipsilateral inhibitory pathway as well, as the lateral nucleus of the trapezoid body mediates excitatory input via the contralateral cochlea. In the medial portion of the complex, where neurons are sensitive to sounds of low frequency, these opposing inputs result in individual neurons becoming attuned to a fixed time delay between the arrival of sound at each ear. In the lateral portion of the complex, where neurons are sensitive to higher frequencies, the opposing inputs result in neurons becoming sensitive to differences in the intensity of sound reaching each ear. Therefore the entire auditory pathway, including the auditory cortex, must be intact for sound localization to take place. Similarly, auditory structures as far as the level of the inferior colliculus are required for frequency discrimination, even though neurons at all levels of the auditory pathway are frequency selective. Intensity discriminations, on the other hand, can be made after the destruction of the inferior colliculus and higher centers. Such discrimination may involve the

collateral pathways that relay auditory signals to the brainstem reticular formation. These pathways are probably also involved in the reflex reaction to a sudden sound.

DISORDERS

A common auditory pathway deficit is vestibular schwannoma. The patient experiences loss of sound

localization, diminished speech discrimination, tinnitus, imbalance, and diminution of the stapedius reflex. Sensorineural deafness can be caused by toxins (e.g., arsenic, lead, quinine) and by antibiotics such as streptomycin, which can also damage the cochlea directly. Because of the multisynaptic and highly complex system of crossed pathways, damage to auditory brainstem tracts and nuclei by trauma, tumors, or vascular disorders results in only slight hearing impairment.

Acoustic area of temporal lobe cortex

Medial geniculate nucleus

Brachium of inferior colliculus

Inferior colliculus

Midbrain

Correspondence between cochlea and acoustic area of cortex:

- **Low tones**
- **Middle tones**
- **High tones**

Lateral lemnisci

Medulla oblongata

Superior olivary complex

Nuclei of lateral lemnisci

Dorsal cochlear nucleus

Inferior cerebellar peduncle

Ventral cochlear nucleus

Cochlear division of vestibulocochlear nerve

Intermediate acoustic stria

Dorsal acoustic stria

Reticular formation

Trapezoid body (ventral acoustic stria)

Spiral ganglion

Inner   Outer

Hair cells

Plate 1.38

Cranial Nerve and Neuro-ophthalmologic Disorders

CENTRIFUGAL AUDITORY PATHWAYS

In addition to the afferent neural pathways that carry auditory information from the cochlea to the higher centers, there is a parallel, descending, efferent pathway aptly named the *centrifugal pathway*. Within the brain, such connections arise from each of the areas involved in the auditory system, including the primary auditory cortex, inferior colliculi and nuclei of the lateral lemnisci, and project to nuclei one or two levels below their point of origin. Individual connections may be either excitatory or inhibitory, but the centrifugal pathways appear to be activated by the inhibition of transmission of auditory signals through the ascending auditory pathways.

Centrifugal auditory pathways also include efferent projections to the sensory hair cells of the cochlea and to the muscles of the middle ear. The cochlear efferent fibers originate from a group of neurons on the medial side of the contralateral superior olive and pass to the cochlea via the crossed olivocochlear bundle and the cochlear division of the vestibulocochlear nerve. They are joined by a smaller number of fibers, which originate in the ipsilateral superior olive. The olivocochlear efferent pathway is composed of the medial olivocochlear system (MOCS) and the lateral olivocochlear system (LOCS). The MOCS has large cell bodies in the medial and anterior olivary regions and innervates the outer hair cells of the cochlea. The LOCS has small cell bodies in and around the LSO and innervates the afferent dendrites beneath the inner hair cells of the ipsilateral cochlea. The large outer hair cell endings are primarily cholinergic, whereas the axodendritic synapses beneath the inner hair cells contain acetylcholine, dopamine, enkephalins, and other peptides. The efferent fibers produce hyperpolarization in the cochlear hair cells and afferent nerve terminals, thereby decreasing the afferent response produced when sound reaches the cochlea. Fibers innervating the muscles of the middle ear originate in the trigeminal motor nucleus and the facial nucleus (the tensor tympani muscle and the stapedius muscle). By contracting, these muscles decrease the transmission of sound vibrations from the eardrum to the oval window by way of the ossicles (incus, malleus, and stapes).

Several functions have been proposed for the centrifugal auditory pathways. One possibility is that efferent impulses can suppress the auditory nerve afferent responses to sound, thus preventing damage from too strong a stimulus. The middle ear muscles contract during loud noises and self-initiated vocalization, thereby helping to prevent saturation or damage of the cochlear receptors. Sound-activated efferent fibers in the olivocochlear bundle may additionally contribute to the suppression of sensory input that could saturate the central nervous pathways. A related mechanism, possibly also mediated by olivocochlear fibers, is improved auditory discrimination by the attenuation of loud background noise.

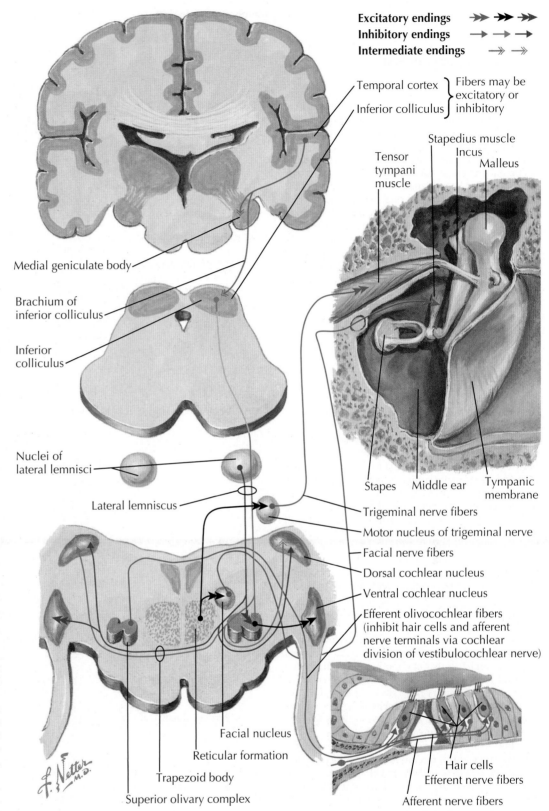

The phenomenon of selective attention to auditory signals is likely also to be an effect of the centrifugal auditory pathways. This "attentional filter" is absent in de-efferented humans. Evidence also shows that habituation to repeated auditory stimuli occurs with inhibition of the cochlear nuclei.

Finally, efferent olivocochlear pathways participate in auditory discrimination. Neurons at higher levels of the auditory pathway tend to respond to transient changes in auditory input rather than to steady signals. Centrifugal inhibition may be a factor in eliminating responses to steady signals, thus accentuating sensitivity to transient ones. Together with the inhibition that takes place within each level of the auditory system, it may also contribute to the processes that sharpen neuronal responses by restricting the ranges of the frequencies to which each neuron responds.

VESTIBULAR RECEPTORS

The *membranous labyrinth* is a specialized structure that converts angular and linear accelerations of the head into neuronal signals. This labyrinth is filled with potassium-rich endolymph and is a system of thin-walled intercommunicating tubes and ducts situated within the petrous part of the temporal bone at the base of the skull. The membranous labyrinth consists of the otolith organ (utricle and saccule) and three semicircular canals. The utricle and saccule contain specialized receptors called maculae that specifically respond to linear acceleration. Connected to the utricle are the three semicircular canals oriented at right angles to each other, which respond to angular acceleration. Within swellings of the canals, called ampullae, are the specialized receptors, the cristae.

The vestibular labyrinth receives dual innervation. The distal axonal processes of the bipolar vestibular afferent neurons have cell bodies housed in the vestibular ganglion of the internal acoustic meatus. The afferent axons terminate on the mechanoreceptive vestibular hair cells that serve as the sensory transducers. The vestibular efferent fibers originate in the brainstem.

Hair cells are specialized epithelial cells that have ciliary tufts protruding from their apical surface. Type I cells are goblet shaped and are enclosed in a nerve chalice (calyx). Synaptic terminals packed with vesicles are in contact with the base of the chalice and are likely presynaptic terminals. Type II hair cells are more common and have small terminal synaptic boutons. They are innervated by thin nerve branches that form synaptic contact with the bottom of the cell. The efferent endings are presynaptic to the hair cell and filled with vesicles. Type I hair cells are thought to be more sensitive than those of type II. Efferent fibers form typical chemical synapses with hair cells or with afferent terminals, which act to increase the discharge rate of afferent fibers and to modulate their response to mechanic stimuli.

The apical ends of both types of hair cells bear a tuft of 40 or more sensory hairs, or stereocilia, whose bases are embedded in a stiff cuticle, and a single, lower kinocilium, which originates from a basal body and has a structure similar to that of a motile cilium. The entire group of hairs is joined together at its free end. The stimulus for the sensory hair cells is shearing displacement of the hair cells. Displacement of the sensory hair bundle in the direction in of the kinocilium is excitatory and results in depolarization of the hair cell and increased firing of the vestibular nerve fibers. In the opposite direction, the response is inhibitory and results in hyperpolarization of the hair cell and reduced firing of the vestibular nerve. Signal transduction in hair cells occurs via a direct gating mechanism in which the hair bundle deflection puts tension on membrane-bound, cation-selective ion channels located near the tip of the hair bundle. This increased tension opens the channel and allows calcium to enter the cell. The increased intracellular calcium promotes adaptation, which may activate molecular motors that adjust the tension of the transduction apparatus.

The *cristae* of the semicircular canals and *maculae* of the utricle and saccule are especially sensitive to angular and linear acceleration, respectively, converting head movements to bending forces on the sensory hairs. The hair cells, the mechanoreceptors in the cristae, are embedded in a gelatinous mass called the cupula, which extends across the ampulla. During angular acceleration, there is displacement of the cupula and resultant bending of the sensory hairs. Because all hair cells in the cristae are oriented in the same direction as their kinocilia, this bending either increases or decreases the discharge rate of all the afferent fibers.

The hairs of the sensory cells found in the maculae of the saccule and utricle are embedded in a gelatinous otolithic membrane, which contains concretions of calcium carbonate called otoconia or otoliths. Because the otoconia are denser than the surrounding fluid, the otolithic membrane tends to move under the influence of linear acceleration. For instance, when the normally horizontal utricular macula is tilted, the pull of gravity tends to make the otolithic membrane slide downward, thus bending the sensory hairs. Because the macula contains hair cells that have two different orientations, this bending increases the discharge rate of some utricular afferent fibers and slows the discharge rate of others. These signals are analyzed by the CNS for information on the position of the head. The macula of the saccule is in a vertical position and is therefore sensitive to vertical acceleration. The saccule may also contribute to the sensing of head position when the head is oriented with one ear down.

The vestibulospinal tracts are discussed in the spinal cord section (see Plate 2.10).

Membranous labyrinth

Vestibular ganglion
Vestibular and cochlear divisions of vestibulo-cochlear nerve
Maculae
Saccule
Utricle
Cochlear duct (scala media)
Superior semicircular canal
Cristae within ampullae
Horizontal semicircular canal
Posterior semicircular canal

Section of crista

Opposite wall of ampulla
Gelatinous cupula
Hair tufts
Hair cells
Nerve fibers
Basement membrane

Section of macula

Otoconia
Gelatinous otolithic membrane
Hair tuft
Hair cells
Supporting cells
Basement membrane
Nerve fibers

Structure and innervation of hair cells

Excitation
Inhibition
Kinocilium
Stereocilia
Cuticle
Basal body
Cuticle
Kinocilium
Stereocilia
Basal body
Hair cell (type I)
Supporting cells
Afferent nerve calyx
Efferent nerve ending
Basement membrane
Myelin sheath
Hair cell (type II)
Supporting cell
Efferent nerve endings
Afferent nerve endings
Myelin sheath

Plate 1.40

Cranial Nerve and Neuro-ophthalmologic Disorders

COCHLEAR RECEPTORS

The *human cochlea* is a spiral channel located within the petrous portion of the temporal bone at the base of the skull. There are three fluid-filled chambers termed scalae: the scala vestibuli, scala media, and scala tympani. The scala media is separated from the scala vestibuli by the vestibular (Reissner's) membrane and from the scala tympani by the stria vascularis, a capillary loop in the upper portion of the spiral ligament. The scala media is filled with potassium-rich endolymph and is continuous with the vestibular labyrinth. The two remaining spaces, the scala vestibuli and the scala tympani, are filled with perilymph. At the basal end of the scala vestibuli is the oval window, which is connected to the auditory ossicles that transmit vibration from the eardrum. At the basal end of the scala tympani is the membrane-covered round window, whose movements provide a compensatory release of the vibratory pressures at the oval window.

The cochlea receives dual innervation: afferent fibers, which originate from cell bodies in the adjacent spiral (cochlear) ganglion, and efferent fibers, which originate in the brainstem. Both types of fibers form synapses with sensory hair cells in the spiral organ of Corti contained within the cochlear duct. Experimental studies have shown that activity in the efferent fibers can inhibit the discharge of cochlear afferent fibers. At the center of the organ of Corti is the tunnel of Corti, flanked by two sets of supporting rods of Corti (pillar cells). When hair cells are activated, impulse transmission is triggered in fibers of the spiral ganglion. The fibers then enter the brainstem as the cochlear nerve.

HEARING

The stapes ossicle bone transmits vibrations to the oval window on the outside of the cochlea. The perilymph vibrates in the scala vestibuli toward the helicotrema, a part of the cochlear apex where the scala vestibuli and scala tympani meet. Within the scala media is the receptor organ, the organ of Corti, which rests on top of the basilar membrane. The vibrations spread through the cochlea and induce vibrations in the basilar membrane, which are then transduced into afferent nerve excitation by the hair cells. The hair cells are arranged in inner and outer groups, and each cell is capped with 50 to 100 hair-like stereocilia that are imbedded in the tectorial membrane. The inner hair cells, about 3500 in number, are arranged in a single row on the inner side of the inner rods of Corti; the 12,000 outer hair cells are longer and are arranged in three rows in the basal coil of the cochlea, and in four or five rows in the apical coil. Physiologic studies suggest that cochlear hair cells behave like their vestibular counterparts; bending of stereocilia in one direction leads to a depolarization of hair cells and an accelerated rate of nerve discharge, whereas bending in the opposite direction produces hyperpolarization and a slowing of discharge.

The cochlear system enables another type of frequency analysis based on the differences in the shape and stiffness of the basilar membrane located between the base and the apex of the cochlea. Specifically, the basilar membrane vibrates most to high frequencies at the base of the cochlea, where the basilar membrane is thinner and narrower, and to low frequencies at the apex. The dimensions of the basilar membrane gradually change, so that for each vibration frequency between the two extremes, a somewhat restricted region of the membrane, and hence a certain group of afferent fibers, responds most vigorously. The cochlea is therefore said to be tonotopically organized: each afferent fiber will respond to some extent to a range of frequencies, but within the range is one frequency to which it will respond most readily.

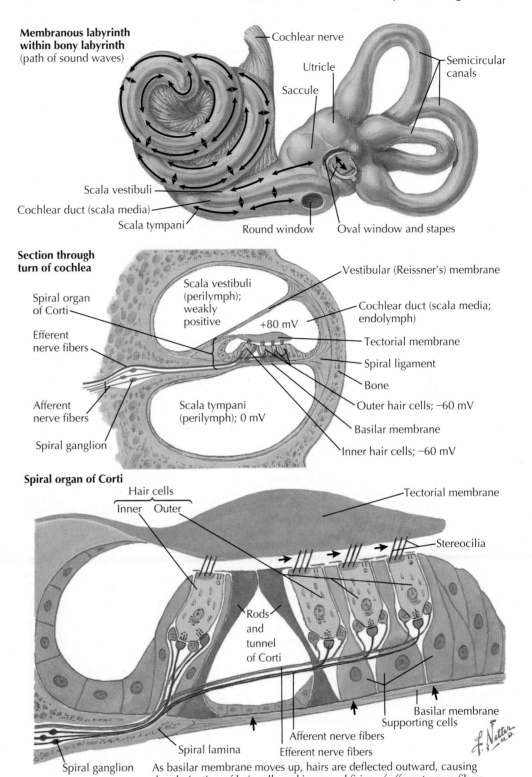

Membranous labyrinth within bony labyrinth (path of sound waves)

Cochlear nerve

Utricle

Saccule

Semicircular canals

Scala vestibuli

Cochlear duct (scala media)

Scala tympani

Round window

Oval window and stapes

Section through turn of cochlea

Spiral organ of Corti

Efferent nerve fibers

Afferent nerve fibers

Spiral ganglion

Scala vestibuli (perilymph); weakly positive

+80 mV

Scala tympani (perilymph); 0 mV

Vestibular (Reissner's) membrane

Cochlear duct (scala media; endolymph)

Tectorial membrane

Spiral ligament

Bone

Outer hair cells; –60 mV

Basilar membrane

Inner hair cells; –60 mV

Spiral organ of Corti

Hair cells

Inner   Outer

Tectorial membrane

Stereocilia

Rods and tunnel of Corti

Basilar membrane

Supporting cells

Afferent nerve fibers

Efferent nerve fibers

Spiral lamina

Spiral ganglion

As basilar membrane moves up, hairs are deflected outward, causing depolarization of hair cells and increased firing of afferent nerve fibers.

DEAFNESS

The cochlea is often the source of deafness, either to a specific pitch or to a broad range of frequencies. Head trauma can produce transient deafness, but severe injury involving a fracture of the petrous part of the temporal bone can cause permanent spiral ganglion or cochlear damage. Intense noise can cause temporary deafness; if it is sustained, permanent cochlear damage will result. The most common cause of deafness in adult life is otosclerosis, a nonneural process that results in the fixation of the stapes to the oval window.

CRANIAL NERVE IX: GLOSSOPHARYNGEAL NERVE AND OTIC GANGLION

GLOSSOPHARYNGEAL NERVE

The glossopharyngeal nerve is closely related functionally and anatomically to the vagus nerve. The two share common nuclei of origin and terminate in the ambiguus and dorsal vagal nuclei. The glossopharyngeal nerve also carries parasympathetic secretomotor fibers from the inferior salivatory nuclei, which are scattered in the reticular formation. The glossopharyngeal nerve contains sensory, motor, and parasympathetic fibers that supply parts of the tongue and pharynx. Its rootlets emerge from the dorsolateral sulcus of the medulla oblongata, rostral to those of the vagus nerve. The rootlets unite, and the nerve joins the vagus nerve and spinal accessory nerve to leave the skull through the central part of the jugular foramen between the inferior petrosal and sigmoid sinuses. As the glossopharyngeal nerve exits, it forms two ganglia, a small superior ganglion and a larger inferior ganglion (petrosal ganglion). The pseudounipolar nerve cells contained in both ganglia transmit multiple afferent impulses: special visceral sensation (taste) from the posterior third of the tongue and part of the soft palate; general visceral sensation (touch, pain, temperature) from the posterior third and adjacent areas of the tongue, fauces and pharynx soft palate, nasopharynx, and tragus of the ear; visceral afferent impulses from the carotid sinus and body; and general somatic afferent impulses from small areas of postauricular skin and the meninges in the posterior cranial fossa via the tympanic branch (Jacobson nerve). The central cell processes subserving taste end in the nucleus of the solitary tract, those concerned with visceral sensation end in the combined dorsal glossopharyngeal-vagal nucleus, and those concerned with general somatic afferents likely end in the spinal tract and nucleus of the trigeminal nerve.

From the jugular foramen, the nerve arches forward between the internal jugular vein and internal carotid artery, then passes deep to the styloid process, and curves behind the stylopharyngeus muscle (which it supplies) to the side of the pharynx. It traverses but does not supply the superior and middle constrictor muscles of the pharynx to enter the base of the tongue. It finally divides into branches that supply the mucous membrane over the posterior third of the tongue, fauces, palatine tonsil, and adjacent part of the pharynx, glands, and vessels in these areas.

The lingual branches convey special and general sensations from the vallate papillae and the tongue behind the sulcus terminalis. These branches are associated with small lingual ganglia. The ganglia act as relay centers for the preganglionic and postganglionic vasomotor and secretomotor neurons. The tympanic branch of the glossopharyngeal nerve arises from the inferior (petrosal) ganglion and ascends through the tympanic canaliculus to the middle ear (tympanic cavity), where it contributes to the tympanic plexus and gives off the lesser petrosal

nerve. The tympanic nerve contains sensory fibers that supply the middle ear, parasympathetic secretory fibers serving the parotid gland, and sympathetic fibers that communicate with the carotid sinus. The inferior ganglion of the glossopharyngeal nerve is also the origin of communications with the auricular vagal branch, the superior vagal ganglion, the superior cervical sympathetic trunk ganglion, and the facial nerve. More distally, the glossopharyngeal nerve also gives off an efferent branch to supply the stylopharyngeus, an afferent carotid

GLOSSOPHARYNGEAL NERVE (IX)

—————— Efferent fibers
—————— Afferent fibers
·············· Parasympathetic fibers

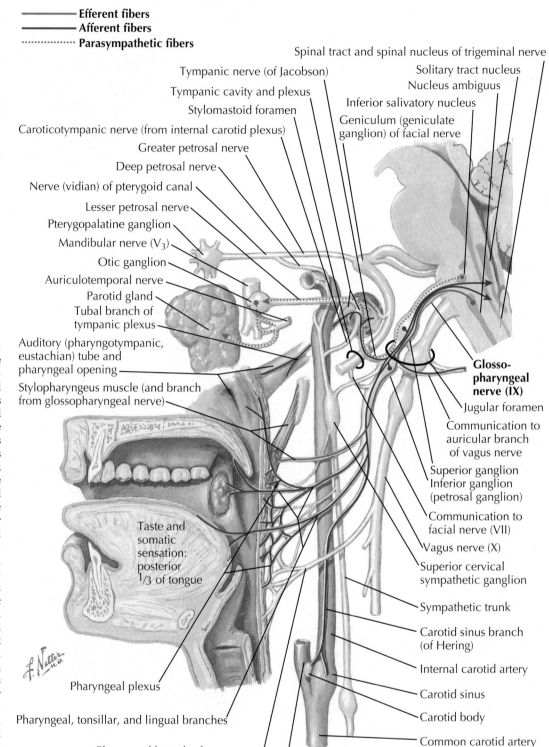

Tympanic nerve (of Jacobson)
Tympanic cavity and plexus
Stylomastoid foramen
Caroticotympanic nerve (from internal carotid plexus)
Greater petrosal nerve
Deep petrosal nerve
Nerve (vidian) of pterygoid canal
Lesser petrosal nerve
Pterygopalatine ganglion
Mandibular nerve (V₃)
Otic ganglion
Auriculotemporal nerve
Parotid gland
Tubal branch of tympanic plexus
Auditory (pharyngotympanic, eustachian) tube and pharyngeal opening
Stylopharyngeus muscle (and branch from glossopharyngeal nerve)

Spinal tract and spinal nucleus of trigeminal nerve
Solitary tract nucleus
Nucleus ambiguus
Inferior salivatory nucleus
Geniculum (geniculate ganglion) of facial nerve

Glossopharyngeal nerve (IX)
Jugular foramen
Communication to auricular branch of vagus nerve
Superior ganglion
Inferior ganglion (petrosal ganglion)
Communication to facial nerve (VII)
Vagus nerve (X)
Superior cervical sympathetic ganglion
Sympathetic trunk
Carotid sinus branch (of Hering)
Internal carotid artery
Carotid sinus
Carotid body
Common carotid artery

Taste and somatic sensation: posterior ¹/₃ of tongue

Pharyngeal plexus
Pharyngeal, tonsillar, and lingual branches
Pharyngeal branch of vagus nerve
External carotid artery

Plate 1.42

Cranial Nerve and Neuro-ophthalmologic Disorders

OTIC GANGLION

Mandibular nerve (V₃) — V_3

Trigeminal ganglion

Otic ganglion

Lesser petrosal nerve

Ophthalmic nerve (V_1)

Chorda tympani nerve

Trigeminal nerve (V)

Maxillary nerve (V_2)

Facial nerve (VII)

Auriculotemporal nerve

Glossopharyngeal nerve (IX)

Superficial temporal artery

Inferior salivatory nucleus

Parotid gland

Pons

Maxillary artery

Medulla oblongata

Inferior alveolar nerve

Tympanic plexus

Lingual nerve

Tympanic nerve (of Jacobson)

Inferior ganglion (IX)

Superior cervical sympathetic ganglion

External carotid artery

Sympathetic trunk

T1 and T2 spinal nerves

Thoracic spinal cord

Internal carotid artery

Dorsal root

Common carotid artery

White   Gray

Ventral root

Sympathetic preganglionic cell bodies in intermediolateral nucleus (lateral horn) of gray matter

Rami communicantes

══════ Sympathetic preganglionic fibers
━ ━ ━ Sympathetic postganglionic fibers
══════ Parasympathetic preganglionic fibers
━ ━ ━ Parasympathetic postganglionic fibers

CRANIAL NERVE IX: GLOSSOPHARYNGEAL NERVE AND OTIC GANGLION (Continued)

sinus branch, and several afferent pharyngeal branches, which unite with similar vagal branches and sympathetic filaments to form a plexus on the surface of the pharynx.

OTIC GANGLION

The otic ganglion lies directly below the foramen ovale between the mandibular nerve and the tensor veli palatini muscle, anterior to the middle meningeal artery. It receives its primary parasympathetic innervation via the lesser petrosal nerve, including the parotid secretory and vasodilatory fibers. After relaying in the ganglion, these fibers reach the gland through the parotid branches of the auriculotemporal nerve (a branch of the trigeminal nerve). Sympathetic innervation of the otic ganglion arises from the middle meningeal plexus, which, in turn, originates from the superior cervical ganglion. The otic ganglion also communicates with the nerve of the pterygoid canal and the chorda tympani. The fibers from the trigeminal-derived medial pterygoid nerve traverse the otic ganglion without relay to supply the tensor veli palatini and tensor tympani muscles.

The pharyngeal reflex or gag reflex is elicited by stimulating the posterior pharyngeal wall and results in bilateral contraction of the pharyngeal muscles and brief elevation of the soft palate. The sensory limb is mediated by the inferior ganglion of the glossopharyngeal nerve (petrosal ganglion). The efferent limb is mediated by the vagus nerve and glossopharyngeal nerve. The vagus nerve originates in the rostral nucleus ambiguus of the medulla, then exits the brainstem dorsolateral to the inferior olive, and exits the skull via the jugular foramen and innervates the stylopharyngeus muscle and superior pharyngeal constrictors. Therefore, if there is a glossopharyngeal nerve lesion, testing for gag reflex produces no response when touching the affected side of the pharynx. If there is vagal nerve damage, the soft palate elevates and pulls toward the intact side.

Lesions of the glossopharyngeal nerve rarely occur in isolation and usually are associated with vagus and spinal accessory nerve dysfunction, manifesting as dysphagia and dysphonia, ipsilateral palatal weakness, loss of gag reflex, ipsilateral vocal cord paralysis, altered taste and oropharyngeal sensation, decreased parotid secretion, and sternocleidomastoid and trapezius weakness. The major causes are trauma, tumors (especially paragangliomas and metastatic lesions to the skull base), extension of mastoid infections, or autoimmune disorders, such as giant cell arteritis.

Glossopharyngeal neuralgia is a disorder characterized by paroxysmal, severe, unilateral pain in the tongue, throat, ear, and tonsils. The pain typically lasts from seconds to a few minutes. It is triggered by chewing, talking, coughing, yawning, swallowing, and eating particular foods. The etiology is often unclear, but some cases may be due to vascular compression of the nerve. There is usually no associated impairment of the glossopharyngeal nerve (e.g., no dysphagia) or any abnormal findings on the neurologic examination. The symptomatic treatment approaches are similar to those employed for trigeminal neuralgia and include anticonvulsants, such as carbamazepine, gabapentin, and phenytoin. The second-line option is rhizotomy or surgical decompression of the nerve.

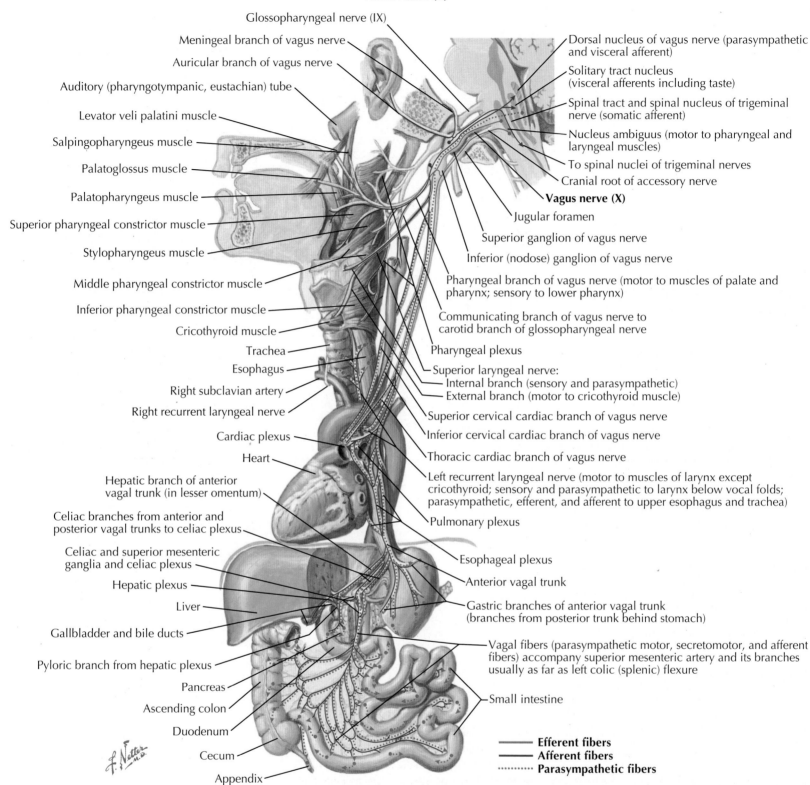

VAGUS NERVE (X)

Glossopharyngeal nerve (IX)

Meningeal branch of vagus nerve

Auricular branch of vagus nerve

Auditory (pharyngotympanic, eustachian) tube

Levator veli palatini muscle

Salpingopharyngeus muscle

Palatoglossus muscle

Palatopharyngeus muscle

Superior pharyngeal constrictor muscle

Stylopharyngeus muscle

Middle pharyngeal constrictor muscle

Inferior pharyngeal constrictor muscle

Cricothyroid muscle

Trachea

Esophagus

Right subclavian artery

Right recurrent laryngeal nerve

Cardiac plexus

Heart

Hepatic branch of anterior vagal trunk (in lesser omentum)

Celiac branches from anterior and posterior vagal trunks to celiac plexus

Celiac and superior mesenteric ganglia and celiac plexus

Hepatic plexus

Liver

Gallbladder and bile ducts

Pyloric branch from hepatic plexus

Pancreas

Ascending colon

Duodenum

Cecum

Appendix

Dorsal nucleus of vagus nerve (parasympathetic and visceral afferent)

Solitary tract nucleus (visceral afferents including taste)

Spinal tract and spinal nucleus of trigeminal nerve (somatic afferent)

Nucleus ambiguus (motor to pharyngeal and laryngeal muscles)

To spinal nuclei of trigeminal nerves

Cranial root of accessory nerve

Vagus nerve (X)

Jugular foramen

Superior ganglion of vagus nerve

Inferior (nodose) ganglion of vagus nerve

Pharyngeal branch of vagus nerve (motor to muscles of palate and pharynx; sensory to lower pharynx)

Communicating branch of vagus nerve to carotid branch of glossopharyngeal nerve

Pharyngeal plexus

Superior laryngeal nerve:
Internal branch (sensory and parasympathetic)
External branch (motor to cricothyroid muscle)

Superior cervical cardiac branch of vagus nerve

Inferior cervical cardiac branch of vagus nerve

Thoracic cardiac branch of vagus nerve

Left recurrent laryngeal nerve (motor to muscles of larynx except cricothyroid; sensory and parasympathetic to larynx below vocal folds; parasympathetic, efferent, and afferent to upper esophagus and trachea)

Pulmonary plexus

Esophageal plexus

Anterior vagal trunk

Gastric branches of anterior vagal trunk (branches from posterior trunk behind stomach)

Vagal fibers (parasympathetic motor, secretomotor, and afferent fibers) accompany superior mesenteric artery and its branches usually as far as left colic (splenic) flexure

Small intestine

——— Efferent fibers
——— Afferent fibers
········· Parasympathetic fibers

CRANIAL NERVE X: VAGUS NERVE

VAGAL NUCLEI

The glossopharyngeal nerve, vagus nerve, and cranial parts of accessory nerves may be considered as a single nerve complex because all have central connections with the dorsal vagal nucleus, solitary tract nucleus, and nucleus ambiguus.

The dorsal vagal nucleus is a mixed nucleus that represents fused visceral afferent and efferent columns of neurons. It consists of a longitudinal column of cells lying beneath the vagal trigone in the fourth ventricle floor, lateral to the hypoglossal nucleus, extending nearly the length of the medulla oblongata. The general visceral afferent fibers ending in the nucleus are the central processes of pseudounipolar sensory cells in the inferior vagal ganglion (nodose ganglion). Extensive peripheral processes of general visceral sensory cells

convey impulses from the heart, aorta, trachea, bronchi, lungs, liver, pancreas, most of the alimentary tract (from the lower pharynx almost to the left colic flexure), and possibly from the kidneys. Preganglionic parasympathetic efferent fibers carrying impulses for the same structures originate in the dorsal vagal nuclei and are distributed through direct vagal branches to the viscera or through branches of the cardiac, celiac, and abdominal plexuses (anterior and posterior vagal trunks). These vagal preganglionic fibers synapse in

Plate 1.44

Cranial Nerve and Neuro-ophthalmologic Disorders

CRANIAL NERVE X: VAGUS NERVE (Continued)

ganglia located near or within the viscera they innervate. Because of this arrangement, vagal parasympathetic postganglionic fibers are relatively short and more limited in their distribution than their sympathetic counterparts. The superior vagal ganglion (jugular ganglion) receives general somatic afferent fibers in the form of pseudounipolar cells involved with sensory impulses conducted through the auricular and meningeal vagal branches, although the fibers in the latter branches may be derived from interconnections between ganglia and upper cervical spinal nerves. Central processes of the superior vagal ganglion cells probably end in the spinal nuclei of the trigeminal nerves.

Sensory fibers that carry taste sensation from the epiglottis, pharynx, and hard and soft palates are in the nodose ganglion. The solitary tract nucleus receives information from these afferent special sensory taste fibers, which travel in the superior laryngeal vagal branches from the mucous membrane of the epiglottis and the epiglottic valleculae. In addition, general visceral sensations from the larynx, oropharynx, linings of the thorax, and abdominal viscera also project to the solitary tract nucleus. The nucleus ambiguus develops from special visceral efferent columns and forms a row of discrete, multipolar neurons located deep in the reticular formation of the medulla oblongata. Its axons emerge in the glossopharyngeal and vagal nerves and in the cranial parts of the accessory nerves. These glossopharyngeal and vagal fibers distribute mainly to the intrinsic laryngeal and pharyngeal muscles (except tensor veli palatini [CN V] and stylopharyngeus [CN IX]), whereas the accessory fibers serve mainly the sternocleidomastoid and the trapezius muscles. The lower precentral gyrus controls vagal motor function.

VAGUS NERVE

The vagus nerve contains both afferent and efferent parasympathetic fibers that are widely distributed to visceral and vascular structures in the neck, thorax, and abdomen; somatic sensory fibers in the auricular and meningeal branches; some special sensory fibers (taste) of the superior laryngeal branch; and special visceral efferent fibers that arise in the nucleus ambiguus and are distributed mainly to laryngeal and pharyngeal muscles.

Each vagus nerve emerges from the lateral medulla oblongata along the posterior sulcus as 8 to 10 rootlets above the rootlets of the glossopharyngeal nerve and cranial parts of the accessory nerve. The rootlets coalesce to form a nerve that exits the skull through the jugular foramen, together with the glossopharyngeal and accessory nerves, the sigmoid sinus, and several other blood vessels. Within or inferior to the jugular foramen, the vagus nerve expands into superior and inferior ganglia.

The superior vagal ganglion (jugular ganglion) communicates with the nearby superior cervical sympathetic trunk ganglion and the facial, glossopharyngeal, and accessory nerves. It gives off a recurrent branch to the meninges of the posterior cranial fossa, an auricular branch that carries somatic sensory impulses from parts of the tympanic membrane and the external acoustic meatus, and a pharyngeal branch that, along with the glossopharyngeal nerve, forms the pharyngeal plexus and sends motor fibers to the muscles of the soft palate and pharynx.

The inferior vagal ganglion (nodose ganglion) connects with the cranial part of the accessory nerve. It also communicates with the superior cervical sympathetic trunk ganglion, the hypoglossal nerve, and the loop between the first and second cervical spinal nerves. It gives off pharyngeal and superior laryngeal branches (which divide into an efferent external ramus supplying motor function to the cricothyroid muscle and an internal ramus that pierces the thyrohyoid to supply sensory fibers to the larynx) and inconstant carotid rami, which assist the glossopharyngeal nerve in innervating the carotid sinus and body.

Below its inferior ganglion, the vagus nerve descends within an ipsilateral carotid sheath, shared with the

internal jugular vein and carotid artery, to the thoracic inlet. The vagus nerve intercommunicates with filaments from the cervical sympathetic trunks or branches so that it is a mixed parasympathetic-sympathetic nerve from the neck downward. Within the neck, the vagus nerve gives off the cardiac rami; these branches join the sympathetic fibers via the cardiac plexus of the heart.

VAGAL NERVE BRANCHES IN THE THORAX

The right and left vagus nerves descend through the body along differing pathways. The right vagus nerve enters the thorax behind the internal jugular vein and in front of the first part of the subclavian artery. Here it

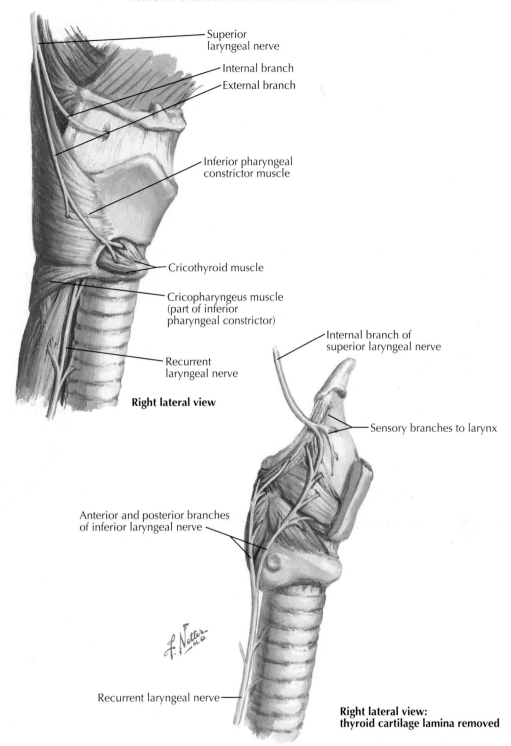

MOTOR AND SENSORY BRANCHES FROM THE VAGUS NERVE

Superior laryngeal nerve

Internal branch

External branch

Inferior pharyngeal constrictor muscle

Cricothyroid muscle

Cricopharyngeus muscle (part of inferior pharyngeal constrictor)

Recurrent laryngeal nerve

Right lateral view

Internal branch of superior laryngeal nerve

Sensory branches to larynx

Anterior and posterior branches of inferior laryngeal nerve

Recurrent laryngeal nerve

Right lateral view: thyroid cartilage lamina removed

CRANIAL NERVE X: VAGUS NERVE (Continued)

gives off the right recurrent laryngeal nerve, which hooks under the artery before ascending to the larynx. The recurrent laryngeal nerves divide into anterior and posterior rami and supply the larynx. The vagus nerve continues posteromedially, behind the right brachiocephalic vein and the superior vena cava, and runs medial to the azygos vein to reach the root of the right lung, where it splits into smaller anterior and larger posterior branches, both of which contribute rami to the anterior and posterior pulmonary plexuses.

The left vagus nerve enters the thorax between the left common carotid and left subclavian arteries, behind the left brachiocephalic vein. It crosses the left side of the aortic arch, giving off the left recurrent laryngeal nerve; thereafter, as on the right side, it participates in the formation of the pulmonary and esophageal plexuses. The left recurrent laryngeal nerve passes underneath the aorta on the outer side of the ligamentum arteriosum and then ascends to the larynx. Both recurrent laryngeal nerves innervate the laryngeal muscles (except the cricothyroids, which are supplied by the external ramus of the superior laryngeal nerve).

The vagal pulmonary branches, along with filaments derived from the second to fifth or sixth thoracic sympathetic trunk ganglia, form anterior and posterior pulmonary plexuses. The pulmonary plexuses become dispersed around the vascular and bronchial structures, and some of their terminal filaments reach the peripheral portion of the lungs. Along the course of the larger bronchi, small ganglia provide relay stations for the preganglionic parasympathetic (vagal) fibers. The sympathetic fibers relay outside the organs, primarily in the sympathetic trunk ganglia. Sympathetic and parasympathetic pulmonary afferent fibers are also present.

The esophageal plexus forms below the lung roots as the vagus nerves break up into two to four parts and travel on the esophagus as it descends through the posterior mediastinum, then divide and reunite to form the esophageal plexus. Filaments from thoracic sympathetic trunks and thoracic splanchnic nerves then join the esophageal plexus. Most of the branches of the right vagus incline posteriorly, whereas most of those from the left vagus incline anteriorly. Above the esophageal hiatus in the diaphragm, the meshes of the esophageal plexus become reconstituted into two or more vagal trunks, which travel by way of the esophageal diaphragm to innervate the abdominal viscera.

VAGAL NERVE DISORDERS

Bilateral supranuclear lesions may result in dysphagia, spastic dysarthria, pseudobulbar palsy, pharyngeal and laryngeal incoordination, and altered sensation with an increased risk of aspiration. Unilateral supranuclear lesions rarely cause vagal dysfunction because the supranuclear control is bilateral, although dysphagia does rarely occur with unilateral precentral gyrus lesions.

Isolated proximal vagus nerve injuries are rare because lesions at or around the jugular foramen, such as those caused by trauma or tumors (e.g., glomus vagale paragangliomas), usually also injure the glossopharyngeal and accessory nerves. Unilateral vagus neuropathy may cause ipsilateral pharyngeal (e.g., dysphagia) and laryngeal (e.g., change in voice) weakness and impaired sensation with inadequate airway protection. Ipsilateral

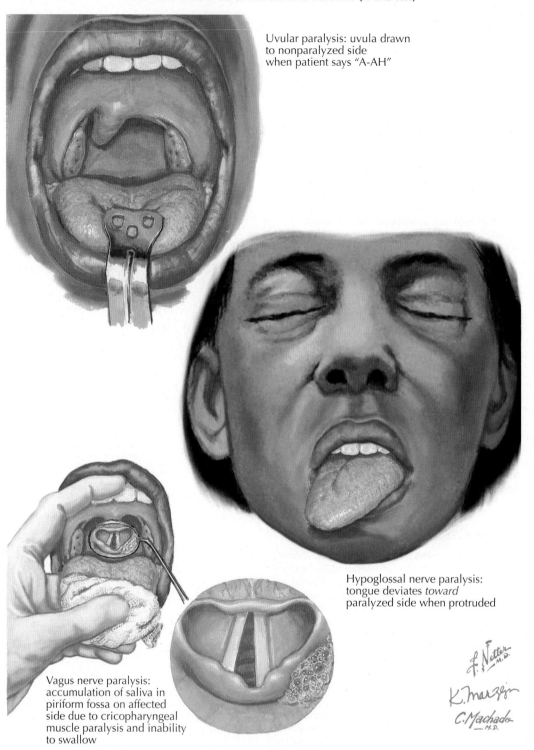

NEUROGENIC DISORDERS OF MOUTH AND PHARYNX (X AND XII)

Uvular paralysis: uvula drawn to nonparalyzed side when patient says "A-AH"

Hypoglossal nerve paralysis: tongue deviates *toward* paralyzed side when protruded

Vagus nerve paralysis: accumulation of saliva in piriform fossa on affected side due to cricopharyngeal muscle paralysis and inability to swallow

soft palate weakness may manifest as nasal regurgitation and nasal speech. Ipsilateral vocal cord paralysis may be the result of superior laryngeal nerve injury (cricothyroid muscle for vocal cord lengthening and laryngeal sensation) or more distal recurrent laryngeal neuropathy (cricoarytenoids and thyroarytenoid muscles for adduction, abduction, and shortening of vocal cords). Recurrent laryngeal nerve lesions affect all laryngeal muscles except for the cricothyroid, which is innervated by the superior laryngeal nerve. Superior laryngeal neuropathy leads to loss of high vocal pitches, a weak voice, and aspiration due to altered laryngeal sensation. Causes

include thyroiditis, local neck infections, or surgery; however, a reasonable proportion of cases are idiopathic. Recurrent laryngeal nerve lesions cause variable symptoms, from slight voice fatigue and breathiness to significantly altered speech, hoarseness, and ineffective cough. When unilateral, they typically cause transient hoarseness. Common causes include thyroid, neck, and lung tumors; thoracic surgery; and rarely thyroiditis. Diabetes, amyloidosis, and other acquired etiologies of polyneuropathy may cause vagal neuropathy, usually accompanied by symptoms and signs of more widespread sensorimotor polyneuropathy.

Plate 1.46

Cranial Nerve and Neuro-ophthalmologic Disorders

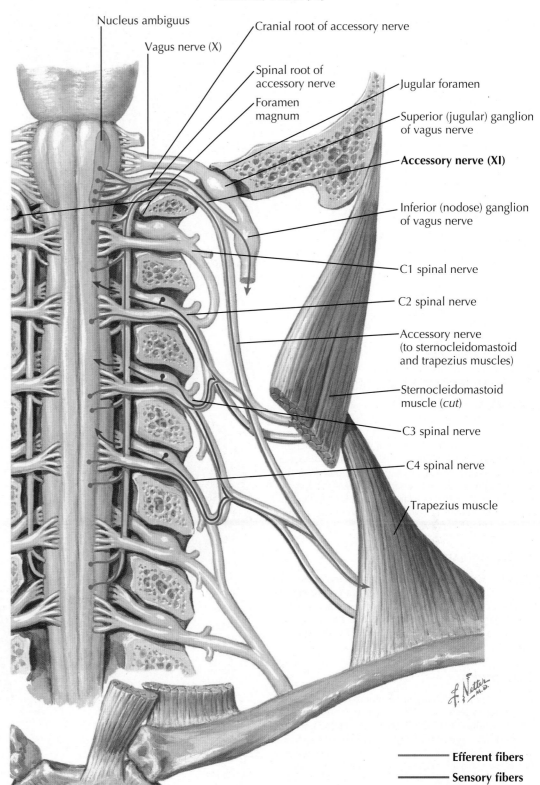

ACCESSORY NERVE (XI)

Nucleus ambiguus

Vagus nerve (X)

Cranial root of accessory nerve

Spinal root of accessory nerve

Foramen magnum

Jugular foramen

Superior (jugular) ganglion of vagus nerve

Accessory nerve (XI)

Inferior (nodose) ganglion of vagus nerve

C1 spinal nerve

C2 spinal nerve

Accessory nerve (to sternocleidomastoid and trapezius muscles)

Sternocleidomastoid muscle (*cut*)

C3 spinal nerve

C4 spinal nerve

Trapezius muscle

—— **Efferent fibers**

—— **Sensory fibers**

CRANIAL NERVE XI: ACCESSORY NERVE

The *spinal nucleus of the accessory nerve* is an elongated strand of motor neurons (special visceral efferent column) that extends caudally from the lower medulla oblongata to the dorsolateral part of the ventral gray column of the upper five to six cervical cord segments. The spinal nucleus gives rise to a series of rootlets, which emerge laterally from the cord via the lateral funiculus about midway between the anterior and posterior cervical roots and coalesce to form the *spinal root of the accessory nerve.* This structure ascends in the subarachnoid space behind the denticulate ligament and enters the skull through the *foramen magnum* behind the vertebral artery. Arching upward and outward, the spinal root unites over a short distance with the *cranial root of the accessory nerve* to leave the skull through the *jugular foramen* in the same dural and arachnoid sheath as the vagus nerve.

The cranial root is the smaller of the two portions of the accessory nerve. Although it is discussed in this section, it is often considered as a part of the vagus nerve rather than the accessory nerve proper because the cranial component rapidly joins the vagus nerve and serves the same function as other vagal fibers. The cranial nerve root fibers, classified as special visceral efferent, arise mainly from neurons in the caudal half of the *nucleus ambiguous* of the medulla, with probable minor contributions from the *dorsal vagal nucleus.* The fibers of the cranial root emerge as four to six rootlets from the dorsolateral sulcus, posterior to the olive and caudal to the vagal roots. As mentioned, the cranial root briefly joins the larger spinal root before exiting the jugular foramen. Although the cranial root communicates by one or two filaments with the superior vagal ganglion, most of its fibers continue as the *internal branch of the accessory nerve,* which joins the vagus nerve at or near its inferior ganglion and provides most of the motor fibers to the pharynx and larynx. Cranial root fibers travel in *pharyngeal branches* of the vagus

nerve to supply the muscles of the soft palate (except the tensor veli palatini) and contribute motor fibers to the pharyngeal plexus. They additionally supply all intrinsic laryngeal muscles (except the cricothyroid) via the *recurrent laryngeal vagal branches.*

COURSE OF ACCESSORY NERVE

The cranial and spinal root fibers separate distal to the jugular foramen to form the *internal* and *external branches*

of the accessory nerve. The internal branch joins the vagus nerve as described earlier. The external accessory branch innervates the sternocleidomastoid and trapezius muscles. This branch usually passes between the internal carotid artery and the internal jugular vein and runs obliquely downward and backward over the transverse process of the atlas and deep to the styloid process, occipital artery, and posterior belly of the digastric muscle before piercing the deep surface of the *sternocleidomastoid muscle.* It passes through and supplies this muscle

CLINICAL FINDINGS IN CRANIAL NERVE XI DAMAGE

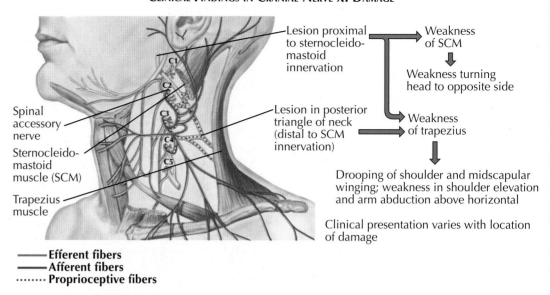

Lesion proximal to sternocleido-mastoid innervation → Weakness of SCM → Weakness turning head to opposite side

Lesion in posterior triangle of neck (distal to SCM innervation) → Weakness of trapezius

Drooping of shoulder and midscapular winging; weakness in shoulder elevation and arm abduction above horizontal

Clinical presentation varies with location of damage

Spinal accessory nerve

Sternocleido-mastoid muscle (SCM)

Trapezius muscle

—— **Efferent fibers**
—— **Afferent fibers**
········ **Proprioceptive fibers**

CRANIAL NERVE XI: ACCESSORY NERVE (Continued)

and emerges from the midpoint of the posterior sterno-cleidomastoid border. The external branch then descends across the posterior cervical triangle and crosses over the levator scapulae muscle to disappear under the trapezius muscle about 2 cm above the clavicle. Along its course, the external branch receives branches from the second, third, and fourth cervical nerve roots.

SUPRANUCLEAR INNERVATION

The trapezius and sternocleidomastoid muscles receive supranuclear innervation from the lower precentral gyrus. The corticobulbar fibers supplying the trapezius are primarily crossed. The corticobulbar fibers controlling the sternocleidomastoid muscle are thought to terminate mainly in the ipsilateral nuclei.

DISORDERS

Proximal spinal accessory nerve lesions cause weakness of the sternocleidomastoid and the trapezius muscles. Damage within the posterior triangle of the neck spares the sternocleidomastoid, resulting in isolated trapezius weakness. Because of the muscle's insertional configuration, sternocleidomastoid impairment manifests as weakness of turning the head to the opposite side. Involvement of the trapezius muscle manifests as drooping of the shoulder and mild upper scapular winging away from the chest wall, with slight lateral displacement. Weakness in shoulder elevation and arm abduction above horizontal is typical. Most individuals with accessory neuropathies also present with shoulder and neck pain.

The most common site of isolated accessory neuropathy is in the neck. The close association of the accessory nerve with the superficial cervical lymph nodes makes it vulnerable to iatrogenic damage during lymph node biopsy or radical neck dissection. The accessory nerve can

Mild shoulder drop

Spinal accessory (CN XI) nerve lesions cause weakness of trapezius muscle on involved side and present with mild shoulder droop. Weakness of shoulder elevation and scapular winging most pronounced on arm abduction.

Normal
Scapular winging

Trapezius muscle

Spinal accessory nerve (CN XI)

Scapula

also be directly compressed by swollen lymph nodes or other solid tumors. Rarely, accessory neuropathy occurs after blunt or penetrating neck trauma or from radiation injury with treatment of neck tumors. Damage can also occur after carotid endarterectomy or jugular vein cannulation because of the nerve's proximity to large neck vessels. Accessory neuropathy is sometimes seen as part of brachial plexitis (Parsonage-Turner syndrome).

Intrinsic spinal cord lesions, posterior fossa meningiomas, or metastases near the jugular foramen or

foramen magnum may injure the intraspinal and intracranial portions of the accessory nerve but usually also affect the glossopharyngeal and vagal nerves. At times, adjacent structures such as the hypoglossal nerve or sympathetic chain fibers may be involved, resulting in unilateral tongue weakness or Horner syndrome, respectively. Disorders of the anterior horn cell, including amyotrophic lateral sclerosis, syringomyelia, and poliomyelitis, may involve the nuclei of the accessory nerve.

Plate 1.48   Cranial Nerve and Neuro-ophthalmologic Disorders

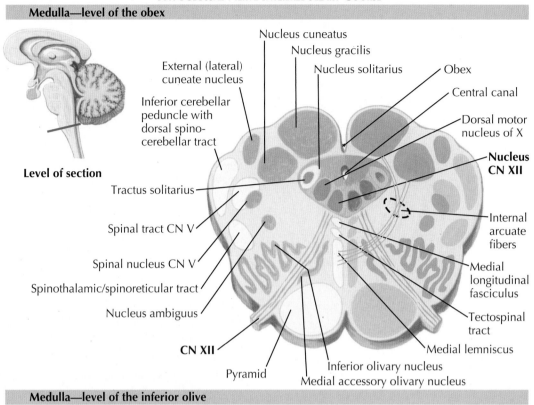

HYPOGLOSSAL NERVE INTERMEDULLARY COURSE

Medulla—level of the obex

Nucleus cuneatus
Nucleus gracilis
Nucleus solitarius
Obex
External (lateral) cuneate nucleus
Central canal
Inferior cerebellar peduncle with dorsal spino-cerebellar tract
Dorsal motor nucleus of X
Nucleus CN XII
Level of section
Tractus solitarius
Internal arcuate fibers
Spinal tract CN V
Medial longitudinal fasciculus
Spinal nucleus CN V
Spinothalamic/spinoreticular tract
Tectospinal tract
Nucleus ambiguus
Medial lemniscus
CN XII
Inferior olivary nucleus
Pyramid
Medial accessory olivary nucleus

Medulla—level of the inferior olive

External cuneate nucleus
Nucleus cuneatus
Nucleus solitarius
Tractus solitarius
Dorsal motor nucleus of X
Nucleus CN XII
Fourth ventricle
Choroid plexus
Inferior cerebellar peduncle
Level of section
Spinal tract CN V
Spinal nucleus CN V
Medial longitudinal fasciculus
CN X
Spinothalamic/spinoreticular tract
Tectospinal tract
Nucleus ambiguus
Inferior olivary nucleus
Medial lemniscus
Dorsal accessory olivary nucleus
CN XII
Pyramid
Medial accessory olivary nucleus

JOHN A. CRAIG —AD

CRANIAL NERVE XII: HYPOGLOSSAL NERVE

The hypoglossal nerve is the motor nerve of the tongue. Nerve fibers arise from the hypoglossal nucleus, which is a column of cells beneath the hypoglossal trigone of the fourth ventricle floor in the medulla oblongata. The nucleus extends from the pontomedullary junction to the caudal-most portion of the medulla oblongata. The main nucleus is composed of subnuclei that are likely associated with the individual muscles they innervate. Hypoglossal nerve fibers leave the nucleus and travel anterolaterally through the medullary reticular formation and the medial portion of the inferior olive and then course laterally to the medial longitudinal fasciculus, medial lemniscus, and pyramid. The nerve splits into two before exiting the medulla between the inferior olivary complex and the pyramid, medial to CNs IX, X, and XI, and then passes through the dura mater and hypoglossal canal of the skull. As the nerve roots enter the upper neck, the two roots coalesce to form a single nerve that runs near the internal carotid artery, internal jugular vein, and CNs IX, X, and XI before passing over the internal and external carotid arteries and beneath the stylohyoid, mylohyoid, and digastric muscles. After passing between the mylohyoid and hypoglossal muscles, the nerve divides into many branches. These

branches convey general somatic efferent innervation to the tongue supplying most of its extrinsic (hyoglossus, styloglossus, genioglossus, and chondroglossus) and all its intrinsic muscles (transverse and vertical lingual muscles, as well as the superior and inferior longitudinal muscles). The other branches of the hypoglossal nerve are derived from the cervical plexus and are not

connected with the hypoglossal nuclei and serve to provide motor innervation to the infrahyoid (strap) muscles. These nerve branches include the superior root of the ansa cervicalis, the meningeal branch, and nerves to the thyrohyoid and geniohyoid muscles. These are derived from the anterior rami of the first and second cervical nerves. The inferior root of the ansa cervicalis

HYPOGLOSSAL NERVE (XII)

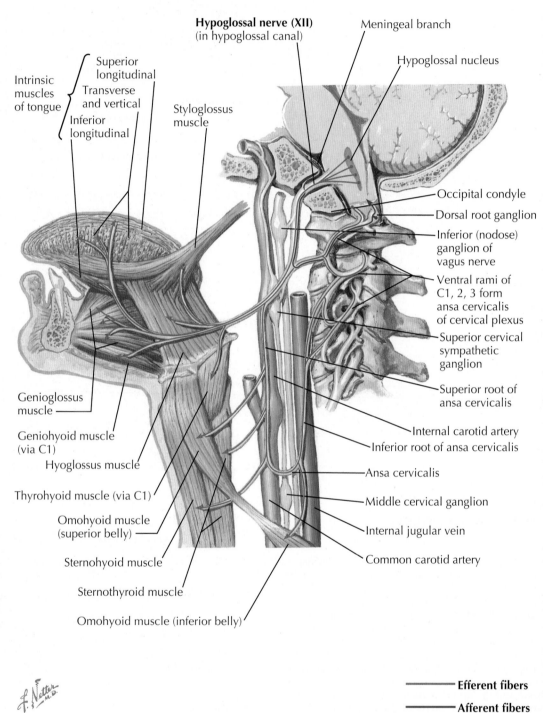

Hypoglossal nerve (XII) (in hypoglossal canal)

Meningeal branch

Hypoglossal nucleus

Intrinsic muscles of tongue

Superior longitudinal
Transverse and vertical
Inferior longitudinal

Styloglossus muscle

Occipital condyle

Dorsal root ganglion

Inferior (nodose) ganglion of vagus nerve

Ventral rami of C1, 2, 3 form ansa cervicalis of cervical plexus

Superior cervical sympathetic ganglion

Superior root of ansa cervicalis

Genioglossus muscle

Geniohyoid muscle (via C1)

Hyoglossus muscle

Thyrohyoid muscle (via C1)

Omohyoid muscle (superior belly)

Sternohyoid muscle

Sternothyroid muscle

Omohyoid muscle (inferior belly)

Internal carotid artery

Inferior root of ansa cervicalis

Ansa cervicalis

Middle cervical ganglion

Internal jugular vein

Common carotid artery

———— Efferent fibers

———— Afferent fibers

CRANIAL NERVE XII: HYPOGLOSSAL NERVE (Continued)

gives off branches to the omohyoid, sternothyroid, and sternohyoid muscles and is derived from the anterior rami of the second and third cervical nerves.

Supranuclear control of the tongue is mediated by the corticobulbar fibers, which originate in the lower portion of the precentral gyrus. The fibers controlling the genioglossus muscles (tongue protrusion) are crossed, but other tongue muscles have bilateral supranuclear control.

DISORDERS OF THE HYPOGLOSSAL NUCLEUS AND NERVE

Supranuclear lesions affecting the corticobulbar fibers above their decussation result in weakness of the contralateral half of the tongue. In these cases, the tongue will deviate away from the side of the lesion due to overaction of the unaffected genioglossus muscle. Bilateral upper motor neuron lesions affecting the corticobulbar tracts cause significant tongue dysfunction and spastic dysarthria.

Lesions of the hypoglossal nucleus or peripheral nerve result in ipsilateral tongue weakness, causing deviation toward the side of the lesion, ipsilateral atrophy,

fasciculations, and increased furrowing. It is best to allow the tongue to rest on the floor of the mouth when assessing for fasciculations. Dorsal medullary lesions causing bilateral lower motor neuron lesions of the tongue are extremely rare but are seen on occasion with tumors or syringobulbia. The medial medullary syndrome (Dejerine anterior bulbar syndrome) is caused by occlusion of the anterior spinal artery supplying the

medial lemniscus, hypoglossal nerve, and ipsilateral pyramids. Hypoglossal nuclear lesions may also result from intramedullary processes such as cavernomas, multiple sclerosis, syringobulbia, and tumors. These lesions may present with lower motor neuron hypoglossal palsy accompanied by contralateral hemiplegia and contralateral loss of position and vibratory sensation. Anterior horn cell disorders, such as amyotrophic

Plate 1.50

Cranial Nerve and Neuro-ophthalmologic Disorders

DISORDERS OF HYPOGLOSSAL NUCLEUS AND NERVE

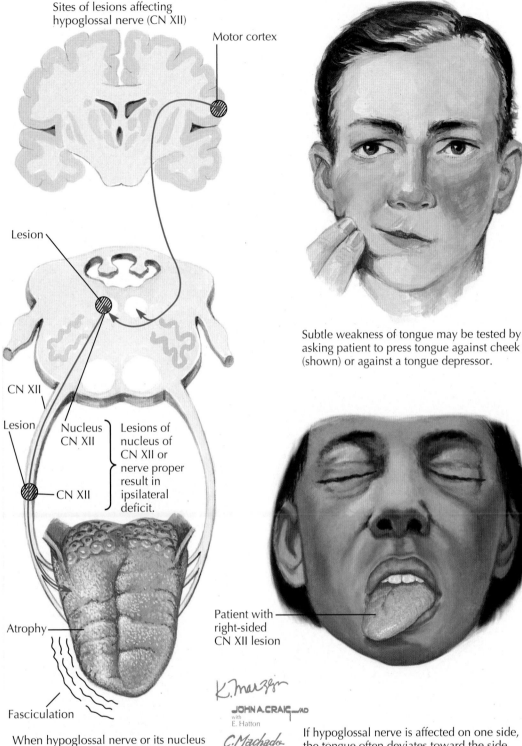

Sites of lesions affecting hypoglossal nerve (CN XII)

Motor cortex

Lesion

CN XII

Lesion

Nucleus CN XII

CN XII

Lesions of nucleus of CN XII or nerve proper result in ipsilateral deficit.

Atrophy

Fasciculation

Subtle weakness of tongue may be tested by asking patient to press tongue against cheek (shown) or against a tongue depressor.

Patient with right-sided CN XII lesion

When hypoglossal nerve or its nucleus is damaged, atrophy and fasciculation of the tongue are noted on evaluation.

If hypoglossal nerve is affected on one side, the tongue often deviates toward the side of the lesion on protrusion (due to imbalance of genioglossus contraction).

CRANIAL NERVE XII: HYPOGLOSSAL NERVE (Continued)

lateral sclerosis, also frequently affect the hypoglossal nuclei.

Because of the proximity of the hypoglossal canal (traversed by CN XII) to the jugular foramina (traversed by CNs IX, X, and XI), basilar skull lesions may damage all four cranial nerves simultaneously, resulting in weakness of the sternocleidomastoid, trapezius, tongue, and pharyngeal and laryngeal muscles, accompanied by loss of taste on the posterior third of the tongue and hemianesthesia of the palate, pharynx, and larynx (Collet-Sicard syndrome). Occipital pain and ipsilateral hypoglossal nerve injury may occur with occipital condyle syndrome, which is usually the result of tumors or chronic inflammatory lesions. Isolated hypoglossal neuropathy may also occur as the result of carotid aneurysm, vascular entrapment, dissection, local infection, rheumatologic disease, neck radiation, or tumors.

Extraaxial intracranial lesions of the hypoglossal nerve are typically caused by neoplasm at the basal meninges or skull base. Examples of neoplasms that cause hypoglossal neuropathy include metastatic bronchial or breast carcinoma, lymphoma, meningioma, chordoma, and cholesteatoma. As mentioned, proximity of the hypoglossal and jugular foramina leads to frequent co-involvement of

other lower cranial nerves (IX, X, XI). Jugular foramen lesions, such as glomus jugulare tumor (a rare hypervascular malignancy that arises from the paraganglionic tissue), can compress the hypoglossal nerve. Infectious and/or granulomatous processes that cause basal meningitis, such as tuberculosis and sarcoidosis, may affect multiple CNs, including the hypoglossal nerve. Primary bony processes (e.g., platybasia and Paget disease) have rarely been reported to affect the hypoglossal nerve. The close spatial relation between the hypoglossal nerve and the carotid artery makes this nerve vulnerable to primary carotid pathology within the neck and is occasionally damaged in the setting of internal carotid artery dissection, neck surgery, or carotid endarterectomy. Nasopharyngeal cancer and radiation therapy may damage the hypoglossal nerve in the neck.

SPINAL CORD: ANATOMY AND MYELOPATHIES

SPINAL CORD IN SITU

SPINAL CORD

The spinal cord is the downward continuation of the central nervous system (CNS) from the medulla oblongata. It extends from the upper border of the atlas to end in a tapering extremity, the *conus medullaris,* opposite the lower border of the first lumbar vertebra, or at the level of the intervertebral disk between the upper two lumbar vertebrae. From the conus, a slender, median, fibrous thread, the *filum terminale,* continues downward as far as the back of the coccyx. The dura mater and arachnoid (and therefore the subarachnoid space) extend down to the level of the second sacral vertebra. Although generally cylindric, the spinal cord is slightly flattened anteroposteriorly and shows *cervical* and *lumbar enlargements* that correspond to segments involved in supplying nerves to the upper and lower limbs. The nerve supply to the upper limb involves the fourth cervical to second thoracic spinal cord segments, and that to the lower limb, the third lumbar to third sacral spinal cord segments.

MENINGES

The cord is surrounded by dura, arachnoid, and pia mater, which are continuous with the corresponding layers of the cerebral meninges at the foramen magnum. The *spinal dura mater,* unlike the cerebral, consists only of a meningeal layer that is not adherent to the vertebrae; it is separated from the boundaries of the vertebral canal by an epidural space containing fatty areolar tissue and many veins. The spinal and cranial *subarachnoid spaces* are continuous and contain cerebrospinal fluid (CSF). The *pia mater* closely invests the cord; on each side, it sends out a series of 22 triangular processes, the *denticulate ligaments* that are attached to the dura mater and thus anchor the cord (see Plate 2.2). The spinal cord is considerably smaller than the vertebral canal; the meninges, the CSF, and the epidural fatty tissue and veins combine to cushion it against jarring contacts with its bony and ligamentous surroundings.

SPINAL NERVES

There are 31 pairs (8 cervical, 12 thoracic, 5 lumbar, 5 sacral, and 1 coccygeal) of symmetrically arranged *spinal nerves,* attached to the cord in linear series by anterior and posterior nerve rootlets, or filaments, which coalesce to form the nerve roots. Each posterior spinal nerve root possesses an oval enlargement, the *spinal (sensory) ganglion.*

In early embryonic life, the cord is as long as the vertebral canal, but as development proceeds, it lags behind the growth of the vertebral column. Consequently, the cord segments move upward in relation to the vertebrae, and the nerve roots, originally horizontal, assume an increasingly oblique direction from above downward as they proceed to their exit foramina. In the adult, except in the upper cervical region, the cord segments lie at varying distances above the

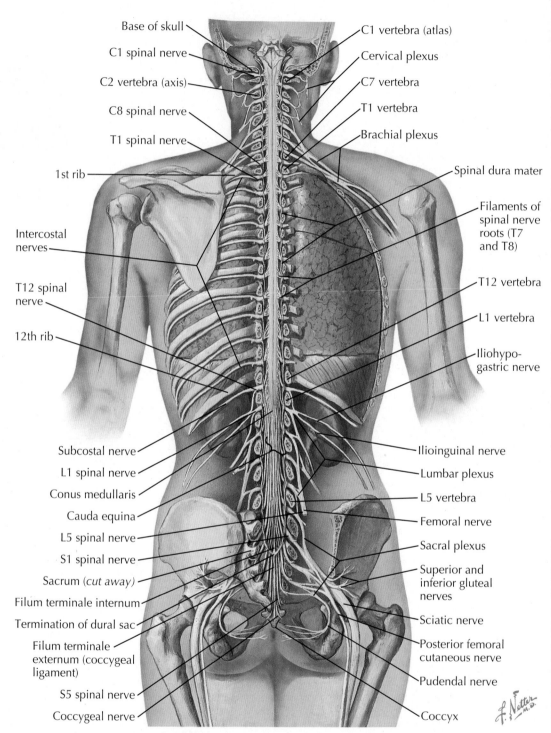

corresponding vertebrae. For clinical purposes, it is customary to localize them in relation to the vertebral spinous processes. In the lower cervical region, the vertebral spines are one lower in number than the corresponding cord segments; in the upper thoracic region, two lower in number; and in the lower thoracic region, three lower in number. For example, the fourth thoracic spinous process is approximately level with the sixth thoracic cord segment. The lumbar, sacral, and coccygeal segments of the cord are crowded together

and occupy the space approximately opposite the ninth thoracic to the first lumbar vertebrae. These alterations of the cord segments relative to the vertebral segments explain why the cervical enlargement (C4 to T2) lies approximately opposite the corresponding vertebrae, whereas the lumbar enlargement (L3 to S3) lies opposite the last three thoracic vertebrae. The nerve roots attached to the lower part of the cord descend to their points of exit as the *cauda equina,* named for their resemblance to the tail of a horse.

Plate 2.2

Spinal Cord: Anatomy and Myelopathies

SPINAL MEMBRANES AND NERVE ROOTS

MENINGES

The spinal cord is enveloped by meninges, which, at the level of the foramen magnum, are directly continuous with those surrounding the brain.

The external, tough, fibrous *dura mater* continues downward as far as the second sacral vertebra, where it ends blindly. It is separated from the wall of the vertebral canal by an *epidural space* containing fatty areolar tissue and a plexus of veins. A peridural membranous layer adjacent to the periosteum and situated between the bony wall of the spinal canal and the dura mater is sometimes described, but reports are inconsistent. The dura ensheathes the anterior and posterior spinal nerve roots, which lie close together when they pierce it; then the roots unite almost immediately to form a spinal nerve, and the dural sheath fuses with the epineurium. Between the dura mater and arachnoid is a potential *subdural space,* which normally contains the merest film of lymph-like fluid.

The spinal *arachnoid* is loose and tenuous and ends at the level of the second sacral vertebra. It is separated from the pia mater by the *subarachnoid space,* which is traversed by delicate mesothelial septa and contains CSF. The spinal nerve roots, up to the points at which they penetrate the dura mater, are loosely enclosed in arachnoid.

The *pia mater* is a thin layer of vascular connective tissue that intimately invests the spinal cord and its nerve roots. Below the conus medullaris, it is continuous with the slender *filum terminale* that descends amid the cauda equina, pierces the terminal parts of the dura and arachnoid, and ends by blending with the connective tissue behind the first segment of the coccyx. On each side, the pia is attached to the dura by 22 pointed processes, the *denticulate ligaments.*

NERVE ROOTS

The spinal cord is a segmented structure, and this is indicated by the regular attachments of the pairs of *spinal nerves.* As explained earlier, the cord and vertebral segments coincide in early embryonic life, but the vertebral canal eventually becomes longer than the cord so that most of the spinal nerves run obliquely downward to their points of exit.

The nerve filaments, or rootlets, are attached to the cord along its anterolateral and posterolateral regions. The *anterior (ventral) filaments* emerge in two or three irregular rows. They are composed predominantly of efferent fibers, which are the axons of cells in the anterior columns, or horns, of gray matter, and they carry motor impulses to the voluntary muscles.

In the thoracic and upper lumbar regions, the filaments also contain preganglionic sympathetic fibers, which are the axons of lateral columnar, or cornual, cells. The *posterior (dorsal) filaments* are attached in a regular series along a shallow groove, the posterolateral sulcus, and are collections of the central processes of nerve cells located in the spinal ganglia of the related dorsal nerve roots. The lateral cell processes pass on in spinal nerves and their branches to peripheral receptors, and they convey afferent impulses back to the spinal cord from somatic, visceral, and vascular sources.

The spinal cord shows an *anterior median fissure* and a shallow *posterior median sulcus* from which a *median septum* of neuroglia extends forward for 4 to 6 mm. The cord is divided into symmetric halves by the fissure, sulcus, and septum. The lines of attachment of the anterior and posterior nerve filaments are used to demarcate the white matter in each half of the cord into *anterior, lateral,* and *posterior columns,* or *funiculi.*

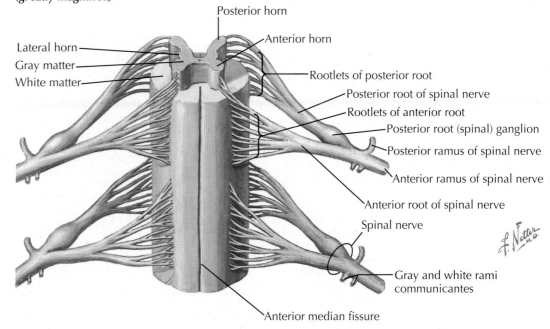

Posterior view

Anterior root of spinal nerve
Posterior root of spinal nerve
Posterior root (spinal) ganglion
White and gray rami communicantes to and from sympathetic trunk
Anterior ramus of spinal nerve
Posterior ramus of spinal nerve
Dura mater
Arachnoid mater
Mesothelial septum in posterior median sulcus
Pia mater overlying spinal cord
Rootlets of posterior root
Denticulate ligament

Membranes removed: anterior view (greatly magnified)

Posterior horn
Anterior horn
Lateral horn
Gray matter
White matter
Rootlets of posterior root
Posterior root of spinal nerve
Rootlets of anterior root
Posterior root (spinal) ganglion
Posterior ramus of spinal nerve
Anterior ramus of spinal nerve
Anterior root of spinal nerve
Spinal nerve
Gray and white rami communicantes
Anterior median fissure

ARTERIES OF SPINAL CORD AND NERVE ROOTS

The spinal cord is supplied by multiple *radicular arteries*, which form the *anterior spinal* and two *posterior spinal arteries*.

The *radicular arteries* arise from the lateral spinal arteries, which traverse the intervertebral foramina at each vertebral segment. Regardless of their origin, the many small radicular arteries pass medially to supply the anterior and posterior nerve roots. Most do not reach the spinal cord. However, some of the larger arteries reach the dura mater, where they give off small *meningeal branches* and then divide into *ascending* and *descending branches* to form the spinal arteries. The larger radicular arteries, which supply both the nerve roots and the spinal cord, are called *radiculomedullary arteries* to distinguish them from those radicular arteries that supply only the nerve roots.

The *anterior spinal artery* lies within the pia and runs the entire length of the spinal cord in the midline. It usually originates in the upper cervical region at the junction of the two *anterior spinal branches* that arise from the intracranial portion of the vertebral artery. Six to ten feeders—the *anterior radiculomedullary arteries*—contribute to it throughout its length, branching upward and downward. Occasionally, in the thoracic region, the anterior spinal artery narrows to such a degree that it is discontinuous. Blood from the anterior spinal artery is distributed to the anterior two-thirds of the substance of the spinal cord via *central* (or *sulcocommissural*) *branches* and *penetrating* branches from the *pial plexus*.

The *cervical* and *first two thoracic segments of the spinal cord* are supplied by radiculomedullary arteries that arise from branches of the *subclavian artery*. Variation is common, and the branches may arise from either the right or the left (often alternately) to join the anterior spinal artery at an angle of 60 degrees to 80 degrees. Not uncommonly, one anterior radiculomedullary branch arises from the vertebral artery and accompanies the C3 nerve root, one branch arises from one of the branches of the costocervical trunk (often the deep cervical artery) and accompanies the C6 root, and one branch arises from the superior intercostal artery and accompanies the C8 root.

The *midthoracic region of the spinal cord* (T3 to T7) usually receives only one radiculomedullary artery,

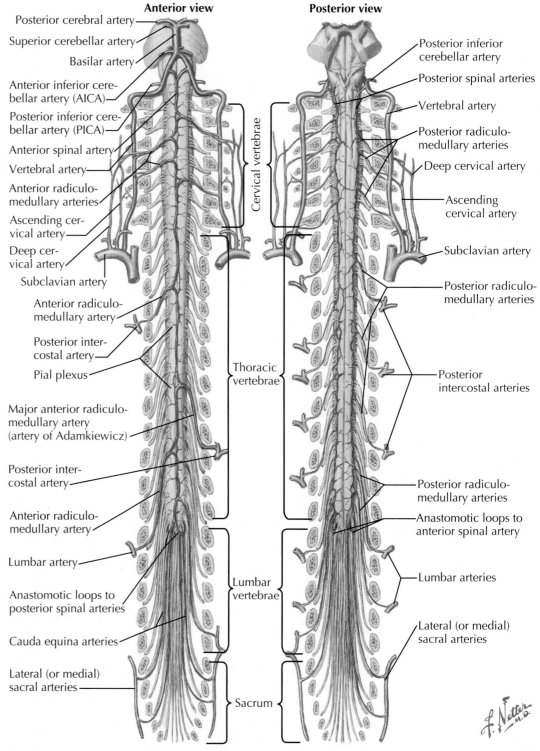

ARTERIES OF SPINAL CORD

Anterior view

Posterior cerebral artery
Superior cerebellar artery
Basilar artery
Anterior inferior cerebellar artery (AICA)
Posterior inferior cerebellar artery (PICA)
Anterior spinal artery
Vertebral artery
Anterior radiculomedullary arteries
Ascending cervical artery
Deep cervical artery
Subclavian artery
Anterior radiculomedullary artery
Posterior intercostal artery
Pial plexus
Major anterior radiculomedullary artery (artery of Adamkiewicz)
Posterior intercostal artery
Anterior radiculomedullary artery
Lumbar artery
Anastomotic loops to posterior spinal arteries
Cauda equina arteries
Lateral (or medial) sacral arteries

Cervical vertebrae
Thoracic vertebrae
Lumbar vertebrae
Sacrum

Posterior view

Posterior inferior cerebellar artery
Posterior spinal arteries
Vertebral artery
Posterior radiculomedullary arteries
Deep cervical artery
Ascending cervical artery
Subclavian artery
Posterior radiculomedullary arteries
Posterior intercostal arteries
Posterior radiculomedullary arteries
Anastomotic loops to anterior spinal artery
Lumbar arteries
Lateral (or medial) sacral arteries

Note: All spinal nerve roots have associated **radicular** or **segmental radiculomedullary arteries**. Most roots have radicular arteries. Both types of arteries run along roots, but radicular arteries end before reaching the anterior or posterior spinal arteries; the larger radiculomedullary arteries continue on to supply a segment of these arteries.

which accompanies the T4 or T5 nerve root. Consequently, this section of the cord is characterized by its poor blood supply, and the anterior spinal artery may not be continuous at this level.

The *thoracolumbosacral part of the spinal cord* (T8 to the conus medullaris) derives its main arterial supply from the artery of Adamkiewicz, which arises from a left *intercostal* (or *lumbar*) *artery* in 80% of individuals. In 85% of instances, it reaches the cord with a nerve

root between T9 and L2; in the 15% of cases in which it reaches the cord between T5 and T8, it is supplemented by a radiculomedullary artery (the artery of the conus medullaris) arising more inferiorly. The *artery of Adamkiewicz* has a large anterior and a smaller posterior branch. On reaching the anterior aspect of the spinal cord, the *anterior branch* ascends a short distance and then makes a hairpin turn to give off a small ascending branch and a larger descending branch, which drops to

Plate 2.4

Spinal Cord: Anatomy and Myelopathies

ARTERIES OF SPINAL CORD: INTRINSIC DISTRIBUTION

- Posterior spinal arteries
- Anterior spinal artery
- Anterior radiculomedullary artery
- Posterior radiculomedullary arteries
- Branch to vertebral body and dura mater
- Spinal branch
- Posterior branch of posterior intercostal artery
- Posterior intercostal artery
- Paravertebral anastomoses
- Prevertebral anastomoses
- Thoracic (descending) aorta

Section through thoracic level: anterosuperior view

- Sulcal (central) branches to right side of spinal cord
- Right posterior spinal artery
- Peripheral branches from pial plexus
- Posterior radiculomedullary artery
- Sulcal (central) branches to left side of spinal cord
- Anterior radiculomedullary artery
- Left posterior spinal artery
- Pial arterial plexus
- Anterior and posterior radicular arteries
- Posterior radiculomedullary artery
- Anterior spinal artery
- Anterior radiculomedullary artery
- Pial arterial plexus

Arterial distribution

Although the anterior and posterior radiculomedullary arteries may contribute to their respective longitudinal spinal arteries at the same segmental level (as shown here for simplicity), this is usually not the case.

ARTERIES OF SPINAL CORD AND NERVE ROOTS (Continued)

the level of the conus medullaris, where it forms an anastomotic circle with the terminal branches of the two posterior spinal arteries.

The *cauda equina* is accompanied and supplied by one or two branches from the *lumbar, iliolumbar,* and *lateral* and *median sacral arteries.* These branches also ascend to contribute to the anastomotic arterial circle around the conus medullaris.

The *central (sulcocommissural) branches* of the anterior spinal artery pass back into the anterior median fissure to supply the central parts of the spinal cord. At the anterior commissure, the branches turn alternately right and left to supply the corresponding halves of the cord, except in the lumbar enlargement, where the left and right branches arise from a common trunk. The terminal branches ascend and descend within the cord, supplying overlapping territories. There are 5 to 8 central arteries for each centimeter length of the spinal cord in the cervical region, 2 to 6 in the thoracic region, and 5 to 12 in the lumbosacral area. Branches from each central artery overlap with those from adjacent arteries. The central arteries supply the anterior commissure and adjacent white matter of the anterior columns, anterior horns, bases of the posterior horns, Clarke's columns, corticospinal tracts, spinothalamic tracts, anterior parts of the gracile and cuneate fasciculi, and the region around the central canal.

The *posterior spinal arteries* are paired arteries coursing on the posterolateral aspects of the entire length of the spinal cord, although they may become discontinuous at times. Each originates from the intracranial portion of the corresponding *vertebral artery* and receives contributions from 10 to 23 *posterior radiculomedullary arteries.* The posterior spinal arteries distribute blood to the posterior third of their respective sides of the cord.

In the cervicothoracic region, the posterior spinal arteries receive one, and sometimes two, tributaries at each segment. Between the T4 and T8 levels there are usually two or three posterior radiculomedullary branches, whereas in the thoracolumbar region there are several feeders, one of which may be the posterior radicular branch of the artery of Adamkiewicz.

PIAL ARTERIAL PLEXUS

Small pial branches arise from the spinal arteries and ramify and interconnect on the surface of the cord to form a *pial plexus. Penetrating branches* of the plexus are radially oriented to supply the outer part of the substance of the cord; they follow the principal sulci of the cord (the posterior median sulcus and the posterior intermedian sulcus) to reach the anterior and posterior horns. The peripheral pial branches supply the outer portions of the posterior horns, most of the posterior columns, and the outer portion of the white matter of the periphery of the spinal cord.

There is some degree of overlap in the distribution of the peripheral and central arteries at the capillary level, but they do not anastomose at the arterial level, and hence both types are, in effect, *end arteries.*

VEINS OF SPINAL CORD, NERVE ROOTS, AND VERTEBRAE

Two plexuses of veins, external and internal, extend along the entire length of the vertebral column and form a series of moderately distinct rings around each vertebra. The plexuses anastomose freely with each other; receive tributaries from the vertebrae, ligaments, and spinal cord; and are relatively devoid of valves. Consequently, changes in the intrathoracic or CSF pressure may produce variations in the volume of blood, especially in the internal vertebral venous plexuses.

The *external vertebral plexus* consists of anterior and posterior parts, which anastomose freely. The veins forming the *anterior external plexus* lie in front of the vertebral bodies, from which they receive venous tributaries and through which they communicate with the basivertebral veins. The *posterior external plexus* is a network located over the vertebral laminae and extending around the spinous, transverse, and articular processes. In the upper cervical region, the posterior plexus communicates with the occipital veins and, via these, with the mastoid and occipital emissary veins. The posterior plexus also communicates with the vertebral and deep cervical veins, and a few channels pass through the foramen magnum to the dural sinuses in the posterior cranial fossa.

The *internal vertebral plexus* is formed by networks of veins lying in the epidural space within the vertebral canal. The networks are arranged in anterior and posterior groups, which are interconnected by many smaller oblique and transverse channels. The *anterior internal plexus* consists of longitudinal veins lying on the posterior surfaces of the vertebral bodies and intervertebral disks found on each side of the posterior longitudinal ligament. Interconnecting branches lie between the ligament and the vertebral bodies and receive the basivertebral veins. The longitudinal veins in the *posterior internal plexus* are smaller than their anterior counterparts. They are located on each side of the median plane in front of the vertebral arches and ligamenta flava. They anastomose with the veins of the posterior external vertebral plexus via small veins that pierce the ligaments and pass between them.

The *basivertebral veins* resemble the cranial diploë and tunnel through the cancellous tissue of the vertebral bodies. They converge to form a comparatively large, single (occasionally double) vein that emerges through the posterior surface of the vertebral body to end, via openings guarded by valves, in the transverse interconnections of the anterior internal vertebral plexus. The basivertebral veins also drain into the anterior external plexus through openings in the front and sides of the vertebral body.

The *veins of the spinal cord* resemble the related arteries in their distribution and form a tortuous plexus in the pia mater. Intrinsic veins from the anteromedial region of the spinal cord and radial veins from the anterior funiculus drain into the *anterior median spinal (longitudinal) vein*, sometimes duplicated. Capillaries and venules from the rest of the spinal cord drain by radial veins into the *coronal veins* on the posterior and lateral surface of the spinal cord. These superficial veins drain, in turn, by the *anterior* and *posterior medullary veins*, sometimes called radicular veins, which accompany the nerve roots and radicular or radiculomedullary arteries. The medullary veins unite with radicular veins draining the nerve roots and with branches from the anterior and posterior internal vertebral plexuses to form the *intervertebral veins*. Above, the spinal veins communicate with veins draining the medulla oblongata and the inferior surface of the cerebellum through the foramen magnum.

The *intervertebral veins* drain most of the blood from the spinal cord and from the internal and external vertebral venous plexuses. They accompany the spinal nerves through the intervertebral foramina and end in the vertebral, posterior intercostal, subcostal, lumbar, and lateral sacral veins. Their orifices are usually protected by valves.

External vertebral venous plexus

Internal vertebral (epidural) venous plexus (Batson's veins)

Basivertebral vein

Internal vertebral (epidural) venous plexus

Intervertebral vein

External vertebral venous plexus

External vertebral venous plexus

Segmental medullary/radicular veins

Basivertebral vein

Internal vertebral (epidural) venous plexus

Intervertebral vein

Internal vertebral (epidural) venous plexus

External vertebral venous plexus

Anterior median spinal vein

Basivertebral vein

Anterior sulcal (central) vein

Internal vertebral (epidural) venous plexus

Anterior segmental medullary/radicular vein

Intervertebral vein

Posterior segmental medullary/radicular vein

Pial venous plexus

Posterior sulcal (central) vein

Posterior coronal spinal vein

Internal vertebral (epidural) venous plexus

Plate 2.6

Spinal Cord: Anatomy and Myelopathies

Sections through spinal cord at various levels

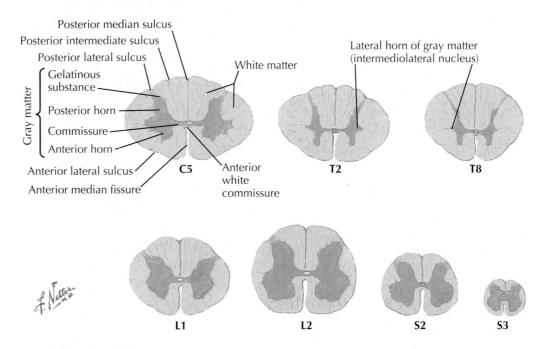

Principal fiber tracts of spinal cord

▬ **Ascending pathways**
▬ **Descending pathways**
▬ **Fibers passing in both directions**

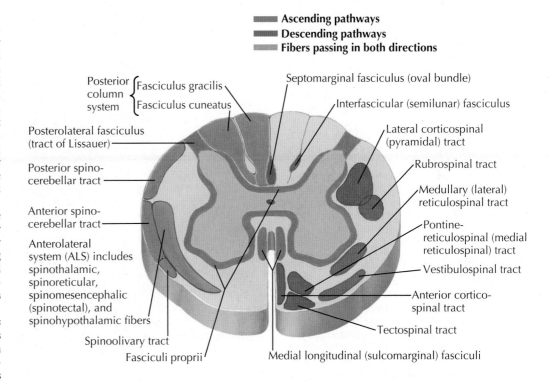

PRINCIPAL FIBER TRACTS OF SPINAL CORD

The spinal cord consists of a core of *gray matter,* surrounded by an outer fiber layer, the *white matter.* The gray matter consists of the cell bodies and dendrites of spinal neurons and the axons and axon terminals issuing from them or ending upon them (see Section 1, Normal and Abnormal Development, in Part I). The white matter consists of the axons of longitudinally running fiber tracts. The outlines of the gray and white matter are different at different spinal levels. The white matter is relatively massive in the cervical region and declines progressively in bulk in the lower levels. The gray matter is most highly developed in the cervical and lumbar enlargements, where it is made up of the neurons involved in the sensory and motor functions of the arms and the legs.

The schematic cross section in the lower part of the illustration shows the location of the principal fiber tracts within the spinal white matter. As indicated by the colors, the tracts can be divided into ascending (blue) and descending (red) pathways linking the spinal cord with the brain, and propriospinal (purple) pathways made up of fibers interconnecting different levels within the spinal cord itself.

The *ascending pathways* include the *fasciculus gracilis* and *fasciculus cuneatus* (part of the medial lemniscus system), which convey fine discriminative sensation from the lower and upper parts of the body, respectively. Less discriminative, higher-threshold sensations are carried by the *anterior* and *lateral spinothalamic tracts;* the latter is particularly important in conveying the sensations of pain, itch, and temperature. Other ascending pathways, which are more closely involved in reflex activity and motor control, include the *posterior* and *anterior spinocerebellar tracts* and the *spino-olivary, spinotectal,* and *spinoreticular tracts.*

The *descending pathways* are divided into two groups. The first group includes the *corticospinal tracts* and the *rubrospinal tract.* It terminates preferentially in the posterolateral regions of the spinal cord, which contain the neurons controlling the distal muscles of the limbs. Damage to these pathways results in loss of fine-fractionated

control of the extremities. The second group includes the *medial* and *lateral reticulospinal tracts* (RSTs), the *tectospinal tract,* the *lateral* and *medial vestibulospinal tracts,* and the *interstitiospinal tract* (from the interstitial nucleus of Cajal and pretectal area) that runs in the medial longitudinal fasciculus and terminates preferentially in the anteromedial regions of the spinal cord. These regions contain the neurons controlling axial and proximal limb muscles and regulate posture and righting. In addition to their motor action, both sets of descending pathways also include fibers that modulate sensory transmission by spinal pathways.

PROPRIOSPINAL PATHWAYS

Some of the propriospinal pathways consist of afferent fibers, which enter the spinal cord via the posterior roots and then ascend or descend in the *oval bundle, comma tract, posterolateral fasciculus* (of Lissauer), *fasciculus gracilis,* or *fasciculus cuneatus* to terminate on spinal neurons at other levels of the spinal cord. Other propriospinal fibers originate from interneurons in the spinal gray matter itself. Collectively, propriospinal fibers are important in mediating spinal reflexes and coordinating activity at different levels of the spinal cord.

SOMESTHETIC SYSTEM OF BODY

Neural pathways conveying somatosensory information to the cerebral cortex can be divided into two major systems: posterior and anterolateral. The posterior pathways are involved in mediating fine tactile and kinesthetic sensations, whereas the anterolateral pathways conduct impulses for pain and temperature and for touch and deep pressure.

The *posterior funiculus*, made up of the *fasciculus gracilis* and the *fasciculus cuneatus*, carries fibers that signal discriminative touch or pressure, muscle length and tension, and joint position. Some afferent fibers, principally those from quickly adapting cutaneous receptors, ascend the entire length of the spinal cord to synapse directly with neurons in the *gracile* and *cuneate nuclei*, which relate to the lower and upper parts of the body. Other fibers leave the posterior columns and either activate spinal neurons for reflex purposes or project upward in the posterolateral funiculus. In humans, most of these secondary ascending fibers also end in the gracile or cuneate nuclei, although a small number of axons sometimes terminate in the upper cervical segments. All of the above nuclei send their axons via the *medial lemniscus* to the contralateral *ventral posterolateral (VPL) nucleus* of the thalamus, which projects to the *somatosensory regions* of the cerebral cortex.

The relay neurons in the gracile, cuneate, and VPL nuclei and the neurons of the primary somatosensory cortex are activated by a single sensory modality over a restricted receptive field. The receptive fields of neurons within each nucleus are arranged in an orderly fashion and give rise to a somatotopic representation of the body surface. Thus a high degree of specificity and order is maintained throughout the pathway.

ANTEROLATERAL FUNICULUS

Two somatosensory pathways ascend in the anterolateral spinal white matter: the lateral and anterior spinothalamic tracts and the smaller spinoreticulothalamic pathway. The *spinothalamic tracts* arise from neurons in the regions of the posterior horn of the spinal cord that correspond to laminae I, IV, V, and VI of Rexed (see Plate 2.13). Most axons cross in the anterior white commissure at about the level of their cell bodies and ascend in the contralateral lateral and anterior funiculi, although a few fibers ascend ipsilaterally. The spinothalamic axons end principally in the *VPL nucleus* and in the *posterior nuclear group* and *intralaminar nuclei*. Some spinothalamic neurons (especially those in lamina I) respond only to strong, noxious stimuli, but most of these neurons are excited by the activity of a wide variety of afferent fibers related to touch, pressure, vibration, and temperature sense. All spinothalamic neurons have large, unilateral receptive fields and transmit information about a wide variety of peripheral stimuli but with less specificity than is shown by neurons in the posterior spinal pathways.

The *spinoreticulothalamic pathway* (not shown) begins with neurons in the regions corresponding to laminae I and V to VIII, which ascend in the lateral and anterior funiculi to activate neurons in the *brainstem reticular formation*, which, in turn, project to the *intralaminar nuclei* of the thalamus. The spinoreticulothalamic neurons respond to the same stimuli as spinothalamic neurons but tend to have large, bilateral receptive fields. This fact, together with the nonspecific nature of the intralaminar nuclei, suggests that this pathway is involved with poorly localizable pain sensation and is more important in generalized arousal reactions than in discriminative processing of sensation.

LESIONS

Because the principal pathways of the posterior and anterolateral columns cross in the medulla and in the spinal cord, and because each pathway transmits specific modalities, damage from spinal cord lesions presents specific and characteristic deficits. *Posterior column destruction* results in ipsilateral loss of discriminatory touch and vibration sense, as well as loss of position sense below the level of the lesion. *Anterolateral column interruption* produces contralateral loss of pain and temperature sense accompanied by diminished touch sense below the lesion.

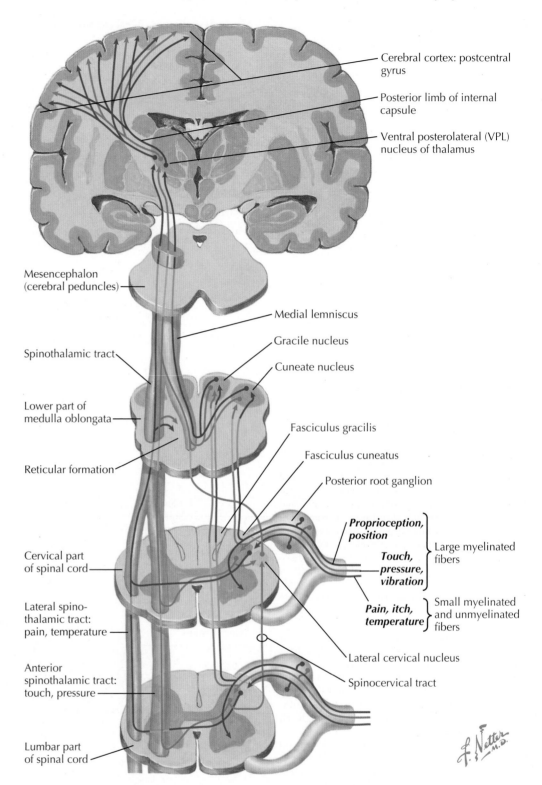

Cerebral cortex: postcentral gyrus

Posterior limb of internal capsule

Ventral posterolateral (VPL) nucleus of thalamus

Mesencephalon (cerebral peduncles)

Medial lemniscus

Spinothalamic tract

Gracile nucleus

Cuneate nucleus

Lower part of medulla oblongata

Fasciculus gracilis

Fasciculus cuneatus

Reticular formation

Posterior root ganglion

Proprioception, position

Large myelinated fibers

Touch, pressure, vibration

Cervical part of spinal cord

Pain, itch, temperature

Small myelinated and unmyelinated fibers

Lateral spino-thalamic tract: pain, temperature

Lateral cervical nucleus

Anterior spinothalamic tract: touch, pressure

Spinocervical tract

Lumbar part of spinal cord

Plate 2.8

Spinal Cord: Anatomy and Myelopathies

CORTICOSPINAL (PYRAMIDAL) SYSTEM: MOTOR COMPONENT

The corticospinal tract arises from wide regions of the cerebral cortex including the motor, premotor, and cingulate motor regions and the postcentral somatosensory areas, and it is involved in multiple functions. It contributes to the control of somatosensory inputs and to motor activity. The motor component of the *corticospinal (pyramidal) tract* originates primarily in the cells of layer V in the primary motor cortex of the precentral gyrus (area 4) and projects to motor neurons and interneurons concerned with motor control throughout the CNS. Only the direct connections, by which cortical neurons excite motor neurons in the motor nuclei of the brainstem and spinal cord, are shown. Other illustrations show the projections of the motor cortex to the basal ganglia, thalamus, red nucleus (see Plate 2.9), reticular formation (see Plate 2.11), and intermediate spinal gray matter (see Plate 2.12).

The *direct motor component* of the pyramidal tract from the motor cortex to, particularly, arm and hand motor neurons is a late evolutionary feature present in dexterous primates and especially in humans. It runs from the precentral gyrus through the posterior limb of the internal capsule and into the midbrain, where it gives slips to the oculomotor, trochlear, and abducens nuclei. It then enters the pons, where it gives off fibers to the trigeminal motor and facial nuclei, which control the muscles of the face. From the pons, the tract continues through the medullary pyramids, giving off fibers to the nuclei of the ninth, tenth, eleventh, and twelfth cranial nerves. The major part of the remaining fibers in the tract then crosses to the opposite side of the brainstem at the *pyramidal decussation,* and the crossed fibers continue to all levels of the spinal cord as the *lateral corticospinal tract.* A smaller group of uncrossed fibers continues to the cervical spinal cord as the *anterior (direct) corticospinal tract.* The fibers end by synapsing with motor neurons in the anterior horn of the spinal cord (see Plate 2.13). The direct corticomotoneuronal input allows a rich repertoire of movements based on the activation of different outputs to hand and finger muscles, effectively bypassing more rigid spinal segmental networks.

The significant projection from the hand area of the primary sensory cortical representation (area 3b) is to the spinal posterior horn and completely avoids the anterior horn, whereas the opposite is true for the characteristic pattern of projections from the hand area of primary motor cortex, which avoid the dorsal horn, but terminate heavily in lamina VII and among the motor nuclei of lamina IX (see Plate 2.12).

The pyramidal tract exhibits a *somatotopic organization* throughout its course in the brain. The homunculus at the top of the illustration indicates the orderly topographic arrangement of areas within the precentral gyrus, from which muscles in various parts of the body can be activated. The area controlling the face lies most laterally, with the areas related to the hand, arm, trunk, and hip following, in order, toward the midline. The areas representing the leg continue downward along the medial aspect of the cortex. Within each area, movements involving distal muscles are represented posteriorly and proximal muscles anteriorly. The initial somatotopic organization at the cortex persists in the arrangement of fibers as they descend the brain, but recent work suggests in fact that there is little separation within the lateral corticospinal tract in the spinal cord and that incomplete spinal injury results in diffuse damage to the tract. The control of voluntary movements

probably relates, however, to distributed networks that are capable of modification rather than to discrete representations. There appears to be considerable plasticity of representations and cell properties in the primary motor cortex, probably related to the horizontal neuronal connections in the cortex. The primary motor cortex is not a simple static motor control structure but contains a dynamic substrate that participates in motor learning. The upper motor neurons show both convergence and divergence in relation to their target motor neuron pools.

Lesions of the motor cortex may produce discrete pareses, depending on the type and size of the lesion

and its somatotopic location. Irritative lesions of the cortex can lead to abnormal movements and ultimately to jacksonian seizures as the irritative focus spreads. Damage to the internal capsule produces contralateral paralysis, along with cranial nerve involvement.

In general, pyramidal tract disturbances produce an initial flaccid paralysis and areflexia, followed by spastic paralysis and hyperactive reflexes. Brainstem lesions cause paralysis contralateral to the lesion, accompanied by ipsilateral or contralateral cranial nerve deficits, depending on the level of the lesion. Spinal cord damage to the tract is usually accompanied by alterations in the autonomic and sensory systems.

Lateral aspect of cerebral cortex to show topographic projection of motor centers on precentral gyrus

Horizontal section through internal capsule to show location of principal pathways

Anterior aspect of brainstem showing decussation of pyramids

Rubrospinal Tract

The *red nucleus* (so-called because of its reddish color in the fresh brain) is situated in the ventral midbrain. It receives many fibers from the contralateral cerebellum and the ipsilateral cerebral cortex and, in turn, has a major projection to the spinal cord, the rubrospinal tract. Knowledge of the rubrospinal tract in humans is limited. It seems to arise predominantly from the large neurons of the caudal part of the red nucleus, is arranged somatotopically, and extends the entire length of the spinal cord, influencing alpha and gamma motor neurons. The predominant target of its action is the motor apparatus controlling the distal muscles of the contralateral limbs, although the tract also acts to inhibit the action of cutaneous and muscle afferent fibers on spinal neurons. Within the brainstem, fibers branch from the rubrospinal tract to terminate in the facial nucleus (control of facial muscles), the lateral reticular nucleus (cerebellar afferent relay), and the gracile and cuneate nuclei (control of afferent input) (see Plate 2.7). In addition to being the source of the rubrospinal tract, the red nucleus sends fibers to the ipsilateral inferior olive (cerebellar afferent relay) and medial reticular formation (see Plate 2.11).

As shown in the illustration, *rubrospinal fibers decussate* almost immediately on leaving the red nucleus to descend through the lateral part of the brainstem to the spinal cord. In the cord, the tract lies in the *posterolateral funiculus,* just anterior to the lateral corticospinal tract. The distal branches of the rubrospinal fibers terminate in the intermediate regions and anterior horn (laminae V, VI, and VII) of the spinal gray matter (see Plate 2.12).

The rubrospinal tract influences the motor neurons in the anterior horns, primarily through its action on inhibitory or excitatory interneurons, but in primates some fibers end directly on anterior horn motor neurons. The predominant pattern of rubrospinal action is to facilitate flexor motor neurons and thus excite limb flexor muscles and to inhibit the corresponding extensor muscles via interneurons. However, several rubrospinal fibers have the opposite action. This allows a wide variety of movements to be executed by the selective activation of appropriate groups of rubrospinal neurons. The rubrospinal tract may thus be responsible for much of the relatively fine control of the extremities—discriminative movement that is retained when the pyramidal tract is damaged. In animals, lesions involving both the pyramidal and rubrospinal tracts result in a much greater deficit in distal movement than that obtained from a lesion of either tract alone.

Rubrospinal control of *afferent input* to the spinal cord takes the form of presynaptic inhibition acting at the central posterior horn terminals of fibers from Golgi tendon organs and cutaneous receptors.

The two major sources of the input that controls the activity of rubrospinal neurons are the *cerebellum* and the *cerebral cortex.* The cerebellar projection to the red nucleus consists primarily of fibers from the interposed (emboliform and globose) nuclei, which cross in the

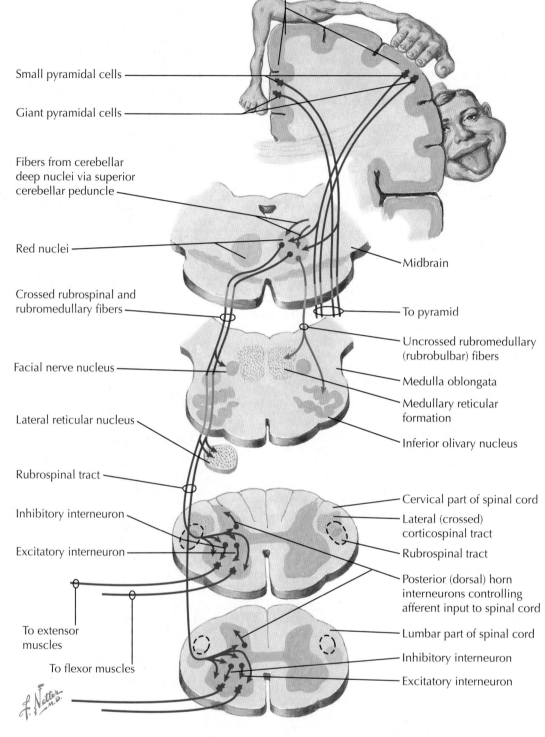

decussation of the superior cerebellar peduncle (brachium conjunctivum) to excite the red nucleus neurons of the opposite side. Neurons of the red nucleus are also excited by branches of small pyramidal cells from the ipsilateral motor cortex (see Plate 2.8). Afferents from the motor and premotor cerebral cortex synapse on their distal dendrites and from the cerebellum on their proximal dendrites and cell bodies. In addition, activity in pyramidal tract axons from giant neurons in the same cortical region exerts an opposite, inhibitory effect on rubrospinal neurons via inhibitory interneurons. The input and the output of the red nucleus are

somatotopically organized. Thus rubrospinal fibers projecting to the lumbar part of the spinal cord originate from neurons in the lateral part of the nucleus. This same region receives input from regions of the cerebellar deep nuclei and motor cortex related to control of the lower limbs. Conversely, the medial part of the red nucleus, which contains neurons projecting to cervical levels of the spinal cord, receives input from cerebellar and cerebral regions responsible for control of the arms. This pattern of organization allows for the selective activation of individual extremities by different groups of rubrospinal neurons.

Plate 2.10

Spinal Cord: Anatomy and Myelopathies

VESTIBULOSPINAL TRACTS

The vestibular system is involved in the control of balance. The *vestibular nuclei* consist of four major groups of neurons—the *superior, medial, lateral,* and *inferior vestibular nuclei*—situated in the posterolateral part of the pons and medulla oblongata. Three of these neuronal groups—the medial, lateral (Deiters), and inferior (descending) vestibular nuclei—make up the major central termination of the vestibular afferent fibers that supply the otolithic organs (utricle and saccule) of the labyrinth. Vestibular afferent fibers supplying the semicircular canals end primarily in the superior, medial, and lateral vestibular nuclei, but many fibers also terminate in the vestibulocerebellum. In addition to these vestibular afferent impulses, the vestibular nuclei also receive input from the spinal cord, cerebellum, reticular formation, and higher centers.

The known output pathways from the vestibular nuclei include projections to the spinal cord, oculomotor nuclei, cerebellum, and reticular formation. Vestibular activity also reaches the thalamus, superior colliculus, and other higher centers, but the exact pathways are not known.

Plate 2.10 shows the projections of vestibular neurons to the spinal cord via the *lateral vestibulospinal tract* (LVST) and *medial vestibulospinal tract* (MVST). These two tracts, which lie in the anterior and anteromedial funiculi (see Plate 2.12), act primarily on the motor apparatus that controls the proximal muscles and therefore are important in the regulation of postural equilibrium.

The LVST is uncrossed and originates primarily from the *lateral vestibular nucleus*. Some of its constituent fibers extend the entire length of the spinal cord, whereas others extend only part of this distance; they may branch to innervate several regions as they descend. The lateral nucleus is *somatotopically organized*: neurons projecting to the lower (hindlimb) levels of the spinal cord are in the posterior and distal portion of the nucleus, and neurons ending at higher levels are situated more anteriorly and rostrally. The former region receives a heavy projection from the cerebellar vermis, whereas the latter region receives a heavy input of vestibular afferent fibers. The LVST ends in lamina VIII and parts of lamina VII; it acts on alpha and gamma neurons.

The predominant action of the LVST is to produce the contraction of extensor (antigravity) muscles and the relaxation of flexor muscles. In the case of neck, trunk, and some lower limb extensor muscles, contraction is produced in part by direct (monosynaptic) excitation of motor neurons. The excitation of other limb extensor muscles and the inhibition of flexor

muscles are mediated by pathways that include spinal interneurons.

The MVST, which projects bilaterally to the cervical cord, is involved in reflex adjustments of the head and axial muscles to vestibular stimulation. It contains fibers that originate primarily in the *medial vestibular nucleus* and produce direct inhibition of motor neurons controlling neck and axial muscles. The tract seems to

stop in the midthoracic region. The two vestibulospinal tracts are important factors in *vestibular reflex reactions* that are triggered by the movement of the head in space. Particularly significant in this regard is the strong vestibular action on the neck muscles, which helps to stabilize the position of the head. However, these tracts and the RSTs (see Plate 2.11) also appear to play a much wider role in the control of the proximal musculature.

Excitatory endings → → → →
Inhibitory endings → →
Ascending fibers in medial longitudinal fasciculi

Superior
Medial
Lateral
Inferior } Vestibular nuclei

Somatotopic pattern in lateral vestibular nucleus

Rostral
Upper limb
Trunk
Anterior
Posterior
Lower limb
Caudal

To cerebellum

Vestibular ganglion and nerve

Motor neuron (controlling neck muscles)

Medial vestibulospinal fibers in medial longitudinal fasciculi

Excitatory endings to back muscles

Lower part of cervical spinal cord

Lateral vestibulospinal tract

Excitatory interneuron
Inhibitory interneuron

To flexor muscles
To extensor muscles

Inhibitory ending
To axial muscles
Excitatory ending
Lateral vestibulospinal tract

To axial muscles
Inhibitory ending

Lumbar part of spinal cord

Inhibitory interneuron
Excitatory synapse

To flexor muscles
To extensor muscles

Fibers from cristae (rotational stimuli)
Fibers from maculae (gravitational stimuli)

RETICULOSPINAL AND CORTICORETICULAR PATHWAYS

The reticulospinal pathways are important in controlling motor activity and in regulating the flow of afferent signals in the spinal cord. They consist of a series of descending fiber connections that originate in two regions of the brainstem and project to the spinal cord via two different *reticulospinal tracts* (RSTs). Both regions of origin are in the medial, magnocellular part of the brainstem reticular formation. The more rostral region is in the nucleus reticularis pontis caudalis and nucleus reticularis pontis oralis of the *pontine reticular formation;* the more caudal region is in the nucleus gigantocellularis, in the rostromedial part of the *medullary reticular formation.*

Pontine reticulospinal fibers project to the spinal cord via the medial RST only. This tract traverses the anterior funiculus ipsilaterally and extends along the entire length of the spinal cord, sending terminal branches to innervate the gray matter of the anterior horn (see Plate 2.12). It excites large numbers of spinal motor neurons of all types, especially flexor motor neurons and motor neurons controlling proximal (trunk and axial) muscles. The pontine system also has a strong, indirect influence on lumbar motor neurons, relayed by spinal interneurons (see bottom of illustration).

The *medullary reticulospinal system* has a more complex pattern of projection. Most fibers originating from the gigantocellular nucleus project to the spinal cord via the *ipsilateral lateral RST,* which is part of the lateral anterolateral funiculus. In addition, some medullary reticular neurons project via the *contralateral lateral RST,* and some join the *medial RST.* Within the spinal gray matter, terminations of medullary reticulospinal fibers cover an exceptionally wide area, encompassing most of the anterior horn and the basal portion of the posterior horn (see Plate 2.12).

The physiologic action of the medullary reticulospinal system on spinal motor neurons is twofold and quite complex. Stimulation of the *rostral part* of the *gigantocellular nucleus* produces *excitation* of motor neurons, whereas stimulation of its *caudal-anterior part* produces *inhibition.* Actions on axial motor neurons are mediated by direct connections, whereas those on limb motor neurons are relayed by spinal interneurons. Stimulation in the caudal-anterior area also produces inhibition of spinal interneurons and inhibition of afferent transmission to the spinal cord. The exact pathways are unknown but appear to involve reticulospinal fibers descending in the posterolateral funiculus (not shown in illustration).

Reticulospinal fibers are involved in the control of certain voluntary and reflex movements, the integration of sensory input to guide motor output, and the coordination of bilateral movements. They can influence both diffuse motor activity and more focused goal-directed movements. The RSTs include descending autonomic fibers that terminate on sympathetic and parasympathetic preganglionic neurons and allow the hypothalamus to influence the autonomic outflow.

Input to the *medial brainstem reticular formation* originates from many sources. Most major sensory systems send collateral branches to one of its regions, and the most pronounced sensory input to the source of reticulospinal fibers comes from the cutaneous and high-threshold muscle receptors of the body. Physiologic studies demonstrate that the great majority of both pontine and medullary reticulospinal neurons receive strong excitatory input from structures involved in

motor control, including the motor or premotor cerebral cortex, themselves a part of an extensive corticoreticular system originating from all parts of the cortex, the cerebellar fastigial nucleus, and the superior colliculus. The resulting *corticoreticulospinal connections* constitute an extrapyramidal pathway by which motor regions of the cortex can act on the spinal motor apparatus. This descending motor pathway reorganizes after corticospinal tract injury in animals. This may involve locally rewired and compensatory plasticity of reticulospinal axons. In

humans, its role in normal motor function and recovery is uncertain, but there are stronger connections to the hand than arm in healthy subjects, and the reverse in stroke subjects. The physiologic role of the projections from sensory regions of the cerebral cortex to reticulospinal neurons is even less certain, but such pathways may be involved in the regulation of sensory input to the spinal cord through reticular-evoked presynaptic inhibition of spinal afferent fibers or through postsynaptic inhibition of spinal sensory interneurons.

Reticulospinal and Corticoreticular Pathways

Thickness of blue line indicates density of cortical projection

Excitatory endings

Inhibitory endings

Parietal
Frontal
Orbito-frontal

6 4 3, 1, 2

Occipital
Temporal

Medial pontine reticular formation

Pons

Receives input from multiple sensory systems via lateral reticular formation

Medial medullary reticular formation

Medulla oblongata

Lateral reticulospinal tract (partially crossed); excites and inhibits axial (neck and back) motor neurons and modulates afferent input to spinal cord

Motor neurons (alpha and gamma)

Trigeminal motor nucleus

Receive excitatory fibers from pontine, inhibitory fibers from medullary reticular formation

Facial nerve nucleus

Exerts strong drive over medullary reticulospinal tract

Medial (anterior) reticulospinal tract; produces direct excitation of motor neurons

Cervical part of spinal cord

Posterior (dorsal) horn interneurons regulating sensory input to spinal cord

Excitatory interneuron

Inhibitory interneuron

Lumbar part of spinal cord

Plate 2.12

Spinal Cord: Anatomy and Myelopathies

SPINAL ORIGIN OR TERMINATION OF MAJOR DESCENDING TRACTS AND ASCENDING PATHWAYS

The spinal neurons receive input from, and send projections to, many parts of the brain (see Plate 2.6). The sections illustrated show the regions of the spinal gray matter, within which axons of the four major descending pathways terminate, and the locations within the spinal gray matter of neurons that project to the thalamus and cerebellum (see Plate 2.13).

The *descending pathways* shown in parts A, B, C, and D have a variety of actions on spinal circuitry, including the modulation of somatosensory input and the production of motor output. Actions on the sensory apparatus are typically mediated by descending fibers that terminate upon neurons in the posterior horn (laminae I to VI) of the spinal cord. As shown in part A, the specific spinal projections from the somatosensory cortex concerned with sensory control end almost entirely in the posterior horn. Some projections from the brainstem reticular formation, which also has a strong action on the sensory apparatus, also terminate in the posterior horn (part C). Conversely, the vestibulospinal tracts (part D), which have only a weak action on sensory processes, have relatively few terminals in the posterior horn. The rubrospinal tract (part B), which has some inhibitory effect on spinal afferents, terminates in intermediate regions and in the rostral part of the anterior (ventral) horn.

The projections from the brain to the spinal cord have been divided into lateral and medial systems. The *lateral descending systems* include the lateral (crossed) corticospinal tract fibers originating in the motor cortex (part A) and the rubrospinal tract (part B) (see Plates 2.8 and 2.9). These tracts terminate predominantly in the lateral parts of laminae V, VI, VII, and IX, which are concerned with the control of the *distal musculature* of the limbs.

The *medial descending systems* include the RSTs (part C) and vestibulospinal tracts (part D) (see Plates 2.10 and 2.11). These tracts end most heavily in laminae VIII and IX_M, which are involved in controlling neck and trunk muscles. Endings are also present in the medial parts of laminae VI, VII, and IX, which control the proximal muscles of the limbs. Thus the medial systems act predominantly upon *axial* and *proximal muscles*. The functional role of the *anterior (direct) corticospinal tract* is uncertain, although its endings in lamina VIII suggest that it may be involved in the cortical control of axial muscles.

CONNECTIONS TO ASCENDING PATHWAYS

Ascending projections from the spinal cord to the brain arise from many parts of the spinal gray matter. In general, however, projections to sensory structures tend to originate in the posterior horn, which is the receiving area for somatosensory input arriving via the posterior roots. The illustration shows the *anterior* and *lateral* divisions of the *spinothalamic tract,* which are continuous with each other. One division originates primarily from neurons in lamina I, which respond chiefly to painful stimuli; the other originates from neurons located mainly in laminae IV to VI, which receive information related to a variety of somatosensory stimuli. Lamina IV also gives rise to projections to other sensory areas, such as the cuneate, gracile, and lateral cervical nuclei. Laminae V to VIII give origin to the spinoreticular tract.

Termination of major descending tracts

A. Corticospinal tracts

Right side of cord — Left side of cord

Lateral (crossed) corticospinal tract
Anterior (direct) corticospinal tract

⠿ Fibers from left motor cortex
⠿ Fibers from left sensory cortex

B. Rubrospinal tracts

Right side of cord — Left side of cord

Right rubrospinal tract

⠿ Fibers from left red nucleus

F. Netter M.D.

C. Reticulospinal tracts

Lateral reticulospinal tract   Medial reticulospinal tract

⠿ Fibers from left pontine reticular formation
⠿ Fibers from left medullary reticular formation

D. Vestibulospinal tracts

Medial vestibulospinal fibers in medial longitudinal fasciculus
Lateral vestibulospinal tract

⠿ Fibers from left lateral (Deiters) nucleus
⠿ Fibers from left medial and inferior nuclei (only to cervical and thoracic levels)

Afferent connections to ascending pathways

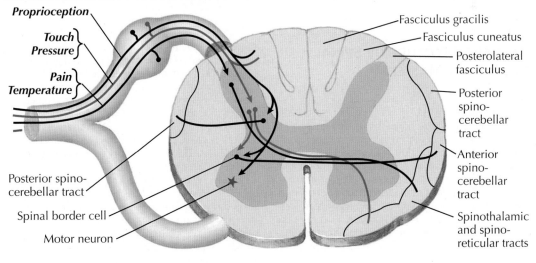

Proprioception
Touch / Pressure
Pain / Temperature

Fasciculus gracilis
Fasciculus cuneatus
Posterolateral fasciculus
Posterior spinocerebellar tract
Anterior spinocerebellar tract
Spinothalamic and spino-reticular tracts

Posterior spinocerebellar tract
Spinal border cell
Motor neuron

Ascending projections to areas involved in motor control tend to arise from laminae VI to IX, which are related to motor movements. The illustration shows two ascending pathways related to motor activity, both of which terminate in the cerebellum. The *posterior spinocerebellar tract* originates from Clarke's column, a group of neurons located in lamina VI, and ascends in the ipsilateral posterolateral funiculus. The *anterior spinocerebellar tract* originates from spinal border cells at the edge of lamina VII and ascends via the contralateral anterolateral funiculus. As shown, neurons projecting in both tracts receive input from muscle proprioceptors; some also receive indirect cutaneous input. In addition to neurons projecting to the cerebellum, the anterior horn also contains neurons projecting to other structures related to motor control, such as the inferior olive and the reticular formation.

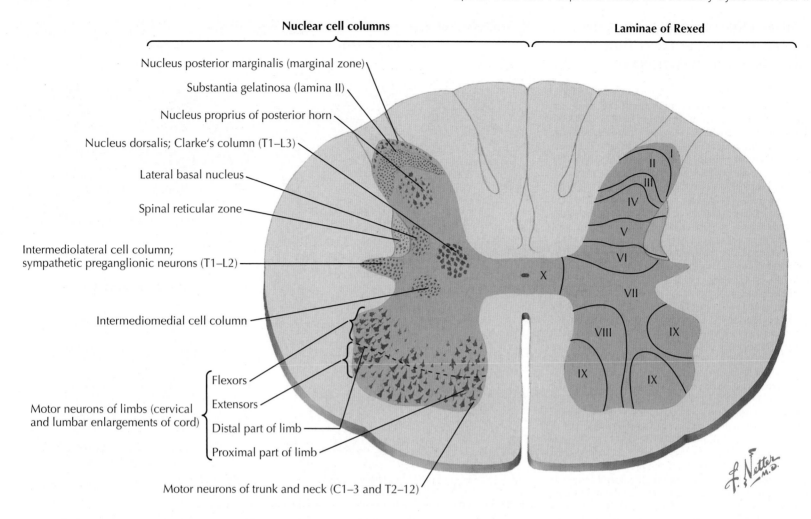

Nuclear cell columns   **Laminae of Rexed**

Nucleus posterior marginalis (marginal zone)

Substantia gelatinosa (lamina II)

Nucleus proprius of posterior horn

Nucleus dorsalis; Clarke's column (T1–L3)

Lateral basal nucleus

Spinal reticular zone

Intermediolateral cell column;
sympathetic preganglionic neurons (T1–L2)

Intermediomedial cell column

Flexors

Extensors

Motor neurons of limbs (cervical
and lumbar enlargements of cord)

Distal part of limb

Proximal part of limb

Motor neurons of trunk and neck (C1–3 and T2–12)

Cytoarchitecture of Spinal Cord Gray Matter

The gray matter of the spinal cord can be broadly divided into a *posterior (dorsal) horn* and an *anterior (ventral) horn,* which are further subdivided according to the size and structure of their component neuronal cell bodies. The left side of the illustration shows some of the clearly recognizable groups of neurons; the right side shows a more systematic subdivision of the spinal gray matter into 10 laminae, which were originally described by Rexed in the spinal cord of the cat but which are useful in discussing human functional neuroanatomy.

POSTERIOR HORN

Many neurons in the six laminae of the posterior horn receive direct synaptic input from spinal afferent fibers that enter the spinal cord via the posterior roots and are thus involved in sensation and in the generation of reflex responses to external or proprioceptive signals (see Plate 2.12).

Lamina I of the posterior horn is a thin layer of large cells, which gives origin to the pathway relaying information about painful stimuli to the thalamus. *Laminae II and III* make up the *substantia gelatinosa,* a tightly packed mass of tiny neurons believed to play a role in regulating afferent input to the spinal cord. *Lamina IV* is a collection of larger neurons (sometimes referred to as the *nucleus proprius of the posterior horn)* that projects to three sensory structures: the lateral cervical nucleus, the posterior column nuclei, and the thalamus. Thus the connections of laminae I to IV indicate their importance in sensation.

Laminae V and VI contain neurons of medium to large size, many of which receive input from afferent fibers carrying proprioceptive information, as well as other sensory information also relayed by neurons in lamina IV. These neurons probably represent an intermediate stage in the transformation of sensory input to motor output. Laminae V and VI are also the sites of origin of ascending projections to higher centers. In spinal segments T1 to L3, lamina VI contains a group of large cells known as *Clarke's column,* which projects to the cerebellum via the posterior spinocerebellar tract.

The *anterior horn* contains the cell bodies of the motor neurons supplying the somatic muscles. These cell bodies are clustered into two distinct groups, referred to by Rexed as lamina IX and IX$_M$. Lamina IX$_M$ contains the motor neurons supplying the muscles of the trunk and neck, whereas lamina IX contains motor neurons supplying the limbs. Lamina IX can be further divided into groups of motor neurons supplying flexor and extensor muscles in the proximal and distal parts of the limbs.

The anterior horn also contains *laminae VII and VIII.* These regions contain interneurons involved in reflex pathways and motor control, as well as neurons that project to motor regions of the brain. The neurons of lamina VIII are particularly related to lamina IX$_M$ and thus participate in movements of the muscles in the trunk and neck. Conversely, neurons of lamina VII are particularly related to lamina IX and therefore participate in movements of the limb muscles. Laminae VII and IX are both highly developed in the spinal enlargements that control the arms and the legs whereas only laminae VIII and IX$_M$ are found in the high cervical or thoracic segments that control the neck and trunk.

In the thoracic and sacral segments, the *intermediolateral cell column,* which is not considered part of either the posterior or the anterior horn, contains the neurons of origin of preganglionic autonomic fibers. *Lamina X,* the small area of gray matter around the central canal, contains neurons that project to the opposite side of the spinal cord, including those in the anterior and posterior commissural nuclei.

Plate 2.14

Spinal Cord: Anatomy and Myelopathies

SPINAL EFFECTOR MECHANISMS

The illustration shows a schematic representation of the structure of the spinal motor nuclei and their segmental connections.

MOTOR NEURONS

Except for muscles innervated by the cranial nerves, each somatic muscle receives its motor supply from a column of motor neurons arranged longitudinally in the anterior horn of the spinal cord. Motor neurons fall into three classes. The large *alpha motor neurons* supply the extrafusal fibers of the muscle, and each motor neuron may innervate several to more than 1000 fibers distributed throughout the muscle. A single motor neuron and all the muscle fibers that it innervates are called a *motor unit*. The small *gamma motor neurons* (fusimotor neurons) innervate the intrafusal muscles of the spindles, thus regulating proprioceptive feedback of information about muscle length. The intermediate-sized *beta motor neurons* project to both extrafusal and intrafusal muscle fibers; their activity causes contraction and adjusts length feedback to compensate for that contraction. The beta motor neurons are divided into dynamic and static, depending on the type of intrafusal muscle fibers that they innervate and their physiologic effects.

Motor nuclei may extend longitudinally over several segments of the spinal cord. Despite this, the nuclei supplying different muscles tend to be arranged in an orderly, somatotopic pattern (see Plate 2.13). In the upper cervical and the thoracic segments, which innervate only axial muscles, the anteromedial group is the only group of somatomotor neurons present; in the cervical and lumbar enlargements of the spinal cord (lower part of illustration), additional motor columns supplying limb muscles appear more laterally in the anterior horn. Moving from the rostral to the caudal end of the two enlargements, the motor nuclei supplying the proximal limb muscles appear first, lying adjacent to the anteromedial column. They are followed by the nuclei supplying the more distal muscles, which tend to lie more posteriorly and laterally. Nuclei supplying the extensor muscles also tend to lie anteriorly and laterally to those supplying the flexor muscles. Even the small movement of an extremity involves activity in the medial and lateral cell columns extending over several spinal cord segments.

PROPRIOCEPTIVE AND EXTEROCEPTIVE FIBERS

Motor neurons can be influenced by both the proprioceptive and the exteroceptive fibers that enter the spinal cord. Upon entering the spinal cord (upper part of illustration), these fibers may give off ascending and descending branches that send terminal branches into the posterior or anterior horn over several segments, which approximately match the extent of the corresponding motor nucleus. Further afferent fiber branches may continue rostrally to various sensory relay nuclei (see Plate 2.7).

The most numerous *proprioceptive fibers* are those carrying information from muscle spindles (groups Ia and II fibers), and from Golgi tendon organs (group Ib fibers). The Ia fibers are unique in that they enter the anterior horn motor nuclei and establish direct connections with motor neurons. These connections form

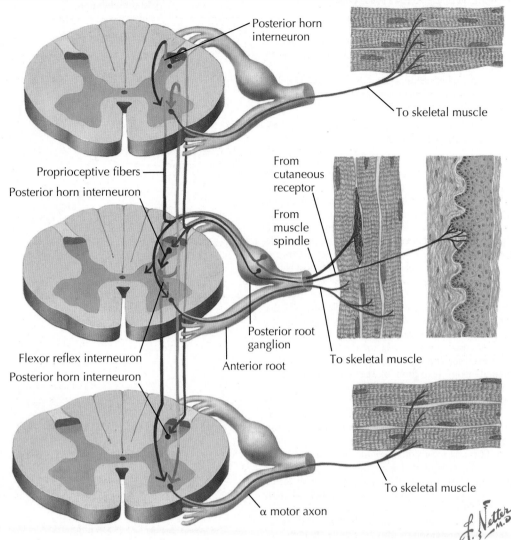

Spinal effector mechanisms

Posterior horn interneuron

To skeletal muscle

Proprioceptive fibers

Posterior horn interneuron

From cutaneous receptor

From muscle spindle

Flexor reflex interneuron

Posterior horn interneuron

Posterior root ganglion

Anterior root

To skeletal muscle

To skeletal muscle

α motor axon

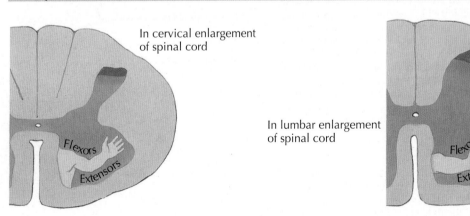

Representation of motor neurons

In cervical enlargement of spinal cord

Flexors

Extensors

In lumbar enlargement of spinal cord

Flexors

Extensors

the basis of the *muscle stretch reflex* (see Plate 2.15). One Ia afferent fiber from a spindle in a given muscle produces direct excitation in virtually every motor neuron supplying that muscle and in a smaller proportion of motor neurons supplying closely related synergistic muscles. This selectivity may be explained by the fact that the terminal field of the Ia fiber is approximately coextensive with the motor nucleus of its muscle and overlaps slightly with synergist motor nuclei located nearby.

The principal reflex elicited by *exteroceptive fibers* is the *flexor withdrawal reflex* (see Plate 2.15). The distribution of motor effects in this reflex is much broader than that of the stretch reflex, comprising most of the flexor muscles of the limb, as well as crossed activation of the contralateral extensor muscles. This distribution does not derive from the projection pattern of the afferent fibers, however, but rather from the divergent projection of chains of interneurons in the posterior and anterior horns that subserve the withdrawal reflex.

SPINAL REFLEX PATHWAYS

The intrinsic circuitry within the spinal cord influences the reflex activity of motor neurons. It is important to emphasize that these circuits are ordinarily under the control of higher centers (see Plates 2.8–2.11), but knowledge about them is an important step toward understanding motor behavior.

MUSCLE STRETCH REFLEX

Parts A and B show some of the connections made by groups Ia and II (not shown) afferent fibers from muscle spindle receptors. These afferent fibers are responsible for the muscle stretch reflex, in which the stretching of a muscle elicits a contraction of that muscle and its close synergists and a relaxation of its antagonists (see Plate 2.14). When the muscle is stretched, its spindle receptors are activated, thus causing increased firing of the spindle afferent fibers. The direct monosynaptic excitation of the motor neurons by these spindle afferent fibers contributes to the contraction of the stretched muscle and its synergists (part B). Relaxation of the antagonist muscles is produced by a disynaptic inhibitory pathway involving an interneuron. The stretching of an extensor muscle leads to a reflex contraction of the extensors acting at that particular joint and to a simultaneous relaxation of the antagonistic flexor muscles.

Excitation and inhibition of motor neurons (part B) are mediated by axosomatic or axodendritic synapses. Muscle spindle afferents, as well as other afferents, may also activate the circuits that modulate the action of afferent fibers by means of *presynaptic afferent inhibition* (part A). Here, Ia fibers from either the flexors or the extensors activate an inhibitory neuron, which forms an axoaxonic synapse with a muscle spindle afferent fiber that terminates on an extensor motor neuron. The action of these synapses blocks or decreases the excitation of a motor neuron by muscle spindle afferents.

Recurrent inhibition is another type of neural interaction that controls the activity of motor neurons (part C). It is produced by the collaterals of motor neurons that excite inhibitory interneurons known as Renshaw cells. When the motor neurons discharge, the Renshaw cells are activated by the motor neuron collaterals and fire a train of action potentials. The firing of the Renshaw cells causes inhibition of motor neurons of the same muscle and of other related, synergistic muscles. In addition to limiting the firing rate of motor neurons, this inhibition is also thought to restrict motor activity to the most intensely excited motor neurons.

TENDON ORGAN REFLEX

Reflex actions evoked by Ib afferent fibers from Golgi tendon organs are shown in part D. These fibers are activated by active (strong) tension in a muscle. When thus activated, the Ib fibers excite spinal interneurons, which inhibit the motor neurons that supply the particular muscle from which the Ib fibers originate and simultaneously excite the motor neurons that supply antagonist muscles. Thus the tendon organ reflex action is opposite to that produced by muscle spindle afferent fibers. The tendon organ reflex was once thought to play a role in protecting the muscles from excessive tension, but the excitatory influence of types Ia and II afferents during brief muscle contractions exceeds any inhibitory effects from the tendon organs. The tendon organ discharge may provide a "force feedback" signal

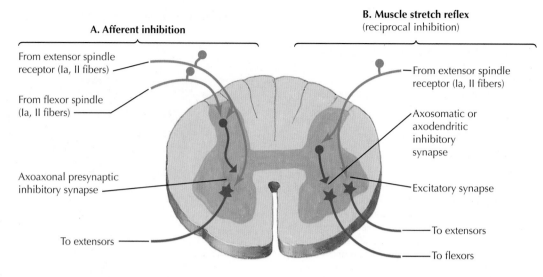

A. Afferent inhibition

From extensor spindle receptor (Ia, II fibers)

From flexor spindle (Ia, II fibers)

Axoaxonal presynaptic inhibitory synapse

To extensors

B. Muscle stretch reflex (reciprocal inhibition)

From extensor spindle receptor (Ia, II fibers)

Axosomatic or axodendritic inhibitory synapse

Excitatory synapse

To extensors

To flexors

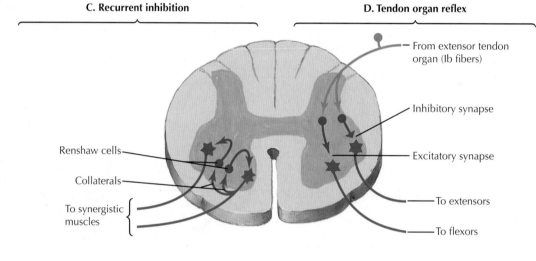

C. Recurrent inhibition

Renshaw cells

Collaterals

To synergistic muscles

D. Tendon organ reflex

From extensor tendon organ (Ib fibers)

Inhibitory synapse

Excitatory synapse

To extensors

To flexors

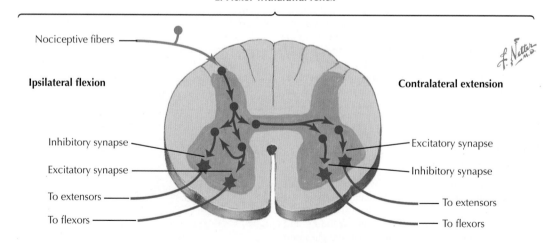

E. Flexor withdrawal reflex

Nociceptive fibers

Ipsilateral flexion

Inhibitory synapse

Excitatory synapse

To extensors

To flexors

Contralateral extension

Excitatory synapse

Inhibitory synapse

To extensors

To flexors

whose inhibitory action opposes the excitatory "length feedback" signal provided by muscle spindle afferents during periods when the muscle is actively generating tension.

FLEXOR WITHDRAWAL REFLEX

Complex pathways are involved in the familiar flexor withdrawal reflex evoked by a painful stimulus (part E). Such a stimulus activates nociceptive afferent fibers, which produce the firing of chains of neurons in the posterior horn of the spinal cord. These neurons, in turn, activate the interneurons in the anterior horn that excite flexor motor neurons and inhibit extensor motor neurons on the side of the painful stimulus. At the same time, commissural neurons activate circuits that excite extensor motor neurons and inhibit flexor motor neurons on the opposite side. The resulting reflex response is flexion or withdrawal of the stimulated limb and extension of the opposite limb.

Plate 2.16

Spinal Cord: Anatomy and Myelopathies

SPINAL CORD DYSFUNCTION

A spinal cord lesion should be considered in any patient with numbness or weakness of one or more extremities, particularly if there is pain in the neck or back and sphincter dysfunction. Various combinations of symptoms and signs point to (1) extradural extramedullary, (2) intradural extramedullary, or (3) intradural intramedullary spinal cord lesions. *Spinal trauma* (see Section 3) may lead to neurologic dysfunction, depending on whether the spinal cord has been affected (for example, by compression, contusion, transection, hemorrhage, or shear injury) and on the site and extent of spinal cord involvement.

MOTOR IMPAIRMENT

The degree of motor dysfunction depends on the extent of the spinal cord lesion. *Complete lesions* destroy all function below the affected level. *Incomplete lesions* cause partial weakness, atrophy, and hyporeflexia at the affected level, usually in combination with a distal upper motor neuron lesion, which may predominate and cause weakness, spasticity, and hyperreflexia. A search for subtle signs of a distal upper motor neuron lesion is imperative in any patient with an apparently isolated spinal nerve root lesion, particularly in the cervical region.

In contrast to a complete peripheral nerve lesion, in which motor function is completely lost in the distribution of that nerve, a complete nerve root lesion typically causes weakness (paresis), sometimes severe, but not total paralysis of the various muscles innervated by that nerve root. This is because each muscle is innervated by multiple nerve roots arising from more than one spinal level.

The diaphragm is innervated by the C3, C4, and C5 segments; therefore a lesion high in the cervical spinal cord threatens respiratory function. Shoulder abduction is a good test of C5 function. In the presence of normal function of the deltoid muscle, weak elbow flexors, predominantly the biceps brachii muscles, suggest a C6 lesion. The elbow and wrist extensors, subserved primarily by the triceps brachii and extensor carpi radialis and ulnaris muscles, are innervated by

C7. Function of the pronator teres muscle is also helpful in identifying a lesion at C7.

Lesions at C8 predominantly affect the intrinsic muscles of the hand, which are also innervated by T1.

The abdominal musculature can be tested clinically for lesions that affect thoracic nerves; a positive Beevor sign indicates weakness below T9 or T10.

The hip flexors and adductors are innervated by L2 and predominantly by L3. The quadriceps femoris muscle is a

good marker of L4 function. L5 innervates the ankle dorsiflexors and great toe extensors, and the ankle plantar flexors are innervated by S1 and S2. The lowest segments of the spinal cord (S2, S3, and S4) control the anal sphincter.

SENSORY IMPAIRMENT

Sensory examination often provides the most significant information in localizing a spinal cord lesion.

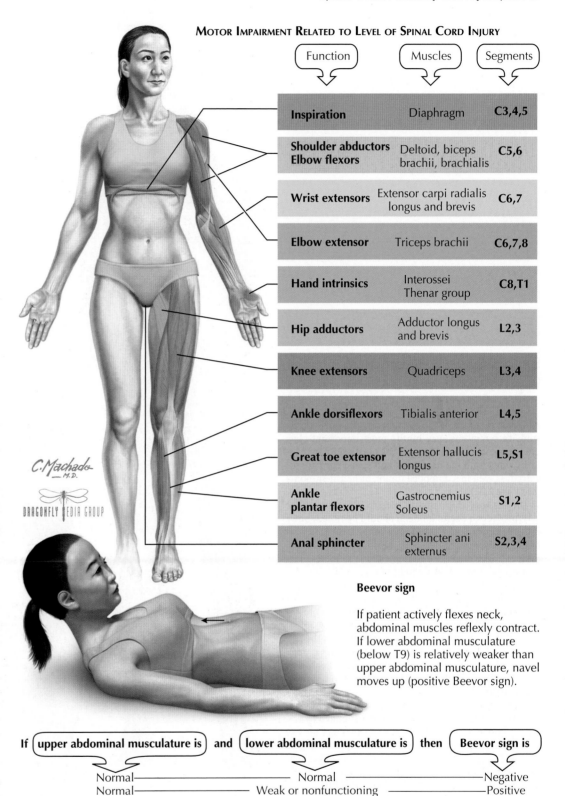

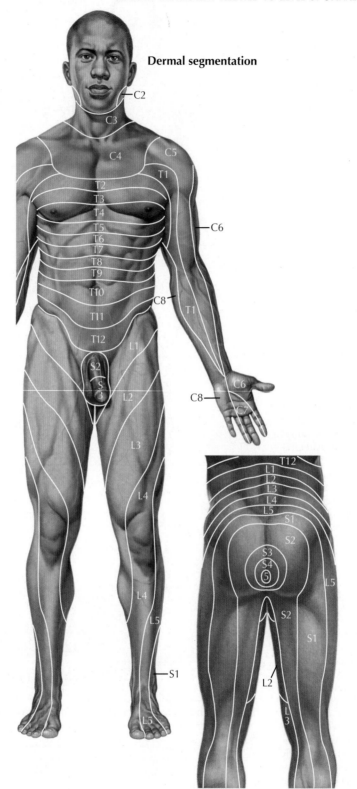

SENSORY IMPAIRMENT RELATED TO LEVEL OF SPINAL CORD INJURY

Dermal segmentation

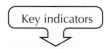
Key indicators

Cervical segments

C5—Anterolateral shoulder
C6—Thumb
C7—Middle finger
C8—Little finger

Thoracic segments

T1—Medial arm
T3—3rd, 4th interspace
T4—Nipple line, 4th,
       5th interspace
T6—Xiphoid process
T10—Navel
T12—Pubis

Lumbar segments

L2—Medial thigh
L3—Medial knee
L4—Medial ankle
       Great toe
L5—Dorsum of foot

Sacral segments

S1—Lateral foot
S2—Posteromedial thigh
S3, 4, 5—Perianal area

SPINAL CORD DYSFUNCTION (Continued)

However, if results of the examination are normal, the patient's symptoms may be the most important clue. The segmental distribution may be most useful in diagnosis when both the nerve root and spinal cord are involved, as seen in a dumbbell tumor, or neurilemmoma (see Plate 2.22).

The sensory dermatomal pattern shown in Plate 2.17 provides a useful guide. It should be noted, however, that segmental maps may differ depending on how they were obtained (e.g., by stimulation or section of individual roots or injection of local anesthetic into individual dorsal root ganglia). The C1 root has no significant sensory component; thus a lesion high in the cervical spinal cord at its most proximal limit affects C2, which involves the posterior part of the scalp. Because the descending spinal tract of the trigeminal (V) nerve extends into the upper cervical spinal cord, lesions at this level may produce changes in pain and temperature sensation over the temple and forehead, possibly with a diminished corneal reflex.

Segments C5 to T1 innervate the arm and hand, with the anterolateral aspect of the shoulder supplied by C5. The thumb and index finger are good markers for C6, the middle finger for C7, and the ring and little fingers for C8. T1 innervates the medial upper arm adjacent to the axilla. The nipple line is innervated by T4 and the area over the abdomen at the umbilicus by T10.

In the lower extremities, L3 and L4 segments innervate the anterior thigh and pretibial regions, respectively. The second, third, and fourth toes are innervated by L5, the fifth toe is innervated by S1, and the posterior medial thigh is innervated by S2. The saddle area of the buttocks is innervated by segments S3, S4, and S5.

Paresthesias in the buttocks are an important sign of possible spinal cord dysfunction. Because segments S3, S4, and S5 are the lowest and most peripheral segments in the spinal cord, an *extramedullary lesion* at any level may first compress these fibers and affect pain and temperature sensation. If the saddle area of the buttocks is not examined for pain and temperature sensation, an early spinal cord lesion may not be suspected. In

contrast, if an *intramedullary lesion* is present, the buttocks region is the last to be affected, with resultant sacral sparing.

Because the various ascending spinal tracts decussate at different levels of the spinal cord, several relatively specific patterns of dissociated sensory loss may be recognized clinically. *Brown-Séquard syndrome* implies a hemisection or unilateral lesion of the spinal cord. This is characterized by ipsilateral diminution of touch,

vibration, and position sense, and contralateral loss of pain and temperature sensation. Because the descending motor fibers decussate at the distal medulla, damage to these nerve fibers causes ipsilateral loss of function, with associated weakness and hyperreflexia (see Plate 2.18).

The *anterior spinal artery syndrome*, resulting from compression of this artery, occlusion of its feeders, trauma, or marked hypotension, affects the anterior

Plate 2.18

Spinal Cord: Anatomy and Myelopathies

INCOMPLETE SPINAL CORD SYNDROMES

Spinal cord orientation

Posterior columns (position sense)

Lower limb
Trunk
Upper limb } Lateral corticospinal tract (motor)

Lower limb } Lateral spinothalamic tract
Trunk } (pain and temperature); fibers
Upper limb } decussate before ascending

Anterior spinal artery

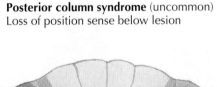

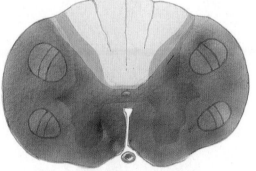

Posterior column syndrome (uncommon)
Loss of position sense below lesion

Anterior spinal artery syndrome
Bilateral paralysis and dissociated sensory
loss below lesion (analgesia but preserved
position sense)

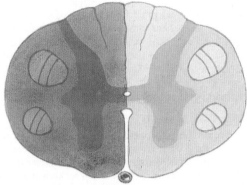

**Brown-Séquard syndrome (lateral cord
hemisection)** Ipsilateral paralysis and loss of
position sense; contralateral analgesia

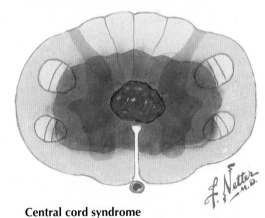

Central cord syndrome
Parts of 3 main tracts involved on both sides;
upper limbs more affected than lower limbs

SPINAL CORD DYSFUNCTION (Continued)

two-thirds of the spinal cord bilaterally, causing loss of pain and temperature sensation at approximately one to two segments below the level of the lesion, accompanied by paraplegia. However, because the posterior columns are preserved, touch, vibration, and position sense are normal bilaterally. The rare *posterior spinal artery syndrome* is characterized by loss of position sense but preserved pain appreciation and motor function below the lesion.

Intramedullary central cord *lesions,* such as with certain tumors, after injury, or in *syringomyelia,* affect decussating spinothalamic fibers in the central gray matter of the spinal cord. It is probably the most common form of incomplete spinal cord injury. When the lesion is in the cervical region, this produces a cape-like loss of pain and temperature sensation, with preservation of posterior column function. Pain and temperature sensation is preserved below the involved levels because the lateral spinothalamic tract is not affected by this central spinal cord syndrome. A concomitant lower motor neuron lesion commonly causing atrophy and fasciculations of the hands and arms is usually seen at the level of the dysfunction.

AUTONOMIC IMPAIRMENT

In addition to its somatic components, the spinal cord also contains autonomic nerve fibers, carried in the intermediolateral columns. A lesion at any level may cause sphincter dysfunction. Spinal cord lesions may damage the upper motor neuron pathways that control the bladder and rectum, but incontinence does not develop unless there is a severe bilateral lesion.

Other signs of autonomic dysfunction include *erectile dysfunction* in men; *postural hypotension; changes in sweating,* with anhidrosis below the level of the lesion; and *Horner syndrome,* which includes ipsilateral miosis, ptosis, and decreased facial sweating secondary to damage to sympathetic fibers at C8–T1. A variety of gastrointestinal disturbances may also occur.

OTHER ABNORMALITIES

Café-au-lait spots may suggest the presence of a *meningioma* or a *neurofibroma.* A tuft of hair or dimple in the midline, particularly in the lower spine, may point to an underlying *congenital vertebral defect.* In rare cases, a cutaneous angioma may overlie or be segmentally related to a spinal cord or dural *arteriovenous fistula.*

Although *scoliosis* is usually idiopathic, it rarely is the first sign of an evolving spinal cord tumor. *Pes cavus*

may be seen with distal spinal cord lesions. A *short neck* may suggest Klippel-Feil syndrome, which is sometimes associated with other cervical spine lesions.

Spinal cord dysfunction can be identified early if the patient's history and the results of neurologic examination are carefully assessed, with particular attention to the distribution of motor, reflex, and sensory changes associated with autonomic dysfunction and the presence of various skeletal and cutaneous changes.

ACUTE SPINAL CORD SYNDROMES

Spinal injury (see Section 3) may lead to a neurologic deficit from spinal cord involvement, but this is generally recognized by the context in which the deficit develops. The recognition of disease processes that can cause acute spinal cord damage is important. If the disorder is diagnosed early, some patients with spinal cord damage can be treated successfully. However, when the subtleties of the clinical picture are not recognized, the course may be disastrous, often culminating in lifelong paraplegia.

The common cause in the patient with a potentially reversible condition is the presence of a mass lesion that has reached a critical size. Because the spinal cord lies within the bony spinal canal, an obstructive extradural or intradural extramedullary process causes compression of the cord and its vessels. If treatment is initiated before severe damage to spinal cord tissue causes total paraplegia, useful recovery is possible.

The acute onset of *back pain* in any patient, and particularly in a patient with cancer, should alert the physician to the potential for an impending spinal disaster. Often, however, the patient is not seen until further symptoms have developed.

PREDISPOSING CAUSES

Metastatic Deposits

The most common cause of an acute spinal cord syndrome, particularly in patients in the middle to late decades of life, is epidural spinal cord compression from metastatic cancer. Most patients have a known preexisting malignancy, but a spinal metastatic lesion may be the first indication of a primary tumor elsewhere, and particularly of prostate, breast, or lung cancer; other common causes are non–Hodgkin lymphoma and plasmacytoma or multiple myeloma (see Plate 2.21). Patients have leg weakness and an impaired gait and frequently complain also of ascending numbness and paresthesias. A spinal sensory level may be present but may be one to several levels below that where the cord is compressed. A "saddle" sensory loss may be present with cauda equina lesions. Depending on the site of spinal involvement, muscle stretch reflexes may be exaggerated if the spinal cord is compressed or lost with cauda equina lesions. Bladder and bowel involvement occur later, most often with urinary retention. Magnetic resonance imaging (MRI) of the entire spine is mandatory; computed tomography (CT) myelography provides similar and sometimes complementary information.

Infarction

Occlusion of the anterior spinal artery affects the anterior two-thirds of the spinal cord (see Plates 2.18 and 2.20). Spinal cord infarction is usually precipitous. The clinical findings include paraparesis or paraplegia in combination with dissociated sensory loss, that is, loss of pain and temperature sensation, with preservation of position and vibration sense. During the acute stage, tone is flaccid and muscle stretch reflexes are lost; spasticity and hyperreflexia develop subsequently. Sphincter control is lost. Back pain, often at a segmental level, may be present.

Although in many cases spinal cord infarction may be idiopathic, in other instances it relates to aortic dissection that compromises the artery of Adamkiewicz (major anterior radiculomedullary artery), emboli from aortic atheroma, profound hypotension, or various types of arteritis. It may also occur as a complication of cardiac or aortic surgery.

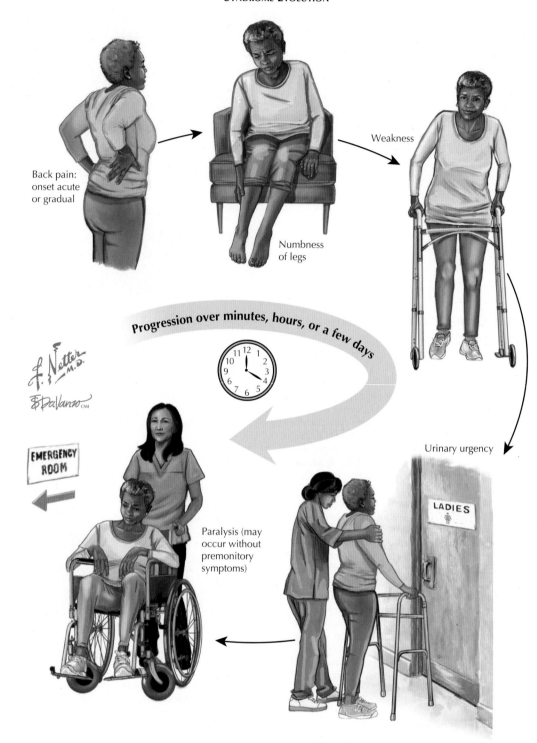

SYMPTOMS OF ACUTE SPINAL CORD
SYNDROME EVOLUTION

Back pain: onset acute or gradual

Numbness of legs

Weakness

Progression over minutes, hours, or a few days

Urinary urgency

LADIES

EMERGENCY ROOM

Paralysis (may occur without premonitory symptoms)

Spinal MRI or CT myelography is indicated to exclude other (compressive) lesions, including spontaneous epidural hematoma. The MRI may also confirm that infarction of the spinal cord has occurred. Spinal angiography may help confirm the diagnosis. Aortic dissection must be excluded. Treatment is based on the underlying pathology. The prognosis for recovery of useful function is poor.

Epidural Abscess

This lesion has a fairly characteristic clinical setting (see Plate 2.20). The vast majority of patients are febrile, and most are acutely ill, sometimes becoming disoriented but always complaining of severe back and nerve root pain. Examination demonstrates exquisite tenderness on percussion over the affected spinal process and signs of spinal cord impairment. Weakness, sensory changes, and bladder or bowel dysfunction occur with progression. If the abscess remains untreated, paralysis develops and may not be reversible.

There is often an apparent predisposing source of infection; staphylococci and gram-negative bacilli are the predominant causative organisms. Risk factors include epidural catheter placement (e.g., for anesthesia),

Plate 2.20

Spinal Cord: Anatomy and Myelopathies

ACUTE SPINAL CORD SYNDROMES: PATHOLOGY, ETIOLOGY, AND DIAGNOSIS

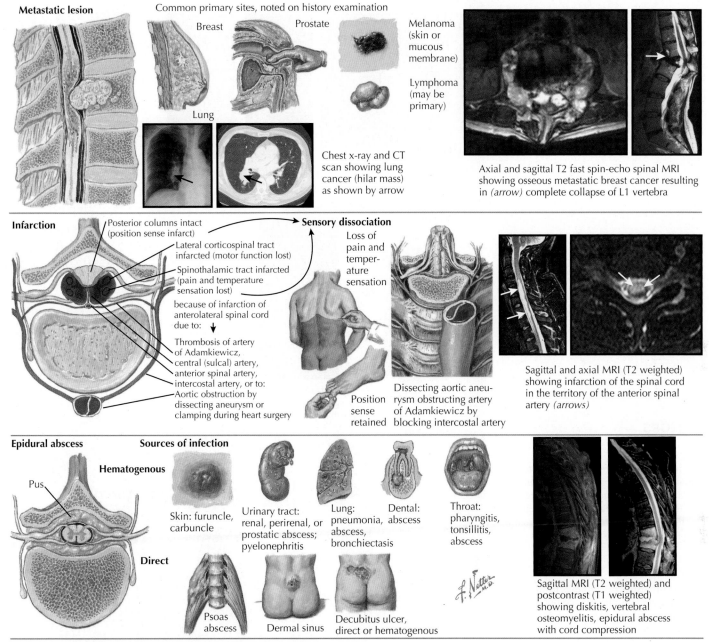

Metastatic lesion

Common primary sites, noted on history examination

Breast

Prostate

Melanoma (skin or mucous membrane)

Lymphoma (may be primary)

Lung

Chest x-ray and CT scan showing lung cancer (hilar mass) as shown by arrow

Axial and sagittal T2 fast spin-echo spinal MRI showing osseous metastatic breast cancer resulting in (arrow) complete collapse of L1 vertebra

Infarction

Posterior columns intact (position sense infarct)

Lateral corticospinal tract infarcted (motor function lost)

Spinothalamic tract infarcted (pain and temperature sensation lost)

because of infarction of anterolateral spinal cord due to:

Thrombosis of artery of Adamkiewicz, central (sulcal) artery, anterior spinal artery, intercostal artery, or to: Aortic obstruction by dissecting aneurysm or clamping during heart surgery

Sensory dissociation

Loss of pain and temperature sensation

Position sense retained

Dissecting aortic aneurysm obstructing artery of Adamkiewicz by blocking intercostal artery

Sagittal and axial MRI (T2 weighted) showing infarction of the spinal cord in the territory of the anterior spinal artery (arrows)

Epidural abscess

Pus

Sources of infection

Hematogenous

Skin: furuncle, carbuncle

Urinary tract: renal, perirenal, or prostatic abscess; pyelonephritis

Lung: pneumonia, abscess, bronchiectasis

Dental: abscess

Throat: pharyngitis, tonsillitis, abscess

Direct

Psoas abscess

Dermal sinus

Decubitus ulcer, direct or hematogenous

Sagittal MRI (T2 weighted) and postcontrast (T1 weighted) showing diskitis, vertebral osteomyelitis, epidural abscess with cord compression

Transverse myelitis Cause and specific pathologic process undetermined. Diagnosis by exclusion of other causes.

ACUTE SPINAL CORD SYNDROMES (Continued)

spinal surgery, paraspinal injections, impaired immunity, alcoholism, diabetes mellitus, and intravenous drug use.

Spinal MRI is important in confirming the diagnosis and localizing the lesion, but CT myelography may also be revealing. Surgery should be performed early to open and drain the area. Antibiotic therapy is administered according to the pathogen isolated in cultures from the abscess or blood, to eradicate the causal organism.

Transverse Myelitis

This syndrome of acute segmental spinal cord dysfunction results from inflammatory disease. Initial symptoms include limb weakness, loss of all sensation below the lesion, and sphincter involvement. Nerve root pain

and back pain are common. Early in the course, muscle stretch reflexes are either depressed or absent; spasticity and hyperreflexia subsequently develop.

The disorder may have an autoimmune basis. It occurs in multiple sclerosis, sometimes as the presenting feature; in neuromyelitis optica (a disorder limited to the optic nerve and spinal cord and characterized by the presence of specific circulating antibodies against the aquaporin-4 antigen or less commonly to myelin oligodendrocyte glycoprotein); and in various connective tissue diseases. It has been described after COVID-19. In many instances it is idiopathic. The diagnosis is one of exclusion in a patient who has a complete acute spinal cord syndrome. Involvement of all sensory modalities in acute transverse myelitis differentiates this disorder from spinal cord infarction, in which dissociated

sensory loss is present. Spinal MRI shows gadolinium-enhancing signal abnormality, with involvement over one or more segments of the spinal cord. In neuromyelitis optica, these changes extend over at least three or more vertebral segments.

Treatment is of the underlying disorder. For neuromyelitis optica, three medications are approved by the US Food and Drug Administration based on trials demonstrating a reduced annual relapse rate or time to first relapse. Eculizumab is a complement inhibitor, inebilizumab is a humanized anti-CD19 antibody that depletes B cells, and satralizumab is an interleukin-6 receptor antagonist. Patients with idiopathic transverse myelitis often make a partial recovery with time but may be left with a significant residual disability. Recovery is unlikely if improvement fails to occur within about 3 months.

Primary

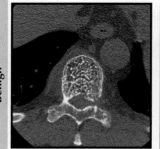
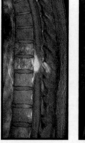
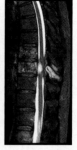

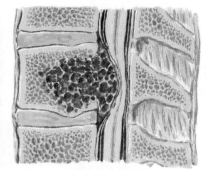

Axial CT scan and MRIs (sagittal T1 postcontrast and T2) of vertebral hemangioma

Hemangioma

Benign

Primary

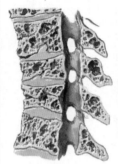

Multiple myeloma

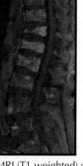

MRI (T1 weighted) of lumbar spine in patient with multiple myeloma and multiple compression fractures of spine

Malignant myeloma cells in biopsy specimen of bone marrow

γ spike on serum electrophoresis

Bence-Jones protein in urine in 60% of cases (precipitates at 45°C to 60°C, redissolves on boiling, and reprecipitates on cooling to 60°C to 45°C)

55°C   100°C   55°C

Metastatic

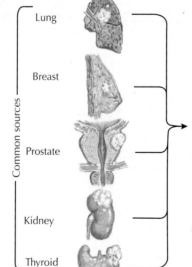

Common sources

Lung

Breast

Prostate

Kidney

Thyroid

Malignant

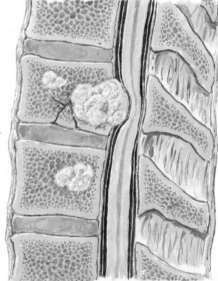

Spinal Tumors

Tumors involving the spine are usually classified as either extradural or intradural. The intradural tumors are further divided into extramedullary and intramedullary lesions. The anatomic location of the tumor provides a clue to the pathologic diagnosis, but accurate diagnosis is based on histologic studies.

EXTRADURAL TUMORS

Extradural tumors are usually *metastases* to the vertebrae that subsequently invade the epidural space. Almost any neoplasm can spread to the spine, but spinal metastases most commonly occur from a primary tumor in the lung, breast, or prostate. The tumor metastasizes through the arterial circulation or Batson's venous plexus, although direct extension from lung cancer or lymphoma is possible. Primary bone tumors, such as *osteogenic sarcoma* and *giant cell tumor,* are also seen, as are benign *hemangiomas* of bone. In most cases, pain is the first symptom of a vertebral tumor. Spinal cord compression, with associated symptoms, usually develops late and may be slowly progressive, but a rapidly growing tumor may cause acute neurologic deterioration secondary to infarction of the spinal cord.

A patient with a known primary cancer in whom spinal pain develops must be assumed to have a metastasis. A bone scan reveals a lesion earlier than plain radiographs but may fail to reveal neoplasms without increased blood flow or new bone formation. Furthermore, bone scanning is not informative about thecal sac compression. Spinal MRI is the preferred imaging modality and has largely replaced CT myelography. Epidural tumor deposits are often multiple, so the entire spine should be imaged.

Epidural tumors must be treated before serious spinal cord dysfunction develops, but treatment is controversial. High-dose corticosteroids (dexamethasone) and

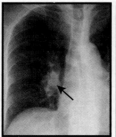
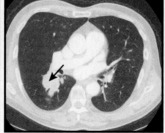
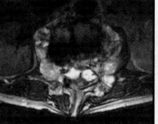
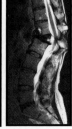

Lung cancer as seen on chest radiograph and CT scan *(arrows)*   Metastatic breast cancer involving the spine, shown on axial and sagittal T2 fast spin-echo spinal MRI. There is osseous metastatic breast cancer resulting in collapse of L1 vertebra.

Plate 2.22

Spinal Cord: Anatomy and Myelopathies

EXTRAMEDULLARY AND INTRAMEDULLARY SPINAL CORD TUMORS

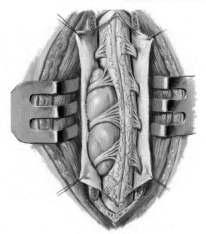

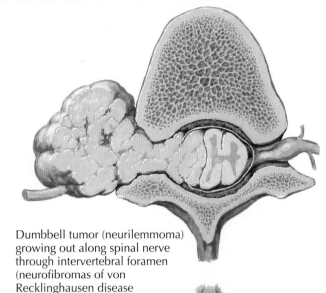

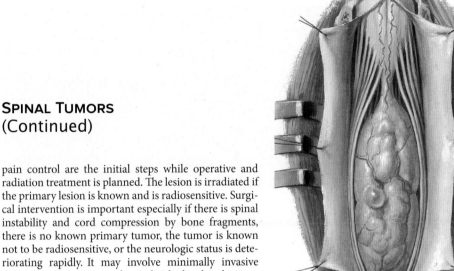

Intradural extramedullary tumor
(meningioma) compressing spinal
cord and deforming nerve roots

Dumbbell tumor (neurilemmoma)
growing out along spinal nerve
through intervertebral foramen
(neurofibromas of von
Recklinghausen disease
may act similarly)

SPINAL TUMORS
(Continued)

pain control are the initial steps while operative and
radiation treatment is planned. The lesion is irradiated if
the primary lesion is known and is radiosensitive. Surgical intervention is important especially if there is spinal
instability and cord compression by bone fragments,
there is no known primary tumor, the tumor is known
not to be radiosensitive, or the neurologic status is deteriorating rapidly. It may involve minimally invasive
decompressions or complex individualized techniques
and lead to pain relief and improvement in neurologic
deficits and quality of life. Radiation therapy is usually
administered postoperatively.

INTRADURAL TUMORS

Intradural extramedullary tumors include the benign
meningiomas and nerve sheath tumors *(neurilemmomas)*
and the *neurofibromas* associated with neurofibromatosis. Local and radicular pain is an early symptom. A spinal cord deficit results from compression of the spinal
cord, usually develops gradually, and leads to sensory
complaints, weakness, and sphincter disturbances. Plain
radiographs are not helpful in diagnosis unless a neurilemmoma has caused widening of the intervertebral
foramen by extending through it in the shape of a dumbbell. MRI allows the entire thecal sac and adjacent bone
and soft tissue to be studied (also see Plate 2.23). CT
myelography is sometimes helpful. These tumors can be
completely resected. Nerve roots in the thoracic region
may be sectioned to provide better exposure, but damage
to radicular arteries must be avoided.

Intramedullary tumors may involve just a short segment of the spinal cord or extend almost to its full
length. They are the most difficult tumors to diagnose
and treat. Diagnosis is confirmed by spinal MRI, which
provides good visualization of the spinal cord and

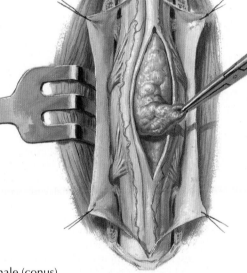

Tumor of filum terminale (conus)
compressing cauda equina.
Enlarged vessels feed tumor.

Intramedullary tumor causing
widening of spinal cord

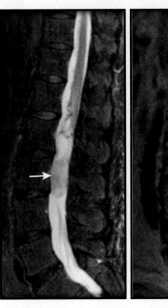

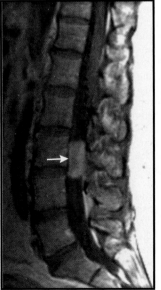

Filum ependymoma. Sagittal T2 fast spin-
echo *(left)* and T1 postgadolinium *(right)*
images of lumbar spine. Intradural
extramedullary enhancing mass posterior
to L3 vertebral body.

NEUROIMAGING (MRI) CHARACTERISTICS OF SPINAL TUMORS

Extradural tumors

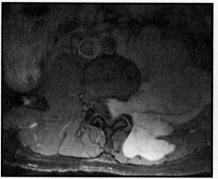
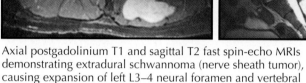

Lymphoma invading spinal canal via intervertebral foramen, compressing dura mater and spinal cord

Axial postgadolinium T1 and sagittal T2 fast spin-echo MRIs demonstrating extradural schwannoma (nerve sheath tumor), causing expansion of left L3–4 neural foramen and vertebral body scalloping

Intradural extramedullary tumors

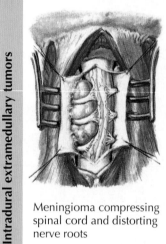
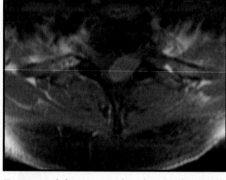

Meningioma compressing spinal cord and distorting nerve roots

T1 postgadolinium axial and sagittal MRIs showing intradural extramedullary mass in left aspect of spinal canal at the T1–T2 level *(arrow)*. Signal characteristics are most characteristic of a meningioma.

Intramedullary tumors

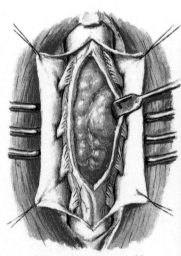
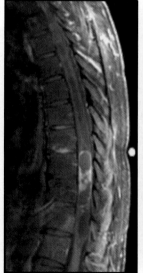
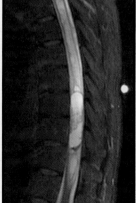

Astrocytoma exposed by longitudinal incision in bulging spinal cord

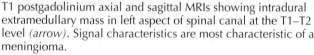

Sagittal T1 postgadolinium and T2 MRI of spinal astrocytoma

SPINAL TUMORS
(Continued)

adjacent structures, with enhancement by gadolinium, or by CT myelography, especially when MRI cannot be undertaken. The cord may be expanded, and cystic changes are sometimes present (Plates 2.22 and 2.23). However, demonstrating a swollen spinal cord with even the most sensitive radiographic studies does not confirm the diagnosis of intramedullary tumor. If the diagnosis is in doubt and the patient is deteriorating, the spinal cord should be explored surgically.

The two most common intramedullary tumors are *astrocytomas* and *ependymomas*. Astrocytomas are infiltrative, and total excision is not possible; however, there is frequently a well-demarcated plane around ependymomas, permitting their excision. Intramedullary metastatic deposits also occur, and improved imaging has resulted in their being recognized with increasing frequency. Surgery on the spinal cord demands the most meticulous technique. If the tumor is not completely excised, radiation therapy may be indicated.

Intradural tumors of the lumbar spine involve the conus medullaris, filum terminale, and cauda equina. Both ependymomas and astrocytomas may arise from the conus medullaris. These tumors produce early deficits of sphincter and sexual function and are difficult to remove without incurring significant neurologic deficit. Ependymomas of the filum terminale (see Plate 2.22) cause pain, often without significant neurologic findings, and can be cured by surgical excision.

The diffuse myxopapillary ependymoma, which involves the roots of the cauda equina, is difficult to excise and should receive postoperative radiation therapy. A neurilemmoma or a meningioma can be successfully removed. Lipoma of the cauda equina arises from fetal rests and is associated with spina bifida occulta. Excision of this tumor is difficult, but meticulous microsurgery can reduce the tumor and preserve neurologic function.

Plate 2.24

Spinal Cord: Anatomy and Myelopathies

SYRINGOMYELIA

Syringomyelia is a condition in which a tubular cavity, or syrinx, usually in the central area of the spinal cord, gradually expands and produces neuronal and tract damage.

When congenital, the syrinx develops most frequently in the cervical and upper thoracic segments. Serial sections of pathologic material show that it arises as a diverticulum from the central canal of the spinal cord. It may then dissect into the posterior or anterior gray matter on one side or enlarge symmetrically into a large, fluid-filled cavity, which, in turn, causes transverse enlargement of the spinal cord. Anterior horn neurons and pain and temperature fibers crossing in the central gray matter are destroyed. Long tracts, first the pyramidal and later the posterior column, may be compressed. In some cases, the syrinx extends from the cervical area into the posterolateral medulla, producing syringobulbia. Lumbar extension is rare.

Pathogenesis. The pathogenesis of syringomyelia is poorly understood. Almost all patients with congenital syringomyelia have an associated type I Arnold-Chiari malformation, which may itself produce symptoms of medullary or upper cervical compression. Other associated developmental defects include basilar impression, the Dandy-Walker syndrome, and atresia of the foramen of Magendie. Some patients have hydrocephalus. It has been suggested that the presence of an Arnold-Chiari malformation means that flow of CSF from the fourth ventricle is diminished, and increased pressure forces fluid into the central canal, producing a gradually expanding syrinx. A communication between the fourth ventricle, central canal, and the syrinx is not always evident, but abnormalities in the hindbrain and CSF dynamics may still be present.

Some cavities are caused by spinal cord trauma and may develop months or even years after injury. Spinal arachnoiditis and intramedullary tumors are also associated with syrinx formation, as occasionally are infectious or inflammatory states. Such *secondary or acquired* cavitation may occur anywhere in the spinal cord, depending on the site of the original pathology, and does not communicate with the central canal.

Clinical Findings. Syringomyelia is rare, with a prevalence of 8 per 100,000 persons. The syrinx may be asymptomatic, being discovered incidentally on spinal cord imaging. Symptoms usually appear late in the second through the fifth decades. Average age at onset is 30 years. The disease progresses at a variable rate; some patients become quadriplegic in 10 years, whereas others have a more benign course with long periods of stabilization. By 20 years, however, probably 50% of patients require use of a wheelchair.

The classic sign of cervical syringomyelia is *dissociated anesthesia,* or loss of pain and temperature sensation in a cape-like distribution, with preservation of light touch sensation and proprioception. Fibers carrying pain, itch, and temperature sensation cross in the central gray matter near the central canal and then form the spinothalamic tract in the anterolateral portion of the spinal cord. These fibers are damaged near the central canal or in the posterior horn before they cross. Fibers carrying light touch and proprioception information do not cross and course rostrally in the posterior columns. Centrally generated pain is sometimes problematic and has a segmental distribution.

Trophic changes occur, and Charcot's joints may be present. When the cavity expands into the anterior horn, atrophy and motor weakness become apparent. Fasciculations may be seen, and kyphoscoliosis resulting from

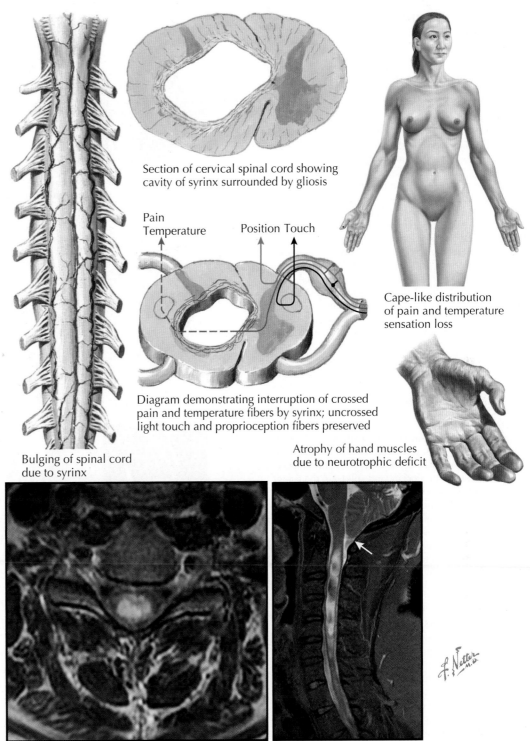

Section of cervical spinal cord showing cavity of syrinx surrounded by gliosis

Pain
Temperature
Position Touch

Cape-like distribution of pain and temperature sensation loss

Diagram demonstrating interruption of crossed pain and temperature fibers by syrinx; uncrossed light touch and proprioception fibers preserved

Bulging of spinal cord due to syrinx

Atrophy of hand muscles due to neurotrophic deficit

Axial and sagittal T2-weighted MRI showing syringomyelia and Chiari malformation, with cerebellar tonsils extending below the foramen magnum *(arrow)*

paraspinal muscle weakness is common. Thus presentation is with a progressive central cord syndrome. As the lesion expands further, it compresses the corticospinal and spinothalamic tracts. Progressive spastic paraparesis with a sensory level then becomes apparent.

Diagnosis. Syringomyelia is readily diagnosed with the use of spinal MRI and CT myelography. The spinal cord may be expanded, and the intramedullary cavity and an Arnold-Chiari malformation may be seen.

Treatment. The cause of the syrinx dictates the appropriate treatment. In most cases, an Arnold-Chiari malformation is present, and decompression of the area with suboccipital craniectomy and upper cervical laminectomy may be sufficient. In patients with no cervicomedullary abnormality, syringostomy may be considered. A plastic tube is placed into the syrinx cavity to provide communication to the subarachnoid space. If the tube remains patent, the process may stabilize. Syringoperitoneal or syringopleural shunting may also be worthwhile. Symptomatic hydrocephalus is treated with ventriculoperitoneal shunting.

In cavitation associated with intramedullary tumor, radiation may be required if total removal is not possible. Posttraumatic syringomyelia is treated surgically if it causes increasing neurologic deficits or intolerable pain.

SUBACUTE COMBINED DEGENERATION

Subacute combined degeneration of the spinal cord refers to degeneration of the posterior and lateral spinal columns. This may result from vitamin B_{12} deficiency, usually because of addisonian *pernicious anemia,* with atrophy of gastric parietal cells and absence of intrinsic factor. The same neurologic picture may appear in any condition in which vitamin B_{12} absorption is impaired or its dietary intake is insufficient. Cases have been reported in strict vegans and in patients who have sprue, Crohn disease, fistula of the small intestine, or fish tapeworm infestation, or who have had a bowel resection or gastrectomy. Vitamin B_{12} deficiency may also lead to mental changes. Early manifestations are subtle and include fatigue, irritability, and mild depression. Delirium, dementia, and paranoid psychosis are major cerebral manifestations. Rarely, seizures or visual blurring occur. A glove-and-stocking anesthesia, although uncommon, reflects peripheral neuropathy.

Subacute combined degeneration may also result from *nitrous oxide* abuse, which leads to inactivation of vitamin B_{12}. A similar syndrome is seen with *copper deficiency,* which may be a consequence of total parenteral hyperalimentation, copper deficiency in enteral feeding, malabsorption, gastrectomy, gastric bypass surgery, short bowel syndrome, or excessive zinc ingestion, which inhibits the intestinal absorption of copper.

Pathogenesis. The earliest neuropathologic lesion in this disorder is myelin swelling in the thoracic and lower cervical posterior columns. Later, demyelination and axonal destruction occur, and still later, the lateral columns and spinocerebellar tracts are involved. Ascending secondary degeneration may be seen in the posterior columns, and descending degeneration may be seen in the corticospinal tract. Small foci of demyelination are scattered throughout the cerebral white matter and optic (II) nerve. Secondary degeneration of association tracts may be present. Mild changes in peripheral nerves and damage to cortical neurons have been described.

Clinical Findings. Fatigue, weight loss, abdominal distress, diarrhea, and sore tongue are the most common general symptoms of pernicious anemia. Examination reveals glossitis and a lemon-yellow tint to the skin.

The most common neurologic symptoms relate to *involvement of the posterior columns.* Tingling, burning, and numbness of the distal extremities are the earliest symptoms. Depending on the site of initial demyelination, the feet or hands may be involved first, or paresthesias may occur simultaneously in all four extremities. Occasionally, the Lhermitte sign is present. Because of proprioceptive loss, imbalance, which worsens in the dark, may be an early sign.

Stiffness is often the first sign of *lateral column dysfunction* but usually occurs after the onset of paresthesias. Later, overt spasticity develops, and if the disease remains untreated, paraplegia with bowel and bladder incontinence ensues.

The cardinal neurologic sign is diminution of vibration sense. Position sense is affected to a lesser degree, but the Romberg sign is often positive. Involvement of the posterior columns and spinocerebellar tract may cause severely disabling sensory ataxia. With extensive spinal cord damage, a sensory level may be noted, usually in the middle or lower thoracic segment. Hyperreflexia, spasticity, clonus, and the Babinski sign signify lateral column damage. A

Degeneration of posterior columns, and corticospinal and direct spinocerebellar tracts, chiefly in midthoracic spinal cord

Numbness, tingling, or pins-and-needles sensation in hands and/or feet

Ataxia, especially in darkness

C4

C6

Copper deficiency (MRI shows posterior column changes)

Patient sways markedly with eyes closed (positive Romberg sign)

Glossitis common in pernicious anemia

Vibration sense lost

Position sense lost

hyperactive bladder may be an associated finding. In severe untreated cases, paraplegia with flexor spasms may develop.

Diagnosis. Subacute combined degeneration is diagnosed clinically by recognition of posterior and lateral column involvement. Determination of the serum vitamin B_{12} level and testing for autoantibodies to intrinsic factor are usually sufficient for confirming a diagnosis of pernicious anemia. It has long been recognized that neurologic signs and symptoms may precede the appearance of anemia. The red blood cell count and the mean corpuscular volume, however, are often abnormal in the face of normal hemoglobin and hematocrit values.

Treatment. For patients with a permanent impairment of vitamin B_{12} absorption (e.g., with pernicious anemia or gastrointestinal resection), treatment will need to be continued indefinitely. Loading doses of intramuscularly administered vitamin B_{12} are given several times per week for several months, followed by a maintenance dosage of at least $1000\ \mu g$/month for life. When the cause of the vitamin B_{12} deficiency is reversible (e.g., diet, nitrous oxide exposure, certain malabsorption syndromes), treatment can be stopped when the vitamin deficiency is completely reversed and its cause eliminated. In patients with copper deficiency, supplementation may halt disease progression and correct hematologic disturbances, but neurologic dysfunction may be irreversible; ingestion of zinc should be discontinued or strictly limited.

Mild paresthesias and mental changes of recent onset may completely resolve with treatment, but when symptoms have been present for several months, complete recovery is unlikely.

Plate 2.26

Spinal Cord: Anatomy and Myelopathies

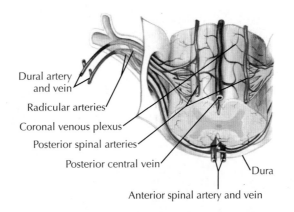

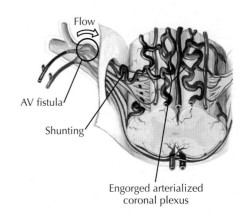

Spinal Dural Fistulas and Arteriovenous Malformations

Spinal dural fistulas (also called arteriovenous malformations [AVMs]) consist primarily of an abnormal arteriovenous communication without intervening capillaries. They may occur at any level but are most common in the thoracolumbar region, where generally only one or two arterial feeding vessels are present. These are a radicular or dural branch of a segmental artery that does not supply the spinal cord itself. The AVM nidus is typically a low-flow shunt drained by a vein that joins the posterior coronal venous plexus. The coronal plexus is arterialized by the fistula and becomes dilated, coiled, and elongated. The increased venous pressure (resulting from the abnormal arteriovenous communication) leads to a reduced arteriovenous pressure gradient across the cord and thus to reduced blood flow. The resulting ischemia/hypoxia leads to a progressive myelopathy.

Symptoms typically develop gradually after age 40 years and progress slowly. They consist of some combination of back or radicular pain, weakness, sensory disturbances, and impaired sphincter function. Neurogenic claudication may be present. Examination commonly reveals mixed upper and lower motor neuron deficits, sensory abnormalities, and reflex changes in the legs. Without treatment, the gait becomes progressively more impaired until the patient must use a wheelchair. A discrete or vague sensory level is sometimes present. A bruit may be audible over the spine.

Intradural AVMs may occur at any level but are more common in the cervical region. There may be one or multiple feeding vessels, which arise from a radiculomedullary vessel supplying the anterior spinal artery or from one of the branches to the spinal cord. The nidus may be intramedullary, in the pia (i.e., extramedullary), or both intramedullary and extramedullary. These are high-volume, high-pressure shunts with rapid blood flow, from which spontaneous intraparenchymal or subarachnoid hemorrhage may occur. Symptoms develop usually during early adult life. Patients, often young adults, present with sudden back pain and a neurologic deficit in the limbs, perhaps accompanied by impaired consciousness when hemorrhage has occurred, or with a progressive myelopathy. When the lesion is located cervically, both upper and lower extremities may be affected. Recurrent hemorrhages lead to clinical deterioration.

Cavernous angiomas or malformations are rare, isolated, or multiple lesions that can spontaneously hemorrhage and are best shown by MRI. Spinal arteriography is normal.

In patients with spinal dural fistulas, MRI demonstrates serpentine filling defects of reduced signal in the subarachnoid space, corresponding to blood flow in the dilated, tortuous coronal venous plexus. Sometimes cord signal is increased from edema or venous congestion. Low cord signal may reflect an intradural nidus.

The spinal cord is supplied via radiculomedullary arteries, which supply the anterior spinal and posterior spinal arteries.

In a dural AVM, the nidus is usually a low-flow AV shunt located within dura of intervertebral foramen. Supplied by a radicular artery and drained via a single vein into the coronal plexus on the posterior, or less commonly, the anterior surface of the cord. Coronal plexus is "arterialized" and becomes coiled, dilated, and elongated.

JOHN A. CRAIG—AD

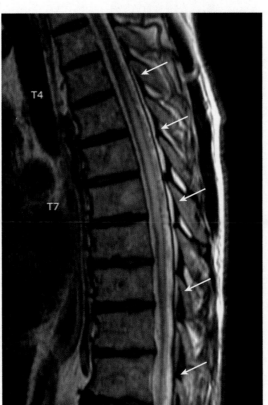

Sagittal T2 MRI shows increased T2 signal in the central cord representing edema and/or gliosis. Multiple signal voids behind the spinal cord are secondary to tortuous vessels from the malformation.

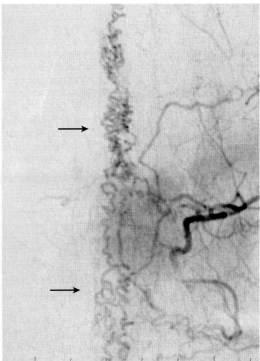

Spinal angiogram of radicular artery, left T6, with arteriovenous fistula filling multiple draining veins at the dural level. These join to form a complex medullary venous plexus.

CT myelography may demonstrate serpentine linear defects, but its use has largely been supplanted by MRI. Selective spinal arteriography defines the precise site of the nidus, its arterial feeders, and the normal blood supply to the spinal cord. Endovascular occlusion of feeding vessels is often undertaken during the procedure and may obliterate the lesion or, at least, reduce its size so that it is easier to remove surgically. Intramedullary lesions may be inoperable, but embolization can occlude feeding vessels and the nidus, reducing flow and allowing lesion thrombosis. It is important to maintain the vascular supply to the spinal cord to prevent damage from subsequent ischemia. After non-operative obliterative procedures, feeding vessels may recanalize or new feeders can open, requiring further treatment.

Early detection and treatment can improve gait disturbances and sometimes bladder or bowel dysfunction, and a previously progressive course can be arrested.

CERVICAL SPONDYLOSIS

The pathologic process in cervical spondylosis is a gradually progressive degeneration of intervertebral disks, with subsequent changes in vertebrae and meninges. Disk degeneration may result from desiccation of the nucleus pulposus that begins in the fifth decade and progresses rapidly thereafter. At the same time, the annulus fibrosus may weaken to allow bulging of the nucleus pulposus. Disk material extrudes when portions of the annulus rupture. Osteophytes (bony spurs) appear on the margins of the vertebral bodies, zygapophyseal joints, and articular cartilages, probably as a result of trauma and disk degeneration. If osteophytes or protruding disks project posteriorly or posterolaterally, they may compress the spinal cord or cervical nerve roots. As disks degenerate and bulge posteriorly, so-called spondylotic bars may be formed, which also may compress the spinal cord or neural foramina. The anteroposterior diameter of the spinal canal is also important. The average sagittal diameter is about 17 mm, whereas the average spinal cord diameter is 10 mm. The canal narrows about 2 mm with maximal neck extension. In most patients, large cervical bars or osteophytes are necessary to produce spinal cord compression, but in those with an already narrowed canal (spinal stenosis), compression may occur with lesser degenerative changes.

Finally, as disk spaces narrow secondary to degeneration, the cervical spine shortens. This can produce infolding of the ligamentum flavum, which narrows the anteroposterior diameter of the spinal canal. The vertebral column shortens, but the length of the spinal cord remains unchanged, resulting in traction on the lower cervical nerve roots.

When spinal cord compression occurs, pathologic examination shows flattening and distortion of the cord. Several indentations may be present, depending on the number of spondylotic bars. Demyelination of the lateral and posterior columns and neuronal damage at the points of compression are the primary microscopic findings.

Clinical Findings. Cervical spondylotic radiculomyelopathy or myelopathy is the commonest myelopathy of later life. Its onset is usually insidious. *Paresthesias* of the hand may occur early, and the patient may experience numbness and tingling in a radicular distribution, as well as *radicular pain.* Weakness and atrophy in the upper extremities vary, depending on the spinal cord segments or nerve roots compressed. Because the fifth and sixth cervical segments are most frequently compressed, stretch reflexes of the biceps and triceps, respectively, may be diminished. In the lower extremities, a *spastic paraparesis* is common, but one leg may be more severely involved than the other. Vibration and position sense are often diminished in the feet. The gait is spastic and sometimes ataxic because of impaired position sense. Sphincter disturbances (especially urinary urgency, frequency, or retention) and sensory levels are seen only in later stages. The spastic paraparesis is insidious and slowly progressive in some cases and more acute in onset in others; muscle fasciculations, atrophy, and weakness of the upper extremities may develop in conjunction with it, sometimes simulating motor neuron disease when sensory or sphincter disturbances are absent.

Diagnosis. Spinal MRI or CT myelography is required to establish the presence of spinal cord compression, confirm the cause, and exclude other pathologic processes. Narrowing of the anteroposterior sagittal

Weakness of lower limb evidenced by circumduction of leg in walking

Paresthesias and/or paresis of upper limb may occur

Ankle clonus

Babinski sign

Loss of vibration sense

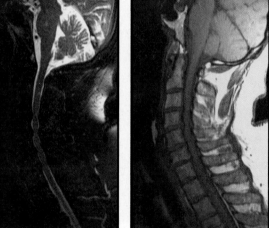
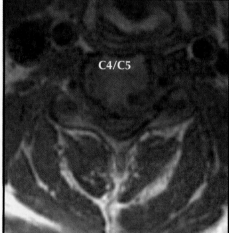

Left to right, T2-weighted sagittal, T1-weighted sagittal, and T1-weighted axial MRIs showing degenerative disease with spinal cord compression. Idiopathic spinal stenosis with disk protrusion anteriorly and hypertrophy of ligamentum flavum posteriorly, most extreme at C4–5.

C4/C5

diameter to 11 mm or less in any area of the cervical spine increases the risk of cord compression. Multilevel disease is common. CSF is normal or shows a mild to moderately elevated protein content.

Treatment. Nonoperative treatment may involve analgesics and immobilization of the neck, for example, in a cervical collar. Local injection of anesthetics or corticosteroids is sometimes helpful. Most nerve root syndromes subside spontaneously. Surgical treatment of cervical spondylosis may be indicated for severe radicular pain

unresponsive to other measures, progression of a significant neurologic deficit, or sphincter disturbances. Some patients improve after surgery, but only stabilization can be realistically expected.

Spinal cord decompression may be done through either an anterior or a posterior approach, and it is not clear which approach is best. About 75% of patients stabilize or improve after surgery, whereas up to 25% may worsen or progress. There is no agreement on factors that predict the surgical outcome.

Plate 2.28

Spinal Cord: Anatomy and Myelopathies

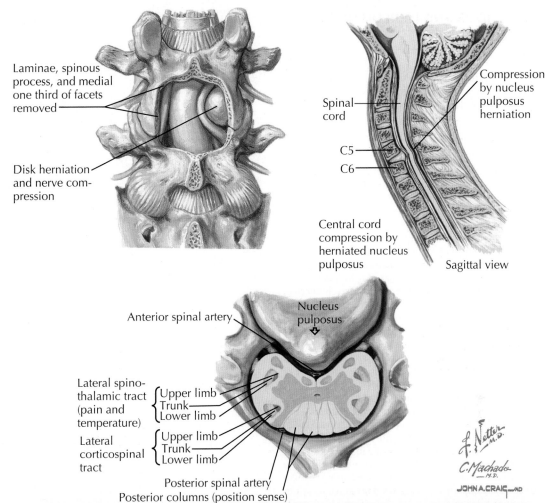

Laminae, spinous process, and medial one third of facets removed

Disk herniation and nerve compression

Spinal cord

Compression by nucleus pulposus herniation

C5

C6

Central cord compression by herniated nucleus pulposus

Sagittal view

Anterior spinal artery

Nucleus pulposus

Lateral spino-thalamic tract (pain and temperature)
Upper limb
Trunk
Lower limb

Lateral corticospinal tract
Upper limb
Trunk
Lower limb

Posterior spinal artery

Posterior columns (position sense)

CERVICAL DISK HERNIATION CAUSING CORD COMPRESSION

Cervical disk disease is a common disorder, accounting for 1% to 2% of all hospital admissions in the United States. (Lumbar disk disease is considered separately in Section 4.) Its etiology is multifactorial. It is sometimes attributed to preceding injury or exertion, but, in most instances, no specific precipitant can be identified.

With age, the nucleus pulposus of the disk dehydrates, placing more stress on the annulus fibrosus (outer lining). Tears in the annulus may permit a sudden herniation of the nucleus—a *ruptured disc.* Alternatively, chronic annular bulging or nuclear herniation may lead to the formation of extensive bony spurs (osteophytes), typically located along the anterior portion of the disk interspace or posteriorly within the nerve root foramen. Osteophytes or ruptured disks produce symptoms only if they compress the spinal cord or nerve roots against posteriorly located structures, including the posterior nerve root foramen and ligamentum flavum.

Clinical Findings. The first manifestation of cervical disk disease is often cervical radiculopathy, with symptoms and signs referable to compression of a cervical nerve root. Cervical and unilateral arm pain, frequently acute in onset, is a common symptom of cervical disk disease, and patients often complain also of numbness, paresthesias, or, less commonly, weakness in the involved arm in a radicular distribution. Examination may show sensory, motor, or reflex abnormalities depending on the involved nerve roots. Gait disturbances, leg weakness, or sphincter disturbances suggest an associated compressive myelopathy.

Diagnosis. Spinal MRI is the imaging modality of choice, but CT myelography may be required in those with a normal MRI when a strong clinical suspicion of the diagnosis remains. Electrodiagnostic studies (needle electromyography to detect signs of denervation

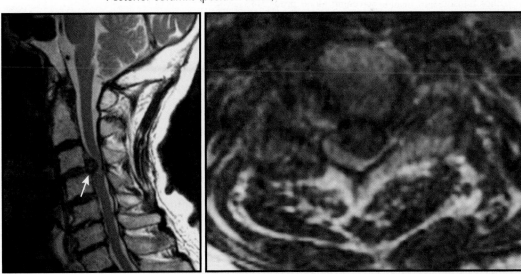

Sagittal and axial (T2) MRI showing disk extrusion at C3–4 extending to C3 vertebral body, severe spinal stenosis, and deformation of the cervical spinal cord *(arrow)*

in muscles) are helpful in indicating the functional significance of any anatomic abnormalities seen on imaging studies.

Treatment. Many patients with cervical radiculopathy respond to *conservative treatment,* including short-term use of a soft cervical collar to immobilize the neck, mild analgesics, physical therapy, and muscle relaxants as required. A brief course of oral steroids is sometimes worthwhile. Many believe that cervical traction is also helpful, provided imaging reveals no contraindication.

If symptoms persist after 4 to 6 weeks, further testing, including spinal MRI, is indicated. If imaging shows compression of the clinically appropriate nerve root, *surgical therapy* is often undertaken. Surgery is also often performed if patients have clinical evidence of myelopathy and imaging evidence of spinal cord compression. Some neurosurgeons strongly advocate an anterior approach, and others, a posterior approach in treatment. In skilled hands, either route leads to excellent relief of symptoms in many patients.

INFECTIOUS AND HEREDITARY MYELOPATHIES

Several infectious myelopathies merit brief comment. *AIDS-associated vacuolar myelopathy* is discussed in the section on infections of the nervous system.

HUMAN T-CELL LYMPHOCYTIC VIRUS-1 MYELOPATHY

This disorder, also known as tropical spastic paraparesis/ human T-cell lymphocytic virus-1 (HTLV-1)–associated myelopathy (TSP/HAM), may be acquired as a sexually transmitted disease, particularly in the Caribbean, eastern South America, equatorial Africa, and southern Japan, where HTLV-1 is endemic. Transmission is by semen, blood or its products, and breast milk. Only a small proportion of HTLV-1 carriers develop the myelopathy after a latent period that may be many years. The mid- to lower thoracic cord is most severely affected, especially the lateral columns and corticospinal tracts. Patients typically present in the middle fourth to fifth decades with a slowly progressive spastic paraparesis and paraparesthesis. Bladder disturbances, impotence, and constipation also develop. Cerebral, cerebellar, and cranial and peripheral nerve dysfunction may occur, as may HTLV-1–associated systemic disorders.

MRI may show spinal atrophy and sometimes the presence of cerebral periventricular white matter lesions. The CSF may contain a mononuclear pleocytosis or elevated protein concentration, with oligoclonal bands. Anti–HTLV-1 antibodies are present in CSF, and polymerase chain reaction is positive for the virus. There is no effective treatment for HTLV-1–related myelopathy other than symptomatic measures. Preventive measures to reduce transmission include screening blood products, sexual education, and use of formula rather than breast milk of infected mothers.

SCHISTOSOMAL MYELOPATHY

Millions of persons worldwide are infected with schistosomes, parasitic blood flukes that are transmitted to humans in contact with fresh water. Neurologic involvement is relatively uncommon in schistosomiasis, but an inflammatory myeloradiculopathy may occur, especially with *Schistosoma mansoni* and *S. haematobium* infection (cerebral involvement is more common with *S. japonicum* infection). *Schistosoma* organisms are found in tropical areas such as the Caribbean and Middle East, the Nile and Amazon River basins, and Lake Victoria in east central Africa. Infective larvae (cercariae) are released into fresh water by infected snails (the intermediate host). After they penetrate the skin of humans, the parasite migrates to selected vascular beds, depending on species. After reproduction of adult male and female parasites, eggs are deposited in various tissues and eventually exit the body in urine or feces; in the right context, the eggs open to release free-swimming larvae *(miracidia)* that infect snails. Involvement of the human nervous system probably occurs by transport of eggs into the CNS circulation by collateral veins or by aberrant migration of adult worms.

Spinal cord involvement, often at the level of the conus medullaris, often follows an initial radiculopathy and may progress acutely or subacutely. Patients may present with back or root pain, paraparesis, sensory abnormalities, and bladder dysfunction. Expanding granulomatous inflammation may lead to a progressive myelopathy; in some instances, an acute transverse myelitis leads to a catastrophic deficit.

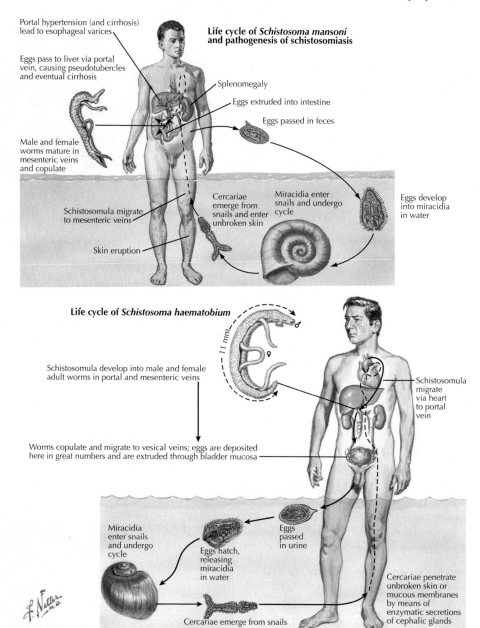

Life cycle of *Schistosoma mansoni* and pathogenesis of schistosomiasis

Portal hypertension (and cirrhosis) lead to esophageal varices

Eggs pass to liver via portal vein, causing pseudotubercles and eventual cirrhosis

Splenomegaly

Eggs extruded into intestine

Eggs passed in feces

Male and female worms mature in mesenteric veins and copulate

Cercariae emerge from snails and enter unbroken skin

Miracidia enter snails and undergo cycle

Eggs develop into miracidia in water

Schistosomula migrate to mesenteric veins

Skin eruption

Life cycle of *Schistosoma haematobium*

Schistosomula develop into male and female adult worms in portal and mesenteric veins

11 mm

Schistosomula migrate via heart to portal vein

Worms copulate and migrate to vesical veins; eggs are deposited here in great numbers and are extruded through bladder mucosa

Miracidia enter snails and undergo cycle

Eggs hatch, releasing miracidia in water

Eggs passed in urine

Cercariae penetrate unbroken skin or mucous membranes by means of enzymatic secretions of cephalic glands

Cercariae emerge from snails

The diagnosis should be suspected in any recent traveler to an endemic area. An eosinophilia in the blood, and sometimes the CSF, is suggestive but may not be present. Enlargement and gadolinium enhancement of the thoracolumbar spinal cord may be evident on MRI. Serologic tests may reveal evidence of schistosomal exposure. Rapid diagnosis and early treatment with praziquantel and high-dose corticosteroids improve the ultimate prognosis.

HEREDITARY SPASTIC PARAPLEGIA

This term refers to a group of clinically heterogeneous hereditary disorders in which a progressive spastic weakness affects the lower extremities. Patients differ according to the mode of inheritance and genetic locus (when known). Age at onset and the severity of symptoms also vary widely. Corticospinal tract and posterior column involvement occurs from a dying-back process affecting the distal ends of long axons, causing the motor and sensory deficits. The disorder occurs most often with autosomal dominant inheritance, but autosomal recessive and X-linked inheritance also occur. Many different genes and genetic loci have been identified.

Patients with the "pure" form of the disorder present with progressive spasticity, hyperreflexia, and weakness of the lower extremities. Vibratory sensation is sometimes mildly decreased. Occasionally patients experience sphincter disturbances manifested by a spastic bladder with urgency and frequency. In the *complicated form*, other findings include cognitive impairment, aphasia, dysarthria, dysphagia, pale optic discs, nystagmus, cataracts, upper extremity weakness, motor neuronopathy, sphincter disturbances, and muscle wasting; neuroimaging may reveal cerebellar or cerebral atrophy, hydrocephalus, white matter changes, and a thin corpus callosum.

A positive family history is one of the most important diagnostic clues. Genetic screening may be supportive, but, in many cases, the genetic abnormality has yet to be identified. MRI helps to exclude other structural causes of the patient's symptoms and sometimes reveals marked spinal atrophy. No specific therapy is available. Management is therefore supportive, and treatment is symptomatic.

SPINAL TRAUMA

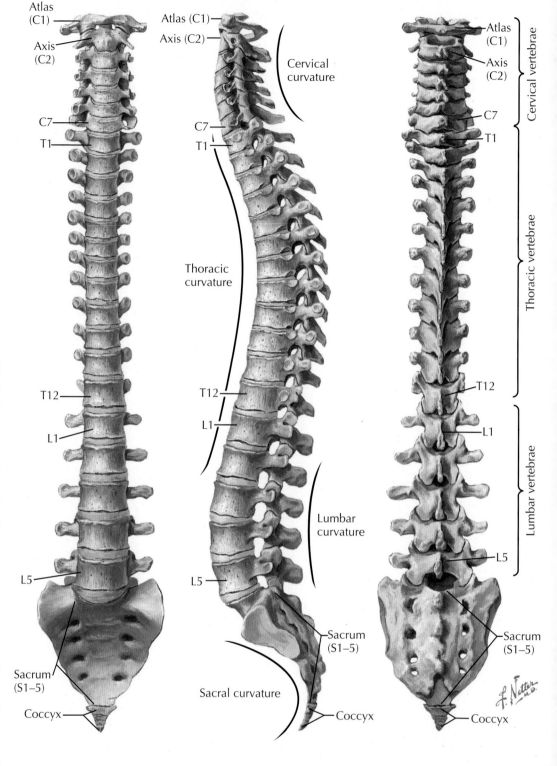

Anterior view

Atlas (C1)
Axis (C2)
C7
T1
T12
L1
L5
Sacrum (S1–5)
Coccyx

Left lateral view

Atlas (C1)
Axis (C2)
Cervical curvature
C7
T1
Thoracic curvature
T12
L1
Lumbar curvature
L5
Sacrum (S1–5)
Sacral curvature
Coccyx

Posterior view

Atlas (C1)
Axis (C2)
C7
T1
Cervical vertebrae
T12
Thoracic vertebrae
L1
Lumbar vertebrae
L5
Sacrum (S1–5)
Coccyx

Spinal Column

The spinal column is built from alternating bony vertebrae and fibrocartilaginous disks, which are intimately connected by strong ligaments and supported by powerful musculotendinous masses. The individual bony elements and ligaments are depicted in Plates 3.2 to 3.10. There are 33 vertebrae (7 cervical, 12 thoracic, 5 lumbar, 5 sacral, and 4 coccygeal), although the sacral and coccygeal vertebrae are usually fused to form the sacrum and coccyx.

All vertebrae conform to a basic plan, but individual variations occur in the different regions. A typical vertebra consists of an anterior, more or less cylindric *body,* and a posterior *arch* composed of two *pedicles* and two *laminae,* the latter united posteriorly to form a *spinous process.* These processes vary in shape, size, and direction in the various regions of the spine. On each side, the arch also supports a *transverse process* and *superior* and *inferior articular processes;* the latter form synovial joints with corresponding processes on adjacent vertebrae, and the spinous and transverse processes provide levers for the many muscles attached to them. The increasing size of the vertebral bodies from above downward is related to the increasing weights and stresses borne by successive segments. The sacral vertebrae are fused to form a solid wedge-shaped base—the keystone in a bridge whose arches curve down toward the hip joints. The *intervertebral disks* act as elastic buffers to absorb the numerous mechanical shocks sustained by the spinal column.

Only limited movements are possible between adjacent vertebrae, but the sum of these movements confers a considerable range of mobility on the vertebral column. Flexion, extension, lateral bending, rotation, and circumduction are all possible, and these actions are freer in the cervical and lumbar regions than in the thoracic. Such differences exist because the disks are thicker in the cervical and lumbar areas, the splinting effect produced by the thoracic cage is lacking, the cervical and lumbar spinous processes are shorter and less closely apposed, and the articular processes are shaped and arranged differently.

At birth the spinal column presents a general posterior convexity, but later the cervical and lumbar regions become curved in the opposite directions—when the infant reaches the stages of holding up its head (3–4 months) and sitting upright (6–9 months). The posterior convexities are *primary curves* associated with the fetal uterine position, whereas the cervical and lumbar

anterior *secondary curves* are compensatory to permit the assumption of the upright position.

Human evolution from a quadrupedal to a bipedal posture was mainly from the tilting of the sacrum between the hip bones, an increase in lumbosacral angulation, and minor adjustments of the anterior and posterior depths of various vertebrae and disks. An erect posture greatly increases the load borne by the lower spinal joints, and, good as these ancestral adaptations were, some static and dynamic imperfections remain and predispose to stress and strain. The length of the vertebral column averages 72 cm in the adult male and

7 to 10 cm less in the female. The *vertebral canal* extends through the entire length of the column and provides excellent protection for the spinal cord, the cauda equina, and their coverings. The spinal vessels and nerves pass through *intervertebral foramina* formed by notches on the superior and inferior borders of the pedicles of adjacent vertebrae, bounded anteriorly by the corresponding intervertebral disks and posteriorly by the joints between the articular processes of adjoining vertebrae. Pathologic or traumatic conditions affecting any of these structures may produce pressure on the nerves or vessels they transmit.

Plate 3.2   Spinal Trauma

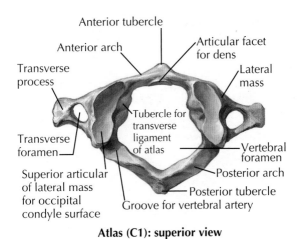

Atlas (C1): superior view

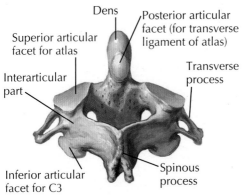

Axis (C2): anterior view

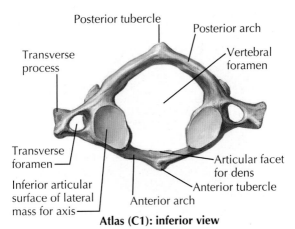

Atlas (C1): inferior view

Axis (C2): posterosuperior view

ATLAS AND AXIS

The atlas and axis are the first and second cervical vertebrae, and both are atypical in relationship to the other vertebrae. They are linked together and to the skull and other cervical vertebrae by a layered pattern of craniocervical ligaments (see Plates 3.4 and 3.5).

The *atlas* (named after the mythical giant who carried the earth on his shoulders) supports the globe of the skull. It lacks a body and forms a ring consisting of shorter anterior and longer posterior arches, with two lateral masses.

The *anterior arch* is slightly curved, with an anterior midline tubercle and a posterior midline facet for articulation with the dens of the axis. The *lateral masses* bear superior and inferior articular facets and transverse processes. The *superior articular facets* are concave and ovoid (often waisted, or reniform) and are directed upward and inward as shallow cups, or foveae, for the reception of the occipital condyles. Nodding movements of the head mainly occur at these atlantooccipital joints. The *inferior articular facets* are almost circular, gently concave, and face downward and slightly medially and backward; they articulate with the superior articular facets on the axis. The *transverse processes* are each pierced by a foramen for the vertebral artery. They provide attachments and levers for some of the muscles involved in head rotation. On the anteromedial aspect of each lateral mass is a small tubercle for the attachment of the transverse ligament of the atlas.

The *posterior arch* of the atlas is more curved than the anterior and has a small *posterior tubercle*, which is a rudimentary spinous process. Just behind each superior articular facet is a shallow *groove for the vertebral artery* and first cervical spinal nerve, the nerve lying between the artery and the bone.

The *axis*, or second cervical vertebra, has a tooth-like process, or *dens*, projecting upward from its body. The dens is really the divorced body of the atlas that has united with the axis to form a pivot around which the

atlas and the skull can rotate. Its anterior surface has an oval *anterior facet*, which articulates with the facet on the back of the anterior arch of the atlas, and a smaller *posterior facet* lower down on its posterior surface, which is separated from the transverse ligament of the atlas by a small bursa. The apex of the dens is attached to the lower end of the apical ligament, and the alar ligaments are attached to its sides.

The *body* of the axis has a lower lip-like projection that overlaps the anterosuperior border of the third

cervical vertebra. The posteroinferior border of the body is less prominent, and attached to it are the tectorial membrane and the posterior longitudinal spinal ligament. The *pedicles* and *laminae* are stout, and the latter end in a strong, bifid *spinous process*. On each side of the body are superior and inferior articular and transverse processes. The *articular processes* are offset because the superior pair is anterior in position to the inferior pair. They articulate with the adjoining processes of the atlas and third cervical vertebra.

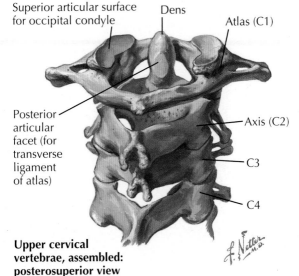

Upper cervical vertebrae, assembled: posterosuperior view

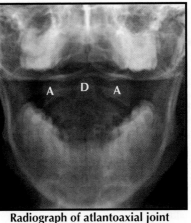

Radiograph of atlantoaxial joint (open mouth odontoid view)

A, Lateral masses of atlas (C1 vertebra)
D, Dens of axis (C2 vertebra)

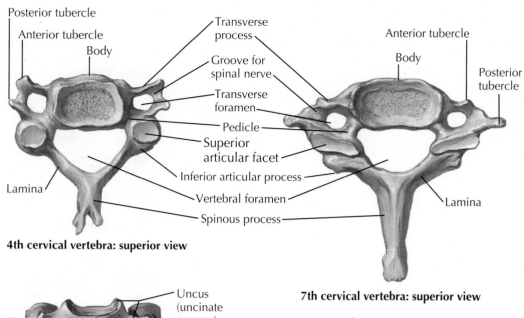

4th cervical vertebra: superior view

Posterior tubercle
Anterior tubercle
Body
Lamina

Transverse process
Groove for spinal nerve
Transverse foramen
Pedicle
Superior articular facet
Inferior articular process
Vertebral foramen
Spinous process

7th cervical vertebra: superior view

Anterior tubercle
Body
Posterior tubercle
Lamina

Uncus (uncinate process)
Interarticular part
Zygapophyseal joint
Intervertebral foramen for spinal nerve

C3
C4
C5

3rd, 4th, and 5th cervical vertebrae: anterior view

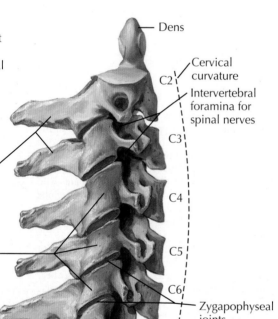

Spinous processes

Articular pillar formed by articular processes and interarticular parts

Dens
Cervical curvature
Intervertebral foramina for spinal nerves
C2
C3
C4
C5
C6
Zygapophyseal joints
Intervertebral joint (symphysis) (*disk removed*)
Costal facets (for 1st rib)
C7
T1

2nd cervical to 1st thoracic vertebrae: right lateral view

CERVICAL VERTEBRAE

The first two cervical vertebrae, the atlas and the axis, are illustrated in Plate 3.2. The other five (C3–7) show the general vertebral features, but cervical vertebrae are easily distinguishable by the presence of foramina in their transverse processes, which (except in the case of a seventh vertebra) transmit the vertebral vessels and nerves (see Plate 3.2).

The cervical *vertebral bodies* are smaller than those of the other movable vertebrae and increase in size from above downward. The superior body surfaces are concave from side to side and slightly convex from front to back, whereas the inferior surfaces are reciprocally curved or saddle shaped.

The cervical spinal canal is comparatively large to accommodate the cervical enlargement of the spinal cord; they are bounded by the bodies, pedicles, and laminae of the vertebrae. The *pedicles* project postero-laterally from the bodies and are grooved by superior and inferior vertebral notches of almost equal depth, which form the intervertebral foramina by connecting with similar notches on adjacent vertebrae. The medi-ally directed *laminae* are thin and relatively long and fuse posteriorly to form short, bifid *spinous processes*. Projecting laterally from the junction of the pedicles and laminae are articular pillars supporting *superior* and *inferior articular facets*.

Each *transverse process* is pierced by a foramen, bounded by narrow bony bars ending in anterior and posterior tubercles; these are interconnected lateral to the

foramen by the so-called *costotransverse bar*. Only the medial part of the posterior bar represents the true trans-verse process; the anterior and costotransverse bars and the lateral portion of the posterior bar constitute the costal element. These elements, especially in the seventh and/or sixth cervical vertebrae, may develop abnormally to form cervical ribs. The upper surfaces of the costo-transverse bars are grooved and lodge the anterior pri-mary rami of the spinal nerves. The anterior tubercles of the sixth cervical vertebra are large and are termed the

carotid tubercles because the common carotid arteries lie just anteriorly and can be compressed against them.

The seventh cervical vertebra is called the *vertebra prominens* because its spinous process is long and ends in a tubercle that is easily palpable at the lower end of the nuchal furrow; the spinous process of the first tho-racic vertebra is just as prominent. The seventh cervical vertebra sometimes lacks a transverse foramen on one or both sides; when present, the foramina transmit only small accessory vertebral veins.

Plate 3.4

Spinal Trauma

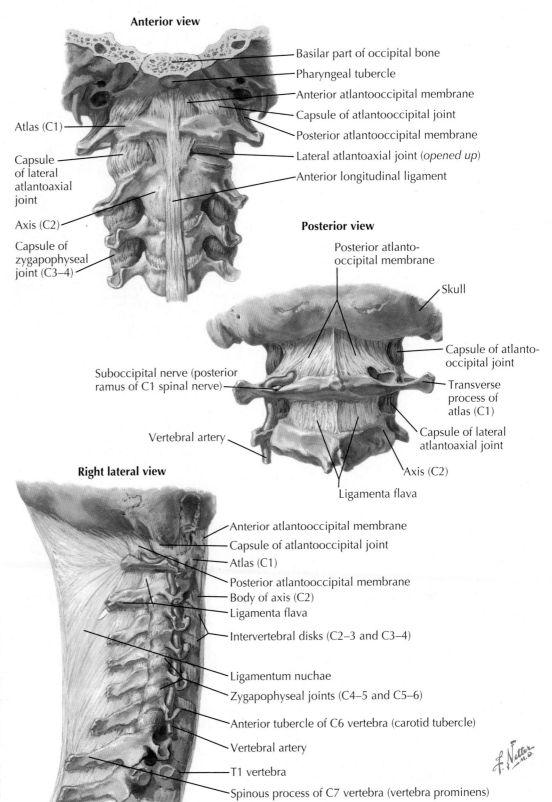

Anterior view

Basilar part of occipital bone
Pharyngeal tubercle
Anterior atlantooccipital membrane
Capsule of atlantooccipital joint
Atlas (C1)
Posterior atlantooccipital membrane
Lateral atlantoaxial joint (*opened up*)
Capsule of lateral atlantoaxial joint
Anterior longitudinal ligament
Axis (C2)
Capsule of zygapophyseal joint (C3–4)

Posterior view

Posterior atlanto-occipital membrane
Skull
Capsule of atlanto-occipital joint
Suboccipital nerve (posterior ramus of C1 spinal nerve)
Transverse process of atlas (C1)
Vertebral artery
Capsule of lateral atlantoaxial joint
Axis (C2)
Ligamenta flava

Right lateral view

Anterior atlantooccipital membrane
Capsule of atlantooccipital joint
Atlas (C1)
Posterior atlantooccipital membrane
Body of axis (C2)
Ligamenta flava
Intervertebral disks (C2–3 and C3–4)
Ligamentum nuchae
Zygapophyseal joints (C4–5 and C5–6)
Anterior tubercle of C6 vertebra (carotid tubercle)
Vertebral artery
T1 vertebra
Spinous process of C7 vertebra (vertebra prominens)

EXTERNAL CRANIOCERVICAL LIGAMENTS

The ligaments uniting the cranium, atlas, and axis allow free movement of the head, and extra security is provided by the action of the surrounding muscles. Ligaments best seen from the external aspect are shown in Plate 3.4.

The *anterior atlantooccipital membrane* is a wide, dense, fibroelastic band extending between the anterior margin of the foramen magnum and the upper border of the anterior arch of the atlas. Laterally, it is continuous with the articular capsules of the atlantooccipital joints. In the midline, it is reinforced by the upward continuation of the anterior longitudinal ligament.

The *posterior atlantooccipital membrane* is broader and thinner than the anterior one and connects the posterior margin of the foramen magnum with the upper border of the posterior arch of the atlas. On each side, it arches over the groove for the vertebral artery, leaving an opening for the upward passage of the artery and the outward passage of the first cervical spinal nerve.

Articular capsules surround the joints between the occipital condyles and the superior atlantal facets. The capsules are rather loose, allowing nodding movements of the head, and are thin medially; laterally, they are thickened and form the *lateral atlantooccipital ligaments*, which limit lateral tilting of the head.

The *anterior longitudinal ligament* extends from the base of the skull to the sacrum. Its uppermost part

reinforces the anterior atlantooccipital membrane in the midline. The part between the anterior tubercle of the atlas and the anterior median ridge on the axis may have lateral extensions—the *atlantoaxial ligaments*.

The *ligamentum nuchae* is a dense fibroelastic membrane stretching from the external occipital protuberance and crest to the posterior tubercle of the atlas and the spinous processes of all the other cervical vertebrae. It provides areas for muscular attachments and

forms a midline septum between the posterior cervical muscles. The ligamentum nuchae is better developed in quadrupeds than in humans.

The *ligamenta flava* contain a high proportion of yellow elastic fibers and connect the laminae of adjacent vertebrae. They are present between the posterior arch of the atlas and the laminae of the axis but absent between the atlas and skull.

Intervertebral disks are lacking between the occiput and atlas and between the atlas and axis.

Upper part of vertebral canal with spinous processes and parts of vertebral arches removed to expose ligaments on posterior vertebral bodies: posterior view

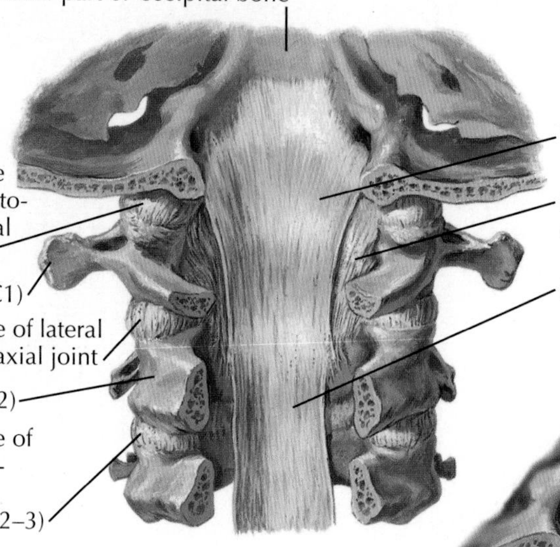

Clivus (surface feature) of basilar part of occipital bone

Tectorial membrane

Capsule of atlanto-occipital joint

Deeper (accessory) part of tectorial membrane

Atlas (C1)

Posterior longitudinal ligament

Capsule of lateral atlantoaxial joint

Axis (C2)

Capsule of zygapophyseal joint (C2–3)

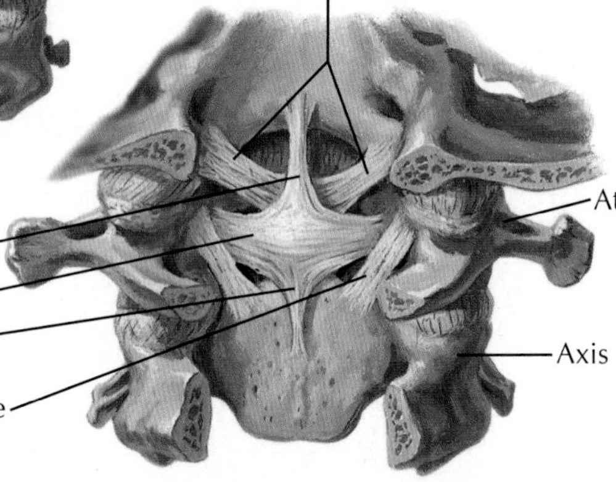

Alar ligaments

Cruciate ligament {
Superior longitudinal band
Transverse ligament of atlas
Inferior longitudinal band
}

Atlas (C1)

Axis (C2)

Deeper (accessory) part of tectorial membrane

Principal part of tectorial membrane removed to expose deeper ligaments: posterior view

Atlas (C1)

Apical ligament of dens

Alar ligament

Posterior articular facet of dens (for transverse ligament of atlas)

Axis (C2)

Anterior tubercle of atlas

Alar ligament

Synovial cavities

Dens

Transverse ligament of atlas

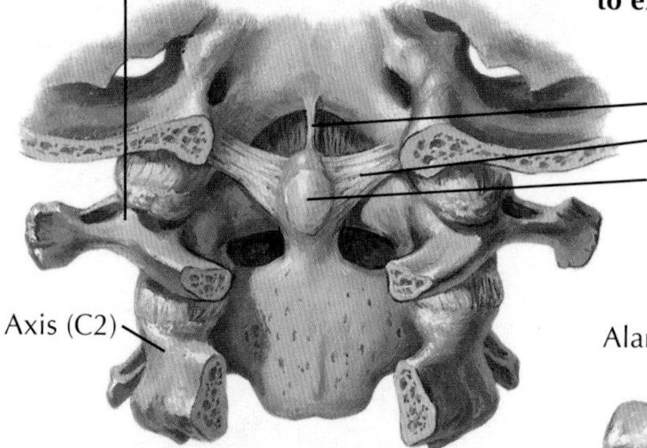

Cruciate ligament removed to show deepest ligaments: posterior view

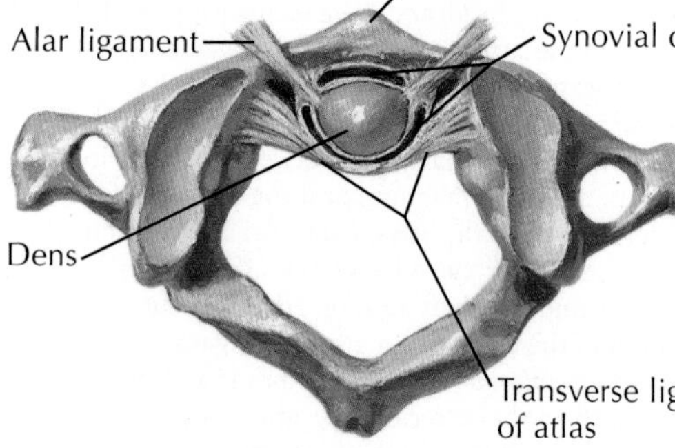

Median atlantoaxial joint: superior view

INTERNAL CRANIOCERVICAL LIGAMENTS

The ligaments on the posterior aspects of the vertebral bodies contribute added strength to the craniocervical region, and some are specifically arranged to check excessive movements, such as rotation at the median and lateral atlantoaxial joints.

The broad, strong *tectorial membrane* lies within the vertebral canal. It prolongs the *posterior longitudinal ligament* upward from the posterior surface of the body of the axis to the anterior and anterolateral margins of the foramen magnum, where it blends with the dura mater. It covers the dens and its ligaments and gives added protection to the junctional area between the medulla oblongata and spinal cord.

The *median atlantoaxial pivot joint* lies between the dens of the axis and the ring formed by the anterior arch and transverse ligament of the atlas (see Plate 3.2).

The *transverse ligament of the atlas* is a strong band passing horizontally behind the dens and attached on each side to a tubercle on the medial side of the lateral mass of the atlas. From its midpoint, bands pass vertically upward and downward to become fixed, respectively, to the basilar part of the occipital bone between the tectorial membrane and the apical ligament of the dens and to the posterior surface of the body of the

axis: the *superior* and *inferior longitudinal fascicles.* These transverse and vertical bands together form the *cruciform ligament.*

The *apical ligament* is a slender cord connecting the apex of the dens to the anterior midpoint of the foramen magnum, lying between the anterior atlantooccipital membrane and the upper limb of the cruciform ligament.

The *alar ligaments* are two fibrous bands stretching upward and outward from the superolateral aspects of the dens to the medial sides of the occipital condyles.

They check excessive rotation at the median atlantooccipital joint.

Lateral atlantoaxial joints are formed between the almost-flat inferior articular facets on the lateral masses of the atlas and the superior articular facets of the axis. They are synovial joints with thin, loose articular capsules. An *accessory ligament* extends from near the base of the dens to the lateral mass of the atlas, close to the attachment of the transverse ligament. It assists the alar ligaments in restricting atlantoaxial rotation.

Plate 3.6

Spinal Trauma

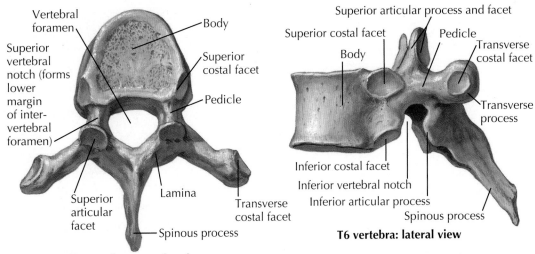

Vertebral foramen — Body

Superior vertebral notch (forms lower margin of intervertebral foramen)

Superior costal facet

Pedicle

Superior articular facet

Lamina

Spinous process

Transverse costal facet

T6 vertebra: superior view

Superior articular process and facet

Superior costal facet

Body

Pedicle

Transverse costal facet

Transverse process

Inferior costal facet

Inferior vertebral notch

Inferior articular process

Spinous process

T6 vertebra: lateral view

THORACIC VERTEBRAE

The 12 thoracic vertebrae are intermediate in size between the smaller cervical and larger lumbar vertebrae. The *vertebral bodies* are heart shaped and are slightly deeper posteriorly than anteriorly. They are easily recognized by costal facets on both sides of the bodies and on all the transverse processes (except those of the eleventh and twelfth thoracic vertebrae), which articulate, respectively, with facets on the heads and tubercles of the corresponding ribs.

The *spinal canal* is smaller and more rounded than those in the cervical region and conform to the reduced size and more circular shape of the spinal cord in the thoracic region. They are bounded by the posterior surfaces of the vertebral bodies and by the pedicles and laminae forming the vertebral arches. The stout *pedicles* are directed backward; they have very shallow superior and much deeper inferior vertebral notches. The *laminae* are short, relatively thick, and partly overlap each other from above downward. The typical thoracic *superior articular processes* project upward from the junctions of the pedicles and laminae, and their facets slant backward and slightly upward and outward. The *inferior articular processes* project downward from the anterior parts of the laminae, and their facets face forward and slightly downward and inward. The processes and facets in the cervicothoracic and thoracolumbar junctional areas show gradual transitional changes.

Most of the thoracic *spinous processes* are long and are inclined downward and backward. Those of the upper and lower thoracic vertebrae are more horizontal. The *transverse processes* are also relatively long and extend posterolaterally from the junctions of the pedicles and laminae. Except for those of the lowest two or, occasionally, three thoracic vertebrae, the transverse processes have small oval facets near their tips, which articulate with similar facets on the corresponding rib tubercles.

Adjacent vertebral bodies are connected by *intervertebral disks* and by *anterior* and *posterior longitudinal ligaments*; the transverse processes, by *intertransverse ligaments*; the laminae, by *ligamenta flava*; and the spinous processes, by *supraspinal* and *interspinal ligaments*. The joints between the articular processes are surrounded by fibrous *articular capsules*.

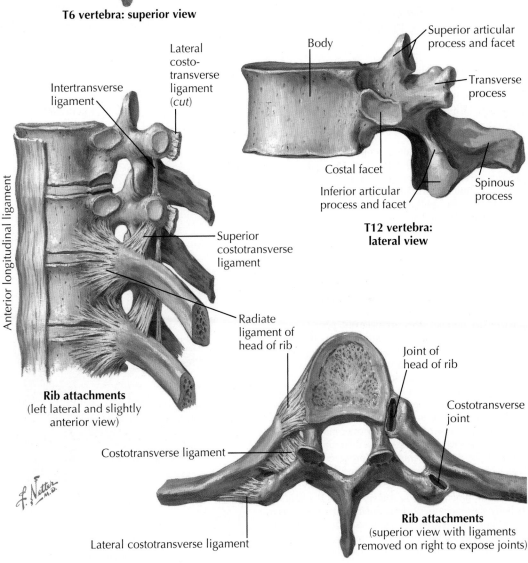

Anterior longitudinal ligament

Intertransverse ligament

Lateral costotransverse ligament (*cut*)

Superior costotransverse ligament

Radiate ligament of head of rib

Rib attachments
(left lateral and slightly anterior view)

Body

Superior articular process and facet

Transverse process

Costal facet

Inferior articular process and facet

Spinous process

T12 vertebra: lateral view

Joint of head of rib

Costotransverse joint

Costotransverse ligament

Lateral costotransverse ligament

Rib attachments
(superior view with ligaments removed on right to expose joints)

COSTOVERTEBRAL JOINTS

The ribs are connected to the vertebral bodies and transverse processes by various ligaments. The *costocentral joints* between the bodies and rib heads have *articular capsules,* and the second to tenth costal heads, each of which articulates with two vertebrae, are connected to the corresponding intervertebral disks by *intra-articular ligaments. Radiate (stellate) ligaments* unite the anterior aspects of the rib heads with the sides of the vertebral bodies above and below, and with the intervening disks.

The *costotransverse joints* between the facets on the transverse processes and on the tubercles of the ribs are also surrounded by *articular capsules.* They are reinforced by a (middle) *costotransverse ligament* between the rib neck and the adjoining transverse process, a *superior costotransverse ligament* between the rib neck and the transverse process of the vertebra above, and a *lateral costotransverse ligament* interconnecting the end of a transverse process to the nonarticular part of the related costal tubercle.

Vertebral body
Vertebral foramen
Pedicle
Transverse process
Mammillary process
Superior articular process
Lamina
Spinous process
Accessory process

L2 vertebra: superior view

Annulus fibrosus
Nucleus pulposus

Intervertebral disk

LUMBAR VERTEBRAE AND INTERVERTEBRAL DISKS

The five lumbar vertebrae are the largest in the spine. The *vertebral bodies* are wider from side to side than from front to back, and the upper and lower surfaces are kidney shaped and almost parallel, except in the case of the fifth vertebral body, which is slightly wedge shaped.

The *pedicles* are short and strong and arise from the upper and posterolateral aspects of the bodies; the superior vertebral notches are therefore less deep than the inferior notches. The *laminae* are short, broad plates that meet in the midline to form the quadrangular and almost horizontal *spinous processes*. The intervals between adjacent laminae and spinous processes are relatively wide.

The *articular processes* project vertically upward and downward from the junctional areas between the pedicles and the laminae. The superior facets are gently concave and face posteromedially to embrace the inferior facets of the vertebra above, which are curved and disposed in a reciprocal fashion. This arrangement permits some flexion and extension but very little rotation. The *transverse processes* of the upper three lumbar vertebrae are long and slender, whereas those of the fourth, and especially of the fifth, are more pyramidal.

Near the roots of each transverse process are small *accessory processes*; other small, rounded *mammillary processes* protrude from the posterior margins of the superior articular processes. The former may represent the true transverse processes (or their tips) because many of the so-called transverse processes are really costal elements. In the first lumbar vertebra, these elements occasionally develop into lumbar ribs.

The *fifth lumbar vertebra* is atypical. It is the largest, its body is deeper anteriorly, its inferior articular facets face almost forward and are set more widely apart, and the roots of its stumpy transverse processes are continuous with the posterolateral parts of the body and with the entire lateral surfaces of the pedicles.

The *intervertebral disks* are interposed between the adjacent vertebral bodies from the axis to the sacrum and are immensely strong fibrocartilaginous structures that provide powerful bonds and elastic buffers. They consist of outer concentric layers of fibrous tissue—the *annulus fibrosus* (the fibers in adjacent layers are arranged obliquely but in opposite directions, to assist in resisting torsion)—and a central springy, pulpy zone, the *nucleus pulposus*. The blood and nerve supplies to the disks are inconspicuous. If the annular fibers give way as a result of injury or disease, the enclosed turgid

Vertebral canal
Superior articular process
Mammillary process
Transverse process
Pars inter-articularis
Accessory process
Spinous process of L3 vertebra
Vertebral body
Lamina
Inferior articular process

L3 and L4 vertebrae: posterior view

Superior articular process
Transverse process
Mammillary process
Pedicle
Inferior articular process
Spinous process
Vertebral body
Intervertebral disk
Inferior vertebral notch
Intervertebral (neural) foramen
Superior vertebral notch
Lamina
Articular facet for sacrum

Lumbar vertebrae, assembled: left lateral view

nucleus pulposus may prolapse and press on related nervous and vascular structures.

In health and maturity, the intervertebral disks account for almost 25% of the length of the vertebral column; they are thinnest in the upper thoracic region and thickest in the lumbar region. In the vertical section, the lumbar disks are rather wedge shaped, with the thicker edge anteriorly. The forward convexity of the lumbar spine is due more to the shape of the disks than to disparities between the anterior and posterior depths

of the lumbar vertebrae. The more defined wedge shape of the lumbosacral disk helps to minimize the effects of the marked lumbosacral angulation.

As age advances, the nucleus pulposus undergoes changes: its water content decreases, its mucoid matrix is gradually replaced by fibrocartilage, and it ultimately comes to resemble the annulus fibrosus. The resultant loss of depth in each disk is small, but overall it may amount to a decrease of 2 to 3 cm in the height of the spinal column.

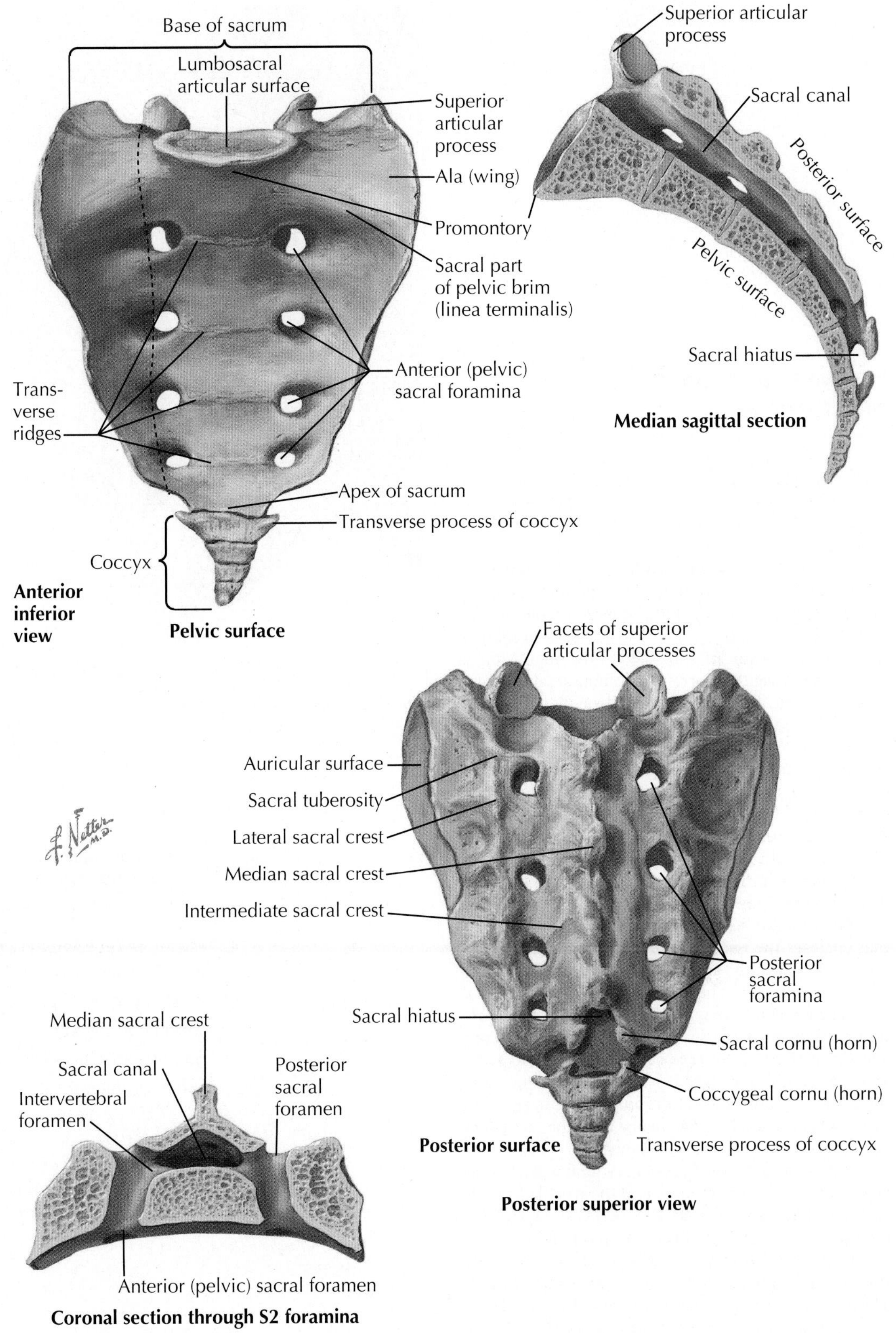

Plate 3.8

Spinal Trauma

Base of sacrum

Lumbosacral
articular surface

Superior
articular
process

Ala (wing)

Promontory

Sacral part
of pelvic brim
(linea terminalis)

Anterior (pelvic)
sacral foramina

Trans-
verse
ridges

Apex of sacrum

Transverse process of coccyx

Coccyx

**Anterior
inferior
view**

Pelvic surface

Superior articular
process

Sacral canal

Posterior surface

Pelvic surface

Sacral hiatus

Median sagittal section

SACRUM AND COCCYX

The *sacrum* consists of five fused vertebrae and is wedge shaped from above down and from front to back. It forms most of the posterior pelvic wall and is fixed between the hip bones at an angle so that its curved pelvic surface is inclined downward and forward.

The broader *base* of the sacrum faces anterosuperiorly toward the abdomen; its elevated central third is the upper part of the first sacral vertebral body and bears a smooth oval area for the attachment of the lumbosacral intervertebral disk. Its projecting anterior border is the sacral *promontory.* On each side, the costotransverse elements of the first vertebra are fused to form a wing-shaped lateral mass (sacral *ala*), separated from the pelvic surface by a curved line, which is the sacral portion of the arcuate pelvic brim. The articular processes are fused, like most of the other components of the sacral vertebrae, but the *superior articular processes* of the first vertebra remain and project upward for articulation with the inferior articular processes of the fifth lumbar vertebra. They are flattened and face almost directly backward to assist in preventing subluxation (spondylolisthesis) of the last lumbar vertebra at the angulated lumbosacral junction.

The narrow *apex* is the lower end of the sacrum and articulates with the coccyx. The pelvic surface is concave both vertically and horizontally and shows four *transverse ridges* indicating the lines of fusion between the bodies of the original five vertebrae. On either side of the ridges, four *pelvic sacral foramina* permit the passage of the anterior rami of the first four sacral nerves and their associated vessels.

The convex posterior surface shows irregular *median, intermediate,* and *lateral sacral crests* representing, respectively, the fused spinous, articular, and transverse processes. The areas between the median and intermediate crests are the fused laminae, and there are four pairs of *posterior sacral foramina* for the passage of the posterior rami of the upper four sacral nerves. The laminae of the fifth and, occasionally, the fourth vertebra fail to unite and thus leave a *hiatus,* which is exploited for the injection of epidural anesthetics. The hiatus is bounded on each side by a *cornu,* a relic of the inferior articular process, and transmits the small fifth sacral and coccygeal nerves.

The parts of the sacrum lateral to the sacral foramina are produced by the fusion of the costal, transverse, and

Facets of superior
articular processes

Auricular surface

Sacral tuberosity

Lateral sacral crest

Median sacral crest

Intermediate sacral crest

Sacral hiatus

Posterior
sacral
foramina

Sacral cornu (horn)

Coccygeal cornu (horn)

Posterior surface

Transverse process of coccyx

Posterior superior view

Median sacral crest

Sacral canal

Intervertebral
foramen

Posterior
sacral
foramen

Anterior (pelvic) sacral foramen

Coronal section through S2 foramina

pedicular elements of the five vertebrae. The upper, broader parts of their lateral surfaces bear uneven *auricular,* or ear-shaped, surfaces for articulation with similar surfaces on the iliac parts of the hip bones. This canal surrounds and protects the terminations of the dural and arachnoid sheaths and the subarachnoid space, which end at about the level of the second sacral vertebra and enclose the sacral and coccygeal roots of the cauda equina and the lower intrathecal portion of the filum terminale. The dura mater is separated from the walls of the canal

by fibrofatty tissue, fine arteries, and nerves and sacral internal vertebral venous plexuses.

COCCYX

The small, triangular coccyx is formed by the fusion of four (occasionally, three or five) rudimentary tail vertebrae. Its base articulates with the sacral apex, and its apex is a mere button of bone. Most of the features of a typical vertebra are lacking.

LIGAMENTS OF SACRUM AND COCCYX

Because the lumbosacral and sacroiliac joints transmit the entire weight of the body to the hip bones and thence to the lower limbs, their ligaments are most important.

The *lumbosacral junction* is mechanically imperfect because of its angulation and the consequent sloping platform provided for the fifth lumbar vertebra by the first sacral vertebra (Plate 3.9). The tendency to subluxation (spondylolisthesis) is resisted by the impingement of the almost sagittally arranged lumbosacral articular processes, and this bony check is strongly augmented by the last *intervertebral disk,* the *anterior* and *posterior longitudinal ligaments,* the *ligamenta flava,* and the *supraspinal* and *interspinal ligaments.* These ligaments are further reinforced by the erector spinae and other muscles and by the *iliolumbar ligaments,* which are strong bands uniting the transverse processes of the fourth and fifth lumbar vertebrae and the posterior parts of the iliac crests and sacral alae. The iliolumbar ligaments are really the expanded lower margins of the anterior and middle layers of the thoracolumbar fascia that encloses the quadratus lumborum muscles. They blend below with the anterior sacroiliac ligaments.

The *sacroiliac joints* between the auricular surfaces of the sacrum and ilia are synovial in type. Movements are limited, however, because of the interlocking elevations and depressions on the opposed articular surfaces, the way the sacrum is wedged between the hip bones, and the restraining influence of the anterior, posterior, and interosseous sacroiliac ligaments and the accessory sacrotuberal and sacrospinal ligaments.

The *anterior sacroiliac ligament* is a thin, wide, fibrous layer reinforcing the anterior part of the articular capsule and stretching from the ala and pelvic surface of the sacrum to the adjoining parts of the iliac bone.

The *posterior sacroiliac ligament* consists of more superficial, longer bundles and deeper, shorter bundles. The fibers of the long posterior sacroiliac ligament interconnect the posterior superior iliac spine and the lateral parts of the third and fourth sacral segments; its outer fibers interdigitate with those of the sacrotuberal ligament. The short posterior sacroiliac ligament interconnects the medial surface of the iliac bone to the lateral parts of the first and second sacral segments and is often considered to be a part of the interosseous ligament.

The *interosseous sacroiliac ligament* is formed by short, thick bundles of fibers interconnecting the sacral and iliac tuberosities—the rough areas behind and above the auricular surfaces of both bones. It is the most powerful bond between the bones and, indeed, is one of the strongest ligaments in the body. It lies deep

to the posterior sacroiliac ligament and is not shown in Plate 3.9.

The *sacrotuberal* and *sacrospinal ligaments* act as accessory ligaments of the sacroiliac joints because they assist in regulating joint movements. The downward thrust at the lumbosacral junction tends to push the upper part of the sacrum down, with coincident upward tilting of its lower part as the sacrum seesaws on a transverse axis through the middle of the sacroiliac joints. The illustration shows how these accessory

ligaments anchor the lower sacrum and coccyx to the ischial tuberosity and spine, thus limiting the seesaw movement.

The *sacrum* and *coccyx* are connected by a small, fibrocartilaginous *intervertebral disk* and by thin bands on the anterior, posterior, and lateral sides of the junction: the *anterior, posterior,* and *lateral sacrococcygeal ligaments.* The posterior ligament has a superficial part, which partly fills in the sacral hiatus, and a deep part, which represents the posterior spinal longitudinal ligament.

Posterior view labels
- Iliolumbar ligament
- Iliac crest
- Supraspinous ligament
- Posterior superior iliac spine
- Posterior sacroiliac ligaments
- Iliac tubercle
- Posterior sacral foramina
- Greater sciatic foramen
- Anterior superior iliac spine
- Sacrospinous ligament
- Sacrotuberous ligament
- Lesser sciatic foramen
- Acetabular margin
- Ischial tuberosity
- Tendon of long head of biceps femoris muscle
- Deep } Posterior sacrococcygeal ligaments
- Superficial }
- Lateral sacrococcygeal ligament

Posterior view

Anterior view labels
- Anterior longitudinal ligament
- Sacral promontory
- Iliolumbar ligament
- Anterior sacroiliac ligament
- Iliac fossa
- Iliac crest { Outer lip / Intermediate zone / Iliac tubercle / Inner lip }
- Anterior sacral foramina
- Greater sciatic foramen
- Anterior superior iliac spine
- Sacrotuberous ligament
- Sacrospinous ligament
- Anterior inferior iliac spine
- Ischial spine
- Arcuate line
- Lesser sciatic foramen
- Iliopectineal line
- Iliopubic eminence
- Superior pubic ramus
- Pecten pubis (pectineal line)
- Obturator foramen
- Ischiopubic ramus
- Pubic tubercle
- Anterior sacrococcygeal ligaments
- Coccyx
- Pubic symphysis

Anterior view

F. Netter m.d.

Plate 3.10

Spinal Trauma

Mechanism

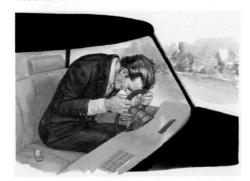

Head-on collision with stationary or moving object. Occupant not restrained by seat belt: head strikes steering wheel, windshield, or roof. Head hyper-flexed on trunk.

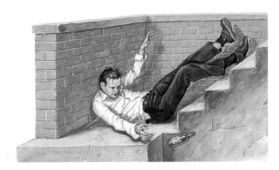

Blow to back of head from falling against hard surface when balance is compromised

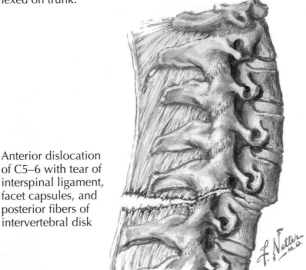

Anterior dislocation of C5–6 with tear of interspinal ligament, facet capsules, and posterior fibers of intervertebral disk

X-ray film (lateral view) showing bilateral interfacet dislocation at C5–6

BIOMECHANICS OF SPINE AND SPINAL CORD INJURIES: DISTRACTIVE FLEXION

Distractive flexion refers to acute, severe flexion of the neck with associated rotation and is one of the most commonly seen spinal injuries. The posterior ligaments are injured initially, manifested as a widening of the distance between two spinous processes. With increasing degrees of force, the facet capsules are disrupted, and there is shearing through the posterior longitudinal ligament, the disk space, and the anterior longitudinal ligament.

In the first phase of injury, the posterior ligaments fail, allowing the facets to displace anteriorly. In the second phase, there is unilateral facet dislocation as the interspinous ligament, facet capsule, and posterior longitudinal ligaments give way. With further force, the second facet capsule ruptures and bilateral facet dislocation occurs.

Approximately one-third of spinal cord injuries occur as a result of distractive flexion forces, and the injuries are typically complete, especially with bilateral facet dislocation (see Plates 2.16–2.20).

Radiographically, unilateral or bilateral facet dislocations are typical, with associated vertebral body subluxation. The difference between these injuries is readily distinguishable radiographically. With a unilateral facet dislocation, there is approximately 25% anterior subluxation of one vertebral body on another. With bilateral facet dislocation, there is greater than 50% anterior subluxation. These injuries are generally highly unstable, are associated with significant neurologic deficits, and commonly require internal reduction and stabilization.

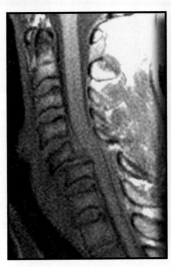

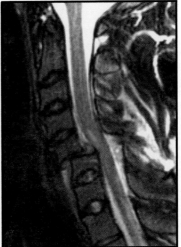

MRI of the cervical spine demonstrating subluxation of C4–6 consistent with bilateral facet dislocation. There is an associated small acute traumatic disk herniation as well as hyperintense signal cord at the level of the injury.

Traction will usually reduce a unilateral facet dislocation. If there are fractures of the facet, once realignment has been accomplished, treatment with a halo may allow for stable healing. Bilateral locked facets are rarely reduced with traction and can be treated through an anterior or posterior surgical approach. On occasion, both anterior and posterior surgical approaches are required to achieve reduction and stabilization.

There is, however, one significant caveat in the use of traction with facet dislocations. It has been reported that up to 25% of these patients will have an associated traumatic herniated disk at the level of injury. Realigning the spine in the face of an anterior compressive mass, such as a traumatic herniated disk, could potentially result in additional spinal cord compression and further spinal cord injury (SCI). It has thus been recommended that patients with facet dislocations and an incomplete SCI syndrome undergo magnetic resonance imaging (MRI) to look for a traumatic herniated disk before realignment is attempted.

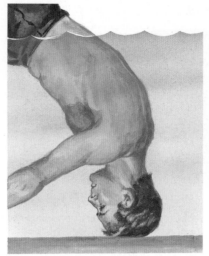

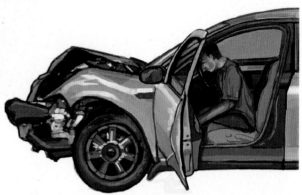

Mechanism. Vertical blow on head as in diving or surfing accident, being thrown from car, or football injury.

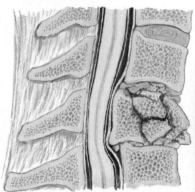

Burst fracture with characteristic vertical fracture through vertebral body

Radiograph showing fracture of C5

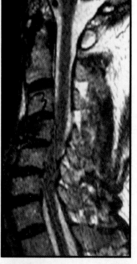

Sagittal MRI of a C4 burst fracture showing swelling of the spinal cord from C4–6

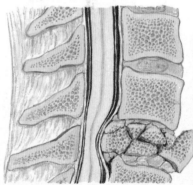

More severe trauma explodes vertebral body. Posteriorly displaced bone fragments frequently produce spinal cord injury.

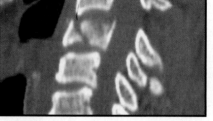

Sagittal reconstructed CT in a patient with a C4 burst fracture demonstrating an anterior fracture line with retropulsion of bone into the spinal canal

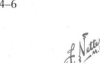

BIOMECHANICS OF SPINE AND SPINAL CORD INJURIES: COMPRESSIVE FLEXION

Compressive flexion injuries occur when there is a combination of axial loading (vertical compression) associated with acute severe flexion of the neck. Such an injury may occur in patients diving into shallow water or being thrown from a moving vehicle. With lesser degrees of force, there is typically only compression of the anterior aspect of a vertebral body; however, as the forces increase, the vertebral body "bursts," and retropulsion of bony fragments into the spinal canal results in severe neurologic injury.

Initially, as force is progressively applied, there is blunting of the anterosuperior aspect of the vertebral body, with the subsequent development of oblique fracture lines through the centrum of the body. Eventually, there is fragmentation of the centrum with peripheral displacement of the bony fragments.

This biomechanical mechanism reinforces the three-column theory of spinal stability. The anterior column extends from the anterior longitudinal ligament to the midpoint of the vertebral body. The middle column includes the posterior half of the vertebral body and the posterior longitudinal ligament. The posterior column includes pedicles, lamina, facets, and spinous processes along with all supporting ligaments. Any injury involving two of the three columns is generally unstable.

Compressive failure of the anterior aspect of the vertebral body rarely leads to neurologic injury.

However, with ligamentous failure and posterior movement of the vertebral body, the incidence of complete SCI significantly increases (see Plates 2.16–2.20). Approximately one-third of spine injuries result from compressive flexion, with a high occurrence at the midcervical levels.

Traction is rarely indicated unless there is an associated facet dislocation or other injury that might be amenable to realignment. An MRI scan will clearly show the degree and extent of spinal canal compromise as well as blood and/or edema within the spinal cord.

Compressive flexion injuries comprise approximately one-third of cervical spine injuries and most commonly occur at the C4–5 and C5–6 levels.

Anterior vertebral body compression and minor burst fractures may be treated with external orthoses such as the halo. These types of fractures will heal stably in more than 70% of patients. Burst fractures with greater than 3 mm retropulsion and significant canal compromise usually require anterior and, on occasion, posterior operative decompression and stabilization as well. Such is also the case if there has been significant associated ligamentous disruption.

Plate 3.12

Spinal Trauma

Individual (usually elderly) falls forward, striking chin or face, causing forceful hyperextension and backward thrust of neck

Osteophytes compressing spinal cord. Hyperextension injury results in cord contusion, self-destructive edema, and intramedullary hemorrhage with rapidly developing quadriplegia.

Radiograph (lateral view) showing osteophytes

Typical CT findings in a patient with central cord syndrome. On axial view the spinal canal is reduced to 7 mm (normal, 15 mm) by a large osteophyte.

Lower limb
Trunk
Upper limb

Section of cervical spinal cord showing orientation of fibers in lateral corticospinal tracts

F. Netter M.D.

Central cord syndrome. Central hemorrhage may damage medial part of lateral corticospinal tract and anterior horn cells, resulting in paralysis of upper limbs, leaving lower limbs intact.

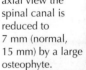
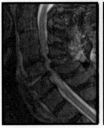
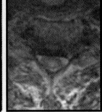

Sagittal *(left)* and axial *(right)* MRIs in a patient with central cord injury. Although there is no acute traumatic injury, the spinal canal is significantly narrowed at C4–6 by anterior osteophytes and posterior in-buckling of the ligamentum flavum.

Biomechanics of Spine and Spinal Cord Injuries: Distractive Extension

Distractive extension injury occurs with acute hyperextension of the spine. In its most minor form, this is termed a "whiplash" injury. In its more severe form, a common scenario for such an injury is the elderly patient with preexisting cervical spondylosis or stenosis who falls, striking the forehead. There is usually no traumatic radiographic abnormality. The spinal cord is pinched between the anterior osteophytes and the in-buckled ligamentum flavum. There are varying degrees of associated injury, including central cord syndrome (see Plates 2.16–2.20). The vertebral injury is rarely unstable, but surgical intervention may be indicated to improve neurologic recovery.

In its more severe forms, the forces producing distractive flexion result in progressive anterior to posterior ligament failure in one or more cervical motion segments. With complete ligamentous failure, the upper vertebrae displace posteriorly, creating significant spinal canal narrowing. When there is no significant bony injury, the ligamentous disruption may be very difficult to detect. With patients in the neutral position, there may very well be no subluxation. Thus MRI is strongly indicated when this mechanism of injury is suspected.

This type of injury pattern occurs in only 1% to 5% of all spine injuries.

COMPRESSIVE EXTENSION

Compressive extension involves axial loading in association with hyperextension. This may produce injuries as minor as a laminar fracture or as severe as the highly unstable "teardrop" fracture. In the latter, the anterior longitudinal ligament is ruptured, avulsing a small bone fragment from the superior aspect of a vertebral body and causing fractures of the lateral masses, pedicles, and lamina.

As force progressively increases, there may be a linear fracture through the facet in association with a pedicle and laminar fracture, bilateral posterior arch fractures, and ultimately ligamentous injury may occur. Most unstable fractures occur at the C6–7 level and account for fewer than 5% of spine injuries.

A comparative study was undertaken of patients with distractive flexion and compressive extension cervical spine injuries. There was no significant difference with respect to severity of injury, level of injury, or neurologic sequelae. Sixteen percent of patients with either type of injury had complete SCI.

CERVICAL SPINE INJURY: PREHOSPITAL, EMERGENCY DEPARTMENT, AND ACUTE MANAGEMENT

PREHOSPITAL MANAGEMENT

Spinal injury may lead to neurologic impairment from *spinal cord involvement*. Initial management of a patient suspected of having an SCI begins at the accident scene, with early, aggressive resuscitation and spinal immobilization. Altered mental status, focal neurologic deficits, intoxication, spinal pain or tenderness, and/or distracting injuries are all potential risk factors for SCI (see Plates 2.16–2.20) and indications for immobilization. Up to 10% of spinal cord injuries occur after the initial traumatic injury, during extrication, transport, or early in the course of management.

The entire spinal column is at risk; 15% of fractures are multiple and involve different spinal segments. The cervical spine can be partially immobilized by a hard cervical collar, but the efficacy of a collar is limited unless used with a hard, full-length backboard. A wide variety of hard cervical collars are available; superiority of one over another has not been shown. Immobilizing the cervical spine is accomplished by simultaneous control of head and trunk motion. This is most reliably accomplished by combining a hard cervical collar with a full-length backboard. Bolsters (or, alternatively, sandbags) on either side of the neck, secured by straps (or tape) across the head, maximally limit movement of the neck; strapping the rest of the body to the backboard prevents truncal movement. This appears to provide the safest and most effective method of spine immobilization for transport.

Airway protection is paramount. If intubation is necessary, in-line cervical traction with efforts to minimize cervical extension should be undertaken, if possible. Immobilization precautions must be taken until spinal injury can be excluded or more definitive spine treatment initiated. It is important, however, to remove the backboard as soon as possible, keeping the patient on a firm padded surface while maintaining spinal alignment. In an insensate patient with SCI, skin breakdown, leading to decubitus ulcers, can begin within 2 hours of lying on a hard backboard. When transfers are necessary, the technique of logrolling should be used to maintain spinal alignment.

In certain patients with preexisting spinal deformities, providing care in the position of greatest comfort for the patient may take precedence over maximum spinal stabilization.

EMERGENCY DEPARTMENT AND ACUTE MANAGEMENT

Initially, it is important to follow advanced trauma life support (ATLS) evaluation and resuscitation protocols, determine the degree and extent of neurologic loss, and prevent any further loss of function. This is accomplished by ensuring an adequate airway and oxygenation; establishing and maintaining a systolic blood pressure greater than 90 mm Hg; conducting serial complete neurologic examinations, spinal alignment, and radiographic identification of the degree and extent of spinal column injury; and ensuring acute stabilization.

The most widely used neurologic examination protocol is that of the American Spinal Injury Association

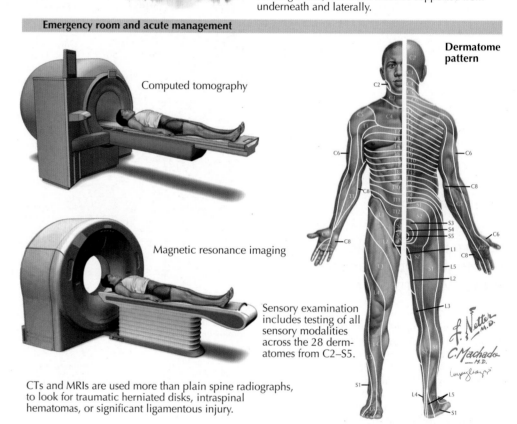

Treatment at site of accident

Patient's head is held securely between attendant's elbow, and shoulders are supported by attendant's hands during lift. Cervical collar applied before lift.

Three-man lift: useful if limited help available for placing patient on board or carrying patient short distances. Head, trunk, and legs must be aligned in straight line, and head must be supported from underneath and laterally.

Emergency room and acute management

Computed tomography

Magnetic resonance imaging

Dermatome pattern

Sensory examination includes testing of all sensory modalities across the 28 dermatomes from C2–S5.

CTs and MRIs are used more than plain spine radiographs, to look for traumatic herniated disks, intraspinal hematomas, or significant ligamentous injury.

(ASIA). Sensory examination includes testing of all sensory modalities across the 28 dermatomes from C2 to S5. The major muscle groups are tested in the arms and legs and graded from 0 (no movement) to 5 (normal active movement against full resistance). The neurologic findings direct the radiographic assessment.

Plain spine radiographs have for the most part been supplanted by computed tomography (CT) scanning with reconstruction. Even if the CT findings are "normal," MRI is always indicated in the presence of SCI to look for traumatic herniated disks, intraspinal hematomas, or significant ligamentous injury.

There continues to be controversy over the pharmacologic treatment of SCI. The National Acute Spinal Cord Injury Studies (NASCIS) demonstrated statistically significant improved neurologic recovery if methylprednisolone was administered within 8 hours of injury. However, the functional significance of this recovery has been questioned, and meta-analysis of published data has failed to confirm any benefit of this approach. If methylprednisolone is to be used, the

loading dose is 30 mg/kg, with a maintenance dose of 5.4 mg/kg/hr for the following 23 hours.

It is important to be vigilant for the presence of neurogenic shock and provide appropriate treatment. With mid-level to high-level cervical SCI, there is loss of sympathetic function and associated loss of vascular tone. This can result in significant pooling of blood in the lower extremities and associated hypotension. Volume resuscitation is ineffective in this setting, and pressors must be used early. Because a patient with an SCI may also have multiple injuries, the distinction between hypovolemic and neurogenic shock must be recognized. In hypovolemic shock, there is tachycardia, cold clammy skin, altered mental status, and low urine output. In neurogenic shock, there is bradycardia, warm dry skin, normal mental status, and normal urinary output.

Once the patient with an SCI has been stabilized, the specific treatment required for the spinal injury is determined. Certain injuries may be treated with traction and bracing, whereas others require surgical intervention.

Plate 3.14

Spinal Trauma

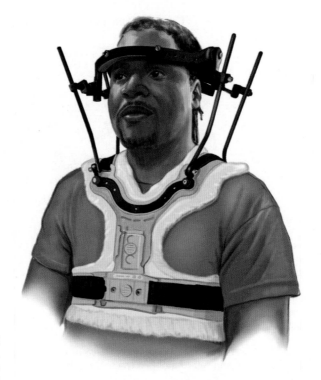

A halo vest is frequently used to treat
many types of bony cervical spine injury.

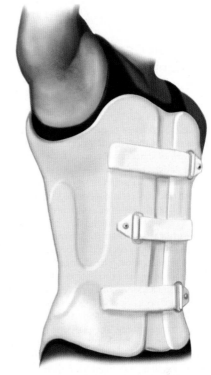

A molded thoracolumbosacral orthosis (TLSO)
vest can be used to treat spine injuries from the
upper thoracic spine to the lower lumbar spine.

TRACTION AND BRACING

Opinions vary on the means and methods of spinal realignment in patients with cervical spine subluxations. Various techniques have been advocated to realign the spine and decompress the spinal canal to preserve or improve neurologic function and recovery. In 1933 Crutchfield first used cranial tongs for spinal realignment. This device or various modifications remained in widespread clinical use for 5 decades. In 1973 Gardner-Wells tongs were introduced, and the ease of their use led to widespread adoption. Gardner-Wells tongs are still used occasionally, and a graphite version compatible with MRI is available. The most common device in clinical use today is the MRI-compatible halo ring. Because the halo device is frequently used as the definitive treatment for many types of cervical spine injury, its use for spinal realignment expedites treatment. Halo ring placement requires both local anesthesia and intravenous sedation to minimize patient discomfort. Four skull pins are needed. The ring should be sized for 1 cm of clearance between the scalp and the ring around the circumference of the head. The frontal pins are typically placed 1 cm above and just lateral to the supraorbital notch to avoid injury to the supraorbital and supratrochlear nerves and the frontal sinus. The patient should be asked to close the eyes as tightly as possible to minimize retracting the forehead skin, which would make subsequent eye closure difficult. The occipital pins are placed several centimeters behind and in line with the tops of the ears.

The pins are first tightened by hand and then with a torque wrench to 6 to 8 lb to engage the outer table of the skull. The torque should be rechecked within the next 48 hours.

Few problems have been associated with acute halo use, with the most significant being pin loosening and pin infection, occurring in up to 25% of instances. This is generally manifested by local pain and discomfort and is helped by careful daily cleaning of the pin sites.

After the halo has been applied, the amount of traction to be used must be determined. A very general guideline is no more than 5 lb of traction per injury level so that 30 to 35 lb may be used for an injury at C6–7. On a practical level, however, for injuries such as bilateral locked facets, up to 80 to 90 lb may be necessary to achieve reduction.

Once traction is instituted, it is important to monitor response by clinical findings and radiographic studies. It is a generally accepted procedure to add cervical traction in increments of 5 to 10 lb every 20 to 30 minutes until

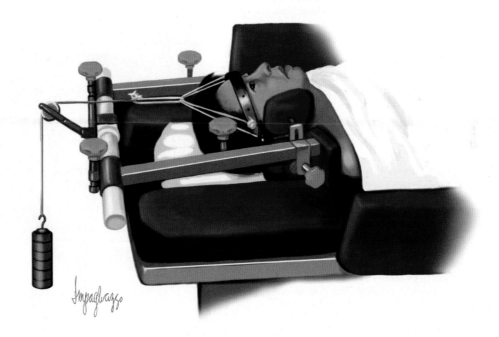

A halo ring can be used to stabilize cervical fractures that will require operative
intervention or to apply traction that can reduce cervical spine subluxations.

reduction is achieved, there is clinical or radiographic evidence of overdistraction, or a maximum weight has been reached. Because there is often significant cervical muscle spasm, it may be necessary to administer muscle relaxants to aid in realignment.

For certain injuries, especially those with a significant ligamentous disruption such as atlantoaxial dislocation, any traction may be contraindicated. A specific concern over bilateral facet dislocation is the possibility of an associated traumatic disk herniation, estimated by some

to be as high as 25%. Realignment of the spine in such a setting could cause significantly increased spinal cord compression. Although not universally agreed, obtaining an MRI before the application of traction is advisable.

Traction is not used for thoracolumbar spine injuries. Those injuries not requiring internal stabilization are generally successfully treated with a thoracolumbosacral orthosis. For injuries involving the lumbosacral junction, a hip extension added to the orthosis provides increased stability.

CERVICAL SPINE INJURY: ANTERIOR INTERBODY FUSION BY GRAFT AND PLATE

ANTERIOR CERVICAL SPINE DECOMPRESSION AND STABILIZATION

Although a significant number of traumatic cervical spine injuries may be treated with external immobilization (i.e., a halo vest or hard cervical collar), certain types require internal stabilization with or without decompression. The types of such injuries that most often require an anterior approach include certain odontoid fractures, traumatic disk herniations (with pain or neurologic deficit), burst fractures, and teardrop fractures.

The surgical approach to the anterior cervical spine has not significantly changed for decades, but the various means of stabilization have changed dramatically. Typically, a transverse incision centered on the medial border of the sternocleidomastoid muscle is made on the right side of the neck. Special precautions, however, may be necessary in a patient with an SCI who has already required tracheostomy. The platysma is divided, and the sternocleidomastoid is sharply dissected from the medial strap musculature down to the prevertebral fascia, which is often swollen and filled with hematoma from the underlying injury. Retractors are used to protect the carotid artery laterally and the esophagus medially. The prevertebral fascia is bluntly dissected off the anterior longitudinal ligament, which may be disrupted from the injury. Even if the injury is obvious, a lateral plain radiograph (or fluoroscopy) is done to confirm the operative level.

If the primary injury is a traumatic herniated disk, the affected disk space is incised and the disk material and end plates of the vertebral bodies above and below are removed in piecemeal fashion using pituitary rongeurs and curettes. Most surgeons use an operating microscope to visualize the posterior aspect of the disk space. Once the disk is removed, the anterior longitudinal ligament (unless already breached by the injury) is removed, and complete decompression of the dura is observed. The spine is then stabilized by using a proper-sized piece of allograft bone. A few surgeons still prefer autogenous bone, but for most patients the discomfort from iliac crest bone harvesting (unless insensate from SCI) outweighs any advantages. The bone is securely wedged between the affected vertebral bodies.

Although stable fusion rates are high with this approach, supplementation with an anterior cervical titanium plate, secured by screws into the affected vertebral bodies, has become popular. This follows the general biologic principle of bone healing: the two elements of most importance in achieving a bony fusion are compression and immobilization. A wide variety of plates are available; all provide for immediate compression and immobilization, with subsequent high fusion rates.

For burst fractures at single or multiple levels, an anterior approach is required to adequately decompress the spinal canal. The approach is the same as for a diskectomy, but all portions of the affected bone are removed. Before the late 1990s, the most common form of reconstruction of the spine after corpectomy was with an iliac strut or fibular graft with or without supplementation by an anterior plate. There has been increasing use of interbody cages, which are intended to provide immediate structural stability. The cage is generally packed with osteoinductive or osteoconductive materials to facilitate fusion.

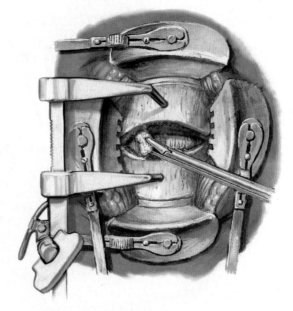

Spine exposed by progressive dissection and self-retaining retractors inserted. Disk, osteophytes, and bone fragments removed piecemeal.

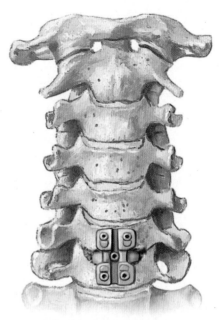

Fusion completed with titanium compression plate and screws

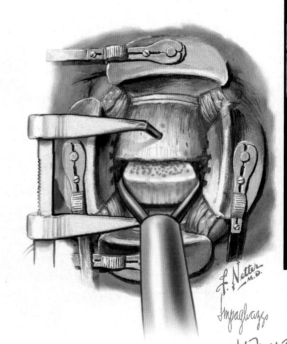

Autogenous bone graft wedged securely in intervertebral space

Lateral cervical radiograph demonstrating anterior cervical interbody fusion and plating at C6–7

Teardrop fractures are unstable anteriorly and posteriorly due to disk and ligamentous injury. Thus both an anterior stabilization (cervical diskectomy and fusion with plate) and posterior stabilization are required.

For unstable odontoid fractures, anterior screw fixation may be quite appropriate. As opposed to posterior fixation, this preserves C1–2 mobility and may be better tolerated. A small incision is made near the C5–6 level and, under biplanar fluoroscopy, a guide is passed up to the C2–3 level. Through the guide, a small pilot hole is drilled into the base of C2. An appropriate-length screw is then passed to the tip of C2. If reduction of the fracture is desired, a lag screw will pull the fracture fragments together. Success of fusion exceeds 90%.

Complications from anterior decompression and stabilization are generally acceptable. Development of new neurologic dysfunction occurs generally in less than 2% of cases. Issues related to carotid or esophageal injury are likewise small. The risk of a significant infection leading to diskitis or osteomyelitis is less than 1%. On rare occasions, there can be failure of the fusion–plate–cage construct, leading to injury to surrounding neck structures, instability, and the need for reoperation.

Plate 3.16

Spinal Trauma

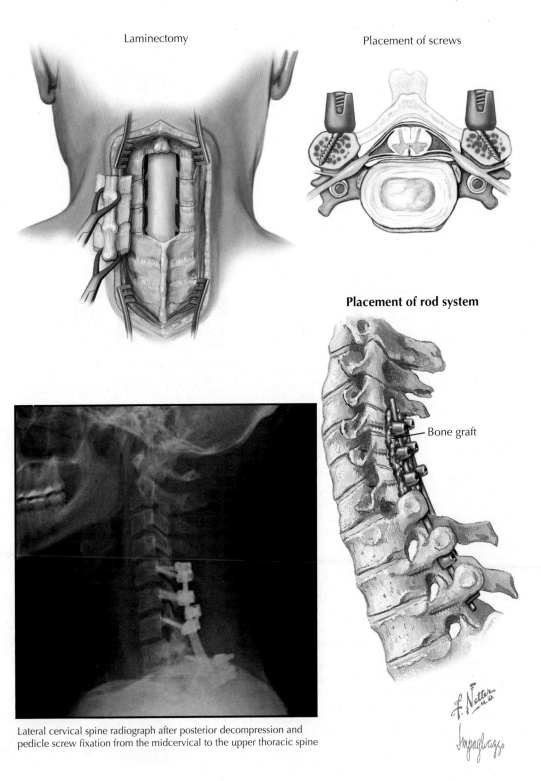

Laminectomy

Placement of screws

Placement of rod system

Bone graft

Lateral cervical spine radiograph after posterior decompression and pedicle screw fixation from the midcervical to the upper thoracic spine

Posterior Cervical Stabilization and Fusion

In the 1940s, posterior cervical spinal stabilization was generally limited to interspinous process wiring and bone fusion. Gallie popularized C1–2 fusion using fine steel wires around the lamina or spines and leaving a bone graft between the spines, tightening the wires over it. Brooks further refined this technique. However, neither of these procedures prevented rotation at the level of the injury, leading to the development of techniques of intrafacetal wiring that eventually evolved into the use of various forms of plates and screws.

Regardless of technique, the goal is to achieve a stable bony fusion in flexion, extension, and rotation as soon as possible. Metallic internal fixation devices provide stability and increase the fusion rate. Plates and screws can be used to temporarily stabilize the cervical spine from the occiput to C7. Screws can be placed into the C2 pedicles, the C1–2 facets, and the C3–7 lateral masses, and various forms of plates are available to add strength to the metal construct. The screws, fixed on each side, can also be connected by a metal rod on each side of the spine (see Plate 3.16).

Operative exposure is common to all levels of the posterior cervical spine, using a midline cervical incision with dissection of the paraspinal musculature and bony exposure at the affected levels. On most occasions, the only bone work necessary is eburnation of the bony surfaces to facilitate fusion. On occasion, a laminectomy may be necessary for spinal decompression, such as for central cord syndrome from spinal stenosis. If there is significant facet subluxation, with "locking" of the facets, it is usually necessary to drill off the superior aspect of the affected inferior facet to allow reduction of the subluxation.

For lateral mass screws, the entry point is 1 mm medial to the center of the lateral mass, angled 20 to 30 degrees rostrally and 20 to 30 degrees laterally. Screw placement needs to be precise to minimize injury to the vertebral artery or nerve roots.

SPINAL CORD INJURY MEDICAL ISSUES

Patients with an SCI are prone to many medical complications requiring vigilance and preventive strategies. The loss of sensation and immobility leads to a high risk for development of decubitus ulcers. The areas at greatest risk are over bony prominences, such as the sacrum. Prevention requires frequent examination of the areas at risk, use of pressure-reduction mattresses (or cushions if the patient can be out of bed), frequent repositioning, and education of family or other caregivers. It is also important to regularly check the skin at the edges of orthoses.

Deep vein thrombosis (DVT) occurs in more than 50% of patients who do not receive prophylactic measures. The first-line preventive measure is mechanical compression devices on the lower extremities, but studies have shown that although this minimizes venous stasis, it is relatively ineffective in preventing DVT when used alone. Thus, unless contraindicated, compression devices should be supplemented with low-molecular-weight heparin, such as enoxaparin, or with unfractionated heparin.

Bladder dysfunction from SCI requires a variety of interventions. In acute cases, an indwelling Foley catheter is appropriate and should be used until the patient is hemodynamically stable. However, because of the risk of infection, the catheter should be removed as soon as medically possible and intermittent catheterization substituted. The prophylactic use of antibiotics acutely or chronically does not reduce infection rates.

SCI has been shown to be an independent risk factor for gastrointestinal (GI) ulcers and upper GI bleeding. There are two forms of pharmacologic prophylaxis: histamine H_2 receptor antagonists and proton pump inhibitors. Based on present evidence, both are equally safe and effective in preventing stress ulceration in patients with an SCI.

Loss of lower GI motility is universal in patients with an SCI and requires early attention. Once enteral nutrition is instituted, bowel movements should be facilitated. This requires the use of oral medications, suppositories, and digital stimulation.

EARLY SPINAL CORD INJURY REHABILITATION

It is important that rehabilitation specialists are involved early in the care of the patient with an SCI. In acute cases, this is intended to maintain range of motion and to begin strengthening exercises, as well as to initiate mobilization, thereby minimizing the risk of joint contracture. In patients with an SCI who have pulmonary problems, respiratory therapists can enhance pulmonary hygiene. Pulmonary interventions, such as suctioning, percussion, vibration, and training of accessory respiratory muscles, reduce the incidence of pneumonia and shorten time in acute care.

One of the primary obstacles to early mobilization is orthostatic hypotension, which limits tolerance to being upright. Nonpharmacologic therapeutic measures include leg compression stockings, abdominal binders, and a tilt table to gradually elevate the patient as tolerated. Pharmacologic treatments typically include adrenergic agents to enhance vascular tone.

SCI creates several psychologic, psychosocial, and family issues. These may include grief and denial reactions, major depression, and, in the most severe cases, decisions to remove life support. It is thus important to provide psychological and social services support to the patient and family.

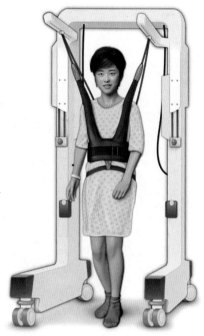

Robotic gait trainers. State-of-the-art robotic gait trainers are routinely utilized in rehabilitation for spinal cord injury.

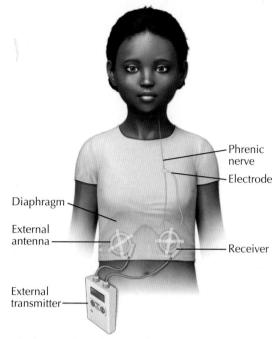

Phrenic nerve
Electrode
Diaphragm
External antenna
Receiver
External transmitter

Diaphragmatic pacing. Diaphragmatic pacing may help restore some breathing control in ventilator-dependent high cervical SCI patients.

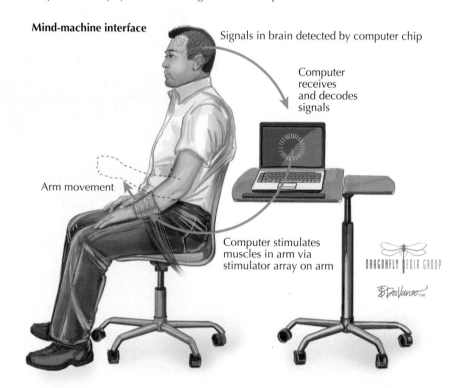

Mind-machine interface

Signals in brain detected by computer chip

Computer receives and decodes signals

Arm movement

Computer stimulates muscles in arm via stimulator array on arm

LONG-TERM REHABILITATION

As soon as the patient with an SCI is medically stabilized, transfer to a long-term rehabilitation facility where active interventions can be instituted to improve lost function is appropriate.

A variety of techniques can be used to stimulate and strengthen affected muscles, all centered around intensive physical therapy. In addition, physical therapy can be augmented by a variety of assistive devices such as robotic gait trainers. Such trainers use various sensors and stimulators, as well as reduced gravity scenarios, to facilitate gait training. Upper extremity function may be augmented by various braces and functional assist devices.

Cutting-edge research with currently limited clinical applicability involves establishing brain-machine interfaces. This technology allows brain signals involving muscle movement to be directly transmitted to muscles via a computer interface to effect movement. Presently, this requires placing sensors directly on the surface of the brain.

Even patients with respirator-dependent, high-cervical SCI may benefit from long-term rehabilitation. Eye movements may be used to control computers. Phrenic nerve stimulation may help provide increased respiratory capacity.

NERVE ROOTS AND PLEXUS DISORDERS

CERVICAL DISK HERNIATION

Cervical disk herniation is a common disorder, accounting for 1% to 2% of all hospital admissions in the United States. Unlike lumbar disk disease, which is approximately six times more common, cervical disk disease is rarely caused by trauma. Furthermore, severe degenerative cervical disk disease often develops in indolent patients.

Etiology. Cervical disk herniation is multifactorial and has been associated with several risk factors that include male sex, advancing age, neck trauma, heavy lifting, and smoking. The nucleus pulposus in the middle of the disk dehydrates with age, placing more stress on the circumferential annulus fibrosus. Tears in the annulus may permit a sudden herniation of the nucleus or *ruptured disk.* Alternatively, chronic annular bulging or nuclear herniation may incite a bony reparative process (spondylosis), leading to the formation of extensive bony spurs (osteophytes). These spurs are generally located along the anterior portion of the disk interspace or posteriorly, within the intervertebral foramen.

Osteophytes or ruptured disks produce neurologic symptoms when they compress the spinal cord or adjacent spinal nerve roots. The cervical nerve roots are most susceptible to injury at the point where they enter the intervertebral foramen (neuroforamen), a space delineated by the uncovertebral joint (anteromedially), the facet joint (posterolaterally), intervertebral disks and the vertebral end plates (medially), and by the pedicles of the vertebral bodies (above and below).

Symptoms. The first manifestation of cervical disk disease is often cervical radiculopathy with symptoms and signs referable to compression of a cervical nerve root. The cervical nerve roots exit above the vertebral body of the same number except for the C8 nerve root, which emerges at the C7–T1 interspace. Thus a lesion of the C5–6 disk produces a C6 radiculopathy. Spondylosis is implicated in cervical nerve root compression about three times more often than acute disk rupture and most frequently involves the C6 or C7 nerve root. The C5 and C8 nerve roots are involved less often, and the T1 root only rarely.

Cervical and unilateral arm pain is the most common symptom of cervical disk herniation, and patients often report numbness or weakness in the involved arm. Occasionally, there may be pain involving the shoulder, occiput, or anterior chest. Cervical tenderness and reduced range of motion in the neck may also be present. Hyperextension and rotation of the neck toward the painful side (Spurling maneuver) decrease the diameter of the neural foramen and may exacerbate radicular symptoms.

Clinical Diagnosis. Neurologic examination with careful attention to motor, reflex, and sensory findings in the upper extremities often reveals a diagnostic constellation of signs. *C5 radiculopathy* usually causes weakness of shoulder external rotation (infraspinatus muscle) and shoulder abduction (supraspinatus and deltoid muscles) with decreased biceps and brachioradialis reflexes and hypalgesia over the lateral shoulder. *C6 radiculopathy* is characterized by diminished sensation over the thumb and index finger; however, the pattern of weakness and

Spurling maneuver. Hyperextension and flexion of neck ipsilateral to the side of lesion cause radicular pain in neck and down the affected arm.

Herniated disk compressing nerve root

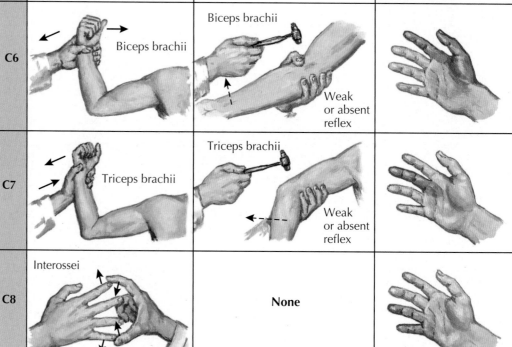

Level	Motor signs (weakness)	Reflex signs	Sensory loss
C5	Deltoid	None	
C6	Biceps brachii	Biceps brachii — Weak or absent reflex	
C7	Triceps brachii	Triceps brachii — Weak or absent reflex	
C8	Interossei	None	

abnormal reflexes may be difficult to distinguish from C5 radiculopathy because of overlap between the C5 and C6 myotomes. Of note, forearm pronation (pronator teres muscle) is more likely to be involved with injury to the C6 root. In *C7 radiculopathy,* weakness is noted in the triceps brachii and extensor muscles of the wrist. The triceps reflex is usually decreased or absent, and sensation over the index and middle fingers is often decreased. *C8 radiculopathy* causes intrinsic hand muscle weakness affecting the finger abductors, adductors, and flexors. The triceps reflex may also be decreased, and sensation may be diminished over the ring and little fingers. The rare *T1 radiculopathy* may be associated with weakness of the intrinsic hand muscles, particularly abduction of the thumb (abductor pollicis brevis muscle) and Horner syndrome (ptosis, miosis, and anhidrosis), which results from disruption of the sympathetic outflow to the face and eye via the root of C8 or T1, or both.

Treatment. Most patients who have symptoms and signs of cervical radiculopathy respond to conservative treatment, including activity modification, use of a soft cervical collar to immobilize the neck for a brief period, mild analgesics, antiinflammatory medications, and muscle relaxants as required. In some cases, cervical traction and epidural steroid injections may also be considered. If symptoms persist beyond 2 to 4 weeks, further testing including cervical magnetic resonance imaging (MRI) and electromyography (EMG) may be indicated. If the findings suggest significant nerve root compression in the setting of progressive neurologic deficits or intractable pain, surgical therapy may be considered. Cervical root decompression may be accomplished by an anterior or posterior approach through the neck. However, epidemiologic data suggest that up to 85% of patients improve with conservative treatment alone.

Plate 4.2

Nerve Roots and Plexus Disorders

RADIOGRAPHIC DIAGNOSIS OF RADICULOPATHY

Herniation of an intervertebral disk, alone or in combination with spondylosis, is the most common cause of surgically remediable lumbar and cervical radiculopathy. In patients with signs and symptoms of radiculopathy, the clinician can often localize the problem to within one or two spinal segments. However, when conservative management has failed or when there are symptoms such as excruciating, unrelenting pain or severe weakness with or without loss of sphincter control, surgical consideration with precise anatomic localization of the disk herniation is necessary. MRI is the most reliable diagnostic procedure in most cases.

MRI effectively demonstrates the bony architecture of the spine, the contours of the intervertebral disk, the paraspinal soft tissues, and the contents of the spinal canal. Various MRI sequences can be used to confirm disk herniation and visualize degenerative or traumatic changes, such as annular tears and end plate edema. Changes that would suggest the presence of a radiculopathy include foraminal narrowing and a decreased amount of adipose tissue surrounding neuroforaminal nerve roots and dorsal root ganglia.

Computed tomography (CT) myelography, a fluoroscopic procedure in which a water-soluble contrast medium is injected into the spinal canal followed by CT imaging of the spine, may also help with localization in that it can further delineate the extradural, bony, and paraspinal tissues. This can be especially helpful in patients who have undergone previous spine surgery, which may result in technical artifacts that obscure the MRI.

The *cervical region* has little, if any, epidural fat, and frequently only a small fragment of disk is enough to cause severe nerve root compression. Because of the lack of epidural fat and the small size of disk herniations, CT is less effective than myelography for diagnosing cervical radiculopathy. In disk herniation, myelography commonly demonstrates displacement of the dural sac, nerve root swelling, or impaired filling or displacement of an axillary sleeve.

When either MRI or CT myelography fails to suggest a clear-cut diagnosis, the other procedure should be considered. CT myelography may be more effective in the setting of prior spine surgery and metal hardware placement or when MRI is contraindicated (e.g., in patients with an internal cardiac defibrillator).

In the cervical region, CT and myelography are complementary. The combination of both studies may clearly show the nature and degree of spinal cord distortion, which is valuable in determining the proper treatment. The diagnosis of cervical spinal nerve root

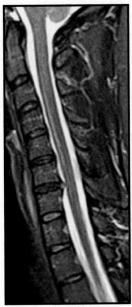
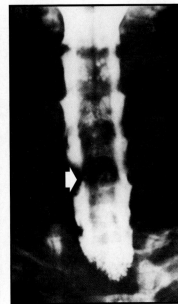

Myelogram (anteroposterior view) showing prominent extradural defect *(arrow)* at C6–7

Central disk herniation, sagittal view

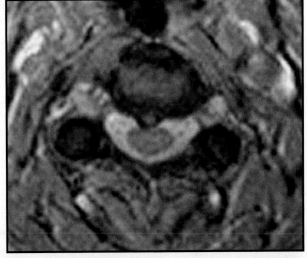

Central disk herniation, axial view

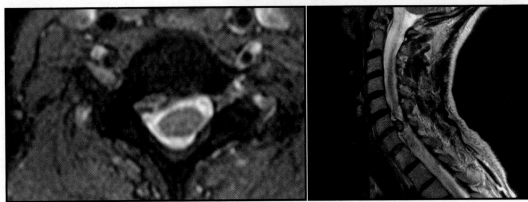

Large, right paracentral disk herniation, C6–7, with associated cord displacement *(left)* and complete right neural foraminal compromise *(right)*

avulsion from traction injury of the arm is best visualized with a combination of CT and myelography, which can identify the diagnostic leakage of cerebrospinal fluid (CSF) into the neuroforaminal and extraspinal space.

Clinical localization of *cauda equina compression* may be difficult. In this case MRI of the lumbosacral (LS) spine is helpful in localizing the compressive lesion. In most patients with cauda equina compression related to disk disease, the MRI will demonstrate

extensive disk material occupying more than one-third of the intraspinal canal space. CT myelogram may also demonstrate a myelographic block, the degree of which can help quantify the severity of neural compression in several different patient positions.

However, MRI is the test of choice because it is more rapidly performed with minimal risk of complications; characterization of the LS spine with MRI in conjunction with the clinical picture may be sufficient for planning surgery.

EXAMINATION OF PATIENT WITH LOW BACK PAIN

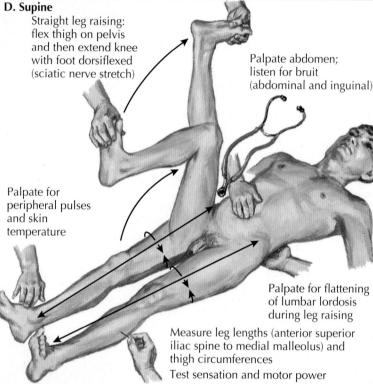

A. Standing

Body build
Posture
Deformities
Pelvic obliquity
Spine alignment
Palpate for:
  muscle spasm
  trigger zones
  myofascial nodes
  sciatic nerve tenderness
Compress iliac crests
  for sacroiliac
  tenderness

Walking on heels
(tests foot and
great toe
dorsiflexion)

Walking
on toes
(tests calf
muscles)

Spinal column
movements:
  flexion
  extension
  side bending
  rotation

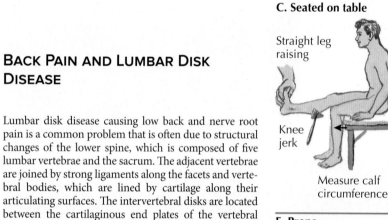

B. Kneeling on chair

Ankle
jerk

Sensation on
calf and sole

C. Seated on table

Straight leg
raising

Knee
jerk

Measure calf
circumference

D. Supine

Straight leg raising:
flex thigh on pelvis
and then extend knee
with foot dorsiflexed
(sciatic nerve stretch)

Palpate abdomen;
listen for bruit
(abdominal and inguinal)

Palpate for
peripheral pulses
and skin
temperature

Palpate for flattening
of lumbar lordosis
during leg raising

Measure leg lengths (anterior superior
iliac spine to medial malleolus) and
thigh circumferences
Test sensation and motor power

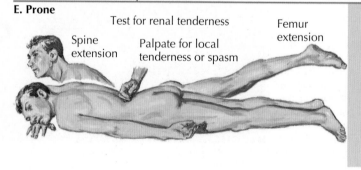

E. Prone

Test for renal tenderness

Spine
extension

Palpate for local
tenderness or spasm

Femur
extension

**F. Rectal and/or pelvic
examination**

**G. MRI and/or CT and/or
myelogram of**
  1. Lumbosacral spine
  2. Abdomen/pelvis

BACK PAIN AND LUMBAR DISK DISEASE

Lumbar disk disease causing low back and nerve root pain is a common problem that is often due to structural changes of the lower spine, which is composed of five lumbar vertebrae and the sacrum. The adjacent vertebrae are joined by strong ligaments along the facets and vertebral bodies, which are lined by cartilage along their articulating surfaces. The intervertebral disks are located between the cartilaginous end plates of the vertebral bodies and normally form a tough fibrocartilaginous structure. With aging, the disk degenerates, fragments, and loses its adherent properties. Over time, mechanic forces may cause the disk fragment to move, usually posterolaterally (point of least ligamentous resistance), where it may compress the nerve root as it exits the spine, resulting in pain and neurologic deficit.

In addition to disk degeneration, a hypertrophic, osteoarthritic process known as spondylosis can also develop over time because of abnormal movement at the facet joint. Enlargement of the facet joints by this spondylotic process narrows the intervertebral foramen, which may cause mechanical pressure on the exiting nerve root. In cases where the anteroposterior diameter of the spinal canal is congenitally narrow with deep lateral recesses, spondylosis can lead to spinal stenosis with possible compression of the dural sac and cauda equina.

Clinical Manifestations. Lumbar spine disease may be manifested as low back pain, radiculopathy, cauda equina syndrome, or spinal stenosis. As an isolated symptom, low back pain is usually self-limited and responds to conservative measures.

Initially, only a detailed history and physical examination may be necessary. However, increasing pain with or without neurologic symptoms in a person who has systemic symptoms raises the question of a destructive lesion and merits further investigation, especially if the response to treatment has been limited. Back pain that is not helped by lying down is nonspecific but may occur with cancer or infection.

The monoradicular syndromes are the classic syndromes of a ruptured disk. Most disk ruptures occur at L5–S1 and L4–5. The herniated disk at L5–S1 usually compresses the S1 root as it passes the interspace on its way beneath the S1 facet. In the same manner, the L4–5 disk compresses the L5 root, and the L3–4 disk compresses the L4 root. Rarely, the disk extrudes laterally into the intervertebral foramen, in which case the L5–S1 disk produces an L5 root syndrome; the L4–5 disk, an L4 root syndrome; and the L3–4 disk, an L3 root syndrome.

Plate 4.4

Nerve Roots and Plexus Disorders

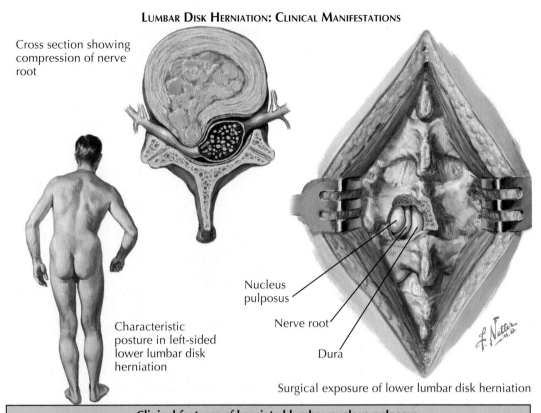

LUMBAR DISK HERNIATION: CLINICAL MANIFESTATIONS

Cross section showing compression of nerve root

Characteristic posture in left-sided lower lumbar disk herniation

Nucleus pulposus

Nerve root

Dura

Surgical exposure of lower lumbar disk herniation

BACK PAIN AND LUMBAR DISK DISEASE (Continued)

Failure to diagnose these problems accurately may result in suboptimal treatment.

The *S1 root syndrome* includes sciatic pain ("sciatica") from the buttock to the posterior thigh, to the posterior or lateral calf and into the foot. When due to disk herniation, it often increases with coughing or sneezing. Numbness and paresthesias commonly occur on the lateral aspect of the foot, the sole, and the heel. With involvement of motor fibers, there may be reduced plantar flexion of the ankle and foot. The ankle jerk is absent.

The *L5 root syndrome* may also present with a sciatic pain that is indistinguishable from that of the S1 root syndrome. Dorsiflexion of the foot and eversion and inversion of the ankle may be weak. The ankle and knee jerks are normal, but the internal hamstring reflex may be diminished or absent. Sensory change develops in the dorsal and medial aspects of the foot and great toe. In the less common *L4 root syndrome*, pain radiates to the lateral and anterior thigh. The quadriceps muscle is weak and atrophied, and the knee jerk is lost. Sensory change occurs in the anterior thigh and pretibial regions. The clinical manifestations of herniation at L4–5 and L5–S1 are summarized in Plate 4.4.

Compression of the cauda equina by a midline disk herniation or tumor may lead to bladder or bowel dysfunction, often with bilateral sciatica, saddle anesthesia, and leg weakness. This is a surgical emergency because deficits may become irreversible if treatment is delayed.

In *lumbar spinal stenosis* (LSS), congenital or acquired narrowing of the spinal canal or intervertebral foramina is caused by several degenerative conditions, including disk bulging or protrusion, bony hypertrophic changes,

or thickening of the ligamentum flavum. In addition to back pain that is relieved by sitting or bending forward, symptoms include pain or other sensory disturbances occurring in one or both legs with exercise that resolves with rest and occasionally presents in a radicular distribution. Such "neurogenic claudication" is distinguished from vascular claudication by the lack of any circulatory abnormality in the legs; the arterial pulses are normal.

Treatment. Most of the monoradicular syndromes, even those with mild neurologic deficit, typically respond to conservative care, which involves a short period of bed rest (generally not more than 2 or 3 days) followed by mobilization and an exercise program. For patients with persistent radiculopathy symptoms that do not improve after 6 weeks, further evaluation with MRI or, less often, CT myelography and possibly EMG should

Clinical features of herniated lumbar nucleus pulposus

Level of herniation	Pain	Numbness	Weakness	Atrophy	Reflexes
L4–5 disk; 5th lumbar nerve root	Over sacro-iliac joint, hip, lateral thigh, and leg	Lateral leg, first 3 toes	Dorsiflexion of great toe and foot; difficulty walking on heels; foot drop may occur	Minor	Changes uncommon in knee and ankle jerks, but internal hamstring reflex diminished or absent
L5–S1 disk; 1st sacral nerve root	Over sacro-iliac joint, hip, postero-lateral thigh, and leg to heel	Back of calf, lateral heel, foot to toe	Plantar flexion of foot and great toe may be affected; difficulty walking on toes	Gastrocnemius and soleus	Ankle jerk diminished or absent

L4–5 Disk Extrusion

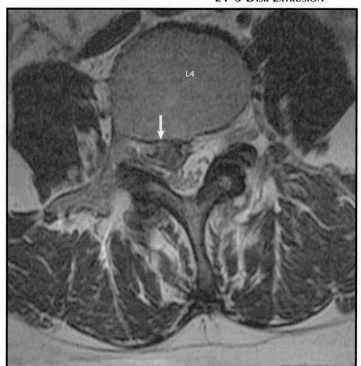

Axial T2-weighted image at L4 shows large paracentral disk extrusion extending into the right lateral recess and neuroforamen.

Back Pain and Lumbar Disk Disease (Continued)

be considered. If a nerve root lesion is identified that correlates with the clinical presentation, then the patient may be referred for surgical evaluation. The surgeon must keep in mind that the important structure is the nerve root. Adequate exposure is essential to expose the root cephalad and caudad to the extruded fragment and to the lateral margin of the spinal canal. This allows maximal exposure of the disk and nerve root, which can be minimally manipulated. The extruded disk is removed, and a foraminotomy is performed. The root is then retracted medially, the annulus is exposed, and the disk is removed from the interspace to reduce the chance of recurrence. The patient is discharged 1 to 3 days postoperatively and can return to a sedentary job in 2 weeks. Diskectomy with use of the operating microscope is also a satisfactory procedure if done at the correct level to adequately expose the root.

If no correlating structural pathology is identified, then continued supportive therapy is recommended unless there is worsening pain or new neurologic deficits.

The *midline disk herniation* is a much more serious problem. The entire cauda equina can be compressed at the level of the rupture and herniation. Because of the danger of irreversible neurologic damage, bilateral sciatica demands more urgent evaluation than unilateral sciatica. Any suggestion of sphincter disturbance should lead to urgent spinal MRI or CT myelography, and, if necessary, decompressive laminectomy with disk removal.

Conservative treatment for LSS includes weight loss, physical therapy (to improve posture, strengthen core abdominal muscles, and increase lumbar flexion), and

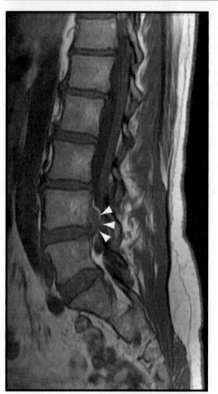

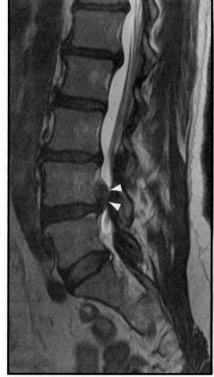

Midline sagittal T2- *(left)* and T1- *(right)* weighted images show disk extrusion extending cephalad from L4–5 interspace.

nonsteroidal antiinflammatory agents. Surgery may be required to relieve symptoms or prevent further deterioration and usually involves single or multilevel decompressive laminectomy, sometimes with lumbar fusion.

The patient who does not improve after surgery should be reevaluated to rule out a recurrent disk fragment and to establish that surgery was done at the correct level. If no surgical lesion is found, the patient should be encouraged to exercise and return to work. Referral to a pain management clinic may be helpful for some patients, but analgesic drugs such as narcotics and tranquilizing medications should be avoided. For those with persistent low back pain in the absence of clinical or radiographic findings, surgery is not indicated.

Plate 4.6

Nerve Roots and Plexus Disorders

LUMBOSACRAL SPINAL STENOSIS

In contrast to patients with a herniated disk, which is usually symptomatic at the level of just one spinal nerve root, some patients develop acute or chronically progressive narrowing of the central spinal canal, known as spinal stenosis. Progressive disk degeneration due to aging, trauma, or other factors can lead to disk protrusion and/or loss of disk height, resulting in pressure on posterior elements of the spine, including the facet joints. Facet joint arthropathy and osteophyte formation along with hypertrophy of the ligamentum flavum often follow. All these processes (facet osteophytes, ligamentum flavum hypertrophy, and disk bulging) can encroach on the central canal and the neural foramina at one or multiple segmental levels, producing the anatomic picture of spinal stenosis, especially at the L3–5 segmental levels.

Spondylolisthesis, in which one vertebral body translates anteriorly or posteriorly with respect to an adjacent vertebral body, can also occur, exacerbating the spinal canal narrowing. The L4–5 level is most commonly involved, followed by L5–S1 and L3–4.

Spinal stenosis typically occurs in older patients and is the most common reason for spinal surgery in patients older than 65 years. However, spinal stenosis may also occur in younger patients due to congenital or developmental bony abnormalities, such as achondroplasia, osteochondrodystrophy, and mucopolysaccharidosis.

Clinical Manifestations. The classic clinical presentation of LSS is neurogenic (or pseudo) claudication, characterized by symptoms of pain or aching in the legs that is exacerbated by walking, standing, and/or maintaining certain postures (especially extension of the spine) and is relieved with sitting or lying. Many patients with LSS are symptomatic only when active. The symptoms are similar to vascular claudication of the leg(s) due to arterial insufficiency exacerbated by walking. Symptoms of neurogenic claudication are reported in most patients with LSS. Other common symptoms include paresthesia, low back pain, and weakness. Symptoms are bilateral in over half of patients but are often asymmetric and can involve an entire lower extremity, including the hip, buttock, thigh, and foreleg.

Unlike patients with vascular claudication, patients with spinal stenosis can pedal long distances on a bicycle or push a grocery cart throughout a store as long as they maintain a fully flexed position. Similarly, patients can walk downhill or down stairs as the spine is in a flexed position. However, walking uphill or up the stairs involves hyperextension of the spine and so is more likely to cause exacerbation of symptoms in patients with LSS. As the degree of canal stenosis increases, spinal nerve roots are continuously compressed so that symptoms and weakness may become constant even at rest.

Diagnosis. The examination of the patient with spinal stenosis is often normal or relatively benign, especially compared with that of patients in whom a herniated nucleus pulposus produces nerve root disease. At rest, patients with spinal stenosis are usually comfortable and have no back pain, muscle spasm, or loss of lumbar lordosis. Straight leg raising does not aggravate symptoms as it does in disk disease. However, hyperextension of the spine precipitates symptoms, which may be relieved by forward flexion. At times, the physician may not consider the patient's symptoms to be serious because testing of strength, deep tendon reflexes, and sensation often fails to reveal any deficit. Furthermore, when there is no change in pulses with exercise testing,

Patient assumes characteristic bent-over posture, with neck, spine, hips, and knees flexed; back is flat or convex, with absence of normal lordotic curvature. Pressure on cauda equina and resultant pain thus relieved.

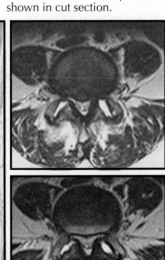

Central spinal canal narrowed by enlargement of inferior articular process of superior vertebra. Lateral recesses narrowed by subluxation and osteophytic enlargement of superior articular processes of inferior vertebra.

Inferior articular process of superior vertebra

Superior articular process of inferior vertebra

Lateral recess

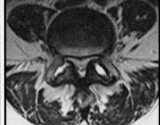

Properly spaced lumbar vertebrae with normal intervertebral disk

Vertebrae approximated due to loss of disk height. Subluxated articular process of inferior vertebra has encroached on foramen. Internal disruption of disk shown in cut section.

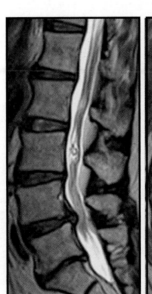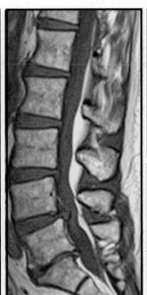

Combined spinal stenosis

the unwary physician may cease the evaluation. The precise mechanism that produces spinal stenosis is not clear but may be related to mechanical compression and nerve root ischemia, among other possibilities.

Plain radiographs of the spine demonstrate spondylosis. MRI usually shows high-grade stenosis of the central canal, whereas CT myelography may demonstrate severe obstruction or complete block. Frequently, multiple levels are involved, usually L2 or L3–5. In contrast to acute disk rupture, L5–S1 is rarely involved.

Treatment. Several studies suggest that clinical outcomes may be better with surgical decompression compared with conservative management, but the quality of evidence is mixed. It should be stressed that in contrast to midline disk herniation, which can also produce bilateral paresthesias, surgery is not urgent. Rather, the patient and surgeon may wish to follow a conservative course of observation until the symptoms produce significant discomfort or interfere with activities of daily life.

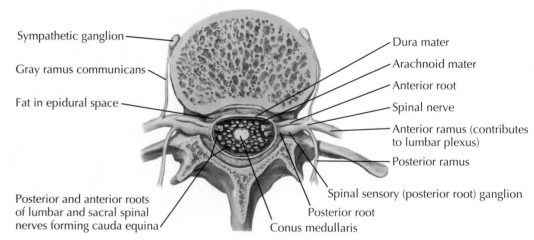

Section through thoracic vertebra

- Body of vertebra
- Dura mater
- Arachnoid mater
- Subarachnoid space
- Pia mater
- Recurrent meningeal branches of spinal nerve
- Pleura
- Lung
- Aorta
- Fat in epidural space
- Sympathetic ganglion
- Anterior root
- Spinal nerve
- White and gray rami communicantes
- Anterior ramus (intercostal nerve)
- Posterior ramus
- Spinal sensory (posterior root) ganglion
- Posterior root
- Lateral horn of gray matter of spinal cord
- Internal vertebral (epidural) venous plexus
- Medial branch
- Lateral branch
} of posterior ramus of spinal nerve

Section through lumbar vertebra

- Sympathetic ganglion
- Gray ramus communicans
- Fat in epidural space
- Posterior and anterior roots of lumbar and sacral spinal nerves forming cauda equina
- Dura mater
- Arachnoid mater
- Anterior root
- Spinal nerve
- Anterior ramus (contributes to lumbar plexus)
- Posterior ramus
- Spinal sensory (posterior root) ganglion
- Posterior root
- Conus medullaris

SPINAL NERVES

The *ventral (anterior)* and *dorsal (posterior) nerve roots* are closely covered by pia mater and loosely invested by arachnoid. As each pair emerges through an interverte-bral foramen, the roots are enclosed in a sheath of dura mater and are surrounded by fatty areolar tissue con-taining a plexus of veins. The roots lie close together as they pierce the dura and unite almost immediately to form a *spinal nerve,* their dural sheaths becoming continuous with the epineurium.

The upper cervical spinal nerves lie horizontally, but all the others assume an increasingly oblique and downward direction as they proceed to their foramina of exit. In the adult, the lumbar, sacral, and coccygeal cord segments lie opposite the last three thoracic and first lumbar vertebrae, and their attached nerve roots descend as a sheath around the filum terminale to constitute the *cauda equina.*

The spinal nerves are connected with adjacent sym-pathetic trunk ganglia by *rami communicantes.* These rami contribute efferent and afferent sympathetic fibers to the spinal nerves, which consist primarily of somatic fibers derived from the ventral and dorsal nerve roots.

Shortly after emerging from the intervertebral foramina, the spinal nerves give off small *recurrent meningeal branches,* which supply the meninges and their vessels; they also supply filaments to adjacent articular and ligamentous structures. They then divide into *ventral (anterior)* and *dorsal (posterior primary)* rami, which contain fibers from both nerve roots and a variable number of sympathetic fibers.

The *ventral rami* supply the anterior and lateral parts of the neck and trunk and make up the nerves of the perineum and limbs. Except in the thoracic region, where they retain their separate identities as intercostal and subcostal nerves, the ventral rami divide and reunite in differing patterns to form the following nerve plexuses: the *cervical plexus,* from the ventral rami of the first four cervical nerves; the *brachial plexus,* from the ventral rami of the lower four cervical and first thoracic nerves; the *lumbar plexus,* from the ventral rami of the first three lumbar nerves and from most of the ventral ramus of the fourth lumbar nerve; the *sacral plexus,* from the remainder of the ventral ramus of the fourth lumbar nerve and from the ventral rami of the fifth lumbar and first three sacral nerves; and the small

sacrococcygeal plexus, from the ventral rami of the fourth and fifth sacral nerves and from the coccygeal nerve. (The plexuses and their branches are described in detail in Plates 4.12 and 4.13.)

The *dorsal rami* turn dorsally and are distributed to the skin, muscle, and other structures of the back of the neck and trunk. Although some dorsal rami join to form loops, their branches do not form true plexuses as do branches derived from the ventral rami. Also, the dorsal rami (except for those from the first and second cervical

nerves) are generally smaller than the corresponding ventral rami. All the dorsal rami, except those from the first cervical, fourth and fifth sacral, and coccygeal nerves, divide into larger *medial* and smaller *lateral* branches. Most medial branches supply the muscles and the skin, whereas the lateral branches end in the mus-cles. However, the lateral branches tend to increase in size from above downward, so that those from the last thoracic, five lumbar, and five sacral nerves provide both muscular and cutaneous filaments.

Plate 4.8

Nerve Roots and Plexus Disorders

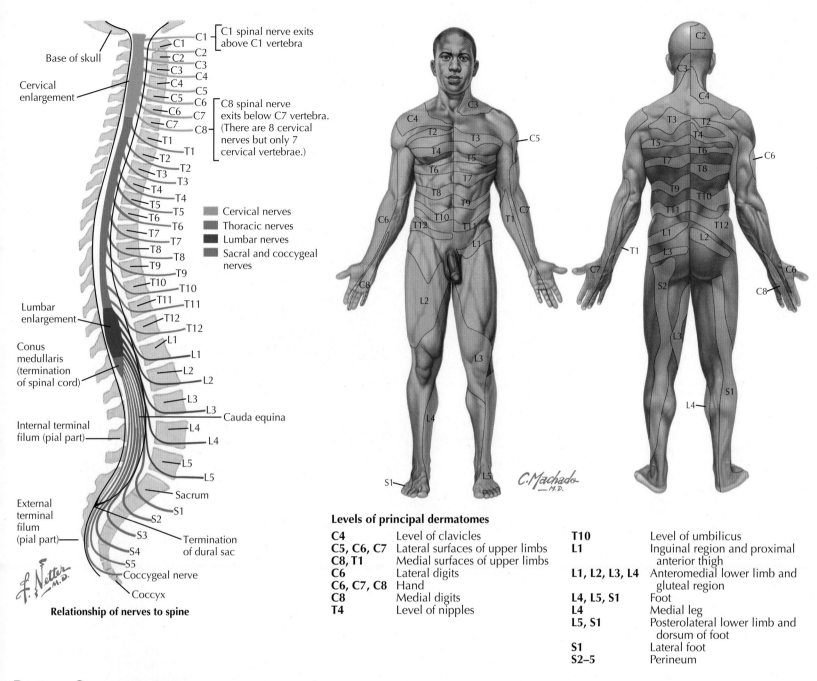

Relationship of nerves to spine

Levels of principal dermatomes

C4	Level of clavicles
C5, C6, C7	Lateral surfaces of upper limbs
C8, T1	Medial surfaces of upper limbs
C6	Lateral digits
C6, C7, C8	Hand
C8	Medial digits
T4	Level of nipples

T10	Level of umbilicus
L1	Inguinal region and proximal anterior thigh
L1, L2, L3, L4	Anteromedial lower limb and gluteal region
L4, L5, S1	Foot
L4	Medial leg
L5, S1	Posterolateral lower limb and dorsum of foot
S1	Lateral foot
S2–5	Perineum

DERMAL SEGMENTATION

The cutaneous area supplied by a single spinal nerve is called a *dermatome*. The cell bodies of the afferent fibers involved are in the dorsal spinal nerve root ganglia and in ganglia on cranial nerves V, VII, IX, and X. One exception should be mentioned: the cell bodies of the trigeminal nerve proprioceptive fibers conveyed from the facial and masticatory muscles are in the trigeminal mesencephalic nucleus and not in the trigeminal ganglion.

The spinal cord is segmental in character, and the spinal nerves are distributed to structures developed from the associated segments, or metameres (see Plate 2.1). In the trunk, the correspondence between neural and bodily segments is clearly apparent because they are arranged in consecutive encircling bands. In the limbs, however, because of plexus formation and interchange of nerve fibers in the nerves supplying them, the segmental distribution is obscured, although the arrangement is explicable embryologically. As the limb

buds develop, they draw out parts of certain segments, together with their mesodermal cores, ectodermal coverings, and corresponding segmental nerves and vessels. Thus the more proximal dermatomes are elongated strips situated along the preaxial (outer) sides of the limbs, and the more distal ones are situated along their postaxial (medial sides). The oblique disposition in the lower limbs is because, during development, the limbs rotate medially around a longitudinal axis.

The fifth cervical to first thoracic metameres and the first lumbar to third sacral metameres contribute, respectively, to the formation of the upper and lower limbs. This is reflected in their innervation and explains why in the neck, trunk, and upper limb the C5 and T1 dermatomes are in parts contiguous, and why in the trunk, perineum, and lower limbs the L1 and L2 dermatomes are in places adjacent to those of S2 and S3—the intervening segments have migrated into the more distal parts of the limbs.

The nerves supplying neighboring dermatomes overlap so that a lesion of one dorsal nerve root produces *hypoesthesia* rather than *anesthesia*. To cause complete cutaneous anesthesia in any area, at least three adjoining spinal nerves or their dorsal roots must be blocked or divided. The exception to this general rule is that a lesion of the dorsal root of C2 produces an area of complete anesthesia in the occipital region of the scalp. The degree of nerve overlap varies for different sensations and is greater for touch than for pain and temperature. Myotomal innervations also overlap so that most of the larger muscles (especially those in the limbs) are innervated by fibers from several ventral nerve roots. Therefore *paresis* occurs if only one or two roots are affected, but *paralysis* results if all innervating roots of a myotome are damaged or destroyed.

Knowledge of the dermatomes enables the clinician to locate lesions affecting the spinal cord or spinal nerves, and the dermatomes of the hand and foot deserve special attention.

THORACOABDOMINAL NERVES

Trapezius muscle
Erector spinae muscle
Medial branch
Lateral branch of
Dorsal (posterior) ramus
Spinal nerve trunk
Meningeal branch
Ventral (anterior) ramus of spinal nerve (intercostal nerve)
Collateral branch
Spinal sensory
(dorsal root) ganglion
External intercostal muscle
Internal intercostal muscle
Dorsal root
Innermost intercostal muscle
Ventral root
Latissimus dorsi muscle
Subcostal muscles
Serratus anterior muscle
Window cut in innermost intercostal muscle
Lateral cutaneous branch
Communicating branch
Internal intercostal muscle
Internal intercostal membranes anterior to external intercostal muscles
Innermost intercostal muscle
Greater and lesser splanchnic nerves
Collateral branch rejoining intercostal nerve
Internal intercostal muscle
Superior costotransverse ligaments
Sympathetic trunk
External intercostal muscle
Gray and white rami communicantes
Transversus abdominis muscle
Slip of costal part of diaphragm
External intercostal membrane
Rectus abdominis muscle
Costal cartilage
External oblique muscle
Linea alba
Anterior cutaneous branch

THORACIC NERVES

The 12 pairs of thoracic nerves resemble other typical spinal nerves in their segmental attachments to the cord by *dorsal* and *ventral nerve roots.* These roots unite to form short *spinal nerve trunks,* which emerge through the corresponding intervertebral foramina, give off recurrent meningeal filaments, establish connections through white and gray rami communicantes with adjacent sympathetic trunk ganglia, and divide into larger *ventral* and smaller *dorsal rami.* (See Plates 7.3 and 7.4 for greater detail of these general arrangements.)

The *dorsal rami* of the thoracic nerves run backward near the zygapophyseal joints, which they supply, and divide into medial and lateral branches. Both sets of branches pass through the groups of muscles constituting the erector spinae and give off branches to them. The terminations of the upper six or seven *medial branches* innervate the skin adjacent to the corresponding spinous processes, but the lower five or six often fail to reach the skin. The terminations of all the *lateral branches* usually pierce the thoracolumbar fascia over the erector spinae muscles and divide into *medial* and *lateral cutaneous branches,* which innervate much of the skin of the posterior thoracic wall and upper lumbar regions.

The *ventral rami* of most of the thoracic nerves, unlike those in other regions, do not form plexuses. They retain their segmental character, and each pair runs separately in the corresponding intercostal spaces as the *intercostal nerves.* The first pair, however, divides into larger and smaller branches; the larger, usually joined by branches from the second pair, participate in the formation of the *brachial plexuses* (Plate 4.13), whereas the smaller branches form the first pair of intercostal nerves. The last (twelfth) pair of ventral rami course below the lowest ribs and are therefore termed the *subcostal nerves.*

The *intercostal nerves* are distributed mainly to structures in the thoracic and abdominal walls. The upper six pairs are limited to the thoracic parietes, whereas the lower five pairs extend from the thoracic into the abdominal walls and contribute fibers to the diaphragm. The intercostal nerves give off *muscular, anterior* and *lateral cutaneous, mammary,* and *collateral branches* and supply filaments to adjacent vessels, periosteum, parietal pleura, and peritoneum.

The upper six pairs supply *muscular branches* to the corresponding intercostal muscles and to the subcostal, serratus posterior superior, and transverse thoracic muscles. The lower five pairs supply the lower intercostal muscles and the subcostal, serratus posterior inferior, transverse, oblique, and rectus abdominal muscles.

Fascicles from the lower intercostal nerves also enter the margins of the diaphragm, but they are sensory. The subcostal nerves supply the pyramidalis muscles.

The *anterior cutaneous branches* supply the front of the thorax. The *lateral cutaneous branches* pierce the internal and external intercostal muscles and end by dividing into branches that extend forward and backward to innervate the skin covering the lateral sides of the thorax and abdomen. The small *lateral branch* of the *first intercostal nerve* supplies the skin of the axilla, and the lateral branch of the second is the *intercostobrachial nerve,* which is distributed to the skin on the medial side of the arm. The *lateral cutaneous branch* of the *subcostal nerve* pierces the internal and external oblique abdominal muscles and descends over the iliac crest to supply the skin of the anterior part of the gluteal region.

The *mammary glands* receive filaments from the lateral and anterior cutaneous branches of the fourth, fifth, and sixth intercostal nerves, which convey autonomic and sensory fibers to and from the glands.

Plate 4.10

Nerve Roots and Plexus Disorders

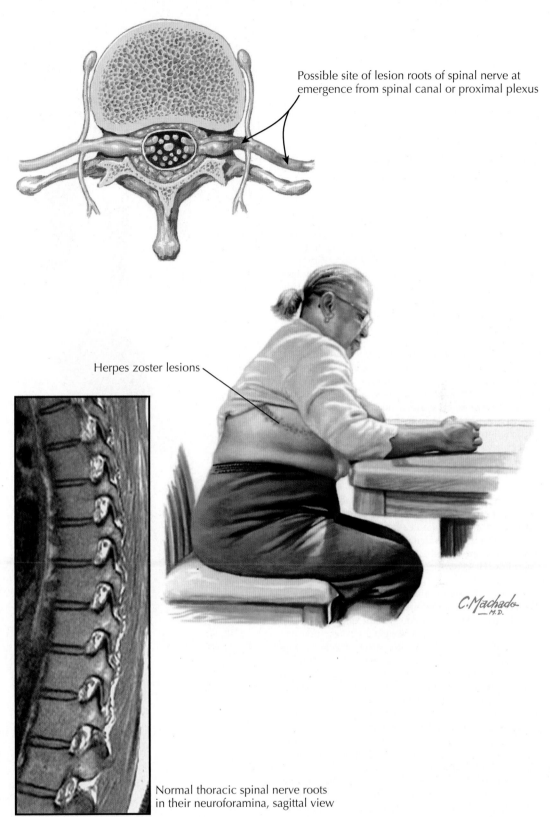

Possible site of lesion roots of spinal nerve at emergence from spinal canal or proximal plexus

Herpes zoster lesions

Normal thoracic spinal nerve roots in their neuroforamina, sagittal view

THORACIC SPINAL NERVE ROOT DISORDERS

The common occurrence of disk herniation and spinal nerve root compression seen at the cervical and lumbosacral levels is not the case at the thoracic levels because of the rib cage, which stabilizes the spine and minimizes the forces leading to disk rupture and spondylosis. Disk herniation at the T1–2 level is more common than at other thoracic levels, resulting in a T1 radiculopathy, which is clinically manifested as numbness and pain in the medial hand and forearm with weakness of thumb abduction. Thoracic nerve roots may also be affected by mass lesions, such as meningiomas and schwannomas. Varicella-zoster reactivation occurs frequently at thoracic spinal root levels, producing a characteristic vesicular rash that follows a radicular pattern from the spine circumferentially around the torso to the abdominal wall. Acute herpes zoster neuropathy is manifested by pain and then anesthesia in a distribution conforming to the involved dermatomal segment. At times, the motor spinal nerve root fibers are also affected, producing weakness in abdominal wall muscles of the affected myotomes. This is clinically manifested as a unilateral bulge of the abdominal wall when contracted, such as during a sit-up maneuver. Postherpetic neuralgia describes the chronic pain and numbness that persist after the rash resolves and is especially prevalent among older individuals. Diabetic thoracic radiculopathy presents with similar symptoms and signs but without rash. Lyme disease can demonstrate neurologic manifestations, such as multifocal radiculitis, which can include the thoracic levels. For disorders affecting the motor fibers at the T9–12 segmental levels, unilateral or bilateral weakness of rectus abdominis muscles and muscle bulging can be seen.

DIABETIC LUMBOSACRAL RADICULOPLEXUS NEUROPATHY

Patients with diabetes mellitus are predisposed to a variety of peripheral nerve disorders, the most common of which is a chronic symmetric distal polyneuropathy with sensory predominance. In addition, a variety of other neuropathic disorders may develop, including an asymmetric polyneuropathy such as mononeuritis multiplex; an acute oculomotor nerve palsy that mimics an aneurysm except for pupillary sparing; compression or entrapment neuropathies; and an acute lumbosacral radiculoplexus neuropathy.

Diabetic lumbosacral radiculoplexus neuropathy is a painful condition that causes severe weakness and muscle wasting of the lower extremities. Several clinical terms have been applied to this syndrome, including diabetic amyotrophy, femoral neuropathy of diabetes, diabetic asymmetric proximal motor neuropathy, and diabetic lumbosacral plexopathy. Differences in terminology have reflected various opinions as to the primary anatomic site of the lesion and underlying pathology. Although the syndrome was initially thought to be limited to the proximal muscles of the thigh, more recent studies have demonstrated that most cases are widespread, affecting both proximal and distal segments in bilateral lower extremities. Pathologic findings on nerve biopsy include microvasculitic changes and inflammation, suggestive of an underlying immune-mediated vasculitis. However, the exact mechanism of injury is still unknown.

Clinical Manifestations. The onset of symptoms is typically focal, beginning with severe pain in the anterior thigh and hip and weakness of the thigh muscles. It is also often accompanied by weight loss. Over time, the symptoms progress to involve distal segments and eventually the contralateral limb. Less commonly, there may be additional thoracic nerve root involvement resulting in truncal pain and paresthesias. The cervical dermatomes are usually not affected, although there may be a concomitant mononeuropathy of the upper limb, such as an ulnar mononeuropathy.

Although the onset of symptoms is often acute, the course may be insidiously progressive in some patients. Pain is the most common initial complaint. In contrast to patients with a disk herniation and radiculopathy who can usually find a comfortable position at night, patients with diabetic lumbosacral radiculoplexus neuropathy often have nocturnal exacerbations. The pain frequently has a dysesthetic quality evoked by touch or exacerbated by clothing, such as garments that fit tightly over the thigh. When thoracic dermatomes are involved, the pain is sometimes severe enough to mimic an abdominal or cardiac crisis.

Weakness without sensory loss may be the first sign in some patients. Involvement of the quadriceps femoris and iliopsoas muscles may compromise climbing stairs or arising from a squatting position. With more distal weakness, the patient may experience gait difficulty due to footdrop.

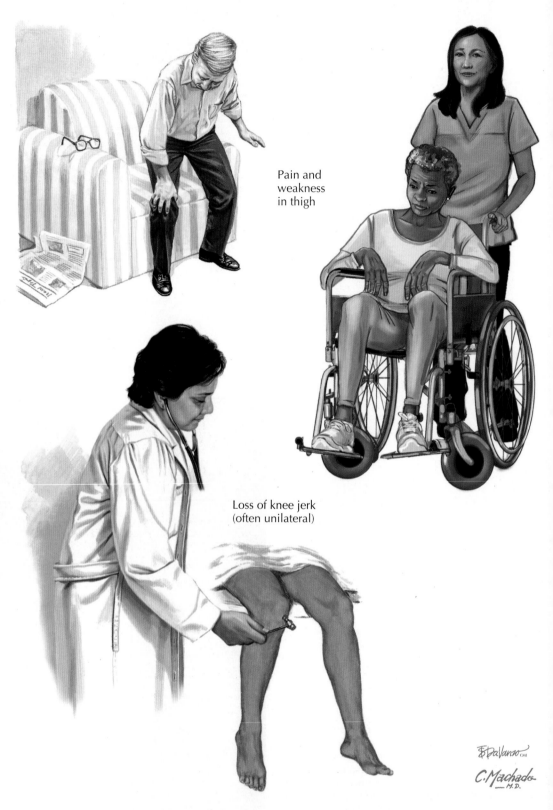

Pain and weakness in thigh

Loss of knee jerk (often unilateral)

Diagnosis. Physical examination confirms the radicular or plexus pattern of motor loss. Deep tendon reflexes, particularly the knee jerk, are often absent. Sensory loss may be difficult to define, although the area of hyperpathia and dysesthesias may sometimes mimic a nerve root distribution. A moderate number of patients show signs of coexisting mild symmetric distal polyneuropathy, although sensory abnormalities in the feet may also be related to distal limb involvement.

Electrodiagnostic studies demonstrate reduced amplitudes of sensory and motor nerve conduction responses with needle examination findings of active denervation and neurogenic motor unit potential changes in the distribution of multiple nerve roots including paraspinal muscles. CSF protein is often elevated. Imaging studies of the LS spine are typically normal.

Course and Treatment. In most cases, improvement occurs spontaneously over a period of 6 to 18 months, but immune-modulating therapy may expedite recovery regarding pain and weakness if initiated early. Symptomatic management with optimal pain control and physical therapy is crucial. Relapse may occur in approximately one in five patients.

Plate 4.12

Nerve Roots and Plexus Disorders

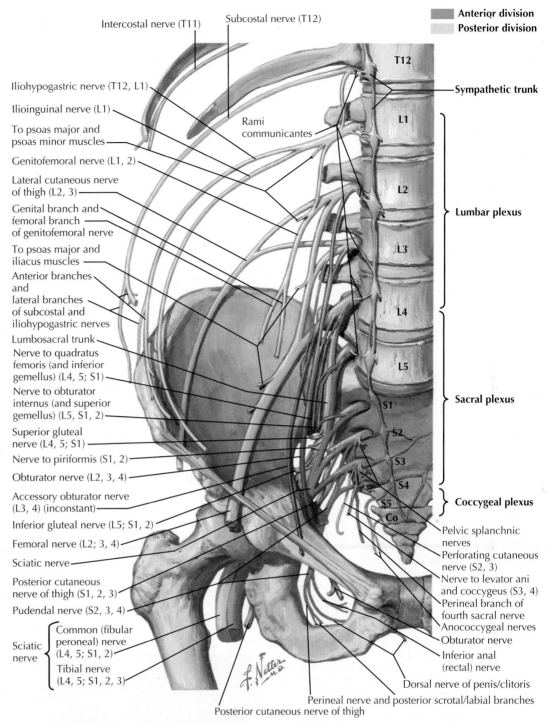

Intercostal nerve (T11)
Subcostal nerve (T12)

Anterior division
Posterior division

Iliohypogastric nerve (T12, L1)

Ilioinguinal nerve (L1)

Rami communicantes

To psoas major and psoas minor muscles

Genitofemoral nerve (L1, 2)

Lateral cutaneous nerve of thigh (L2, 3)

Genital branch and femoral branch of genitofemoral nerve

To psoas major and iliacus muscles

Anterior branches and lateral branches of subcostal and iliohypogastric nerves

Lumbosacral trunk

Nerve to quadratus femoris (and inferior gemellus) (L4, 5; S1)

Nerve to obturator internus (and superior gemellus) (L5, S1, 2)

Superior gluteal nerve (L4, 5; S1)

Nerve to piriformis (S1, 2)

Obturator nerve (L2, 3, 4)

Accessory obturator nerve (L3, 4) (inconstant)

Inferior gluteal nerve (L5; S1, 2)

Femoral nerve (L2; 3, 4)

Sciatic nerve

Posterior cutaneous nerve of thigh (S1, 2, 3)

Pudendal nerve (S2, 3, 4)

Sciatic nerve { Common (fibular peroneal) nerve (L4, 5; S1, 2)

Tibial nerve (L4, 5; S1, 2, 3)

T12
Sympathetic trunk
L1
L2
Lumbar plexus
L3
L4
L5
S1
Sacral plexus
S2
S3
S4
S5
Co
Coccygeal plexus

Pelvic splanchnic nerves

Perforating cutaneous nerve (S2, 3)

Nerve to levator ani and coccygeus (S3, 4)

Perineal branch of fourth sacral nerve

Anococcygeal nerves

Obturator nerve

Inferior anal (rectal) nerve

Dorsal nerve of penis/clitoris

Perineal nerve and posterior scrotal/labial branches

Posterior cutaneous nerve of thigh

LUMBAR, SACRAL, AND COCCYGEAL PLEXUSES

The lumbar, sacral, and coccygeal plexuses are a network of interconnected peripheral nerves that are formed from the ventral rami of the *lumbar, sacral,* and *coccygeal nerves.* Variations in their makeup are common.

The *lumbar plexus* is produced by the union of the ventral rami of L1 to L3 and the superior portion of L4 with a contribution from T12 (subcostal nerve). The plexus lies anterior to the lumbar vertebral transverse processes and is embedded in the posterior part of the psoas major muscle.

The first lumbar nerve receives a fascicle from the subcostal nerve (T12) and divides into upper and lower branches; the upper branch splits into the iliohypogastric and ilioinguinal nerves, whereas the lower branch joins a branch from the second lumbar nerve and becomes the genitofemoral nerve. Except near their terminations, all three nerves run parallel to the lower intercostal nerves and help supply the transverse and oblique abdominal muscles. The *iliohypogastric nerve* gives off a lateral cutaneous branch to the skin on the anterolateral aspect of the buttock and ends as the anterior cutaneous branch to the skin above the pubis. The *ilioinguinal nerve* pierces the internal oblique muscle above the anterior part of the iliac crest and then runs above and parallel to the inguinal ligament to traverse the inguinal canal and supply the skin over the root of the penis, the adjoining part of the femoral triangle, and the upper part of the scrotum (mons pubis and adjacent part of labium majus in the female). The *genitofemoral nerve* penetrates the psoas major muscle and divides into *genital* and *femoral branches.* The genital branch in males passes through the inguinal canal and supplies the cremaster muscle and the skin of the

scrotum; in females, it ends in the mons pubis and labia majora. The femoral branch in both males and females supplies the skin over the upper part of the femoral triangle.

The larger part of the second lumbar nerve, the entire third lumbar nerve, and a branch from the fourth lumbar nerve split into ventral (anterior) and dorsal (posterior) divisions, which unite to constitute, respectively, the *obturator* and *femoral nerves* (see Plates 5.15 and 5.16). The *lateral femoral cutaneous nerve* (see Plate 5.16) is formed by offshoots from the second and third posterior divisions.

The lower part of the ventral ramus of the fourth lumbar nerve joins the ventral ramus of the fifth to form the *lumbosacral trunk.* The trunk and the ventral rami of the first three sacral nerves and the upper part of the fourth sacral ramus constitute the *sacral plexus.*

The *sacral plexus,* by convergence and fusion of its roots, becomes a flattened band that gives rise to many branches before its largest part passes below the piriformis muscle and through the greater sciatic foramen as the *sciatic nerve* (see Plate 5.17). The rami forming the sacral plexus divide into ventral (anterior) and dorsal (posterior) divisions, which subdivide and regroup to become branches of the plexus.

COCCYGEAL PLEXUS

The lower part of the ventral rami of the fourth and fifth sacral nerves and the coccygeal nerves form the small coccygeal plexus. It consists of two loops on the pelvic surface of the coccygeus and levator ani muscles. Branches are given off to these muscles, and fine *anococcygeal nerves* supply the skin between the anus and coccyx.

Note: Usual composition shown.
Prefixed plexus has large C4
contribution but lacks T1.
Postfixed plexus lacks C5 but
has T2 contribution.

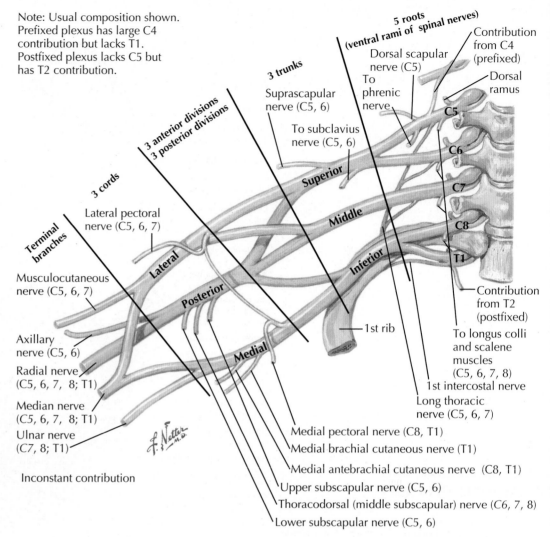

5 roots
(ventral rami of spinal nerves)

3 trunks

3 anterior divisions
3 posterior divisions

3 cords

Terminal branches

Dorsal scapular nerve (C5)

To phrenic nerve

Contribution from C4 (prefixed)

Dorsal ramus

C5

C6

C7

C8

T1

Suprascapular nerve (C5, 6)

To subclavius nerve (C5, 6)

Superior

Middle

Inferior

Lateral pectoral nerve (C5, 6, 7)

Lateral

Posterior

Medial

Musculocutaneous nerve (C5, 6, 7)

Axillary nerve (C5, 6)

Radial nerve (C5, 6, 7, 8; T1)

Median nerve (C5, 6, 7, 8; T1)

Ulnar nerve (C7, 8; T1)

Inconstant contribution

1st rib

Contribution from T2 (postfixed)

To longus colli and scalene muscles (C5, 6, 7, 8)

1st intercostal nerve

Long thoracic nerve (C5, 6, 7)

Medial pectoral nerve (C8, T1)

Medial brachial cutaneous nerve (T1)

Medial antebrachial cutaneous nerve (C8, T1)

Upper subscapular nerve (C5, 6)

Thoracodorsal (middle subscapular) nerve (C6, 7, 8)

Lower subscapular nerve (C5, 6)

BRACHIAL PLEXUS

ROOTS

The brachial plexus is formed by the union of the ventral (anterior) primary rami of C5–8 and the greater part of T1, which constitute the roots of the plexus. Usually, a small branch from C4 joins the C5 root, and one from T2 joins the T1 root; thus C4 and T2 often provide minor contributions to the plexus. However, the contributions are variable in size, especially if so-called prefixation or postfixation exists. A "prefixed" plexus shows a cranial shift and the C4 contribution is large, whereas the contribution from T1 is small and that from T2 is often absent. In a "postfixed" plexus, the condition is reversed: the contribution from T2 is large, that from C5 is small, and that from C4 is often missing. The roots lie between the anterior and middle scalene muscles.

Efferent and afferent (somatic and autonomic) fibers are arranged accordingly within the various trunks, divisions, cords, and terminal branches for distribution to the muscles, skin, vessels, and glands in the upper limbs. Afferent fibers reach the roots of the plexus through the sympathetic rami communicantes.

Trunks

The upper roots (C5, C6) unite to form the *superior trunk*, the C7 root continues alone as the *middle trunk*, and the lower roots (C8, T1) constitute the *inferior trunk* of the plexus. The trunks lie in the lower part of the posterior cervical triangle.

Divisions and Cords. Each trunk divides into three *ventral* (anterior) and three *dorsal* (posterior) *divisions*, which supply the ventral (flexor) and dorsal (extensor) structures in the upper limb. In the axilla, the divisions become regrouped as follows: the *ventral division* of the *inferior trunk* continues as the *medial cord* (C8, T1), the *ventral divisions* of the *superior* and *middle trunks* unite to form the *lateral cord* (C5, C6, C7), and all *three dorsal divisions* of the *trunks* join to produce the *posterior cord* (C5–8, T1). (The terms *medial*, *lateral*, and *posterior* indicate the relationships of the cords to the second part of the axillary artery.)

Branches. Most of the branches of the brachial plexus originate in the axilla from the *cords* located below the level of the clavicle and are termed the *infraclavicular branches*. In contrast, some branches of the plexus arise from the *roots* and *trunks* in the posterior cervical triangle above the clavicle and are referred to as the *supraclavicular branches*. Of note, nerves derived from a cord do not necessarily contain fibers from all its constituent roots; for instance, the axillary nerve arising from the posterior cord (C5–8, T1) contains fibers from only C5 and C6.

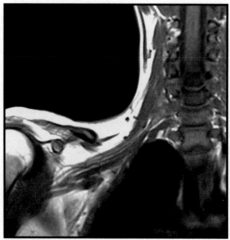

Normal right brachial plexus, T1-weighted coronal view

Supraclavicular branches	
From plexus roots or spinal cord	
To longus colli and scalene mm.	C5, 6, 7, 8
Dorsal scapular	C5
Branch to phrenic	C5
Long thoracic	C5, 6, 7
Spinal accessory	Cervical spinal cord (and C3, 4)
From superior trunk	
Suprascapular	C5, 6
To subclavius m.	C5, 6

Infraclavicular branches	
From lateral cord	
Lateral pectoral	C5, 6, 7
Musculocutaneous	C(4), 5, 6, 7
Lateral root of median	C(5), 6, 7
From medial cord	
Medial pectoral	C8, T1
Medial cutaneous n. of arm	T1
Medial cutaneous n. of forearm	(C8), T1
Ulnar	C(7), 8, T1
Medial root of median	C8, T1
From posterior cord	
Upper subscapular	C5, 6, (7)
Lower subscapular	C5, 6
Axillary (circumflex humeral)	C5, 6
Thoracodorsal	C6, 7, 8
Radial	C5, 6, 7, 8; T1

Plate 4.14

Nerve Roots and Plexus Disorders

BRACHIAL PLEXUS AND CERVICAL NERVE ROOT INJURIES AT BIRTH

Neonatal brachial plexus injuries occur in approximately 0.5 to 2 per 1000 live births. The injury is caused by traction forces during labor and delivery. Predisposing factors include gestational diabetes, occipitoposterior or transverse presentation, the use of oxytocin, instrumented delivery, shoulder dystocia, and macrosomia.

As nerve roots are anchored by the spinal column and cord, traction or propulsive forces can result in stretching of the brachial plexus. Lesion severity depends on the degree of stretch, but axonal injury is the usual result. If the epineurial nerve sheath remains intact, nerve regeneration down to the denervated muscles occurs at a rate of about 1 mm per day. Complete rupture of the nerve sheath, as well as the axons, leads to poor reinnervation. With severe traction injuries, there may be additional damage to spinal nerve roots that include root avulsion. The diagnosis is supported by the clinical examination, which demonstrates reduced movement of the affected arm in a brachial plexus distribution. Electrodiagnostic testing can aid in assessing the extent of nerve injury, underlying nerve pathophysiology (axon loss versus conduction block), and presence of reinnervation. Imaging studies such as CT myelography and MRI may be helpful in diagnosing root avulsion injuries and excluding other potential etiologies.

Neonatal brachial plexus injuries may be classified according to the location of the nerve injury. Upper brachial plexus injuries involve the portion of the plexus supplied by the C5 and C6 roots (Erb palsy), whereas lower injuries involve the portion of the plexus derived from the C8 and T1 roots (Klumpke palsy).

UPPER TRUNK BRACHIAL PLEXUS INJURY (ERB PALSY)

Erb palsy affects muscles supplied by C5 and C6 and is the most common of the brachial plexus injuries, accounting for 90% of cases. An *asymmetric Moro response* is usually the first indication of the injury. The upper extremity assumes the "waiter's tip" position: the shoulder is adducted and internally rotated, the elbow is extended, and the forearm is pronated with the wrist in flexion. A mild sensory loss may develop over the lateral aspect of the shoulder and arm but is difficult to elicit. Associated fractures of the clavicle or humerus must be excluded, and fluoroscopic examination should be carried out to exclude the rare diaphragmatic paralysis caused mainly by a C4 lesion.

LOWER BRACHIAL PLEXUS INJURY (KLUMPKE PALSY)

A pure lower brachial plexus injury is uncommon, and most cases of Klumpke palsy involve the more proximal muscles supplied by C7 or C6. An *absent grasp reflex* is the most prominent clinical feature. There may be involvement of sympathetic fibers from T1, causing Horner syndrome (ptosis, miosis, anhidrosis). A significant sensory deficit is usually present, occasionally resulting in unwitting trauma to fingers. Prognosis for full recovery in these infants is poor. The upper extremity often remains small and distally foreshortened.

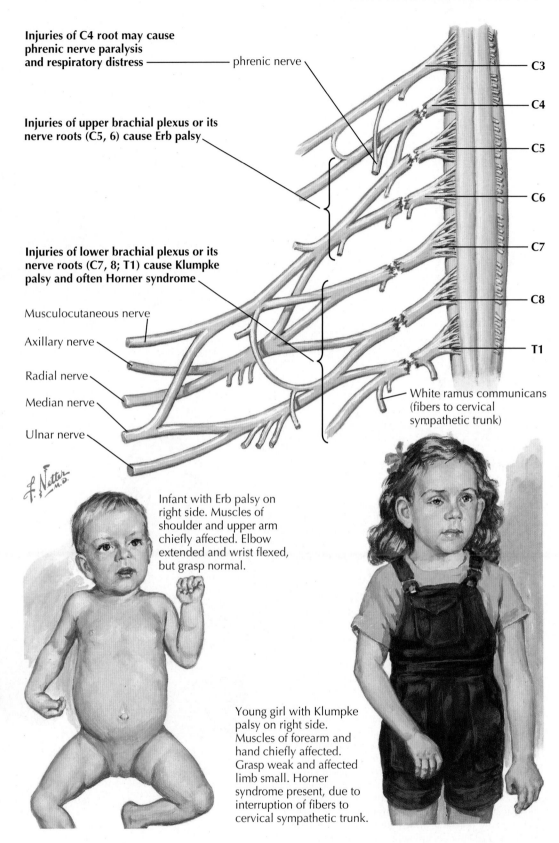

Injuries of C4 root may cause phrenic nerve paralysis and respiratory distress —— phrenic nerve

Injuries of upper brachial plexus or its nerve roots (C5, 6) cause Erb palsy

Injuries of lower brachial plexus or its nerve roots (C7, 8; T1) cause Klumpke palsy and often Horner syndrome

Musculocutaneous nerve

Axillary nerve

Radial nerve

Median nerve

Ulnar nerve

C3
C4
C5
C6
C7
C8
T1

White ramus communicans (fibers to cervical sympathetic trunk)

Infant with Erb palsy on right side. Muscles of shoulder and upper arm chiefly affected. Elbow extended and wrist flexed, but grasp normal.

Young girl with Klumpke palsy on right side. Muscles of forearm and hand chiefly affected. Grasp weak and affected limb small. Horner syndrome present, due to interruption of fibers to cervical sympathetic trunk.

MANAGEMENT

Immediate treatment of neonatal brachial plexus injury is conservative. Once a structural lesion of the neck and brachial plexus has been excluded, physical and occupational therapy should be initiated as soon as possible. Functional positioning, passive range-of-motion exercises, splinting, and sensory stimulation may help lead to significant improvement in the first few months of life. Electrostimulation has also been used to promote functional motor recovery. Surgical intervention should be considered when there is complete arm paresis or no clinical improvement in the first 3 to 6 months. Procedures include surgical exploration, neurolysis, and peripheral nerve transfers. After the child is 5 to 6 years of age, muscle transfers may also be helpful.

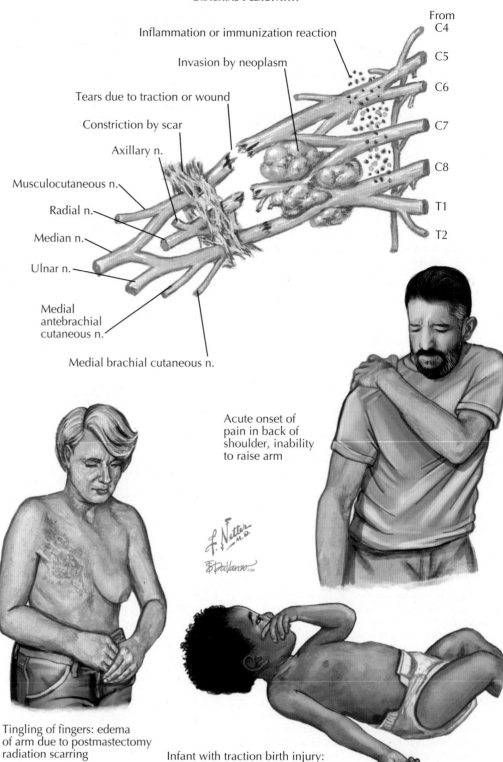

BRACHIAL PLEXOPATHY

Inflammation or immunization reaction

Invasion by neoplasm

Tears due to traction or wound

Constriction by scar

Axillary n.

Musculocutaneous n.

Radial n.

Median n.

Ulnar n.

Medial antebrachial cutaneous n.

Medial brachial cutaneous n.

From C4

C5

C6

C7

C8

T1

T2

Acute onset of pain in back of shoulder, inability to raise arm

Tingling of fingers: edema of arm due to postmastectomy radiation scarring

Infant with traction birth injury: paralysis of right arm (Erb palsy)

BRACHIAL PLEXOPATHY

Trauma is responsible for many acute brachial plexus lesions. The prognosis depends on the severity of the lesion and the distance between the lesion and the muscles innervated by the affected nerve fibers. Thus the likelihood of reinnervation is better for upper trunk/lateral cord lesions and worse for lower trunk/medial cord lesions. However, when the traumatic injury results in spinal nerve root avulsion, reinnervation of the affected brachial plexus segment will not occur. Common nonsurgical traumas to the brachial plexus include gunshot wounds and motorcycle and motor vehicle accidents. Surgical trauma to the brachial plexus can occur in open heart surgery, when rib cage retraction causes fracture of the first thoracic rib at the costovertebral joint and migration of the rib upwards with entrapment of the C8 anterior primary ramus proximal to its point of combination with the T1 segment to form the lower trunk. The clinical presentation is severe pain and numbness in the medial hand with weakness of finger abduction, and finger extension.

Neuralgic amyotrophy (acute brachial plexitis) is an immune-mediated disorder of one or more peripheral nerves within the brachial plexus that is often triggered by an acute infectious illness, immunization, or surgery. It has many potential presentations that range from an individual mononeuropathy to a pan-plexopathy, but it usually affects nerve trunks of the shoulder girdle, upper trunk nerve fibers, and parts of the peripheral nerve trunks of the arm. Winging of the scapula from long thoracic neuropathy, inability to externally rotate the shoulder from a suprascapular neuropathy, and inability to abduct the shoulder from axillary neuropathy are common presentations. Spontaneous improvement occurs in most individuals over 6 to 12 months.

Progressive brachial plexus lesions may result from infiltrative processes that spread from local structures.

This commonly includes malignancies, such as lung (Pancoast tumor) and breast cancers, which tend to involve the lower trunk/medial cord first, producing sensory loss in the fourth and fifth fingers and weakness of intrinsic hand muscles. A progressive brachial plexopathy can also result from radiation therapy that had been administered to the region of the brachial plexus years earlier for treatment of these malignancies.

A slowly progressive lower trunk brachial plexopathy (neurogenic thoracic outlet syndrome) can arise from a fibrous band extending from an elongated C7 transverse process to the first thoracic rib. This anatomic anomaly causes compression of the T1 anterior primary ramus before it merges with the C8 segment to form the lower trunk, producing a classic clinical presentation of numbness of the medial hand and forearm, along with weakness and atrophy of thumb and other intrinsic hand muscles. Progression of weakness is halted by surgical section of the offending fibrous band.

Plate 4.16

Nerve Roots and Plexus Disorders

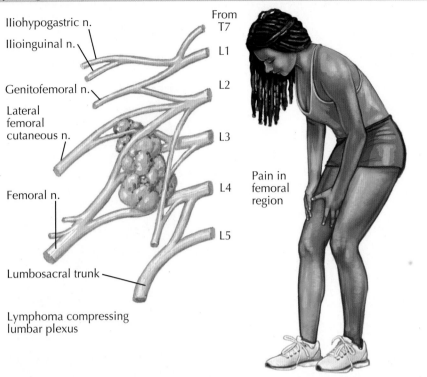

Tumor compressing lumbar plexus

Iliohypogastric n.
Ilioinguinal n.
Genitofemoral n.
Lateral femoral cutaneous n.
Femoral n.
Lumbosacral trunk
Lymphoma compressing lumbar plexus

From T7
L1
L2
L3
L4
L5

Pain in femoral region

Lumbosacral Plexopathy

The clinical presentation of lumbosacral plexopathy varies depending on which portion of the plexus is affected: the lumbar plexus, the sacral plexus, or both. Patients with lesions of the lumbar plexus will note prominent hip flexion weakness, although knee extensors and hip adductors may also be involved. This is often accompanied by pain and sensory loss in the distribution of the inguinal region, most of the thigh, and the medial lower leg. With lesions affecting the sacral plexus, footdrop is a common presenting complaint along with weakness in hip extensors, hip abductors, knee flexors, and foot/ankle movements. Pain and sensory changes may be seen in the posterior thigh, most of the lower leg, and throughout the foot. Lesions affecting both parts of the lumbosacral plexus are uncommon but can lead to extensive weakness and sensory changes involving the entire leg.

In contrast to the brachial plexus, traumatic lesions of the lumbosacral plexus are relatively uncommon because of its protective location within the pelvis. Injuries such as gunshot wounds, falls, and motor vehicle accidents, which often result in pelvic fractures, can cause an acute and diffuse lumbosacral plexopathy via blunt force or nerve avulsion.

Malignancy may also cause an extensive lesion of the lumbosacral plexus. Tumor invasion from lymphoma, metastatic disease, or malignancies arising from neighboring structures (e.g., gynecologic tumors and colorectal cancer) may cause compression or direct infiltration of the plexus. Another cancer-related cause is radiation injury, which is a slowly progressive lesion that occurs several years after radiation treatment for cancers within the pelvis. Radiation injuries typically affect the sacral plexus (lower portion), causing weakness, sensory loss, and sometimes pain in the corresponding distributions.

In diabetic patients, an immune-mediated vasculitic lesion may lead to a syndrome called diabetic lumbosacral radiculoplexus neuropathy, which causes severe pain and muscle weakness in lumbosacral plexus–innervated muscles with corresponding sensory loss (see Plate 4.11). Also known as diabetic amyotrophy, the syndrome may initially mimic a femoral neuropathy but soon progresses to involve more distal segments and eventually the contralateral lower extremity. Nondiabetic patients may experience a similar clinical syndrome, which is also thought to be due to an immune-mediated microvasculitis. Spontaneous recovery over several months typically occurs in both types, although immune-modulating therapies have been shown in small studies to improve pain and weakness.

A more recently described etiology is maternal lumbosacral plexopathy, which occurs primarily in petite women due to compression of the lumbosacral trunk (L5 nerve root with posterior portion of L4) by the

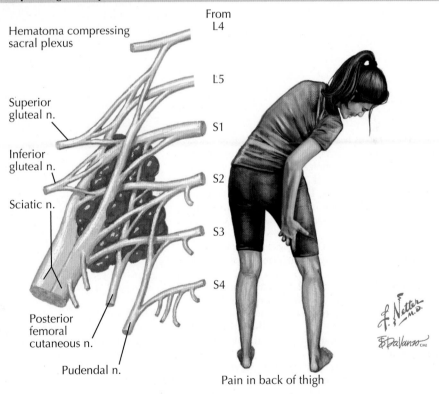

Hematoma compressing sacral plexus

Hematoma compressing sacral plexus
Superior gluteal n.
Inferior gluteal n.
Sciatic n.
Posterior femoral cutaneous n.
Pudendal n.

From L4
L5
S1
S2
S3
S4

Pain in back of thigh

descending fetal head at the pelvic brim. After a difficult or prolonged labor that, in many cases, necessitates a forceps delivery or cesarean section, the patient will notice a footdrop on attempts to stand or walk. Fortunately, the underlying pathophysiology of the lesion is thought to be demyelinating conduction block, and most patients spontaneously recover within 3 months.

Retroperitoneal hematomas in patients receiving anticoagulation or after experiencing blunt trauma may compress the lumbar plexus and result in acute weakness of hip flexors with pain in the groin, hip, or lower abdomen. The hemorrhage is usually seen on CT of the abdomen and pelvis and can be accompanied by a sudden drop in the hematocrit level.

Finally, infection may cause a lumbosacral plexopathy through a compressive mechanism due to an infraabdominal abscess or infiltrative lesion, such as that seen with herpes simplex or cytomegalovirus infections.

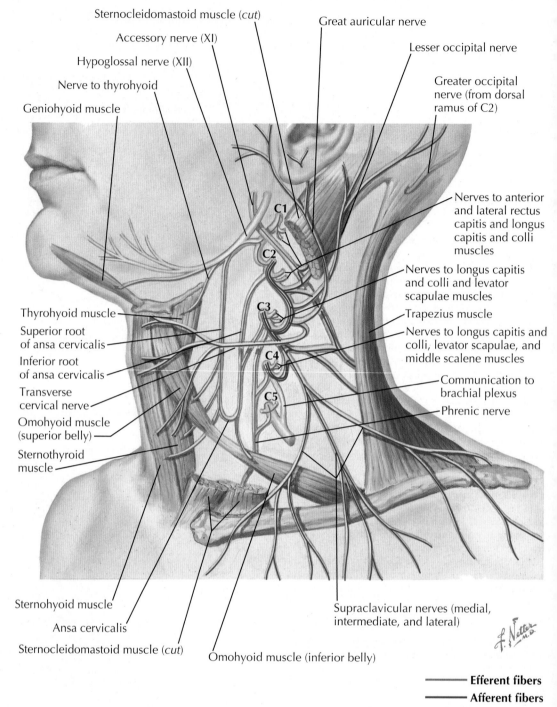

Sternocleidomastoid muscle (*cut*)

Accessory nerve (XI)

Hypoglossal nerve (XII)

Nerve to thyrohyoid

Geniohyoid muscle

Great auricular nerve

Lesser occipital nerve

Greater occipital nerve (from dorsal ramus of C2)

C1

C2

C3

C4

C5

Nerves to anterior and lateral rectus capitis and longus capitis and colli muscles

Nerves to longus capitis and colli and levator scapulae muscles

Trapezius muscle

Nerves to longus capitis and colli, levator scapulae, and middle scalene muscles

Communication to brachial plexus

Phrenic nerve

Thyrohyoid muscle

Superior root of ansa cervicalis

Inferior root of ansa cervicalis

Transverse cervical nerve

Omohyoid muscle (superior belly)

Sternothyroid muscle

Sternohyoid muscle

Ansa cervicalis

Sternocleidomastoid muscle (*cut*)

Omohyoid muscle (inferior belly)

Supraclavicular nerves (medial, intermediate, and lateral)

——— **Efferent fibers**

——— **Afferent fibers**

CERVICAL PLEXUS

The cervical plexus lies deep to the sternocleidomastoid muscle. Its branches convey motor fibers to many cervical muscles and to the diaphragm; sensory fibers received from parts of the scalp, neck, and chest; and autonomic fibers to vessels and glands. The superficial branches perforate the cervical fascia to supply cutaneous structures, whereas the deep branches supply mainly muscles and joints.

The *superficial branches* are the lesser (minor) occipital, great auricular, transverse (cutaneous) cervical, and supraclavicular nerves.

The *lesser occipital nerve* (C2, C3) curves around the accessory (XI) nerve, ascends near the posterior border of the sternocleidomastoid muscle, and then divides into branches that supply the skin on the superolateral aspects of the neck, the upper part of the auricle, and the adjacent area of the scalp.

The *great auricular nerve* (C2, C3) is larger than the lesser occipital and passes obliquely upward over the sternocleidomastoid muscle, lying near the external jugular vein before dividing into anterior and posterior branches. The former passes over or through the parotid gland to supply the skin of the posteroinferior part of the face. The latter supplies the skin over the mastoid process and over the medial and lateral surfaces of the lower part of the auricle.

The *transverse cervical nerve* (C2, C3) runs forward beneath the external jugular vein to divide into superior and inferior branches, which supply the skin over the anterolateral aspects of the neck from the mandible above to the sternum below.

The *supraclavicular nerves* (C3, C4) arise from a common trunk, which descends for a variable distance before dividing into medial, intermediate, and lateral supraclavicular nerves. These supply the skin over the lower neck from near the midline to the acromioclavicular region and above the shoulder. They then pass in front of the clavicle to innervate the skin of the anterior chest wall to the level of the sternal angle and the second rib. The medial and lateral nerves, respectively, send branches to the sternoclavicular and acromioclavicular joints.

The *deep branches* are mainly motor, but they also carry proprioceptive, osseous, articular, and autonomic fibers to and from muscles, bones, joints, and vessels in their areas of distribution. Some motor branches pass *medially* to supply the rectus capitis anterior and rectus capitis lateralis (C1, C2), longus capitis (C1, C2, C3), longus colli and intertransverse (C2, C3, C4) muscles, and the diaphragm through the phrenic nerve. Other muscular branches pass *laterally* to the sternocleidomastoid (C2, C3), trapezius (C3, C4), levator scapulae (C3, C4), and scalenus anterior and scalenus medius (C3, C4) muscles. The branches to the sternocleidomastoid and trapezius muscles are reputedly proprioceptive, but they nevertheless communicate with motor branches of the accessory nerve to these muscles.

A branch from the loop between C1 and C2 joins the hypoglossal (XII) nerve. Some of these fibers continue onward, along with the hypoglossal nerve, to supply the thyrohyoid and geniohyoid muscles, whereas others leave it as a filament running downward, anterolateral to the carotid sheath, the *superior root (descendens hypoglossi)* of the *ansa cervicalis*, or *ansa hypoglossi*. The ansa ("loop") is completed by the *inferior root (descendens cervicalis)* derived from C2 and C3. Branches from the ansa supply the sternohyoid, sternothyroid, and omohyoid muscles.

MONONEUROPATHIES

COMPRESSION NEUROPATHIES

Compression neuropathies occur acutely (e.g., proximal radial nerve palsy, peroneal neuropathy at the fibular head) or more gradually (e.g., median neuropathy at the wrist, ulnar neuropathy at the elbow). Acute compressive neuropathies typically develop at sites where external pressure compresses the nerve against a harder surface, such as the radial nerve at the humerus' spiral groove. Chronic compression neuropathies occur where nerve passes through fibrous tunnels that have a propensity to narrow with time, eventually entrapping the nerve itself.

Acute neuropathies tend to manifest more with predominant motor manifestations; for instance, peroneal neuropathy (footdrop) and radial neuropathy (wristdrop); sensory disturbances are relatively mild. Entrapment neuropathies usually present with paresthesias predating focal weakness by months and often years, as well as overshadowing it. Median neuropathies at the wrist initially are characterized by hand tingling at night or with various hand activities, particularly driving; only later in the course does weakness of the thumb, particularly the abductor pollicis brevis, become evident. Diabetes mellitus, myxedema, or, rarely, hereditary neuropathy with predisposition to pressure palsy makes nerves more susceptible to compression injury.

Peripheral nerves are made up of myelinated and unmyelinated nerve fibers originating from either the anterior horn cell (motor) or the posterior root sensory ganglia and traveling the nerve's entire length. Nerve fibers are organized into *fascicles;* elements contained within the fascicles represent the *endoneurium.* The *perineurium,* a protective sheath of connective tissue, surrounds each fascicle. *Schwann cells* concentrically wrap their cytoplasmic processes around axons many times, creating the myelinated nerve fiber. Each nerve segment is associated with one adjacent Schwann cell. When many Schwann cells are lined up contiguously, the entire nerve fiber becomes myelinated. An *internode* consists of one *myelinated segment. Nodes of Ranvier* represent areas lacking myelin, thus interrupting the internodal sections and containing high concentrations of *voltage-gated sodium channels. Juxtaparanodal* and *paranodal regions* are distinctive myelin folds at internode edges containing high concentrations of *voltage-gated potassium channels.* These areas are integral to conduction of action potentials along the axon.

ACUTE NERVE COMPRESSION

When nerve tissues are subjected to mechanical compression, some of the compressed tissues are displaced to sites of lower pressure. This is especially the case for acute compression neuropathies, such as radial neuropathy at the spiral groove ("Saturday night palsy") and neuropathies secondary to tourniquet compression. With acute nerve compression, damage is concentrated at the compression edges. The predominant injury at this level implies that the pressure gradient itself, rather than the absolute pressure, is the critical factor for acute compression neuropathy.

In the setting of experimental acute compression, the earliest histopathologic change seen within just a few hours is an *invagination of one paranodal segment* into

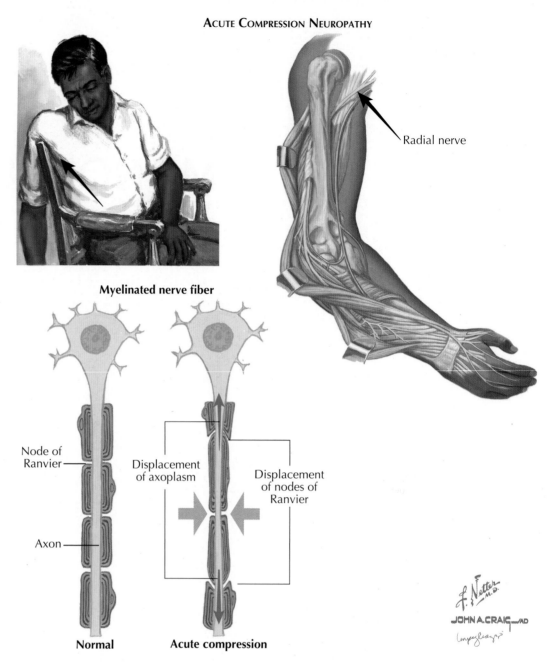

ACUTE COMPRESSION NEUROPATHY

Radial nerve

Myelinated nerve fiber

Node of Ranvier

Axon

Displacement of axoplasm

Displacement of nodes of Ranvier

Normal   **Acute compression**

its adjacent paranode. Directed toward the uncompressed tissue, paranodal myelin, tethered to the axon, may be grossly distorted, resulting in invagination on one side and passive stretching on the other side. Longitudinal movement of the axon relative to the Schwann cell accompanies the paranodal myelin alterations. In extreme cases, myelin lamellae may be ruptured. These findings are reminiscent of intussusception of the bowel, suggesting that the pressure gradient between compressed and uncompressed nerve provides definitive forces causing axoplasm extrusion, similar to toothpaste from a tube.

The sequential events of acute, focal compression initially include an early combined extrusion of endoneurial fluid (i.e., the fluid between fibers), axonal fluid, and cytoskeletal elements and, subsequently, a distortion of myelin and Schwann cell elements. A second slower phase is attributed to further endoneurial and axonal fluid extrusion, paranodal disruption, Schwann cell cytoplasm extrusion, and displacement of other

tissue elements. Additional damage (e.g., of the cytoskeletal network) may occur at more extreme pressures or with protracted compression. Nodes of Ranvier are frequently obscured or lengthened because of displaced paranodal myelin.

Routine nerve conduction studies (NCSs) provide a means to measure the magnitude of conduction block of the nerve or compound muscle action potential (CMAP), as well as focal conduction slowing. These findings correlate with the degree and duration of compression. Focal ischemia may also contribute in some compression neuropathies, particularly in combination with the direct effects of pressure. Transient nerve block, such as when a limb "goes to sleep" for a few seconds, may be related to modest external pressures or may be primarily caused by focal ischemia, because no recognizable structural nerve pathology can be demonstrated. For more severe cases of acute compression, nerve fiber remyelination may occur weeks to months after resolution of the acute compression.

Plate 5.2

Mononeuropathies

CHRONIC NERVE COMPRESSION

The earliest histopathologic change observed in chronic nerve compression is an asymmetric distortion of the large myelinated fiber internodes; there is tapering of the internodes at one side and swelling of the internodes at the other. A modified axoplasm accumulation occurs, possibly caused by interference of axon flow. The direction of tapering (i.e., polarity) reverses on the other side of the compressive lesion. In cases of chronic ulnar neuropathy, the reversal of polarity appears to lie under the aponeurosis of the flexor carpi ulnaris muscle. Similarly, with chronic median neuropathies, the reversal of polarity is under or near the flexor retinaculum over the carpal tunnel. In contrast to the pathologic changes of acute nerve compression, there is no displacement of nodes of Ranvier. In chronic nerve compression, the paranodal axoglial junctions are thought to be disrupted. Subsequently, this results in the thinning of myelin due to demyelination and remyelination. This is mediated by Schwann cell proliferation, currently hypothesized to be triggered by mechanical stress.

Ischemia and endoneurial edema also contribute to the pathology of nerves that sustain chronic compression; modest pressure magnitudes develop. The ischemic hypothesis has focused on the *transperineurial vascular system*. This includes an intrafascicular circulation, composed mostly of capillaries running longitudinally within the endoneurium and an extrafascicular network within the epineurium, composed predominantly of venules and arterioles. The extrinsic vessels penetrate the relatively rigid perineurium to anastomose with the intrinsic circulation, and it is this transperineurial vessel network that may be particularly susceptible to focal compression, especially because these vessels traverse the perineurium at oblique angles.

These transperineurial vessels, especially the venules, are vulnerable to constriction caused by endoneurial edema and elevated (intrinsic) endoneurial fluid pressure. Constriction of these vessels causes venous congestion, endoneurial capillary leakage, and elevated endoneurial fluid pressures. These effects introduce metabolic disturbances to the microenvironment, with subsequent damage to the peripheral nerve anatomy and nerve function. Thus chronic external compression may induce ischemia and endoneurial edema with concomitantly elevated endoneurial fluid pressures. These two effects impair nerve function by altering the metabolic microenvironment as well as contributing to nerve injury by further constricting transperineurial venules. Thus a precarious cycle of venous congestion, ischemia, and metabolic disturbances is initiated that eventually leads to a "miniature compartment syndrome."

In cases of median neuropathy at the wrist (i.e., carpal tunnel syndrome [CTS]), it is thought that carpal tunnel pressures may rise to abnormal levels, increasing the endoneurial fluid pressure and thereby impairing the transperineurial microcirculation. Carpal tunnel pressure and consequently endoneurial fluid pressures probably rise significantly at night in the setting of CTS because the limb venous return is impeded by limb posture and reduced limb movement. *Endoneurial edema* due to other causes (e.g., diabetes) further increases nerve susceptibility to compression.

Moderately elevated pressures also disturb axonal transport. Retrograde axonal transport is critical for communication with the nerve cell body. Fast and slow anterograde axonal transport may also be reversibly impaired after compression. The blocking of axonal

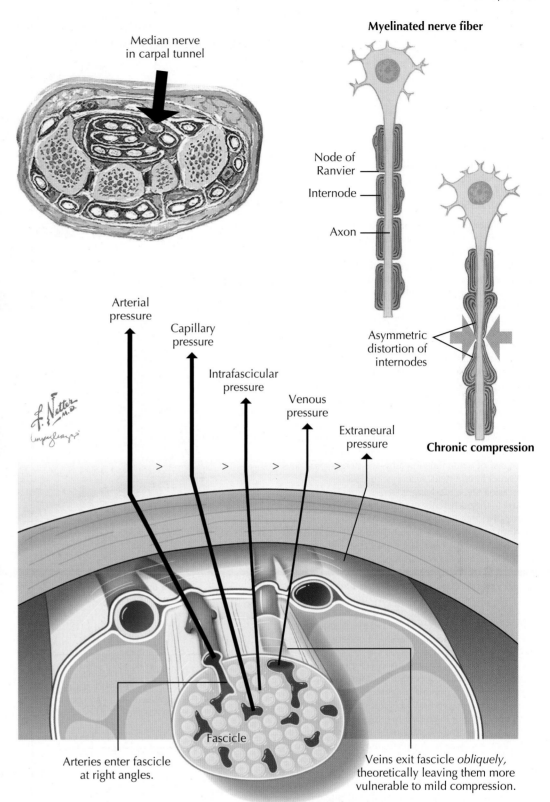

Median nerve in carpal tunnel

Myelinated nerve fiber

Node of Ranvier

Internode

Axon

Asymmetric distortion of internodes

Chronic compression

Arterial pressure

Capillary pressure

Intrafascicular pressure

Venous pressure

Extraneural pressure

Fascicle

Arteries enter fascicle at right angles.

Veins exit fascicle *obliquely,* theoretically leaving them more vulnerable to mild compression.

Pressure gradient necessary for adequate intrafascicular circulation

transport with compression is a graded effect, related to the magnitude and duration of compression. For example, the susceptibility to entrapment in diabetic polyneuropathy may be in part due to the combination of widespread endoneurial edema (diabetes) and focal (entrapment) impairment of axonal flow.

The gliding capacity of a peripheral nerve is another important factor inherent to chronic compression neuropathies. This is particularly relevant at common sites of entrapment, such as the wrist and elbow. Gliding of nerves is necessary during movement of limbs and is made possible by conjunctiva-like adventitia that allows longitudinal excursion of a nerve trunk. Restriction of glide may occur with extraneural and intraneural fibrosis, especially at sites of entrapment, inducing nerve stretch lesions, edema, inflammation, and further fibrosis. Stretch may contribute to nerve injury at common sites of entrapment, although it is unlikely to be the major factor in injury and is likely overshadowed by the consequences of direct pressure and perhaps ischemia.

EVALUATION OF MONONEUROPATHIES

CLINICAL ASSESSMENT

Careful history taking and neurologic examination are essential for evaluation of mononeuropathies. Initially, one should define the precise clinical motor and sensory deficits and next decide whether this fits an individual peripheral nerve's anatomic distribution. This is relatively easily accomplished with acute nerve trauma, such as a laceration or gunshot wound. In contrast, most mononeuropathies have a relatively progressive course characterized first by intermittent paresthesias that may not result in clinically definable functional loss.

Each peripheral nerve has a unique clinical anatomic signature that leads to its motor and sensory deficits when damaged. This is illustrated by the complicated cutaneous sensory and motor distribution of the median, radial, and ulnar nerves in the hand. With this knowledge, clinicians are often able to outline characteristic clinical features of a specific pattern of compromised function appropriate to a mononeuropathy. Frequently, symptoms of a mononeuropathy are stereotypical and sometimes intermittent, such as with CTS.

Occasionally, underlying systemic illnesses may predispose to the occurrence of more than one acute mononeuropathy; that is, mononeuritis multiplex. A sudden footdrop secondary to a fibular (peroneal) nerve lesion is followed in days to weeks by another mononeuropathy, such as a wristdrop from an acute radial nerve lesion, and soon thereafter another nerve becomes acutely compromised. Systemic vasculitides, such as occur in polyarteritis nodosa, are often responsible. Hereditary neuropathy with predisposition to pressure palsy (HNPP) is characterized by recurrent and progressive multiple mononeuropathies with underlying demyelinating polyneuropathy.

Central nervous system disorders can sometimes present with focal sensory and/or motor symptoms or signs that mimic mononeuropathies. Such conditions include transient cerebral ischemic attack (TIA) and intracranial tumor such as a meningioma. Parasagittal cerebral lesions may occasionally manifest primarily with foot weakness. Amyotrophic lateral sclerosis (ALS) can present with focal motor findings mimicking mononeuropathy, such as footdrop suggesting peroneal neuropathy.

Acute neck or low back pain can be the initial feature of an intervertebral disk herniation affecting a single spinal nerve root. Often this discomfort radiates into an arm or a leg and is associated with paresthesias and sometimes weakness confined to the distribution of a nerve root. Clinical history alone may not be sufficient to make a diagnosis. For example, in the setting of footdrop, examination will discriminate between weakness only in the peroneal distribution (foot dorsiflexors and foot evertors) versus additional weakness of foot invertors that would support an L5 root lesion. The distinction is sometimes difficult to make, and NCS and electromyography (EMG) can aid in identifying the specific nerve and muscle involvement.

ELECTRODIAGNOSTIC STUDIES IN COMPRESSION NEUROPATHY

Electromyography (EMG)

Nerve impulse (action potential)

Concentric recording needle

First dorsal interosseous muscle

EMG detects and records electric activity or potentials within muscle in various phases of voluntary contraction.

Normal Needle insertion

Motor unit action potential

Maximal contraction

Abnormal

Fibrillation

Denervation positive waves

Fasciculation

Compression-induced denervation produces abnormal spontaneous potentials.

Nerve conduction studies

Stimulation of ulnar nerve at wrist

Response of hypothenar muscles

|← 0.24 meter →|

Stimulation of ulnar nerve at elbow

Response of hypothenar muscles

|← 0.24 meter →|

Stimulation at wrist

Response

Stimulation at elbow

Response

8 mV

Normal

0.003 second

0.007 second

$0.007 - 0.003 = 0.004$ second for impulse to travel 0.24 meter

0.24 meter $\div$ 0.004 second = 60 meters/second

10 mV/D

3 msD

Wrist

Amp = 13.3 mV

60 m/s

Below elbow

Amp = 12.9 mV

40 m/s

Above elbow

Amp = 8.5 mV

Ulnar nerve in conduction study demonstrating conduction block.

From Preston D, Shapiro B. Electromyography and Neuromuscular Disorders: Clinical-Electrophysiologic Correlations. 2nd ed. Elsevier; 2005.

Often, the degree of weakness is more profound in a mononeuropathy than a nerve root lesion because the affected muscles are solely dependent on that nerve, whereas a nerve root lesion does not affect all fibers going to the affected muscles. For example, with a wristdrop where there is concomitant C6 and C7 root supply, if just the C7 root is affected, the muscles continue to have partial innervation from the C6 root, and thus there is not a total paralysis of the wrist and finger extensors. In contrast, if the radial nerve is damaged, there is no overlapping safety feature of multiple innervations as in nerve root disorders. Here the deficit's severity is directly related to how significant the damage is within that nerve. Often, total paralysis occurs with severe, acute radial nerve damage. Muscle atrophy develops when there is significant peripheral denervation.

Numbness rather than pain is more common with early mononeuropathies. The symptom onset and progression can help in the diagnosis. Because the sensory examination is subjective, the extent of

Plate 5.4   Mononeuropathies

EVALUATION OF MONONEUROPATHIES (Continued)

sensory loss is occasionally difficult to define. Sometimes the patient can provide an accurate assessment by roughly outlining the area in question such as with meralgia paresthetica (see Plates 5.15 and 5.16), where the patient outlines an elliptic loss of sensation on the lateral thigh. These assessments often clarify whether the pattern of sensory loss is specific to a peripheral nerve or nerve root dermatome. Meralgia paresthetica best illustrates this with lateral thigh sensory loss secondary to a lateral femoral cutaneous nerve (LFCN) lesion.

Percussion over an affected nerve can elicit paresthesias within its specific distribution, described as a *Tinel sign.* This can be elicited over the median nerve at the wrist (i.e., CTS), ulnar nerve at the elbow, radial nerve over the spiral groove of the humerus, and fibular (peroneal) nerve at the fibular head.

MONONEUROPATHY: DIAGNOSTIC STUDIES

The clinical neurologic examination may not be sensitive enough to provide the precise diagnosis or localization of a mononeuropathy. Electrodiagnostic studies (NCSs and needle EMG) can aid in more precise anatomic localization of peripheral nerve damage by assessing the integrity of nerve trunks and presence of damage to their innervated muscles. NCS can identify the site of nerve damage, such as the ligamentous thickening over the carpal tunnel (see Plate 5.10), sudden sustained acute pressure over the radial nerve at the humerus (see Plate 5.13), or fibular (peroneal) compression at the knee (see Plates 5.19 and 5.20).

Early signs of CTS are defined initially by abnormal sensory NCS, and later by motor NCS, demonstrating prolongation of the time for nerve conduction across the wrist (distal latency). Motor NCS can be useful in defining proximal nerve compression, such as at the elbow (ulnar nerve), mid-humerus (radial nerve), and knee (fibular [peroneal] nerve). This leads to a diminution of the CMAP proximal to the site of nerve compression (see Plate 5.3). Conduction slowing across a nerve segment provides another means to identify the site of a nerve compression. Here there is focal motor conduction slowing (by 30%–40%; i.e., 10–20 m/sec) across the site of anatomic compromise, as across the fibular head for the fibular (peroneal) nerve.

Needle EMG can define the specially affected muscles. Denervation of a muscle fiber leads to muscle membrane changes that produce fibrillation potentials, spontaneous firing discharges that are seen on needle EMG usually after 3 to 4 weeks. Neighboring healthy motor nerve fibers send nerve branches to denervated muscle fibers. Over time this process leads to changes in the muscle discharges, indicating a reinnervating process.

Patients with a footdrop secondary to a fibular (peroneal) nerve lesion demonstrate denervation findings on needle EMG confined to fibular-innervated muscles. However, if the footdrop is secondary to an L5 root

RADIOLOGIC STUDIES IN COMPRESSION NEUROPATHY

Median nerve lymphoma

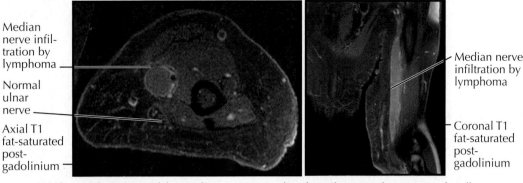

Median nerve infiltration by lymphoma

Normal ulnar nerve

Axial T1 fat-saturated post-gadolinium

Median nerve infiltration by lymphoma

Coronal T1 fat-saturated post-gadolinium

Fusiform enlargement of the median nerve extending from the upper humerus to the elbow. This mass enhanced with gadolinium but without periosteal involvement.

Peroneal nerve schwannoma

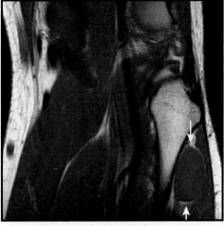

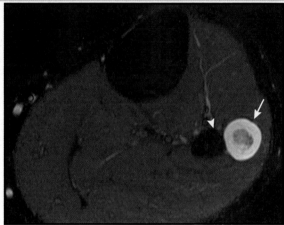

Coronal T1-weighted MRI demonstrates an oval mass of left peroneal nerve *(arrows).*

Axial T1-weighted postgadolinium-enhanced fat-saturated MRI demonstrating enhancing peroneal nerve schwannoma with central myxoid degeneration *(arrow)* near fibula *(arrowhead).*

Median nerve entrapment

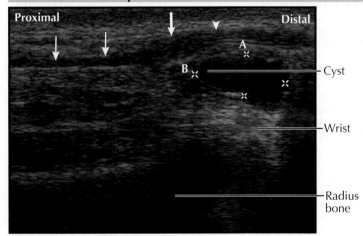

Proximal

A

B

Distal

Cyst

Wrist

Radius bone

Longitudinal ultrasound image of the median nerve within the wrist (Toshiba Nemio XG, 14.0 MHz linear array transducer). The nerve *(arrows)* is compressed from below by a fluid-filled structure *(arrowhead),* consistent with a ganglion cyst *(A, stars).* Compression-related swelling of the median nerve can be appreciated at the proximal end of the cyst *(B). (Ultrasound courtesy Steven Shook, MD.)*

lesion, signs of denervation are demonstrated not only in fibular (peroneal) muscles but also in L5 muscles, innervated by both peroneal and posterior tibial nerves; these include the posterior tibial, the gluteus medius, and the lumbosacral paraspinal musculature. Thus by combining NCS and EMG, the anatomic localization and physiologic state of the nerve lesion can be defined.

Magnetic Resonance Imaging. Magnetic resonance imaging (MRI) studies provide a means to evaluate causes of mononeuropathies, such as tumors or congenital

lesions (Plate 5.4). Some causes of nerve compression, such as fibrous bands, may not be apparent on MRI. In this instance surgical exploration based on the clinical and EMG findings may lead to a diagnosis.

Ultrasound. This modality is gaining an increased presence in some centers for more rapid identification of sites of nerve compression or entrapment.

Skeletal Radiograph. Bony abnormalities can entrap a peripheral nerve. An example is a bony exostosis at the fibular head that entraps the fibular nerve at that site.

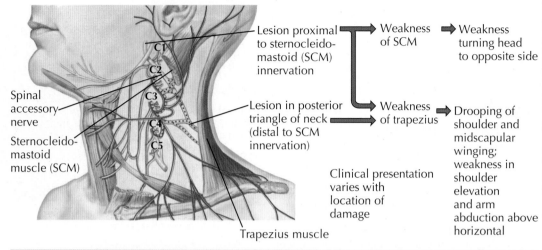

CLINICAL COMPARISON OF WINGED SCAPULA CRANIAL NERVE XI AND LONG THORACIC NERVE PALSY

PROXIMAL NERVES OF THE UPPER EXTREMITY

When evaluating the patient with shoulder pain or weakness, the presence of proximal arm neuropathies needs to be differentiated from fifth cervical nerve root disorders and primary musculoskeletal shoulder disorders.

The clinical demonstration of weakness and atrophy specific to one of the shoulder girdle nerves provides important differential diagnostic clues. Typically, the patient with a primary orthopedic problem, such as a rotator cuff injury, has significant shoulder pain but lacks significant weakness. Although assessment of weakness in a patient with orthopedic injury is clouded by shoulder pain, careful neurologic or orthopedic examination can point to the likely correct diagnosis. In cases of shoulder trauma, orthopedic and mononeuropathies may coexist. In this setting, NCS/EMG and MRI can lead to accurate localization.

The *spinal accessory nerve* is a pure motor nerve derived from the C1–C4 segments. Its cell bodies are found within the lateral anterior gray column's posterolateral anterior horn. The nerve ascends through the foramen magnum and exits the skull via the *jugular foramen,* accompanying the vagus nerve. The spinal accessory nerve innervates two muscles: the trapezius and sternocleidomastoid muscles, which raise the shoulder and turn the head to the opposite side, respectively.

Injury to the spinal accessory nerve can occur because of surgical procedures involving the posterior triangle of the neck, where it is particularly at risk during lymph node biopsy. Spinal accessory nerve injury can lead to scapular winging secondary to loss of some innervation of the trapezius muscle. This form of scapular winging is characterized by lateral scapula deviation with abduction of the shoulder. Weakness of the trapezius can also lead to shoulder drop and impaired shoulder abduction. Very proximal lesions of the spinal accessory nerve will additionally cause weakness of the sternocleidomastoid muscle, leading to weakness of neck flexion and rotation of the head to the opposite side.

The *long thoracic nerve* originates directly from C5 to C7 roots, immediately proximal to the formation of the brachial plexus. It primarily innervates the *serratus anterior* muscle that stabilizes the scapula for pushing movements and allows for elevation of the arm above 90 degrees. There is no cutaneous sensory innervation. *Long thoracic neuropathy* is the most common cause for scapular winging, which can be elicited by extending the arm and pushing against a wall, leading to prominent projection of the inferior medial scapular border away from the chest. Scapular winging caused by weakness of the trapezius (*spinal accessory neuropathy*) or the rhomboid muscle (*dorsal scapular neuropathy*) produces a lateral scapular deviation, in contrast to the long thoracic medial scapula deviation. Causes of long thoracic neuropathy include acute brachial plexus neuritis (neuralgic amyotrophy), mechanical factors, and

Comparison of clinical findings in CN XI and long thoracic nerve damage

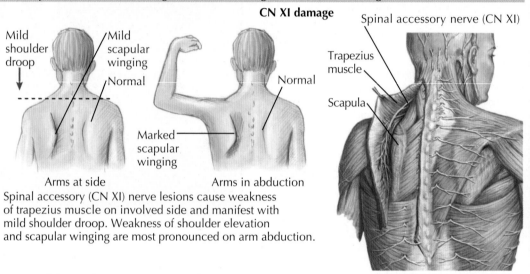

CN XI damage

Spinal accessory (CN XI) nerve lesions cause weakness of trapezius muscle on involved side and manifest with mild shoulder droop. Weakness of shoulder elevation and scapular winging are most pronounced on arm abduction.

Long thoracic nerve damage

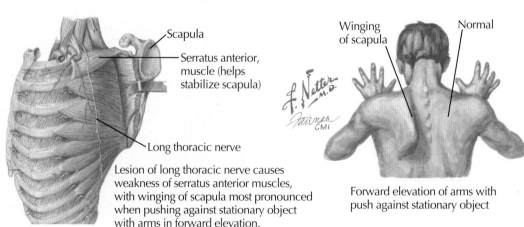

Lesion of long thoracic nerve causes weakness of serratus anterior muscles, with winging of scapula most pronounced when pushing against stationary object with arms in forward elevation.

Forward elevation of arms with push against stationary object

surgical procedures, including mastectomy or thoracotomy. When scapular winging is bilateral, primary muscle disorders such as facioscapulohumeral muscular dystrophy should be considered.

The *dorsal scapular nerve* (C5) arises from the *uppermost element* of the brachial plexus. It pierces the scalenus medius and runs deep to the *levator scapulae,* helping to innervate this muscle. It terminates by supplying the *rhomboid muscles* (C5). These muscles stabilize and rotate

the scapula in a medial-inferior direction as well as elevate the arm (see Plate 5.6). *Rhomboid* weakness presents with scapular winging, most prominently when the arm is raised overhead. The affected patient typically notes difficulty reaching into a back pants pocket or scratching the back. Causes include shoulder dislocation, weightlifting, and entrapment by the scalenus medius muscle.

The *suprascapular nerve* (C5, C6) arises from the *upper trunk* of the brachial plexus. It runs laterally, deep

Plate 5.6

Mononeuropathies

PROXIMAL NERVES OF THE UPPER EXTREMITY (Continued)

to the trapezius, before entering the *supraspinous fossa* through the scapular notch and winding around the lateral border of the scapular spine to reach the *infraspinous fossa*. It supplies both the *supraspinatus* (C5, C6), an initiator of shoulder abduction, and the *infraspinatus* (C5, C6), the predominant external rotator of the arm. This is a pure motor nerve with no cutaneous component. The *suprascapular notch* under the *transverse scapular ligament* is the most common site of entrapment. This affects innervation of both the supraspinatus and infraspinatus. Less commonly, the suprascapular nerve can be injured more distally, at the *spinoglenoid notch,* affecting the infraspinatus alone. Acute-onset *suprascapular neuropathies* result from brachial plexus neuritis, blunt shoulder trauma, or forceful anterior rotation of the scapula. Chronic suprascapular neuropathies may develop subsequent to postfracture callous formation, entrapment at the suprascapular or spinoglenoid notch, compression from a ganglion, or traction from repetitive overhead activities, such as volleyball or tennis.

The *axillary (circumflex humeral)* (C5, C6) and *radial* (C6, C7) nerves are the primary derivatives of the posterior cord of the brachial plexus. Descending behind the axillary vessels, the axillary nerve curves posteriorly and below the *subscapularis* (C5, C6) muscle. It next passes through a *quadrangular space,* bounded above by the *teres minor* (C5), below by the *teres major* (C5–C7), medially by the *triceps brachii* long head, and laterally by the humerus. An *anterior branch* passes to innervate the *deltoid* muscle. The *posterior branch* innervates both the deltoid and the *teres minor muscle.* The axillary nerve terminates as the superior lateral cutaneous nerve of the arm, supplying the upper most portion of the arm immediately below the shoulder.

Axillary neuropathies are characterized by shoulder abduction weakness and diminished cutaneous sensation over the lateral shoulder, an area also having C5 dermatome representation. Weakness of arm external rotation is not always clinically evident because teres minor is not the primary external rotator of the shoulder. Acute axillary neuropathies most typically result from blunt trauma, anterior shoulder dislocations, or humerus fractures or may be a feature of *brachial plexus neuritis.* Axillary neuropathies primarily require differentiation from C5 radiculopathies. EMG is particularly helpful because the *deltoid* and *teres minor* are the only two muscles innervated by this nerve. Denervation confined to these muscles is diagnostic of a primary axillary nerve lesion, whereas the concomitant finding of infraspinatus/supraspinatus and/or rhomboid denervation favors a C5 radiculopathy.

The *musculocutaneous nerve* originates directly from the lateral cord of the brachial plexus, innervating the *biceps brachii, brachialis,* and *coracobrachialis* (C5, C6) muscles. It terminates as the *lateral antebrachial cutaneous* nerve, supplying sensation to the lateral anterior forearm

SUPRASCAPULAR AND MUSCULOCUTANEOUS NERVES

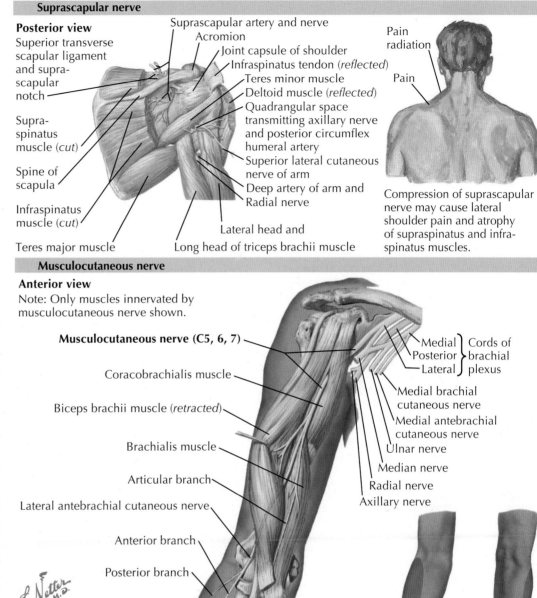

Suprascapular nerve

Posterior view

Superior transverse scapular ligament and suprascapular notch

Suprascapular artery and nerve
Acromion
Joint capsule of shoulder
Infraspinatus tendon (*reflected*)
Teres minor muscle
Deltoid muscle (*reflected*)
Quadrangular space transmitting axillary nerve and posterior circumflex humeral artery
Superior lateral cutaneous nerve of arm
Deep artery of arm and Radial nerve

Supraspinatus muscle (*cut*)

Spine of scapula

Infraspinatus muscle (*cut*)

Teres major muscle

Lateral head and
Long head of triceps brachii muscle

Pain radiation
Pain

Compression of suprascapular nerve may cause lateral shoulder pain and atrophy of supraspinatus and infraspinatus muscles.

Musculocutaneous nerve

Anterior view

Note: Only muscles innervated by musculocutaneous nerve shown.

Musculocutaneous nerve (C5, 6, 7)

Coracobrachialis muscle

Biceps brachii muscle (*retracted*)

Brachialis muscle

Articular branch

Lateral antebrachial cutaneous nerve

Anterior branch

Posterior branch

Medial
Posterior } Cords of
Lateral } brachial
plexus

Medial brachial cutaneous nerve
Medial antebrachial cutaneous nerve
Ulnar nerve
Median nerve
Radial nerve
Axillary nerve

Hypesthesia

Weakness of elbow flexion

Musculocutaneous nerve compression within coracobrachialis muscle causes hypesthesia in lateral forearm and weakness of elbow flexion.

Cutaneous innervation (via lateral antebrachial cutaneous nerve)

Anterior (palmar) view

Posterior (dorsal) view

immediately below the elbow to just proximal to the thumb. Isolated *musculocutaneous neuropathies* have been reported in weightlifting, surgical procedures, and prolonged pressure during sleep. Isolated musculocutaneous neuropathy may also be a feature of brachial plexus neuritis. Patients present with weakness of forearm flexion and supination, with sensory loss of the lateral volar forearm. The biceps reflex is reduced or absent, but, importantly, the brachioradialis reflex (also

C5/C6 but innervated by the radial nerve) is preserved. More distal lesions, primarily affecting the lateral antebrachial cutaneous nerve, may result from attempted cannulation of the basilic vein in the antecubital fossa.

The *thoracodorsal nerve* is derived from the posterior cord of the brachial plexus and innervates the *latissimus dorsi* (C6, C7, C8). Injury to this nerve is uncommon, causing weakness of the latissimus dorsi with impaired arm adduction, extension, and internal rotation.

MEDIAN NERVE

The *median nerve* supports the ability to grip and to pinch the thumb and index fingers. It also provides discriminatory sensory function for the thumb, index, and middle fingers. The median nerve sensory and motor innervations are responsible for fine finger dexterity.

UPPER ARM

The *median nerve* is derived from the C6–C8 cervical nerve roots and the first thoracic (T1) nerve root. Within the axilla, *various fascicles* of these nerve roots join to form the lateral, medial, and posterior cords of the brachial plexus. Subsequently, a significant portion of the lateral and medial cords fuses to form the median nerve adjacent to the axillary artery. As the median nerve travels through the axilla and into the arm, it lies lateral to the brachial artery. Lower, near the coracobrachialis muscle insertion, the nerve moves medially over the brachial artery, descending toward the cubital fossa at the elbow. An anatomic variant, the ligament of Struthers, is sometimes present just above the elbow, characterized by a fibrous band extending from a small supracondylar spur to the medial epicondyle of the humerus and forming the roof of a tunnel for the median nerve and brachial artery as they approach the elbow. Here, the median nerve lies posterior to the bicipital aponeurosis (lacertus fibrosis) and the intermediate cubital vein but superficial to the insertion of the brachialis muscle at the ulna tuberosity.

When performing venipuncture or arterial puncture, the close proximity of the median nerve to the intermediate basilic vein and brachial artery must be considered. Venipuncture should be performed immediately lateral to the bicipital tendon to avoid the brachial artery, which lies just medial to this prominent tendon. There are no significant median nerve motor or sensory branches within the upper arm.

FOREARM

The median nerve enters the forearm between the long and short heads of the biceps muscle. Initially, it innervates the *pronator teres* (PT) muscle (C6, C7) before innervating three other forearm muscles: *flexor carpi radialis* (FCR; C6, C7), *palmaris longus* (C7, C8, T1), and *flexor digitorum superficialis* (FDS; C7, C8). It also provides articular twigs to the elbow and proximal radioulnar joints.

Within the proximal forearm, the *anterior interosseous nerve* (AIN; the primary median nerve motor branch) arises from the primary trunk of the median nerve. It is a pure motor branch coursing distally, superficial to the anterior interosseous ligament, accompanied by the anterior interosseous artery. The AIN innervates the *lateral head of the flexor digitorum profundus* (FDP; C7, C8), a muscle providing tendons that flex the most distal interphalangeal (DIP) joints of the index and middle fingers; the *flexor pollicis longus* (FPL; C7, C8, T1), which flexes the distal phalanx of the thumb, and the *pronator quadratus* (C7, C8, T1), which aids in wrist pronation. Through its innervation of the FDP and the FPL, the AIN provides the essential means for important movements, including flexion of the thumb, distal index and middle fingers.

Anterior view

Note: Only muscles innervated by median nerve are shown.

Musculocutaneous nerve

Median nerve (C5, 6, 7, 8; T1)

Pronator teres muscle (humeral head)

Articular branch

Flexor carpi radialis muscle

Palmaris longus muscle

Pronator teres muscle (ulnar head)

Flexor digitorum superficialis muscle (*turned up*)

Flexor digitorum profundus muscle (lateral part supplied by median [anterior interosseous] nerve; medial part supplied by ulnar nerve)

Anterior interosseous nerve

Flexor pollicis longus muscle

Pronator quadratus muscle

Palmar branch of median nerve

Thenar muscles {
Abductor pollicis brevis
Opponens pollicis
Superficial head of flexor pollicis brevis (deep head supplied by ulnar nerve)
}

1st and 2nd lumbrical muscles

Dorsal branches to dorsum of middle and distal phalanges

Medial
Posterior } Cords of brachial plexus
Lateral

Medial brachial cutaneous nerve

Medial antebrachial cutaneous nerve

Axillary nerve

Radial nerve

Ulnar nerve

Communicating branch of median nerve with ulnar nerve

Common palmar digital nerves

Proper palmar digital nerves

In the distal forearm, the main trunk of the median nerve lies deep to the FDS and superficial to the FDP. Eventually, the primary median nerve trunk becomes more superficial, lying between the tendons of the palmaris longus and the FCR (C6, C7). Here the *median palmar cutaneous branch* originates, arising 3 to 4 cm proximal to the flexor retinaculum and descending over this area to supply the skin of the median palm and the thenar eminence. This is the first median sensory branch that arises before the median nerve enters the hand.

In the forearm, the median and ulnar nerves are occasionally interconnected by fibers passing between these nerves. The most common are the median-ulnar anastomosis (Martin-Gruber syndrome), wherein portions of the median nerve branch off within the forearm to join the ulnar nerve. Typically, when this ulnar nerve variant reaches the hand, these median fibers will subsequently innervate their appropriate median intrinsic muscles. This is important for electromyographers to recognize, especially when looking for ulnar nerve block at the elbow as discussed on the ulnar nerve plates.

Plate 5.8

Mononeuropathies

PROXIMAL MEDIAN NEUROPATHIES

Proximal median nerve lesions are situated near the elbow or the PT muscle, affecting the main median nerve trunk or its anterior interosseous division.

PRIMARY MEDIAN TRUNK

All median nerve function may potentially be compromised with proximal lesions. In contrast to the patient with CTS experiencing finger paresthesias, proximal median trunk lesions present with combined sensory/motor dysfunction, not only affecting the classic three and a half lateral digits but also diminished palmar sensation because of *median palmar cutaneous branch* involvement, a finding not seen in CTS. All median-innervated muscles may be affected.

Supracondylar humerus fractures leading to nerve compression, entrapment, or total laceration are common causes of proximal median nerve lesions. The primary median nerve trunk is usually damaged; however, because of the fascicular characteristics of peripheral nerves, the anterior interosseous component of the median nerve trunk may occasionally be traumatized in isolation at a proximal site. Elbow dislocations, hyperextension of the arm, shoulder injury, lacerations, blunt nerve trauma, arterial or venous puncture, and repetitive pronation/supination are other mechanisms.

Median nerve entrapment can occur just above the elbow at the ligament of Struthers, an uncommon anatomic variant composed of a fibrous band extending from a small supracondylar spur on the humerus to the medial epicondyle. Here the ligament forms the roof of a tunnel, radiographically identifiable in about 2% of the population. Otherwise, median entrapment has occurred with a distal humeral osteoid osteoma and congenital fibromuscular bands. Lipofibromas, hamartomas, neurofibromas, hemangiomas, juvenile cutaneous mucinosis, calcified FDS tendons, and abscesses may also lead to proximal median nerve lesions.

ANTERIOR INTEROSSEOUS NERVE

Patients with anterior interosseous neuropathy present with difficulty with fine motor activities, such as handwriting and placing and turning a key in a lock. This symptom is related to an inability to pinch because of weakness of the FPL *and flexor digitorum profundus* (FDP; C8, T1) muscles, which limits the patient's ability to flex the DIP joints of both the index finger and thumb. The third muscle innervated by the AIN, the *pronator quadratus* (PQ, C8, T1), is clinically silent but provides localizing value with needle EMG. The AIN may be affected alone or in conjunction with other shoulder girdle neuropathies in acute brachial neuritis.

Acute median nerve compression by the bicipital aponeurosis at the elbow presents with acute elbow pain during the course of a maximal and vigorous contraction of the biceps brachii muscle. Examination demonstrates

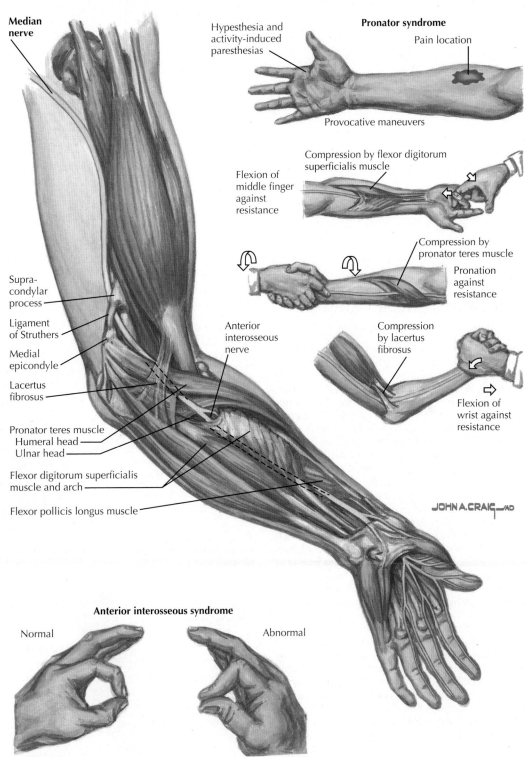

Median nerve

Hypesthesia and activity-induced paresthesias

Pronator syndrome

Pain location

Provocative maneuvers

Flexion of middle finger against resistance

Compression by flexor digitorum superficialis muscle

Compression by pronator teres muscle

Pronation against resistance

Compression by lacertus fibrosus

Flexion of wrist against resistance

Supracondylar process

Ligament of Struthers

Medial epicondyle

Lacertus fibrosus

Anterior interosseous nerve

Pronator teres muscle
Humeral head
Ulnar head

Flexor digitorum superficialis muscle and arch

Flexor pollicis longus muscle

JOHN A. CRAIG—AD

Anterior interosseous syndrome

Normal

Abnormal

Hand posture in anterior interosseous syndrome due to paresis of flexor digitorum profundus and flexor pollicis longus muscles. Affected hand compensates by use of ulnar-innervated adductor pollicis.

severe pain on median nerve palpation at the elbow as well as with triceps contraction when extending the elbow, but there is no neurologic compromise.

EVALUATION

EMG is the primary means for identifying these proximal median nerve lesions as discussed above. Ultrasound and MRI can assist with localization and evaluation for structural abnormalities or injuries in the setting of suspected proximal median neuropathy.

THERAPY AND PROGNOSIS

Surgical exploration may be indicated for acute painful median nerve compression at the elbow. Surgical exploration may uncover an acute median nerve entrapment at the ligament of Struthers, lacertus fibrosis, PT, or FDS that improves with decompression. In more chronic settings, options include local corticosteroid injection, surgical exploration, and conservative management. However, if neurologic signs of progressive median neuropathy develop, surgical exploration becomes an important option.

DISTAL MEDIAN NERVE

Thenar muscles {
Abductor pollicis brevis
Opponens pollicis
Superficial head of flexor pollicis brevis (deep head supplied by ulnar nerve)
}

Median nerve

Communicating branch of median nerve with ulnar nerve

Common palmar digital nerves

Proper palmar digital nerves

1st and 2nd lumbrical muscles

Dorsal branches to dorsum of middle and distal phalanges

Section through wrist at distal row of carpal bones shows carpal tunnel. Increase in size of tunnel structures caused by edema (trauma) or inflammation (rheumatoid disease); ganglion, amyloid deposits, or diabetic neuropathy may compress median nerve.

Palmaris longus tendon
Median nerve
Flexor carpi radialis tendon

Flexor retinaculum
Ulnar artery and nerve

In ulnar bursa {
Flexor digitorum superficialis tendon
Flexor digitorum profundus tendon
}

Flexor pollicis longus tendon in radial bursa

Hamate bone
Capitate bone

Trapezium bone
Trapezoid bone

Carpal tunnel syndrome: sensory loss

Musculocutaneous nerve:
Lateral cutaneous nerve of forearm

Medial cutaneous nerve of forearm

Radial nerve:
Superficial branch

Radial nerve:
Posterior cutaneous nerve of forearm

Superficial branch and dorsal digital branches

Ulnar nerve:
Palmar branch

Median nerve:
Palmar branch
Palmar digital branches

Dorsal branch and dorsal digital branches

Palmar digital branches

Division between ulnar and radial nerve innervation on dorsum of hand is variable; it often aligns with middle or 3rd digit instead of 4th digit as shown.

Median nerve:
Proper palmar digital branches

Anterior (palmar) view

Posterior (dorsal) view

DISTAL MEDIAN NEUROPATHIES

The *median nerve* is the most commonly compromised single peripheral nerve trunk, mainly because of its relation to the carpal tunnel, where it can be compressed. As the median nerve enters the palm, it passes through the central lateral aspect of the relatively restricted anatomic space that is the *carpal tunnel*. If the canal thickens enough to entrap the median nerve over time, *carpal tunnel syndrome* (CTS) develops. Symptoms of CTS range from relatively mild and annoying to severe and debilitating. However, it is highly treatable (see Plate 5.10).

Within the carpal tunnel, the median nerve is bounded anteriorly by the stiff *flexor retinaculum* and posteriorly by the carpal bones. In contrast, the ulnar nerve does not travel through the carpal tunnel; rather, it has a very medial position, reaching the hand through the much less restrictive *Guyon canal*. Because of these different paths, it is relatively uncommon to have both the median and ulnar nerves affected together at the wrist, unless there is a diffuse polyneuropathy, such as found in a patient with diabetes mellitus. Once the median nerve leaves this anatomically defined tunnel, it divides into its *terminal sensory and motor branches*, providing motor and sensory function to 70% of the hand. These branches directly accompany tendons originating from the digital flexor muscles, including the FDS, FDP, and FPL. *The muscular branch arises close to, or is initially united with, the common palmar digital nerve* to the thumb. This curves outward over or through the *flexor pollicis brevis* to supply its superficial head before dividing to innervate the *abductor pollicis brevis* and *opponens pollicis* muscles, all C8, T1–innervated muscles. In addition, this muscular branch usually innervates both the *first and second lumbrical* muscles. Only one thenar muscle, the ulnar-innervated *adductor pollicis* (C8, T1) is not innervated by the median nerve.

Another motor innervation variant within the hand is the *Riche-Cannieu anastomosis*. Here the deep ulnar branch of the ulnar nerve (C8, T1) communicates with the *terminal motor branch of the median nerve*. Because the ulnar nerve has its own clinical presentation, such a variation can rarely lead to diagnostic confusion. Another rare, but important, anatomic variation occurs when the distal median motor nerve branches off earlier than usual within the carpal tunnel, exiting it by directly piercing the flexor retinaculum, rather than leaving the carpal tunnel at its most distal extent near the thenar

eminence. This *anatomic variant* is of potential clinical concern if an incision is made through this area when operating on a patient with CTS symptoms. If unrecognized, the motor function of the thumb may be compromised if this branch is severed.

CARPAL TUNNEL SYNDROME

CTS is the most common adult mononeuropathy; it is three times more common in women, usually

manifesting in middle to late life. CTS rarely occurs in young children. The symptoms of CTS include numbness and tingling in the first three and one-half fingers (thumb, index, middle, and half of ring finger) of one or both hands. Although some patients report that their hand feels "asleep," at times these paresthesias have an annoying, allodynic quality. Some individuals report that *all* their fingers are affected. Rarely, there is a component of dysautonomia with changes in temperature, color, and sweating.

Plate 5.10

Mononeuropathies

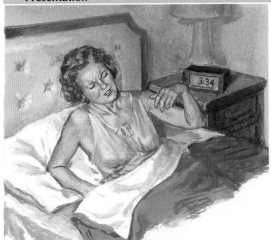

Patient awakened by tingling, pain, or both in sensory distribution of median nerve

DISTAL MEDIAN NEUROPATHIES

Typically, these symptoms occur, or are worse, at night, awakening the patient from sleep. Many patients also note similar symptoms on awakening in the morning. Simple shaking of the fingers and hand can abort symptoms. Occasionally, there is radiation of the pain into the volar forearm; rarely, this will spread into the upper arm.

Repetitive occupational and recreational activities involving the wrist often underlie development of CTS. Some systemic disorders, including diabetes mellitus, rheumatoid arthritis, hypothyroidism, acromegaly, and systemic amyloidosis, predispose adult patients to developing CTS. There is a broader set of possible mechanisms in children, including congenital carpal tunnel canal stenosis, leading to familial CTS. Thickening of the flexor retinaculum occurs in the mucopolysaccharidoses, and here the motor fibers are primarily affected, leading to painless thumb atrophy.

Early on, there may be no specific clinical findings in CTS. Symptoms can sometimes be elicited by tapping over the nerve at the wrist, known as the *Tinel sign*. Initial clinical signs of CTS are usually decreased sensation in the median-innervated fingertips, sparing the palm because the palmar branch of the median nerve does not pass through the carpal tunnel. Two-point discrimination, light touch, and pinprick sensory modalities may be affected with early sensory loss. As the degree of entrapment increases, the motor branches become affected, leading to weakness and then atrophy of the thenar eminence, particularly affecting thumb abduction and opposition.

C6 or C7 cervical radiculopathy may present with clinical symptoms like CTS. The symptoms of radiculopathy tend not to fluctuate and are usually associated with neck or intrascapular pain. Cervical spine MRI is useful in making this diagnosis.

Thenar atrophy may be seen in other disorders, including proximal median nerve lesions, T1 radiculopathy, motor neuron disease (MND), multifocal motor neuropathy, and neurogenic thoracic outlet syndrome. In contrast to numbness in the thumb, index, and middle fingers in median nerve disorders, patients with neurogenic thoracic outlet syndrome have sensory loss in the ulnar nerve distribution because the disorder specifically affects the T1 root and not the median nerve.

When the clinical and electrodiagnostic findings do not support CTS or other neuromuscular disorders, a central

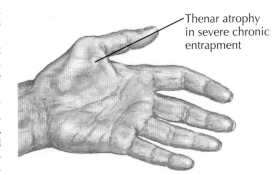

Thenar atrophy in severe chronic entrapment

Gradual numbness of fingers while driving

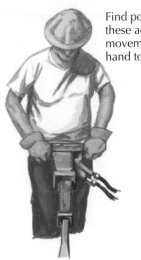

Find possible causes and avoid these actions. Avoid repetitive movements, such as vibrating hand tools.

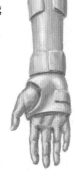

Wrist splint at night can be helpful

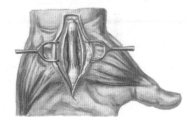

If pain does not improve, wrist surgery to decompress median nerve in the carpal tunnel may be recommended

nervous system lesion should be considered. Syringomyelia or other intramedullary spinal disorders may lead to thenar weakness and atrophy. Rarely, TIAs or a slow-growing intracranial tumor may initially mimic CTS.

DIAGNOSIS AND THERAPY

NCS/EMG studies are the primary means for supporting a CTS diagnosis. These demonstrate delayed conduction across the carpal tunnel, and the sensory components of the study are often abnormal in the early stages of CTS. Although conservative therapy with wrist splints (used while sleeping) is helpful early on, patients with significant CTS changes or those who continue to progress despite conservative management require simple outpatient surgical decompression. This is successful in the vast majority of patients.

ULNAR NERVE

The C8, T1, and occasionally the C7 nerve roots provide the primary segmental derivations for the ulnar nerve. These nerve roots join soon after leaving the spinal cord to form the *lower trunk and medial cord of the brachial plexus,* eventually terminating as either the ulnar nerve or the medial portion of the median nerve within the lower axilla. Here the ulnar nerve lies between the axillary artery and vein; after entering the arm, it lies medial to the brachial artery. After piercing the medial intermuscular septum, midway down the arm, the ulnar nerve descends anterior to the medial head of the triceps brachii muscle. Proximal to the elbow, the *initial ulnar nerve segment* has no branches in the upper arm. Proximal to the elbow, the ulnar nerve inclines posteriorly, passing through a groove between the medial humeral epicondyle and the olecranon to reach the forearm. Here it occupies a superficial plane covered with fascia and skin and is easily palpable and can be rolled between the fingers. This superficial positioning allows for modest bumping to send a shock-like sensation distally into the medial two fingers, giving rise to the description of the elbow's medial epicondyle and adjacent ulnar nerve as the "funny bone."

Within the proximal forearm, the ulnar nerve courses along the length of the medial forearm, lying on the ulnar collateral ligament immediately below the elbow; it subsequently passes between the two heads of the *flexor carpi ulnaris* (C7, C8, T1) and the *medial flexor digitorum profundus* (C8, T1), providing flexion of the fourth and fifth DIP joints, innervating both muscles. The palmar and dorsal cutaneous sensory branches leave the ulnar nerve within the lower forearm. As the flexor carpi ulnaris narrows into its tendon, the nerve and artery emerge from under its lateral edge, where it is covered just by skin and fascia.

Entering the hand through the *Guyon canal,* the ulnar nerve passes anterior and superficial to the flexor retinaculum, almost immediately splitting into its superficial and deep terminal branches. This contrasts with the median nerve, which passes deep to the flexor retinaculum, a potential entrapment site at the carpal tunnel. At the wrist, the ulnar nerve divides into the superficial and deep branches. The *superficial branch* innervates the *palmaris brevis* muscle and then splits into its terminal sensory nerves, providing sensation to the entire fifth digit and medial ring finger. The *deep terminal motor branch* (C8, T1) has a purely motor function, supplying all the hypothenar muscles, including the *abductor digiti minimi, opponens digiti minimi,* and *flexor digiti minimi.* Subsequently, it curves along the palm, providing motor branches to the third and fourth lumbricals, the four dorsal and three palmar interossei, the adductor pollicis, and the deep head of the flexor pollicis brevis.

The *ulnar palmar cutaneous branch* arises 7 cm proximal to the wrist, descends near the ulnar artery, and pierces the deep fascia, supplying the hypothenar eminence; it communicates with the medial cutaneous nerve of the forearm and the palmar cutaneous branch of the median nerve. The *dorsal ulnar branch* arises 5 to 10 cm proximal to the wrist; passes posteriorly, deep to the tendon of flexor carpi ulnaris; pierces the deep fascia; and continues distally along the posteromedial side of the wrist. Here it divides into branches that supply the *palmaris brevis* muscle and, as the *superficial terminal branch,* the skin on the medial side of the back

of the hand and fingers. There are usually two or three *dorsal digital nerves:* one, the *proper palmar digital nerve,* supplying the medial side of the little finger, and the other splitting into a *common palmar digital nerve,* communicating with the adjoining common palmar digital branch of the median nerve before dividing into the two *proper palmar digital nerves* for the adjacent sides of the little and ring fingers. Very rarely, the ulnar

nerve supplies 2.5 rather than 1.5 digits, in which case the areas supplied by the median and radial nerves are reciprocally reduced.

There is a variety of interconnections between the ulnar and median nerve branches, allowing interchanges of fibers from different nerve roots. Their clinical implications are important, allowing explanations for seemingly "nonanatomic" findings.

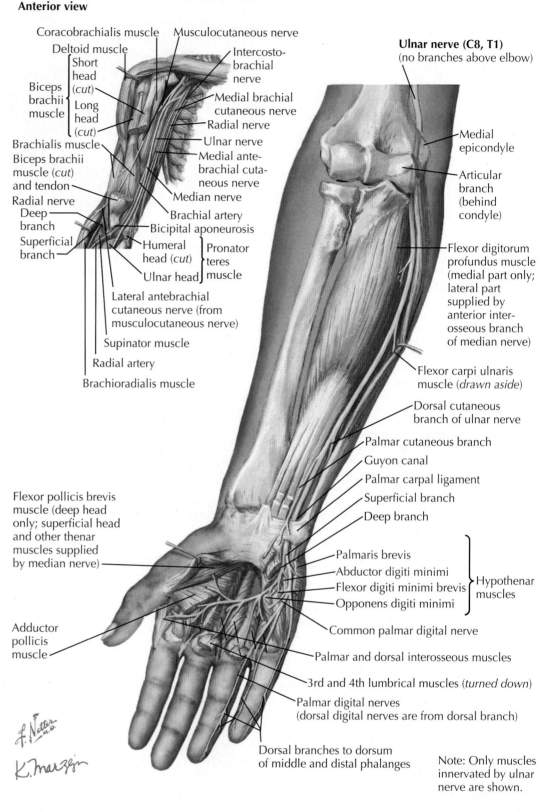

PROXIMAL ULNAR NERVE IN THE AXILLA AND UPPER ARM

Anterior view

Coracobrachialis muscle
Deltoid muscle
Short head (*cut*)
Biceps brachii muscle
Long head (*cut*)
Brachialis muscle
Biceps brachii muscle (*cut*) and tendon
Radial nerve
Deep branch
Superficial branch

Musculocutaneous nerve
Intercosto-brachial nerve
Medial brachial cutaneous nerve
Radial nerve
Ulnar nerve
Medial ante-brachial cuta-neous nerve
Median nerve
Brachial artery
Bicipital aponeurosis
Humeral head (*cut*)
Ulnar head
Pronator teres muscle
Lateral antebrachial cutaneous nerve (from musculocutaneous nerve)
Supinator muscle
Radial artery
Brachioradialis muscle

Ulnar nerve (C8, T1) (no branches above elbow)

Medial epicondyle
Articular branch (behind condyle)
Flexor digitorum profundus muscle (medial part only; lateral part supplied by anterior interosseous branch of median nerve)
Flexor carpi ulnaris muscle (*drawn aside*)
Dorsal cutaneous branch of ulnar nerve
Palmar cutaneous branch
Guyon canal
Palmar carpal ligament
Superficial branch
Deep branch

Flexor pollicis brevis muscle (deep head only; superficial head and other thenar muscles supplied by median nerve)

Adductor pollicis muscle

Palmaris brevis
Abductor digiti minimi
Flexor digiti minimi brevis
Opponens digiti minimi
} Hypothenar muscles

Common palmar digital nerve
Palmar and dorsal interosseous muscles
3rd and 4th lumbrical muscles (*turned down*)
Palmar digital nerves (dorsal digital nerves are from dorsal branch)
Dorsal branches to dorsum of middle and distal phalanges

Note: Only muscles innervated by ulnar nerve are shown.

Plate 5.12

Mononeuropathies

ULNAR MONONEUROPATHIES: POTENTIAL ENTRAPMENT SITES

Ulnar nerve dysfunction occurs at two anatomic loci: primarily the elbow and, less commonly, the wrist. Proximal ulnar lesions at the elbow are the second most common adult mononeuropathy; however, these are less than 10% as frequent as median nerve lesions from CTS. In contrast, ulnar nerve elbow lesions are the most common childhood mononeuropathy.

PROXIMAL ULNAR NERVE LESIONS

Chronic ulnar nerve lesions at the elbow primarily exist at the *cubital tunnel* or *condylar groove*. Patients with these lesions present with symptoms of numbness and tingling and/or sensory loss over the entire fifth and medial fourth fingers. The ulnar nerve does not provide sensory innervation until reaching the wrist; thus medial forearm paresthesias indicate a medial brachial plexus lesion or a C8/T1 radiculopathy. Indolent ulnar damage presents with what is sometimes referred to as the "papal blessing hand," or "Benediction sign," characterized by hyperextension of the fourth and fifth metacarpophalangeal joints and flexion of proximal interphalangeal joints (PIPs). This position is due to unopposed flexion of the PIP and DIP joints because of the loss of function of the ulnar-innervated third and fourth lumbrical muscles, primarily extending the PIP/DIP joints. Unopposed contraction of radial nerve–innervated *extensor digitorum muscles* keeps the proximal phalanxes extended. Although ulnar forearm muscle weakness is rarely apparent to patients, the *medial flexor digitorum profundus* for the fourth and fifth fingers' distal PIP joints is weakened with nerve entrapment at the elbow.

Typically, ulnar nerve entrapment at the elbow occurs at the ulnar *condyle,* presumably after remote elbow trauma *(tardy ulnar palsy),* or just distal to the elbow joint *(cubital tunnel syndrome).* Although chronic ulnar neuropathies are relatively common, a precise etiology is often not identified. Constant pressure from leaning the elbow on a chair arm or desktop may predispose to injury. Uncommonly, idiopathic focal hypertrophic neuropathy, tumors, and hamartomas affect the ulnar nerve. Elbow fractures or dislocations commonly produce acute ulnar nerve compromise. Other acute mechanisms include prolonged external compression from malpositioning in anesthetized patients, hemorrhage in hemophilia patients, intravenous fluid extravasation leading to a compartment syndrome, and burns.

DISTAL ULNAR NERVE LESIONS

Ulnar neuropathies at the wrist or palm are uncommon. Entrapment at the Guyon canal may occur after wrist fractures, with rheumatoid arthritis, or with ganglion cysts. Sensory symptoms may not be present. When sensory loss is demonstrated on the dorsal medial hand, compatible with involvement of the dorsal ulnar cutaneous nerve, the lesion is proximal to the wrist. In contrast, ulnar-innervated muscle weakness confined to the intrinsic hand muscles suggests a pure motor ulnar neuropathy at or distal to the Guyon canal. The most distal pure motor ulnar lesion involves the deep ulnar motor branch within the palm. This is characterized by weakness of the adductor pollicis, the primary thenar muscle not innervated by the median nerve, as well as concomitant weakness of the first dorsal interosseous

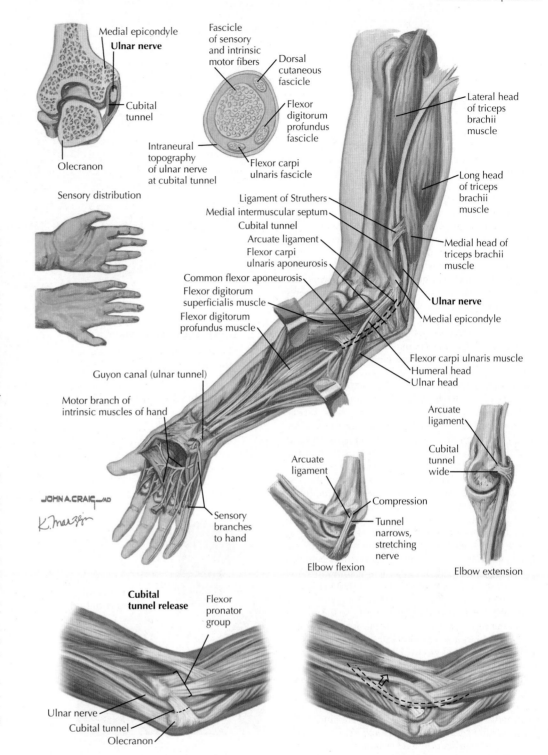

muscle. The preservation of fifth-finger abduction provides the key to localizing the compression site to the lateral palmar hypothenar eminence.

Primary palmar lesions usually result from repetitive hand injury, such as bicycling or occupations using tools that require significant intermittent pressure over the distal ulnar motor fibers at the hypothenar eminence. Typically there is difficulty adducting the thumb and index finger, leading to difficulty placing a key in a lock. When the offending activity is discontinued, significant recovery frequently occurs.

DIFFERENTIAL DIAGNOSIS

Motor neuron disease (MND) is a primary consideration in patients presenting with asymmetric painless atrophy of the hand intrinsic muscles, with no associated sensory deficits. The presence of concomitant median-innervated thenar weakness and atrophy usually occurs in MND because these muscles share C8, T1 innervation. *Lower brachial plexus* lesions characteristically include both motor and sensory dysfunction in components of median, ulnar, and radial peripheral nerves and in C8 and T1 nerve root territories within the arm. *Neurogenic thoracic outlet syndrome* is a T1 extraspinal root lesion mimicking an ulnar neuropathy with greater thenar than hypothenar muscle weakness and atrophy. *C8 radiculopathy* is often accompanied by neck pain and usually affects both ulnar and nonulnar (thenar eminence, FPL, and extensor indicis proprius) innervated muscles and can be associated with medial forearm numbness.

RADIAL NERVE

The *radial nerve* (C5–C8, T1) is primarily derived from the *posterior cord of the brachial plexus.* This is the only nerve trunk that innervates muscles in both the upper arm and forearm. Its primary function is as an extensor of the limb; however, it also contributes to arm flexion through its innervation of the *brachioradialis muscle.* The radial nerve provides cutaneous innervation of *the posterior arm,* forearm, and the dorsal three and half lateral fingers up to the DIP joint.

Within the axilla, the radial nerve lies posterior to the axillary artery and subsequently upon the *subscapularis and latissimus dorsi* muscles while anterior to the teres major muscle. Here it is vulnerable to compression injuries, such as inappropriate positioning of crutches. As the radial nerve exits the axilla and enters the arm, it lies between the brachial artery and the *triceps brachii long head* and innervates the triceps long and medial heads as it passes deep to this muscle.

Proximal to the spiral groove, the *posterior cutaneous nerve of the arm* arises from the radial nerve. The *primary radial nerve trunk* (C5, C6) then passes distally, accompanying the brachial artery within the shallow *radial (spiral) groove of the posterior humerus,* where it is vulnerable to external compression with pressure against the humerus, potentially leading to wrist drop. More distally, the radial nerve takes a medial to posterolateral direction. The *radial posterior muscular branches* innervate the *lateral and medial heads of the triceps muscle* (C6, C7) as well as a long, slender branch to the distal *anconeus muscle* (C6, C7) at the elbow. This small forearm extensor muscle, lying adjacent to the lateral epicondyle of the humerus, sometimes helps localize the primary site of radial neuropathies. If EMG demonstrates anconeus denervation, the lesion site is at or proximal to the spiral groove of the humerus; if the anconeus is unaffected, the injury is distal to the groove. The *posterior cutaneous nerve of the forearm* crosses proximal to the anconeus muscle.

Distal to the spiral groove, adjacent to the lower humerus, the radial nerve lies within the furrow between the medial *brachialis* (C5, C6) muscle and the *brachioradialis* (C5, C6) and the *extensor carpi radialis longus* (C6, C7) laterally, innervating these muscles. There are three cutaneous radial nerve branches originating proximal to the elbow: (1) the *posterior cutaneous and* (2) *lower lateral cutaneous nerves of the arm* and (3) the *posterior cutaneous nerve of the forearm.*

RADIAL NERVE IN FOREARM

As the radial nerve enters the forearm, piercing the *lateral intermuscular septum* descending anterior to the *lateral humeral epicondyle,* it supplies lateral muscular branches, innervating the most proximal *brachioradialis and extensor carpi radialis* muscles. Here the radial nerve bifurcates into its superficial and deep terminal branches. The *superficial sensory radial branch* descends within the forearm deep to the brachioradialis and extensor carpi radialis muscles, eventually emerging in the distal forearm as the *superficial terminal sensory radial branch* (STSRB), descending along the anterolateral side of the forearm. In its upper third, the STSRB branch and the radial artery converge midway down

the lateral forearm, only again to diverge in the distal forearm as the STSRB inclines posterolaterally, deep to the brachioradialis tendon. Here it pierces the deep fascia, subdividing into a *lateral branch* supplying the radial side of the thumb and a *medial branch* splitting into four or five *dorsal digital nerves.* This cutaneous sensory innervation extends just to the DIP joints, whereas the most distal phalanges are supplied, respectively, by the median (digits 1–3.5) and ulnar (digits 4.5 and 5) nerves. The cutaneous hand areas supplied by the radial, median, and ulnar nerves can have individual variations due to intrabranch communication and minor overlap.

The terminal deep muscular radial branch winds posteroinferiorly around the lateral side of the radius

innervating the brachioradialis (C5, C6), extensor carpi radialis longus (C6, C7), and supinator (C5, C6, C7). It enters the *supinator muscle* through the *arcade of Frohse* between its superficial and deep heads, reaching the posterior forearm as the *posterior interosseous nerve* (PIN). This accompanies the posterior interosseous artery between the superficial and deep extensor forearm musculature, innervating the *extensor carpi radialis brevis* (C6, C7), *extensor digitorum and minimi* (C7, C8), *extensor carpi ulnaris* (C7, C8), *abductor pollicis longus* (C7, C8), *extensor pollicis longus* (C7, C8) *and brevis* (C8), and *extensor indicis proprius* (C8). The radial nerve terminates as a small nodule, a pseudoganglion, sending filaments to the distal bones, joints, and ligaments.

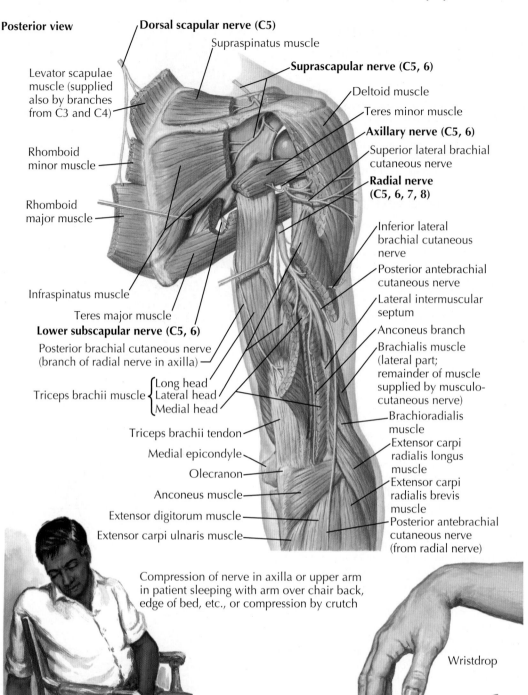

Posterior view

Dorsal scapular nerve (C5)

Supraspinatus muscle

Levator scapulae muscle (supplied also by branches from C3 and C4)

Suprascapular nerve (C5, 6)

Deltoid muscle

Teres minor muscle

Axillary nerve (C5, 6)

Superior lateral brachial cutaneous nerve

Rhomboid minor muscle

Radial nerve (C5, 6, 7, 8)

Rhomboid major muscle

Inferior lateral brachial cutaneous nerve

Posterior antebrachial cutaneous nerve

Lateral intermuscular septum

Infraspinatus muscle

Teres major muscle

Lower subscapular nerve (C5, 6)

Posterior brachial cutaneous nerve (branch of radial nerve in axilla)

Anconeus branch

Brachialis muscle (lateral part; remainder of muscle supplied by musculocutaneous nerve)

Triceps brachii muscle { Long head / Lateral head / Medial head }

Brachioradialis muscle

Extensor carpi radialis longus muscle

Triceps brachii tendon

Medial epicondyle

Olecranon

Extensor carpi radialis brevis muscle

Anconeus muscle

Extensor digitorum muscle

Extensor carpi ulnaris muscle

Posterior antebrachial cutaneous nerve (from radial nerve)

Compression of nerve in axilla or upper arm in patient sleeping with arm over chair back, edge of bed, etc., or compression by crutch

Wristdrop

Plate 5.14

Mononeuropathies

RADIAL NERVE COMPRESSION AND ENTRAPMENT NEUROPATHIES

PROXIMAL RADIAL NEUROPATHIES

These radial compression neuropathies frequently occur at the midhumerus spiral groove and, rarely, the axilla. External compression leads to painless wrist and finger extensor weakness, referred to as wrist drop. Elbow extension is spared, except with axilla lesions, because the radial branches to the triceps originate proximal to the spiral groove. A confounding examination feature is apparent concomitant weakness of ulnar-innervated finger abduction. Because full function of ulnar muscles is promoted by simultaneous wrist extension, finger abduction should be tested by placing the hand and forearm flat on a firm surface, mechanically maximizing ulnar muscle function. In radial neuropathy, sensory signs and symptoms are sometimes overlooked because the motor loss predominates. The brachioradialis reflex is typically diminished or lost, whereas the triceps and biceps reflexes are normal.

Patients unexpectedly assuming a prolonged posture, with an arm resting posteriorly against a hard surface, are liable to develop acute radial nerve palsies. Examples include sleeping with weight on an arm ("honeymooner's palsy"); in patients lying on a hospital gurney, when an arm becomes inadvertently draped over a side rail; or in stuporous individuals seated with an arm draped over the back of a chair. ("Saturday night palsy") (see Plate 5.13). Continued pressure on the radial nerve sequentially produces focal demyelination, conduction block, and clinical weakness. Primary radial nerve lesions are more severe than those found with a C6 or C7 cervical radiculopathy that may have a similar distribution of weakness.

DISTAL RADIAL NEUROPATHIES

The *posterior interosseous nerve* (PIN) is analogous to the anterior interosseous nerve, being a distal, pure motor branch of a major peripheral nerve trunk. The *extensor carpi radialis longus and brevis* (C6, C7) *and brachioradialis* (C5, C6) *muscles* are innervated by radial nerve branches exiting the main trunk before the PIN origin in the upper forearm; therefore finger drop, rather than wristdrop, is the predominant manifestation of a PIN neuropathy. Because the *extensor carpi ulnaris* is affected and the extensor carpi radialis is spared, radial hand deviation occurs during wrist extension. Although the PIN provides no cutaneous innervation, PIN neuropathy is associated with pain near the lateral humerus epicondyle, extending distally as the PIN gives off sensory fibers supplying the interosseous membrane and hand joints near the forearm.

PIN neuropathy can occur with fracture of the proximal radius or with compression by a soft tissue mass or ligamentous structure near or within the supinator muscle. It may develop in patients performing repetitious and strenuous pronation/supination movements, such as recurrent hammering or serving at tennis. Occasionally, instances of this activity lead to intermittent PIN entrapment by the fibrous *arcade of Frohse* at the proximal *supinator muscle* or by a hypertrophied or anomalous supinator.

PREDOMINANT SENSORY RADIAL NEUROPATHIES

The superficial terminal radial sensory branch may be injured in isolation with external pressure at the wrist, as can be seen with handcuff injuries. The distribution of sensory loss is on the posterolateral portion of the hand, particularly the thumb. Symptoms can be elicited by prolonged dorsiflexion of the wrist, leading to temporary entrapment. Sensory symptoms over the posterior forearm from isolated injury to the posterior cutaneous nerve of the forearm can also occur.

In children, more than 50% of radial neuropathies occur secondary to trauma, either by fracture or laceration. Forty percent are due to compression, either intrauterine from prolonged labor in neonates, or due to varied mechanisms similar to those in adults. In addition, benign tumors such as lipomas, ganglia, fibromas, neuromas, and hemangiomas may affect the radial nerve.

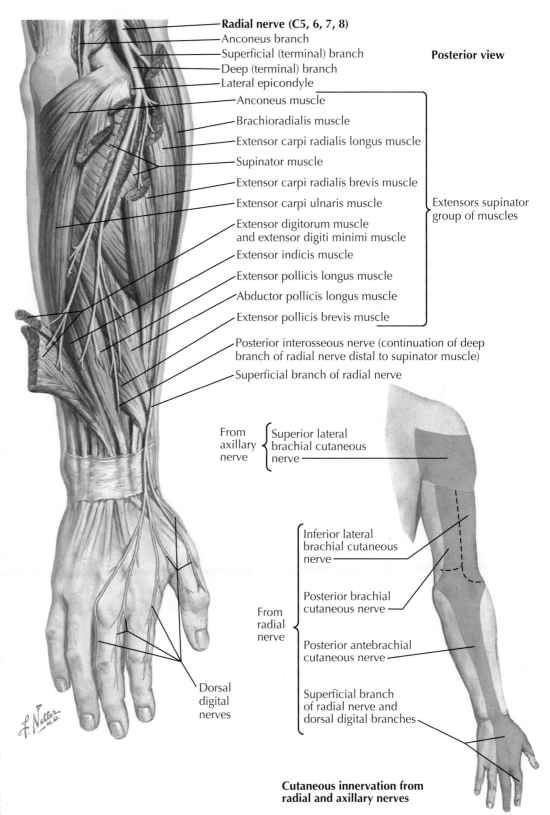

Radial nerve (C5, 6, 7, 8)
Anconeus branch
Superficial (terminal) branch
Deep (terminal) branch
Lateral epicondyle

Posterior view

Anconeus muscle
Brachioradialis muscle
Extensor carpi radialis longus muscle
Supinator muscle
Extensor carpi radialis brevis muscle
Extensor carpi ulnaris muscle
Extensor digitorum muscle and extensor digiti minimi muscle
Extensor indicis muscle
Extensor pollicis longus muscle
Abductor pollicis longus muscle
Extensor pollicis brevis muscle

Extensors supinator group of muscles

Posterior interosseous nerve (continuation of deep branch of radial nerve distal to supinator muscle)
Superficial branch of radial nerve

From axillary nerve { Superior lateral brachial cutaneous nerve

Inferior lateral brachial cutaneous nerve

From radial nerve

Posterior brachial cutaneous nerve

Posterior antebrachial cutaneous nerve

Superficial branch of radial nerve and dorsal digital branches

Dorsal digital nerves

Cutaneous innervation from radial and axillary nerves

FEMORAL AND LATERAL FEMORAL CUTANEOUS NERVES

FEMORAL NERVE

Anatomy. The *femoral nerve* (L2–L4) is the largest branch of the lumbar plexus, initially exiting this plexus and passing inferolaterally beneath the psoas muscle and then coursing within the pelvis between the *iliacus and psoas* (L2, L3) muscles (together forming the iliopsoas muscle) to innervate them. The femoral nerve enters the thigh, descending beneath the inguinal ligament lateral to the femoral vascular sheath and thus lateral to the femoral artery pulse, with the femoral vein placed medially. Muscular branches then supply, in order, the *sartorius, pectineus, and the quadriceps femoris* (all L3, L4 nerve roots). The *anterior femoral cutaneous nerves* supply the skin and fascia over the front and medial sides of the thigh. The *saphenous nerve* communicates with the anterior femoral cutaneous and obturator nerves, then gives off its infrapatellar branch, descends medial to the knee onto the medial foreleg (close to the great saphenous vein), and distally subdivides at the ankle, distributing to the medial arch and dorsum of the foot.

Clinical Findings. Injury to the femoral nerve leads to unilateral knee extension weakness and wasting of the quadriceps muscle. The patellar reflex is diminished or absent. If the nerve is involved proximal to the branches supplying iliopsoas muscle, there is also weakness of hip flexion. Sensory symptoms are variable and usually involve the anteromedial thigh and medial lower leg. Groin and thigh pain may occur. When severe, femoral neuropathy is disabling; total loss of knee extension precludes walking because leg stability is compromised from lack of quadriceps femoris function. With partial lesions, patients first note difficulty descending stairs as the ability to lock the knee to support weight is compromised.

Acute femoral nerve disorders may occur when an expanding mass, particularly a spontaneous hematoma, develops within the *iliopsoas* muscle in an anticoagulated patient. Historically, *diabetes mellitus* was considered a common cause of femoral neuropathy, but most of these likely represent diabetic amyotrophy (i.e., diabetic lumbosacral radiculoplexus neuropathy) with dominant involvement of the femoral nerve. In such cases, careful clinical and EMG examination demonstrates more extensive involvement implicating the plexus or lumbar roots. Autoimmune inflammation of small epineurial vessels (microvasculitis) is thought to be the underlying pathology of diabetic amyotrophy.

Femoral neuropathy may occur in the setting of mononeuritis multiplex due to vasculitis such as polyarteritis nodosa. Femoral neuropathy may occur in patients as the result of pelvic surgery or childbirth requiring a prolonged lithotomy position. Other iatrogenic mechanisms include postoperative hematomas or abscesses, misplaced femoral artery or venous puncture, and direct nerve injury subsequent to nephrectomy or hip arthroplasty. Tumors such as neurofibromas and lymphoma can cause femoral neuropathies. Isolated saphenous nerve injuries may result from knee arthroscopy, from femoral-popliteal artery bypass surgery, and during vein harvesting for coronary artery bypass graft surgery. Gonalgia paresthetica is the term used for damage to the infrapatellar branch of the saphenous nerve that presents with pain over the patella aggravated by squatting or bending the limb at the knee.

Femoral mononeuropathies in children may occur with orthopedic or renal transplant surgery after stretch injuries, or with spontaneous intrapelvic intraneural or extraneural hematomas in patients with hemophilia, perineuriomas, and neurofibromas.

Differential Diagnosis. L2, L3, and L4 nerve root and lumbar plexus lesions can mimic femoral neuropathy. Thigh adductors (innervated by obturator nerve) are spared in femoral mononeuropathy, and their weakness associated with rectus femoris weakness points to lumbar plexopathy or radiculopathy.

Other disorders in the differential diagnosis include early MND and a form of *lumbar plexitis* that occurs in children, similar to acute brachial neuritis (neuralgic amyotrophy) in adults.

Evaluation. NCS/EMG, computed tomography, and MRI are the main diagnostic modalities. Relevant blood studies include serum glucose, erythrocyte sedimentation rate, C-reactive protein, and antineutrophilic cytoplasmic antibodies.

Treatment and Prognosis. Immediate surgical decompression of an iliopsoas hematoma can lessen the likelihood of irreversible weakness. Vasculitic mononeuritis multiplex typically requires immunosuppressive therapies. Physical therapy, particularly utilizing knee bracing for knee stabilization, should be considered for all patients. The degree of axonal damage and subsequent reinnervation determines the patient's outcome.

LATERAL FEMORAL CUTANEOUS NERVE

The LFCN is a pure sensory nerve derived from the L2 and L3 nerve roots, emerging from the *lateral psoas* muscle, passing obliquely over the *iliacus,* to course toward the anterior superior iliac spine. Eventually, it enters the thigh by passing above or through the most lateral portion of the inguinal ligament. The LFCN next passes over or through the proximal *sartorius* muscle, descending deep to the *fascia lata*. After a number of small branches are delivered to the overlying skin, the

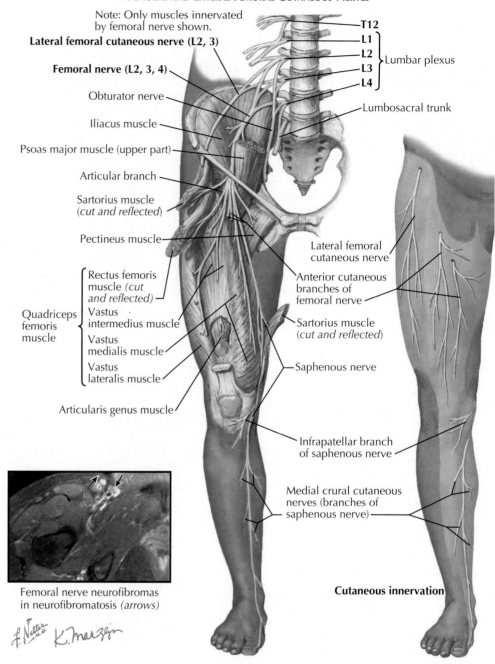

FEMORAL AND LATERAL FEMORAL CUTANEOUS NERVES

Note: Only muscles innervated by femoral nerve shown.

Lateral femoral cutaneous nerve (L2, 3)

Femoral nerve (L2, 3, 4)

Obturator nerve

Iliacus muscle

Psoas major muscle (upper part)

Articular branch

Sartorius muscle (*cut and reflected*)

Pectineus muscle

Rectus femoris muscle (*cut and reflected*)

Quadriceps femoris muscle

Vastus intermedius muscle

Vastus medialis muscle

Vastus lateralis muscle

Articularis genus muscle

T12
L1
L2
L3
L4 } Lumbar plexus

Lumbosacral trunk

Lateral femoral cutaneous nerve

Anterior cutaneous branches of femoral nerve

Sartorius muscle (*cut and reflected*)

Saphenous nerve

Infrapatellar branch of saphenous nerve

Medial crural cutaneous nerves (branches of saphenous nerve)

Cutaneous innervation

Femoral nerve neurofibromas in neurofibromatosis (*arrows*)

Plate 5.16

Mononeuropathies

FEMORAL AND LATERAL FEMORAL CUTANEOUS NERVES (Continued)

LFCN pierces the fascia about 10 cm below the inguinal ligament to innervate the anterolateral thigh.

Damage to this cutaneous nerve is one of the most commonly observed adult mononeuropathies, termed *meralgia paresthetica*. Symptoms include lateral thigh numbness and unpleasant paresthesias described as burning and hypersensitivity when the affected skin is touched by hand or by clothing. Symptoms are usually aggravated by standing or walking. In contrast to patients with lumbar radiculopathy, there is no back pain or symptoms distal to the knee. On neurologic examination, the patient is usually able to circumscribe a well-defined area of skin over the lateral thigh not extending as far as the knee. There is no weakness of femoral-innervated muscles, and the patellar reflex is preserved.

LFCN neuropathies often occur in overweight individuals, especially after recent weight gain, during pregnancy, and as a result of wearing tight belts and tightly fitting pants over the pelvic brim. Other causes include compression with orthopedic appliances, athletic injury from direct blunt trauma to the thigh, and repetitive impact by parallel bars on the thigh of a gymnast. Iatrogenic cases due to iliac bone harvesting or inguinal herniorrhaphy have been reported. Pain that is constant and progressive is not typical of idiopathic LFCN lesions, and the possibility of a mass lesion such as a soft tissue malignant tumor should be considered.

ILIOHYPOGASTRIC, ILIOINGUINAL, AND GENITOFEMORAL NERVES

The iliohypogastric, ilioinguinal, and genitofemoral nerves are primary sensory nerves innervating the lower abdomen, inguinal region, the upper and medial anterior thigh, and part of the genitalia. Each has an L1 origin with occasional T12 and L2 contributions. The *iliohypogastric and ilioinguinal nerves* track laterally, similar to other cutaneous thoracoabdominal nerves. The genitofemoral nerve descends distally through the psoas, emerging to pass under the inguinal ligament, dividing into genital and femoral branches. Its *genital branch* accompanies the ilioinguinal nerve and has a similar cutaneous distribution; it also innervates the cremaster muscle. The *femoral branch* and the *ilioinguinal nerve* innervate small areas of the most proximal anterior thigh. The *ilioinguinal nerve* innervates the skin above the inguinal ligament, the base of the penis and upper scrotum in males, the mons pubis and labium majus in females, and the upper medial thigh. The *iliohypogastric nerve* innervates the distal abdominal wall musculature, its adjacent skin, a small area above the pubis, and a minor portion of the upper buttocks.

The majority of these neuropathies are iatrogenic, occurring during the course of inguinal hernia repair, appendectomy, hysterectomy, or bone harvesting procedure. Blunt trauma and pregnancy are less common associations. Entrapment may occur as the nerves pass through the layers of abdominal wall musculature. Patients describe iliac fossa and inguinal allodynia or hyperesthesia radiating to the genitalia, often exacerbated by walking, hip extension, or maneuvers associated with increased intraabdominal pressure such

as sneezing or coughing. Relief may occur with hip flexion. These neuropathies are often clinically difficult to verify; a local nerve block may confirm the diagnosis and provide therapy. Retroperitoneal lymphoma and intrapelvic and inguinal endometriosis merit differential diagnostic consideration.

OBTURATOR NERVE

Originating within the lumbar plexus and derived from the anterior divisions of the L2, L3, L4 nerve roots, the obturator nerve is constituted within the posterior psoas muscle, thereafter descending through the iliopsoas to emerge medially near the upper sacroiliac joint. The nerve then courses along the pelvis, lying lateral to the ureter and internal iliac vessels, bending anteroinferiorly to follow the lateral pelvic wall. It next passes anterior to the obturator vessels while lying on the obturator internus muscle, to reach the obturator groove, and on to the obturator canal. After giving off a branch to

obturator externus muscle, it divides into anterior and posterior portions and descends into the medial thigh. Here the anterior portion supplies pectineus, adductor longus, adductor brevis, and gracilis before ending in a sensory branch supplying the skin over the medial thigh. The posterior division supplies the obturator externus, adductor magnus (the innervation of which it shares with sciatic nerve), and adductor brevis.

With *obturator mononeuropathy*, weakness is typically confined to large thigh adductors and may present as hip instability. In some cases, sensory loss over the medial thigh is the only discernible deficit. Pathophysiologic mechanisms of obturator mononeuropathies include pelvic and hip fracture, obturator hernia, malignancy, and surgery involving the hip and pelvis. In particular, prolonged lithotomy position can lead to unilateral or bilateral obturator neuropathies from stretching the nerves at the bony obturator foramen. Compression of the nerve by the fetal head against the bony pelvis during difficult labor has been described.

ILIOHYPOGASTRIC, ILIOINGUINAL, GENITOFEMORAL, AND OBTURATOR NERVES

Intercostal nerve (T11)
Iliohypogastric nerve (T12, L1)
Ilioinguinal nerve (L1)
Genitofemoral nerve (L1, 2)
Lateral cutaneous nerve of thigh (L2, 3)
Genital branch and Femoral branch of genitofemoral nerve
Anterior branches and Lateral branches of subcostal and iliohypogastric nerves

T12
Sympathetic trunk
Rami communicantes
L1
L2
L3
L4
L5
S1
S2

Anterior division
Posterior division

Lumbar plexus
Sacral plexus

Iliohypogastric nerve
Ilioinguinal nerve
Genitofemoral nerve
Lateral femoral cutaneous nerve
Femoral nerve
Obturator nerve (L2, 3, 4)
Posterior branch
Articular branch
Anterior branch
Posterior branch
Cutaneous branch
Articular branch to knee joint
Adductor hiatus

L1
L2
L3
L4
Lumbar plexus
Lumbosacral trunk

Obturator externus muscle
Note: Only muscles innervated by obturator nerve are shown.

Adductor brevis muscle
Adductor longus muscle (*cut*)
Adductor magnus muscle (ischiocondylar, or "hamstrings," part supplied by sciatic [tibial] nerve)
Gracilis muscle

Cutaneous innervation

SCIATIC AND GLUTEAL NERVES

GLUTEAL AND PROXIMAL SCIATIC NERVES

The *gluteal nerves* originate from the anterior divisions of the lumbosacral trunk. Both gluteal nerves leave the company of the adjacent sciatic nerve within the buttocks near the sciatic notch. The *superior gluteal nerve,* primarily L5 in origin, emerges above the piriformis muscle to innervate the *gluteus medius and tensor fasciae lata muscles,* both important abductors of the hip. Concomitantly, the *inferior gluteal nerve,* having a predominant S1 origin, emerges below the piriformis muscle, innervating the *gluteus maximus* muscle, the primary extensor of the thigh. The gluteal nerves provide an important clinical localization for the electromyographer because, in the patient presenting with symptoms suggestive of sciatic neuropathy, the absence of denervation in the gluteal muscles provides support for a localization in the sciatic nerve at or distal to the sciatic notch. Conversely, involvement of the gluteal muscles places the lesion at the level of plexus or roots.

SCIATIC AND POSTERIOR FEMORAL CUTANE-OUS NERVES

Anatomy. The sciatic and gluteal nerves share common derivations originating from the anterior rami of the fourth lumbar through the third sacral nerve roots, immediately forming the lumbosacral plexus. The *sciatic nerve* (SN) is a very large single elliptic trunk, 2.0 cm in diameter, that inclines laterally beneath the gluteus maximus muscle while resting on the posterior ischium and the nerve to the quadratus femoris. The *posterior femoral cutaneous nerve,* lying immediately adjacent to the medial edge of the sciatic nerve, provides cutaneous innervation to the posterior thigh. Concomitantly, the sciatic nerve is also accompanied by the inferior gluteal artery (IGA), providing primary blood supply to this nerve. On reaching a point about midway between the ischial tuberosity and the greater trochanter, the SN turns downward over the *gemelli,* the obturator internus tendon, and the *quadratus femoris* muscle, separating it from the hip joint to exit the buttock and enter the thigh beneath the lower border of the *gluteus maximus,* then emerging from the pelvis through the sciatic notch. Here it is found lying just anterior to the piriformis muscle; however, in about 10% to 15% of individuals, part or all of the SN pierces the piriformis muscle.

After passing through the *sciatic notch,* the sciatic nerve descends into the thigh, where it innervates the *semitendinosus* (L5, L4–S2), *semimembranosus* (L5), *biceps femoris* (S1, S2), *and distal part of the adductor magnus* (L5) muscles. The sciatic nerve then descends near the mid-posterior thigh, initially directly posterior to the *adductor magnus,* the distal portion of which it also innervates. It soon travels obliquely over the long head of the *biceps femoris.* Just above the apex of the popliteal fossa, it is overlapped by the contiguous margins of the biceps femoris and *semimembranosus muscles.*

The sciatic nerve trunk has two well-defined divisions, namely, the *lateral fibular (peroneal),* derived from the anterior divisions of the anterior rami of the L4–S2 roots, and *medial tibial,* derived from the posterior divisions of the anterior rami of the L4–S3 nerve roots. The tibial division innervates all posterior thigh muscles, with the exception of the short head of biceps femoris, which is innervated by the fibular division. In approximately 90% of individuals, these two divisions share a common sheath from the pelvis to the popliteal

fossa. However, in 10% of individuals, the anatomic separation of the sciatic divisions occurs higher in the thigh. Rarely, the common fibular and tibial nerves arise independently from the sacral plexus itself, pursuing similar courses until truly separating at the apex of the *popliteal fossa* into its two terminal branches, the common fibular (peroneal) and tibial nerves. Through the sensory branches of the tibial nerve (sural, medial and lateral plantar, and calcaneal) and the superficial fibular (peroneal) nerve, the sciatic nerve supplies sensation to almost the entire foot and the lateral and posterior lower leg (except a small area in the medial foreleg supplied by the saphenous nerve).

Clinical Findings. Acute proximal sciatic neuropathies manifest with distal leg weakness affecting both fibular- and tibial-innervated muscles, leading to

footdrop (secondary to weakness of the *tibialis anterior*) and weakness of eversion (*peroneus longus* muscles), plantar flexion (*gastrocnemius),* and inversion (*tibialis posterior* muscles). More proximal sciatic-innervated *hamstring muscles* are also weakened. The ankle jerk and hamstring muscle stretch reflexes are usually depressed or absent with primary sciatic nerve lesions. Sensory loss and painful dysesthesias of the sole and dorsum of the foot and posterolateral foreleg are common concomitant sensory findings.

The fibular (peroneal) division and tibial division have somewhat different soft tissue anchoring structures; the fibular division's more fixed anchoring makes is more susceptible to stretch injury. Consequently, a proximal sciatic neuropathy often manifests with an isolated footdrop and needs to be differentiated from the

GLUTEAL NERVES

Gluteus maximus muscle (*cut*)
Superior gluteal nerve
Sciatic nerve (*cut*)
Inferior gluteal nerve
Posterior femoral cutaneous nerve (*cut*)
Nerve to obturator internus (and superior gemellus)
Pudendal nerve
Ischial spine
Sacrospinous ligament
Perforating cutaneous nerve
Sacrotuberous ligament
Inferior anal (rectal) nerve
Dorsal nerve of penis
Perineal nerve
Posterior scrotal nerve
Perineal branches of posterior femoral cutaneous nerve
Ischial tuberosity
Semitendinosus muscle
Biceps femoris muscle (long head) (covers semimembranosus muscle)

Iliac crest
Gluteus medius muscle (*cut*)
Gluteus minimus muscle
Piriformis muscle
Superior gemellus muscle
Tensor fasciae latae muscle
Obturator internus muscle
Gluteus medius muscle (*cut*)
Nerve to quadratus femoris (and inferior gemellus) supplying articular branch to hip joint
Greater trochanter of femur
Intertrochanteric crest
Inferior gemellus muscle
Quadratus femoris muscle
Gluteus maximus muscle (*cut*)
Sciatic nerve (*cut*)
Posterior femoral cutaneous nerve (*cut*)
Inferior cluneal nerves

Plate 5.18

Mononeuropathies

SCIATIC AND GLUTEAL NERVES (Continued)

more common fibular (peroneal) neuropathy (FN) at the fibular head. Weakness of the more proximal muscles (hamstrings) and/or foot plantarflexion and inversion (gastrocnemius and tibialis posterior, respectively) helps differentiate between primary sciatic and fibular nerve lesions. Involvement of the *gluteal muscles* seen clinically or confirmed by EMG will point to a proximal *lumbosacral plexus* or L5, S1 nerve root lesion with combined sciatic nerve and gluteal nerve involvement.

Etiology. The sciatic nerve is particularly vulnerable to trauma because it is situated immediately behind the bony pelvis and adjacent to the hip joint, predisposing it to injury from pelvic or femoral fractures and/or posterior hip dislocations. Sciatic neuropathies occasionally occur subsequent to hip arthroplasty and, if incomplete, may have predominant involvement of the fibular (peroneal) division. Similar to femoral neuropathies, sciatic lesions occasionally occur during surgery with the patient in the lithotomy position for a prolonged period of time, presumably from nerve stretch or compression in lean individuals who are anatomically predisposed. In the setting of *acute gluteal compartment syndrome* secondary to an expanding hematoma compressing the SN, there is often severe pain within the buttocks. The sciatic notch and gluteal musculature must be palpated to search for tenderness or fullness compatible with a hematoma or other infiltrating lesion.

Rarely, sciatic neuropathies develop secondary to external pressure, resulting in compression injury in comatose or immobilized patients. Slender individuals may develop SN damage with prolonged involuntary seated positioning on a hard surface such as a bench or a toilet seat (such as during a period of unconsciousness). Likelihood for recovery depends on the degree of axon loss from the injury. Other traumatic mechanisms leading to sciatic neuropathy occur with misplaced injections into the inferior medial quadrant of the buttocks.

Vasculitis, such as polyarteritis nodosa, may cause nerve infarcts leading to a painful sciatic neuropathy.

Various benign nerve sheath or malignant tumors, such as lymphomas, affect the sciatic nerve in rare instances. Iliac artery aneurysms, systemic vasculitis, or endometriosis can cause sciatic neuropathy. Congenital fibrous bands may entrap the SN in the midthigh.

Pediatric sciatic neuropathies are primarily related to trauma or iatrogenic orthopedic or other surgery. Other examples of prolonged extrinsic compression leading to sciatic neuropathy include heel compression in an orthopneic child who has slept with a foot tucked under the buttock, after prolonged lithotomy surgical positioning, and the consequences of sitting in the lotus posture. The precise mechanism of injury is unclear; these are possibly due to ischemia, stretch, or external compression. Interruption of circulation through a persistent sciatic artery at the pelvic notch may predispose to sciatic nerve compression and infarction. A variety of tumors affect SN function in children, including neurofibromas, lymphomas, pelvic neuroblastomas, and chloromas. Various vascular lesions may cause sciatic neuropathy, including hemophilia, arteriovenous malformations, hypereosinophilic or meningococcemia vasculitis, and hematocolpos. The sciatic nerve is at risk during newborn crises when parenteral medications are inadvertently injected into the umbilical artery rather than the umbilical vein. Because the umbilical artery supplies the IGA and the fetal sciatic artery, severe IGA vasoconstriction or thromboembolism

can lead to sciatic nerve ischemia. Congenital iliac anomalies or myofascial bands deep within the thigh are rare causes of pediatric sciatic neuropathy. Occasionally, no specific cause is defined, even in the face of a progressive clinical deficit.

Differential Diagnosis. A *nerve root lesion* at L5, S1 and a *lumbosacral plexus* lesion are the primary differential diagnostic considerations in most sciatic neuropathies, when findings clearly encompass not only fibular but also tibial and or proximal sciatic nerve damage. Diminished sensation over the posterior thigh points to a concomitant posterior femoral cutaneous neuropathy near the greater sciatic foramen. Injury to the *perineal branches of the sacral plexus* nerves leads to sensory loss over the scrotum or labia majora. Hip extension and abduction, dependent on gluteal nerve and

muscle function, are preserved in primary sciatic neuropathies and their involvement should raise suspicion for a primary lesion adjacent to the pelvis, such as a malignant process (lymphoma or schwannoma). Although most patients with diabetic amyotrophy (diabetic lumbosacral radiculoplexus neuropathy) present with pain and weakness in the anterior thigh, onset in the distal leg can occur and can mimic sciatic neuropathy. In such cases, subtle clinical and electromyographic involvement of the muscles supplied by gluteal or femoral nerves helps with the correct localization.

The piriformis syndrome is a poorly defined entity without evidence-based literature to validate the diagnosis to date. Objective clinical or electrodiagnostic evidence of sciatic neuropathy has not been confirmed in most patients in whom piriformis syndrome is suspected.

SCIATIC AND POSTERIOR FEMORAL CUTANEOUS NERVES

Posterior femoral cutaneous nerve (S1, 2, 3)
Inferior gluteal nerves
Perineal branches
Tibial division of sciatic nerve (L4, 5; S1, 2, 3)
Long head (*cut*) of biceps femoris muscle
Adductor magnus muscle (also partially supplied by obturator nerve)
Semitendinosus muscle
Semimembranosus muscle
Tibial nerve
Articular branch
Plantaris muscle
Medial sural cutaneous nerve
Gastrocnemius muscle
Sural nerve
Soleus muscle
Tibial nerve
Medial calcaneal branches
Medial and lateral plantar nerves

Greater sciatic foramen
Sciatic nerve (L4, 5; S1, 2, 3)
Common fibular (peroneal) division of sciatic nerve (L4, 5; S1, 2)
Short head of biceps femoris muscle
Long head (*cut*) of biceps femoris muscle
Common fibular (peroneal) nerve
Articular branch
Lateral sural cutaneous nerve
Sural communicating branch
Lateral calcaneal branches
Lateral dorsal cutaneous nerve

Cutaneous innervation

Posterior femoral cutaneous nerve
Common fibular (peroneal) nerve via lateral sural cutaneous nerve
Medial sural cutaneous nerve
Superficial fibular (peroneal) nerve
Sural nerve
Tibial nerve via medial calcaneal branches

From sciatic nerve

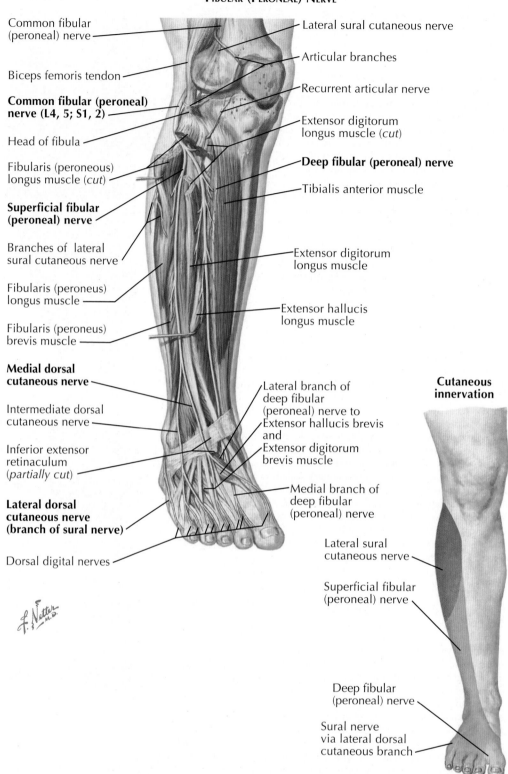

FIBULAR (PERONEAL) NERVE

Common fibular (peroneal) nerve

Biceps femoris tendon

Common fibular (peroneal) nerve (L4, 5; S1, 2)

Head of fibula

Fibularis (peroneous) longus muscle (*cut*)

Superficial fibular (peroneal) nerve

Branches of lateral sural cutaneous nerve

Fibularis (peroneus) longus muscle

Fibularis (peroneus) brevis muscle

Medial dorsal cutaneous nerve

Intermediate dorsal cutaneous nerve

Inferior extensor retinaculum (*partially cut*)

Lateral dorsal cutaneous nerve (branch of sural nerve)

Dorsal digital nerves

Lateral sural cutaneous nerve

Articular branches

Recurrent articular nerve

Extensor digitorum longus muscle (*cut*)

Deep fibular (peroneal) nerve

Tibialis anterior muscle

Extensor digitorum longus muscle

Extensor hallucis longus muscle

Lateral branch of deep fibular (peroneal) nerve to Extensor hallucis brevis and Extensor digitorum brevis muscle

Medial branch of deep fibular (peroneal) nerve

Cutaneous innervation

Lateral sural cutaneous nerve

Superficial fibular (peroneal) nerve

Deep fibular (peroneal) nerve

Sural nerve via lateral dorsal cutaneous branch

FIBULAR (PERONEAL) AND TIBIAL NERVES

FIBULAR (PERONEAL) NERVE

The *common fibular (peroneal) nerve* (CFN) is one of the two major subdivisions of the sciatic nerve, having a lateral, more superficial locus within the sciatic nerve sheath. It is derived from the *posterior* divisions of the fourth and fifth lumbar anterior rami and the first and second sacral nerves. Transcending the thigh, usually within the sciatic trunk, it enters the popliteal fossa, where it and the tibial division bifurcate as separate entities. At the knee, the CFN descends along the lateral popliteal fossa, initially overlapped by the medial biceps femoris tendon; it passes between the biceps tendon and the lateral gastrocnemius head and behind the fibular head to wind around the fibula's bony surface.

This nerve next passes between the two heads of the *fibularis (peroneus) longus* (L5) muscle; here it is particularly vulnerable to being compressed against the fibular bone, leading to footdrop. The CFN divides into the *superficial* and *deep fibular nerves* here. Concomitantly, two superficial sensory nerves take origin. The *lateral sural cutaneous nerve* supplies the skin and fascia on the lateral and adjacent parts of the anteroposterior proximal calf. The *peroneal communicating branch* joins the *sural nerve*, a branch of the tibial nerve, to be distributed with it.

The *superficial fibular nerve* initially descends between the *extensor digitorum longus and brevis* (L5, S1) muscles to innervate the *fibularis (peroneus) longus* (L5) and *brevis* (L5) muscles and to provide sensation to the dorsum of the foot and lateral aspect of the lower half of the calf. The *accessory fibular* (peroneal) nerve, a motor branch of the superficial fibular nerve, is an important *anatomic variation* found in 10% of individuals. This provides partial innervation to the extensor digitorum brevis.

Subsequently, the superficial fibular nerve pierces the deep fascia in the lower leg, dividing into cutaneous nerves. The *medial dorsal cutaneous nerve innervates* the skin on the anterior distal leg; then it travels across the anterior ankle to the dorsum of the foot and across the lower inferior extensor retinaculum. It divides into two *medial dorsal digital nerves;* one supplies the medial and posterior aspects of the foot and great toe, and the other innervates the second and third toes. The *intermediate dorsal cutaneous nerve* courses along the lateral dorsal foot, supplying its adjacent skin and fascia. The *lateral dorsal digital nerves* innervate the skin and fascia of the third through fifth toes.

The *deep fibular (peroneal) nerve* (DFN) originates at the fibular head, passing obliquely downward around the proximal fibular neck, between the *fibularis (peroneus) longus* and *extensor digitorum longus* (L5, S1), muscles that it innervates, to then descend lateral to the *tibialis anterior* (L4, L5) and medial to the *extensor digitorum longus and brevis* (L5, S1) and *extensor hallucis longus* (L5, S1). The *DFN* innervates each of these muscles and the fibularis (peroneus) tertius muscles. The DFN divides at the ankle. Its *medial terminal branch* gives rise to a *dorsal digital nerve*, whose two branches supply the contiguous surfaces of the first two toes. Its *lateral terminal branch* curves outward under the extensor digitorum brevis muscle, which it supplies.

Clinical Findings

Common FN is the most frequent lower extremity mononeuropathy, demonstrated clinically by high stepping ("steppage") gait, owing to weakness of foot dorsiflexion and eversion. Patients have diminished

Plate 5.20

Mononeuropathies

PERONEAL NERVE COMPRESSION

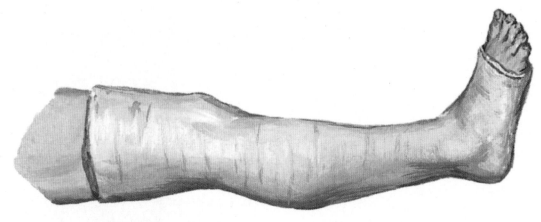

Compression of common peroneal nerve over fibular head may occur by cast, in debilitated patient sitting with legs crossed, or after sleeping on side on hard surface.

FIBULAR (PERONEAL) AND TIBIAL NERVES (Continued)

sensation over the dorsum of the foot and distal half or two-thirds of the lateral calf. Isolated involvement of the deep fibular branch leads to sparing of foot eversion; isolated involvement of the superficial fibular nerve leads to sensory loss confined to the first webspace and weakness of foot eversion.

Most FNs are due to external compression at the fibular head where the nerve is most susceptible as it winds around the fibular neck. Recent weight loss, immobilization, or habitual leg crossing increase the risk of external pressure on the nerve. Occupations requiring prolonged squatting may lead to compression of the nerve between the biceps femoris tendon and lateral gastrocnemius origin. Iatrogenic causes include tightly applied casts at the fibular head, Buck traction, Velcro straps, and intravenous footboards in small children.

Entrapment

Progressive footdrop can develop from a *common or deep fibular nerve* entrapment at the knee. The proximal tendon of the *fibularis longus* can entrap the fibular nerve within the fibular tunnel at the fibular head. Lesions including schwannomas, hemangiomas, bony exostoses, osteochondromas, perineuriomas, and intraneural ganglia or synovial cysts within the popliteal fossa may entrap the fibular nerve. Forcefully stepping into a hole can lead to inversion of the ankle and stretch or avulsion of the CFN at its anatomic fixation to the fibular head, producing a footdrop. A posttraumatic anterior tibial compartment syndrome can lead to deep FN requiring consideration for urgent fasciectomy to release pressure on the nerve trunk. The *lateral cutaneous nerve of the calf* branch of the fibular nerve can be entrapped in the lateral popliteal fossa, leading to popliteal fossa and lateral calf pain, exacerbated when seated and aided by extension of the knee.

TIBIAL NERVE

This is the larger and medial terminal branch of the sciatic nerve. Its fibers are derived from the anterior divisions of the anterior rami of the fourth and fifth lumbar and the first, second, and third sacral nerves. In the distal thigh, after its origin from the sciatic bifurcation, the tibial nerve is overlapped by the semimembranosus and biceps femoris muscles, becoming more superficial in the popliteal

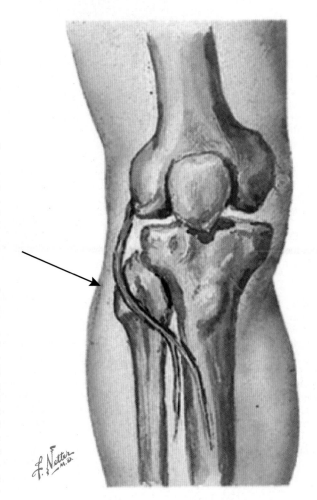

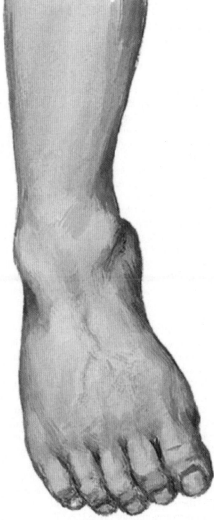

fossa, proceeding into the leg beneath the heads of the *gastrocnemius lateral* (L5, S1), *medial* (S1, S2), and *plantaris* muscles, and descending to be superficial to the *popliteus* muscle and deep to the *soleus* (S1, S2) to travel between the gastrocnemius medial and lateral heads of the tibialis posterior and, subsequently, between the *flexor digitorum longus* (L5, S1) and *flexor hallucis longus* muscles, innervating each of these muscles as well as *plantaris* and *popliteus* muscles. Distally, the nerve lies superficially, descending to the ankle, medial to the Achilles tendon,

curving anteroinferiorly and posteriorly to the medial malleolus. Here it enters the tarsal tunnel, proceeding into the foot deep to the flexor retinaculum between the flexor hallucis longus and flexor digitorum longus tendons. Here it terminates, dividing into the medial and lateral plantar nerves that innervate all intrinsic foot muscles (S1, S2) and provide sensation to the plantar surface of the foot.

The *sural nerve*, a cutaneous branch, arises from the tibial nerve at the popliteal fossa, descends between the gastrocnemius heads, pierces the deep fascia, gives off a

TIBIAL NERVE

Medial sural cutaneous nerve (*cut*)

Articular branches

Plantaris muscle

Gastrocnemius muscle (*cut*)

Nerve to popliteus muscle

Popliteus muscle

Interosseous nerve of leg

Soleus muscle (*cut and partly retracted*)

Flexor digitorum longus muscle

Tibialis posterior muscle

Flexor hallucis longus muscle

Sural nerve (*cut*)

Lateral calcaneal branch

Medial calcaneal branch

Flexor retinaculum (*cut*)

Lateral dorsal cutaneous nerve

Tibial nerve (L4, 5; S1, 2, 3)

Common fibular (peroneal) nerve

Articular branch

Lateral sural cutaneous nerve (*cut*)

Sural nerve (S1, 2) via lateral calcaneal and lateral dorsal cutaneous branches

Saphenous nerve (L3, 4)

Lateral plantar nerve (S1, 2)

Medial plantar nerve (L4, 5)

From tibial nerve

Medial calcaneal branches (S1, 2)

Cutaneous innervation of sole

Note: Articular branches not shown

Common and plantar digital nerves

Superficial branch to flexor digiti minimi brevis muscle and 4th interosseous muscle

Deep branch to adductor hallucis muscle, 2nd, 3rd, and 4th lumbrical muscles and interossei muscles

Abductor digiti minimi muscle

Quadratus plantae muscle and nerve

Nerve to abductor digiti minimi muscle

Lateral plantar nerve
Lateral calcaneal branch of sural nerve

Plantar digital nerves

Common plantar digital nerves

1st lumbrical muscle and nerve

Flexor hallucis brevis muscle and nerve

Abductor hallucis muscle and nerve

Flexor digitorum brevis muscle and nerve

Medial plantar nerve
Medial calcaneal branch

Tibial nerve

Flexor retinaculum (*cut*)

FIBULAR (PERONEAL) AND TIBIAL NERVES (Continued)

small *medial sural cutaneous nerve* (it may be larger and arise directly from the tibial nerve), and is joined by the *fibular communicating branch of the lateral sural cutaneous nerve,* next passing over and lateral to the Achilles tendon. It provides cutaneous innervation to the posterior lateral lower leg, the lateral ankle, and heel. The terminal portion courses forward as the lateral dorsal cutaneous nerve of the foot.

The *medial plantar nerve* can be compared with the median nerve in the hand. It originates under the flexor retinaculum, traveling deep to the *abductor hallucis,* innervating it and subsequently the *flexor digitorum brevis* and *flexor hallucis brevis* muscles (S1, S2). At the tarsometatarsal joints, this nerve ends by dividing into a *proper plantar digital nerve* that supplies the medial great toe and three *common plantar digital nerves* in a fashion similar to the median nerve of the hand.

The *lateral plantar nerve* is homologous with the ulnar nerve in the hand, arising deep to the flexor retinaculum; passing outward to innervate the lateral sole, the *flexor digitorum brevis,* the *quadratus plantae,* and the *abductor digiti minimi* (S1, S2); and ending near the fifth metatarsal bone. Lastly, it divides into two branches: the *superficial branch* that splits into *proper and common plantar digital nerves* that innervate the plantar lateral small toe and the *flexor digiti minimi and interossei* muscles (S1, S2) of the fourth intermetatarsal space. The *common plantar digital nerve* divides into two *proper plantar digital nerves* supplying the fourth and fifth toes. A *deep branch* supplies the *adductor hallucis,* the second to fourth *lumbricals,* and the medial three *interossei muscles* (S1, S2).

Clinical Findings
The tibial nerve is well protected within the entirety of its course from the sciatic notch, through the thigh, within the popliteal fossa, and deep within the calf. It is not at high risk for compression or entrapment. However, traumas such as localized laceration, fracture, and hematoma may involve the tibial nerve. A Baker cyst within the knee joint or a ganglion within the tibiofibular joint occasionally compromises this nerve. Intrinsic nerve tumors may affect the tibial nerve anywhere along its course. Depending on the site of involvement,

there can be calf and/or foot muscle weakness and atrophy as well as sensory loss appropriate to the lesion site. Proximal tibial neuropathy (at or proximal to the gastrocnemius/soleus innervation) will produce weakness of foot plantar flexion and inversion and loss of the ankle reflex. Weakness of intrinsic foot muscles occurs with tibial neuropathy at any level, but these muscles are difficult to evaluate clinically. Sensory loss and pain may be present on the plantar aspect of the foot and heel, as well as the posterior calf if there is concomitant involvement of the sural nerve.

Tarsal tunnel syndrome (TTS) is an uncommon neuropathy of the distal tibial nerve at the ankle. In well-documented cases, entrapment of the tibial nerve and its terminal branches at the ankle (medial and lateral plantar nerves) produces pain on the sole of the foot and atrophy of intrinsic foot muscles. Pain is exacerbated with weight bearing and at night. Although NCS/EMG can confirm TTS, its principal value lies in assessing for more common conditions causing plantar foot pain such as S1 radiculopathy and polyneuropathy. Foot fracture may also lead to distal tibial neuropathy.

Plate 5.22

Mononeuropathies

CUTANEOUS INNERVATION

Anterior (palmar) view   **Posterior (dorsal) view**

Supraclavicular nerves (from cervical plexus: C3, 4)

Axillary nerve Superior lateral cutaneous nerve of arm (C5, 6)

Radial nerve Inferior lateral cutaneous nerve of arm (C5, 6)

Lateral cutaneous nerve of forearm (C5, 6, [7]) (terminal part of musculo-cutaneous nerve)

Radial nerve Superficial branch (C6, 7, 8)

Median nerve palmar branch and palmar digital branches (C6, 7, 8)

Palmar branch

Palmar digital branches

Intercosto-brachial nerve (T2) and medial cutaneous nerve of arm (C8, T1, 2)

Medial cutaneous nerve of forearm (C8, T1)

Ulnar nerve (C8, T1)

Dorsal branch and dorsal digital branches

Proper palmar digital branches

Supraclavicular nerves (from cervical plexus: C3, 4)

Axillary nerve Superior lateral cutaneous nerve of arm (C5, 6)

Radial nerve Posterior cutaneous nerve of arm (C5, 6, 7, 8)

Inferior lateral cutaneous nerve of arm

Posterior cutaneous nerve of forearm (C[5], 6, 7, 8)

Lateral cutaneous nerve of forearm (C5, 6, [7]) (terminal part of musculo-cutaneous nerve)

Radial nerve Superficial branch and dorsal digital branches (C6, 7, 8)

Median nerve Proper palmar digital branches

Lateral femoral cutaneous nerve

Anterior cutaneous branches of femoral nerve

Infrapatellar branch of saphenous nerve

Medial crural cutaneous nerves (branches of saphenous nerve)

Femoral nerve

Obturator nerve

Note: Division is variable between ulnar and radial innervation on dorsum of hand and often aligns with middle of 3rd digit instead of 4th digit as shown.

From tibial nerve
Medial calcaneal branches (S1, 2)
Medial plantar nerve (L4, 5)
Lateral plantar nerve (S1, 2)

Saphenous nerve (L3, 4)

Sural nerve (S1, 2) via lateral calcaneal and lateral dorsal cutaneous branches

Tibial nerve

Posterior femoral cutaneous nerve

From sciatic nerve
Common fibular (peroneal) nerve via lateral sural cutaneous nerve
Superficial fibular (peroneal) nerve
Sural nerve
Tibial nerve via medial calcaneal branches

Sciatic nerve

Lateral sural cutaneous nerve

Superficial fibular (peroneal) nerve

Sural nerve via lateral dorsal cutaneous branch

Deep fibular (peroneal) nerve

Common peroneal nerve

Plates 5.22-5.23

DERMATOMAL AND CUTANEOUS NERVE PATTERNS

Symptoms of numbness, tingling, and pain are very common in neuropathy but may not be helpful in pre-cise localization of the lesion.

Hand numbness is the leading and earliest clinical feature of CTS, resulting from median nerve entrap-ment at the wrist. Symptoms present during the night or on awakening in the morning or that are precipitated by driving or repetitive hand/wrist activities differenti-ate this disorder from central nervous system lesions affecting sensory pathways.

Median nerve lesions primarily affect the *palmar aspects of fingers 1 to 3.5;* the dorsal tips of these fingers are also compromised to the DIP joints. In contrast, *ulnar neuropathies* also manifest with finger numbness but with a different anatomic distribution involving the *medial one and a half fingers,* specifically the entire little (fifth) finger and the medial aspect of the ring (fourth) finger. The *ulnar nerve* is the only nerve in the hand to equally affect the palmar and dorsal portions of the fingers and hand. Owing to peripheral nerve origins, a *medial cord or lower trunk brachial plexus lesion* may also present with numbness mimicking ulnar neuropa-thy. Although a *C8 radiculopathy* has a similar sensory distribution, it is usually accompanied by significant neck pain. The *radial nerve* primarily innervates the dorsum of the proximal thumb, index, middle, and lat-eral half of the ring finger to the DIP joint, as well as the *dorsum of the hand* in continuity with these fingers, thus sparing the fingertips because of their full median

innervation. Thus, when the fingertips are involved, there is either a median or ulnar nerve lesion or a nerve root lesion present.

A cervical radiculopathy involving the C6, C7, or C8 root also leads to numbness developing in the fingers. The C6 and C7 nerve roots are the two most commonly compromised sites at the nerve root level. Often, the history of nerve root impingement is relatively abrupt in onset, commonly preceded by intrascapular or neck pain. Annoying finger numbness may be the only

clinical symptoms of a recent C6, C7, and/or C8 nerve root lesion. In contrast to a peripheral nerve lesion affecting primarily the palmar surface, such as the me-dian nerve in CTS, a C6 or C7 nerve root lesion will compromise sensation of both palmar and posterior finger surfaces.

In the leg and foot, numbness and tingling of the toes may be features of FN or tibial neuropathy or nerve root involvement at the L5 or S1 level. Low back pain with radiation into the buttock and down the leg, often

DERMATOMES

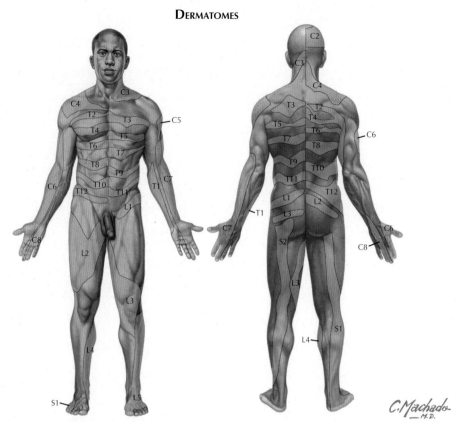

C.Machado
—M.D.

Levels of principal dermatomes

C4	Level of clavicles	T10	Level of umbilicus
C5, C6, C7	Lateral surfaces of upper limbs	L1	Inguinal region and proximal anterior thigh
C8, T1	Medial surfaces of upper limbs	L1, L2, L3, L4	Anteromedial lower limb and gluteal region
C6	Lateral digits	L4, L5, S1	Foot
C6, C7, C8	Hand	L4	Medial leg
C8	Medial digits	L5, S1	Posterolateral lower limb and dorsum of foot
T4	Level of nipples	S1	Lateral foot

Schematic based on Lee MW, McPhee RW, Stringer MD. An evidence-based approach to human dermatomes. Clin Anat. 2008; 21(5):363–373. doi: 10.1002/ca.20636. PMID: 18470936. Note that these areas are not absolute and vary from person to person. S3, S4, S5, and coccyx supply the perineum but are not shown for reasons of clarity. Of note, the dermatomes are larger than illustrated, as the figure is based on best evidence; gaps represent areas in which the data are inconclusive.

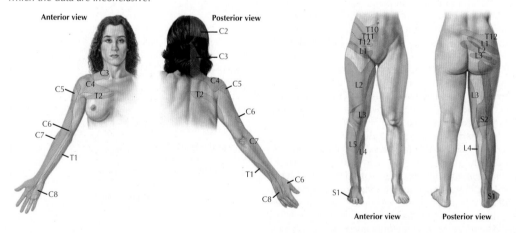

DERMATOMAL AND CUTANEOUS NERVE PATTERNS (Continued)

described as sciatica, is a common accompaniment when a lumbosacral nerve root lesion is responsible for foot numbness and paresthesia. When symptoms in the feet are bilateral, peripheral polyneuropathy becomes the more likely cause of stocking distribution symptoms and also, over time, glove distribution symptoms. When there is global, symmetric, pure sensory loss, the possibility of a disorder primarily affecting the dorsal root ganglion cells (*sensory ganglionopathy*) should be considered.

Mononeuropathy multiplex is a disorder characterized by initial acute onset of a mononeuropathy, followed over time by involvement of another anatomically distinct mononeuropathy, and subsequently additional nerve trunks may be involved to produce a confluent pattern suggesting a generalized peripheral polyneuropathy. Typically, the individual nerve trunk lesion presents as an acute sensory and motor deficit. When related to vasculitis, the underlying mechanism is occlusion of small arterioles, the *vasa nervorum,* that supply the individual nerve, leading to nerve infarction. Two likely etiologies include the arteriopathy associated with diabetes mellitus and systemic vasculitis, such as polyarteritis nodosa.

Hereditary neuropathy with predisposition to pressure palsies (HNPP) affects multiple individual peripheral nerves in a varied sequence associated with an underlying demyelinating peripheral polyneuropathy. HNPP is an autosomal dominant form of demyelination that is secondary to a *PMP22* deletion on the short arm of chromosome 17p11.2.

Some peripheral mononeuropathies manifest predominantly with weakness, particularly the wristdrop of radial nerve lesions or the footdrop of fibular (peroneal) nerve lesions. Sometimes these are mistaken for a stroke. A clear appreciation of each individual peripheral nerve's motor distribution ultimately aids in the correct diagnosis. Rarely, lesions as high as the parasagittal region of the brain may also manifest with isolated foot weakness.

Atrophy of muscles innervated by the involved nerve occurs with chronic denervation. Concomitantly, fasciculations may also be present. Measuring extremity circumference may document significant side-to-side asymmetries and, by inference, muscle atrophy secondary to anterior horn cell, nerve root, or peripheral nerve damage. When encountering a clinical pattern suggesting mononeuropathy, the absence of sensory symptoms or signs should raise concern for an intraspinal lesion such as ALS or syringomyelia.

PERIPHERAL NEUROPATHIES

PERIPHERAL NERVE

The main function of the peripheral nerve is to connect and conduct signals between the central nervous system (CNS) and all the muscles, organs, and glands of the body. Each peripheral nerve is composed of *neurons, axons,* and the supportive cells, vessels, and connective tissue that house and sustain neuronal function.

Peripheral nerves are separated into three structural layers: *epineurium, perineurium,* and *endoneurium.* The *epineurium,* the outermost layer, forms a sheath of fibrous connective tissue surrounding the inner layers and contains many well-collateralized, small *arterioles, capillaries,* and *venules* coursing longitudinally (Plate 6.1, top left) and entering inward radially to supply the perineurium and endoneurium. Compromise of the nerve vasculature can result in infarction of an entire nerve by severe and prolonged limb ischemia or of individual fascicles by widespread inflammation affecting many vessels in autoimmune vasculitis.

The individual fascicles of axons and myelin comprising the endoneurium are separated from the epineurium by thin layers of tightly bound connective tissue derived from fibroblasts called the *perineurium.* The perineurium forms the *blood-nerve barrier,* which is analogous to the blood-brain barrier, formed in the central nervous system by creating tight junctions and regulating the extracellular endoneurial environment.

The innermost layer, the *endoneurium,* is composed of *nerve fiber bundles* containing neuronal cell bodies and their axons, *Schwann cells* producing *myelin* sheaths, and other supportive cells. The *neuronal cell body* contains the nucleus and other important organelles needed to maintain the neuron and produce important *cytoskeletal proteins and neurotransmitters* necessary for *axonal transport* and signal transduction. The peripheral nerve *axon* is the long process of *axoplasm* surrounded by a cell membrane. It extends from the neuronal cell body that conducts electric signals to the target destination.

The *epineurium* and *perineurium* have important roles in maintaining the function and structure of the nerve. They protect the nerve from mechanical compressive and tensile stresses that threaten axons (Plate 6.1, top right). Repetitive physical compression of superficial nerves (e.g., habitual leg crossing compressing the fibular nerve at the fibular head) may exceed the protective capacity, leading first to demyelination. This is followed by axonal loss with continued repetitive or severe compression. The spiral configuration of the nerve fiber bundles (Fontana's bands) within each fascicle helps protect the nerve from traction injuries, in which the nerve may be suddenly extended longitudinally. This type of injury often occurs with sudden, direct blunt trauma to the limb or neck region in the case of the nerves in the brachial plexus, such as with trauma after high-speed collisions. Although the spiral configuration protects the nerves from relatively minor traction injuries, it does not prevent injury from more severe injuries (e.g., nerve root avulsion from the spinal cord).

Individual nerve fibers may be myelinated or unmyelinated (Plate 6.1, bottom). *Myelinated fibers* are axons that have been surrounded by multiple *Schwann cells* longitudinally along their length. The Schwann cells' cytoplasm wraps around a 0.5- to 1.0-mm segment of a single axon, producing *lamellae.* The plasma membrane of the Schwann cells that encircle the axon is

composed of lipids (including cholesterol, cerebrosides, sulfatides, proteolipids, sphingomyelin, glycolipids, and glycoproteins) and proteins. Concentric layers of these membrane materials wrapping around axons form the myelin sheath. The function of the myelin is to "insulate" the axon. The regions where one Schwann cell cytoplasm meets another, between myelinated segments, are small unmyelinated regions named *nodes of Ranvier,* where axons possess high concentrations of

sodium and potassium membrane channels. As a result, the *action potentials* that are generated and propagated along the axon are rapidly transmitted, jumping from node to node, producing saltatory conduction.

In contrast to myelinated fibers, *unmyelinated fibers* consist of smaller caliber axons grouped together and embedded loosely within a Schwann cell cytoplasm. A single Schwann cell and its cytoplasm surround multiple unmyelinated axons in structures named *Remak bundles.*

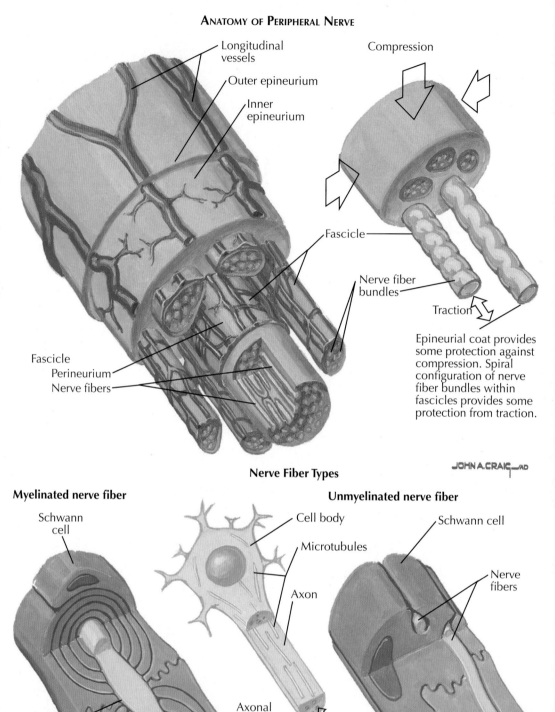

ANATOMY OF PERIPHERAL NERVE

Longitudinal vessels
Compression
Outer epineurium
Inner epineurium
Fascicle
Nerve fiber bundles
Traction
Fascicle
Perineurium
Nerve fibers

Epineurial coat provides some protection against compression. Spiral configuration of nerve fiber bundles within fascicles provides some protection from traction.

JOHN A. CRAIG—AD

Nerve Fiber Types

Myelinated nerve fiber

Schwann cell
Node of Ranvier
Nerve cell axon
Myelin sheath

Cell body
Microtubules
Axon
Axonal transport

Microtubules within axoplasm allow transport of cell products (anterograde and retrograde). Compression may inhibit axonal transport.

Unmyelinated nerve fiber

Schwann cell
Nerve fibers

Plate 6.2

Peripheral Neuropathies

HISTOLOGY OF PERIPHERAL NERVE

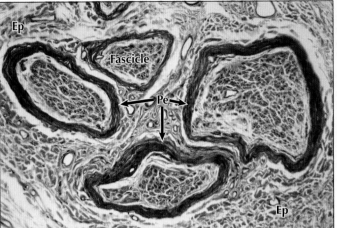

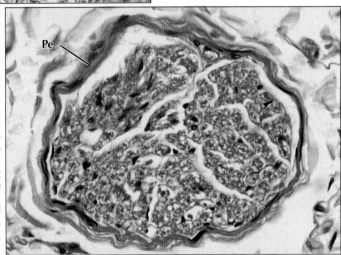

Light micrograph of a peripheral nerve in transverse section. Several fascicles that make up this nerve are enveloped by connective tissue of the epineurium (*Ep*), which merges imperceptibly with surrounding loose connective tissue. A more deeply stained perineurium (*Pe*) encloses the fascicles. Each fascicle consists of large numbers of nerve fibers, which are embedded in a more delicate endoneurium (not well resolved at this magnification). 200×. *Masson trichrome.*

Light micrograph of one peripheral nerve fascicle in transverse section at medium magnification. The perineurium (*Pe*) forms an investment around the fascicle. This small nerve has a single fascicle in the connective tissue, so it lacks an epineurium. The interior has numerous nerve fibers sectioned transversely or obliquely and embedded in loose connective tissue of the endoneurium. Many nerve fibers are surrounded by myelin sheaths, which appear washed out because of lipid content. Within the fascicle are nuclei of occasional fibroblasts, Schwann cells, and capillary endothelial cells between nerve fibers. 280×. *H&E.*

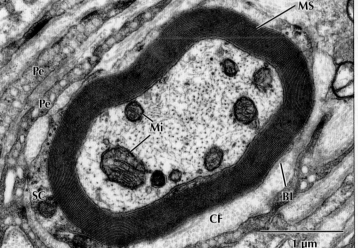

Electron micrograph of a peripheral nervous system nerve fiber in transverse section. The axon is surrounded by a myelin sheath (*MS*) composed of multiple lamellae formed by the plasma membrane of a Schwann cell. A thin rim of Schwann cell cytoplasm (*SC*) envelops the myelin and is invested externally by a thin basal lamina (*BL*). Collagen fibrils (*CF*) of the endoneurium and flattened perineurial cells (*Pe*) are in the surrounding area. The nerve fiber axoplasm contains mitochondria (*Mi*), neurofilaments, and a few microtubules. 30,000×.

From Ovalle W, Nahirney P. Netter's Essential Histology. Saunders; 2008.

PERIPHERAL NERVE (Continued)

Although there is a smaller amount of protective myelin than with myelinated fibers, there are no nodes of Ranvier, and sodium channels are equally dispersed along the entire course of the axon, resulting in slower action potential propagation along the nerve.

Both myelinated and unmyelinated nerve fibers contain the other basic structures of a neuron: dendrites, a cell body, the axon, and the nerve terminals. Several cytoskeletal proteins within the axon provide structure and assist to transport intracellular materials to and from the cell body and nerve terminals. The largest of these proteins are *microtubules,* which transport products forward from the cell body to the nerve terminal (*anterograde transport*) and in reverse from the nerve terminal to the cell body (*retrograde transport*). Other proteins, such as intermediate neurofilaments, help maintain axonal structure.

The structures of the nerve can be identified microscopically. At different magnifications, the definition and various individual components of the nerves can be identified. The upper image shows a light micrograph transverse section of a peripheral nerve at a magnification of 200× (Masson trichrome stain). In this image, four individual nerve fascicles are seen. The epineurium is the connective tissue that envelops and supports the individual fascicles. Each fascicle is surrounded by a barrier of dark-appearing connective tissue, the *perineurium,* which also provides tensile support of the axons. The large myelinated axons within the endoneurium appear as many, small, red, circular "bicycle wheel" structures surrounded by many light blue Schwann cells and their cytoplasms, along with other supportive cells and endoneurial microvessels.

In the middle light micrograph, a transverse section of a single nerve fascicle is seen at medium magnification (280×, hematoxylin and eosin [H&E] stain). In this image, the darker-stained perineurium can be seen forming a surrounding protective barrier for nerve fibers within it. Inside the perineurium are multiple nerve fibers that are sectioned transversely or obliquely. Many of the visible fibers are surrounded by myelin sheath, which stains as a foamy white ring around axons because of the high lipid content. Surrounding the individual axons are dark nuclei of fibroblasts, Schwann cells, and capillary endothelial cells.

The bottom electromicrograph is a transverse section of an individual axon at very high magnification (330,000×). The axon is surrounded by *perineurial* cells and collagen fibrils that constitute the supportive endoneurium. The Schwann cell surrounding the axon is composed of cytoplasm that wraps around the axon in *lamellae forming the myelin sheath.* The thin external basal lamina of the myelin can also be identified. Within the myelin is the axon. Individual organelles, including mitochondria, neurofilaments, and microtubules, can also be seen.

Peripheral nerves are assessed through electrodiagnostic (EDX) testing including electromyography (EMG) and nerve conduction study (NCS). NCS is performed with direct stimulation of large-caliber peripheral sensory or motor nerves, measuring the action potentials generated along the nerve at a site distant from stimulation. EMG further assists localization of nerve injury by assessing characteristics of action potentials in muscle membranes that are transmitted by motor nerves. Many disease states affect peripheral nerves, including genetic disorders such as Charcot-Marie-Tooth (CMT) disease; metabolic disorders occurring with other organ dysfunction, including diabetes mellitus and chronic renal failure; various toxins, including chemotherapeutic medications and certain environmental toxins; and acquired autoimmune disease or as a result of malignancy producing a paraneoplastic disorder.

Individual peripheral nerves may be affected by local factors, such as thickening of the transverse carpal ligament that compresses of the median nerve at the wrist (carpal tunnel syndrome) or extrinsic compression of the common fibular nerve at the fibular head by repetitive crossing of the legs. Muscle weakness occurs with sufficient denervation (loss of motor axons) or with blockage of nerve conduction due to alteration of myelin function.

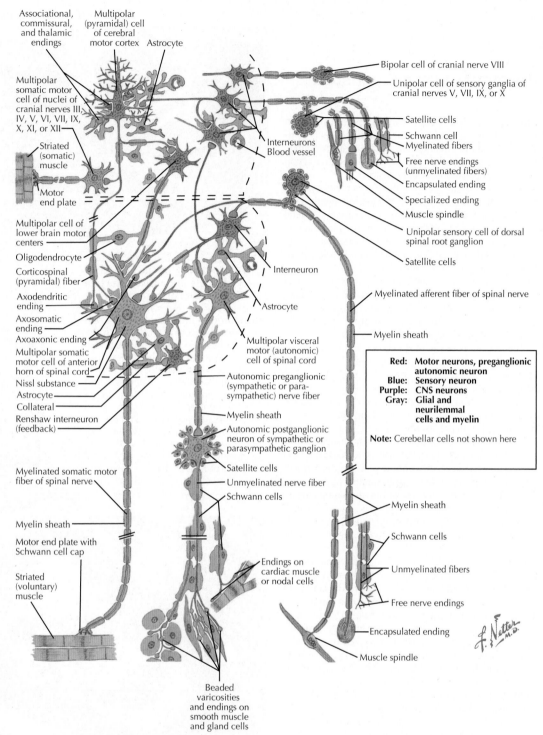

CELL TYPES OF NERVOUS SYSTEM

SENSORY NEURONS

Sensory neurons transmit information from the periphery to the CNS via action potentials. *Cell bodies* of these unipolar neurons generally lie in peripheral ganglia. The *proximal (central) processes* of these cells enter the CNS via cranial nerves or dorsal (posterior) spinal roots and terminate synaptically either on interneurons or, in the case of group I muscle spindle afferents, on skeletal motor neurons. The *distal (peripheral) processes* of sensory neurons, which may be either myelinated or unmyelinated, terminate in one of three ways:

1. In the *free nerve ending*, the peripheral process branches widely and ends without obvious specialization. These endings respond primarily to intense stimuli and are thought to play a role in the perception of pain.
2. In the *encapsulated ending*, an accessory structure envelops the terminal peripheral process, modifying stimuli before they reach the nerve terminus. Examples include Ruffini and Golgi endings and pacinian and paciniform corpuscles. Muscle spindles and Golgi tendon organs are highly specialized encapsulated endings in which the sensory nerve terminal also performs stimulus transduction.
3. In the *taste buds* and the *cochlear* and *vestibular systems*, specialized receptor cells transduce specific chemical or mechanical stimuli into action potentials that reach sensory fibers and central nuclei.

Olfactory and *optic afferent neurons* do not fit into any of these categories. Olfactory stimuli are detected by specialized receptor cells with axons projecting directly to interneurons of the olfactory bulb. The retina, formed by an outgrowth of the brain, contains both receptor cells and interneurons. The optic nerve therefore corresponds more to a central sensory tract than a sensory nerve.

MOTOR NEURONS

All neurons sending efferent axons to the periphery can be described as motor (effector) neurons. These are typically medium to large multipolar cells with long myelinated axons. There are three classes of motor neurons:

1. *Motor neurons supplying skeletal muscles* are located in the anterior horn of the spinal cord and project peripherally via anterior (ventral) spinal

roots. Motor neurons supplying muscles of the face and some muscles of the neck and throat are located in the brainstem motor nuclei and project to their target muscles via cranial nerves V, VII, IX, X, XI, and XII. Two kinds of motor neurons supply skeletal muscles: *alpha motor neurons*, which supply the main extrafusal muscle fibers, and *fusimotor (gamma motor) neurons*, which supply the intrafusal fibers of muscle spindles.

2. *Extraocular motor neurons* are located in cranial nerve III, IV, and VI nuclei. Because human extraocular muscles lack muscle spindles, these are all alpha motor neurons. The contractions of these muscles in various combinations direct eye movements.

3. *The motor innervation of the autonomic nervous system* differs from the innervation of skeletal and extraocular muscles because two neurons are involved. The first, called the *preganglionic neuron*, is located in the intermediate horn of the spinal cord or in the brainstem and sends a thinly myelinated axon to one of the various sympathetic or parasympathetic ganglia. The sympathetic ganglia are located near the spinal cord, whereas parasympathetic ganglia are located close to or within the organ being innervated. Within the ganglion, the preganglionic fiber forms an excitatory (cholinergic) synapse with a ganglionic neuron. The ganglionic neuron then sends an unmyelinated *postganglionic axon* to innervate the target structure.

Plate 6.4

Peripheral Neuropathies

RESTING MEMBRANE POTENTIAL

Rapid transmission of electrical signals along neurons relies on the generation and propagation of electrical charges along the membrane. A complex and constantly occurring series of processes along the axon membrane is necessary for the development of the action potential. The axon membrane potential electrical gradients are responsible for the changes that occur during action potential generation, and the processes occurring at rest provide the foundation for these processes Several structures along the axonal plasma membrane are responsible for the generation of the *resting membrane potential* (RMP)—the sodium (Na^+), potassium (K^+), and chloride (Cl^-) channels and the adenosine triphosphate (ATP)-dependent Na^+-K^+ pump.

The *transmembrane ion concentrations* depend on the passive diffusion of ions from the site of higher concentration to the site of lower concentration through ion channels, as well as the active adenosine triphosphatase (ATPase)-dependent transport of ions against a concentration gradient. At rest, the concentrations of sodium, chloride, and calcium ions are higher extracellularly, whereas the concentrations of potassium ions and impermeable protein anions are higher intracellularly. As a result, sodium and chloride are driven to move from the extracellular to intracellular space and potassium in the opposite direction. With the diffusion of ions across the cell membrane, a separation of charges develops because the nondiffusible negatively charged intracellular ions have a charge opposite that of the diffusible ions. As a result, an electrical potential difference develops between the intracellular and extracellular axon membrane. This electrical potential difference produces an electrical pressure that opposes the physical movement of the ion. The net ionic movement continues until the electrical pressure equals the diffusion pressure, and there is no net movement of ions. The resulting electrical potential across the membrane is called the *equilibrium potential*.

The equilibrium potential of each ion (E_{ion}) is the voltage difference across the membrane that exactly offsets the diffusion pressure of an ion to move down its concentration gradient. This potential is different for each ion and can be defined by the *Nernst equation,* which defines the equilibrium potential, E_m, inside the cell for any ion in terms of its concentration extracellularly $[X_e]$ and intracellularly $[X_i]$:

$$E_m = (61.5\ mV/Z_i)\log_{10}([X_e]/[X_i])$$

The approximate equilibrium potentials of the major ions are:

$K^+ = -90\ mV$, $Na^+ = +50\ mV$, and $Cl^- = -70\ mV$

The contribution of a given ion to the actual resting transmembrane voltage depends on the permeability of the membrane to that ion as a result of the open or closed state of that ion channel. Increased permeability (i.e., opening of the channel) to a particular ion brings the membrane potential toward the equilibrium potential of that ion. If a membrane is permeable to multiple ions that are present in differing concentrations on either side of the membrane, the resultant membrane potential is a function of the concentrations of each of the ions and of their relative permeabilities. The Goldman equation combines these factors for the major ions (Na^+, K^+, and Cl^-) that influence the membrane potential and is used to calculate the RMP.

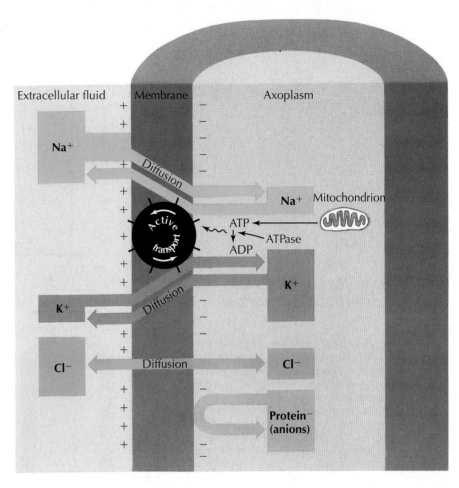

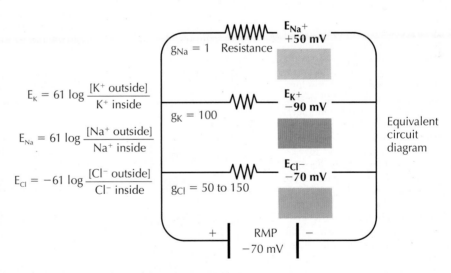

$$E_K = 61\ \log \frac{[K^+\ outside]}{K^+\ inside}$$

$$E_{Na} = 61\ \log \frac{[Na^+\ outside]}{Na^+\ inside}$$

$$E_{Cl} = -61\ \log \frac{[Cl^-\ outside]}{Cl^-\ inside}$$

An electrical circuit model using Ohm's law (E = IR) can be used to demonstrate the contribution of each ion to the RMP. The movement of ions across the membrane is expressed as an ion current. By Ohm's law, this current depends on the driving force of the ion (the difference between the membrane potential and the equilibrium potential of that ion) and conductance of the ion (g). Using this model, the conductance (g) (or the reciprocal of the resistance) for a particular ion is dependent on the ion channel permeability of each ion. The concentration ratios of the different ions are represented by their respective equilibrium potentials (E_{Na}, E_K, E_{Cl}); their ionic permeabilities are represented by their respective conductances. Therefore, at rest, the conductance of the potassium ions is high, whereas sodium conductance is low and chloride conductance is moderate. As a result, the flow of potassium ions is the predominant contributor to the membrane potential at rest. The RMP is the sum of the conductances of all the open channels permeable to each ion.

ION CHANNEL MECHANICS AND ACTION POTENTIAL GENERATION

The role of the neuron is to generate and rapidly transmit electrical signals over relatively long distances. This relies on the membrane potential and the gating of the sodium channels, which play a critical role in action potential generation and propagation.

At rest, the RMP, or the absolute difference in electrical potential between the inside and the outside of the inactive neuron, results predominantly from the membrane permeability to potassium as a result of the open state of the potassium leak channels. This RMP is approximately –70 mV. If an electrical circuit diagram is used to demonstrate the transmembrane potential at rest, with conductance and resistance of Na$^+$, K$^+$, and Cl$^-$ shown in parallel, the contribution of conductance of K$^+$ and Cl$^-$ is responsible for the overall current flow and membrane potential.

When a negatively charged stimulus (physiologic or external) is applied to the extracellular axon membrane, there is a decrease in the value of the RMP as the charge difference between the extracellular and intracellular membranes decreases (called depolarization). If the membrane is depolarized only a small degree, only a few sodium channels are activated, and a local potential is generated. If this charge difference reaches the *excitation threshold* for opening of many voltage-gated sodium channels (approximately –50 to –55 mV), the conductance of sodium rapidly becomes greater than that of K$^+$, and Na$^+$ ions rapidly move from the extracellular to intracellular space, resulting in a movement of the transmembrane potential difference toward the equilibrium potential of sodium (+60 mV). This *depolarization* locally reverses the polarity of the membrane, the inside becoming positive with respect to the outside.

This rapid change in conductance results in the *action potential*. Action potentials are "all-or-none," allowing for rapid transmission of information over long distances along the nerve. The change in sodium conductance is transient and lasts only a few milliseconds. As the sodium channels become inactive and the potassium channels reopen, the sodium conductance decreases and potassium conductance increases, resulting in an increase in flow of potassium out of the cell and *repolarization* of the membrane.

The rate of return of the membrane potential to the baseline slows after sodium conductance has returned to baseline, producing a small residual on the negative component of the action potential, which is called the

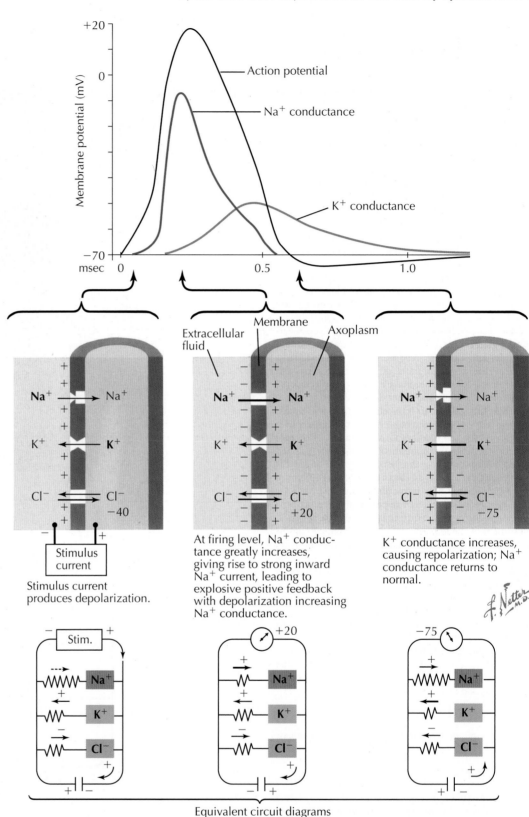

Stimulus current produces depolarization.

At firing level, Na$^+$ conductance greatly increases, giving rise to strong inward Na$^+$ current, leading to explosive positive feedback with depolarization increasing Na$^+$ conductance.

K$^+$ conductance increases, causing repolarization; Na$^+$ conductance returns to normal.

Equivalent circuit diagrams

negative afterpotential. This afterpotential is positive when the membrane potential is recorded with a microelectrode within the cell, but it is negative when recorded with an extracellular electrode. The increase in potassium conductance persists and results in a *hyperpolarization* after the spike component of the action potential—the after-hyperpolarization—which is due to continued efflux of potassium ions, with a greater than resting difference in potential between the inside and the outside of the cell. The after-hyperpolarization

is positive when measured with extracellular electrodes and therefore is called a *positive afterpotential*.

The changes in Na$^+$ and K$^+$ channel activation and inactivation overlap to a degree. As a result, the membrane potential is a function of the ratios of the conductances of the Na$^+$, K$^+$, and Cl$^-$ ions. These can be demonstrated in an electrical circuit diagram, demonstrating current flow relative to the conductances (ion channel permeability) of Na$^+$, K$^+$, and Cl$^-$ in the resting states and after a threshold-reaching stimulus.

Plate 6.6

Peripheral Neuropathies

NEUROPHYSIOLOGY AND PERIPHERAL NERVE DEMYELINATION

Several pathologic changes within the nerves may occur as a result of disease. Nerve injury may affect the components of the nerve to different degrees and produce three stages of severity—neurapraxia, axonotmesis, and neurotmesis. In *neurapraxia,* compression or dysfunction of the myelin without injury to the axon may produce a block of conduction of the action potential across the region of nerve injury. This may occur when external pressure is applied against a single nerve resting against a bony surface. An example of focal neurapraxia is the wristdrop that develops from subacute pressure against the radial nerve passing through the spiral groove within the midhumerus. Some diffuse peripheral nerve disorders, such as Guillain-Barré syndrome (GBS) and chronic inflammatory demyelinating polyradiculopathy (CIDP), may also be characterized by demyelination and neurapraxia in multiple areas along the nerve. In both settings, the axon and supporting structures may remain intact structurally; however, action potential conduction across the abnormal demyelinated axon is slowed or blocked. Conduction of action potentials and the structural integrity of the proximal and distal portions of the region of neurapraxia are maintained. Focal demyelination is the predominant pathologic alteration of this stage. A similar physiologic response may also develop when there is alteration of the cell membrane or channels, such as with local anesthetic.

On neurophysiologic testing with motor NCSs, the pattern of changes in the recorded responses differs when focal neurapraxia occurs to the same degree and at the same site along multiple axons within a nerve compared with differing degrees of focal demyelination among different axons within the nerve. In disorders where *uniform demyelination* occurs at a focal site along a nerve *(conduction block),* stimulation of the nerve distal to the site will elicit a normal compound muscle action potential (CMAP) response, whereas stimulation proximal to the site will elicit a CMAP that is of lower amplitude and area but of similar morphology (Plate 6.6, *A*). In contrast, when *multifocal demyelination* occurs among the axons within the nerve, the *degree of slowing or block varies* among different axons. As a result, stimulation distal to the areas of demyelination will result in a normal CMAP response, but stimulation at a proximal site will elicit a response that is of lower amplitude and area as well as increased in duration (*temporally dispersed;* Plate 6.6, *B*).

With both *axonotmesis* and *neurotmesis* the continuity of the axon is disrupted, and the portion of the axon separated from the anterior horn cell or posterior root ganglion undergoes *wallerian degeneration.* Axonotmesis occurs when axonal continuity is disrupted; however, the connective tissue, including the endoneurium, is preserved. Axonal regeneration and regrowth along the endoneurial tubes are still possible if the connective tissue along the endoneurial tube remains intact. *Neurotmesis* is a more severe stage of injury, where the axon, myelin, and connective tissue sheath, including the epineurium, are disrupted and the two ends of the nerve are separated. In this stage, effective recovery is very

unlikely or impossible, depending on the amount of separation of the two ends of the nerve.

When NCSs are performed during the first week after an axonotmetic or neurotmetic injury and a nerve is stimulated electrically distal to the site of injury, the portion of the axon that is separated from the cell body will temporarily continue to have the ability to propagate an action potential. However, once an entire week

of axonal wallerian degeneration occurs, the disconnected segment of the axon can no longer respond to electrical stimulation to conduct an action potential. Therefore the CMAP amplitude will be reduced or absent with distal and proximal stimulation sites. The motor fibers are more sensitive and lose their ability to conduct at about 7 days, whereas one may still obtain a sensory nerve action potential up to about 10 days.

CONDUCTION BLOCK AND TEMPORAL DISPERSION

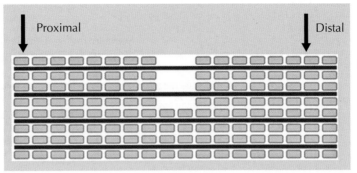

Schematic showing focal demyelination of 50% of axons within a nerve ("conduction block")

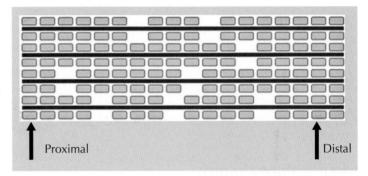

Schematic of segmental and varying degrees of demyelination of axons within a nerve

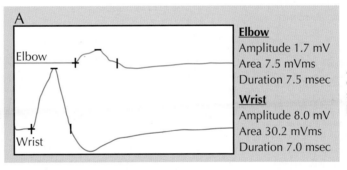

A

Elbow	
Amplitude	1.7 mV
Area	7.5 mVms
Duration	7.5 msec

Wrist	
Amplitude	8.0 mV
Area	30.2 mVms
Duration	7.0 msec

Amplitude and area reduction seen on an ulnar motor nerve conduction study in a patient with a severe partial focal conduction block

Reduction in amplitude and area with an increase in duration, with proximal compared to distal nerve stimulation, on an ulnar motor nerve conduction study (indicative of "temporal dispersion")

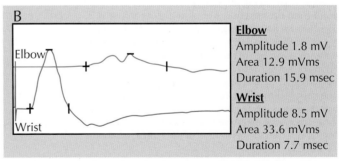

B

Elbow	
Amplitude	1.8 mV
Area	12.9 mVms
Duration	15.9 msec

Wrist	
Amplitude	8.5 mV
Area	33.6 mVms
Duration	7.7 msec

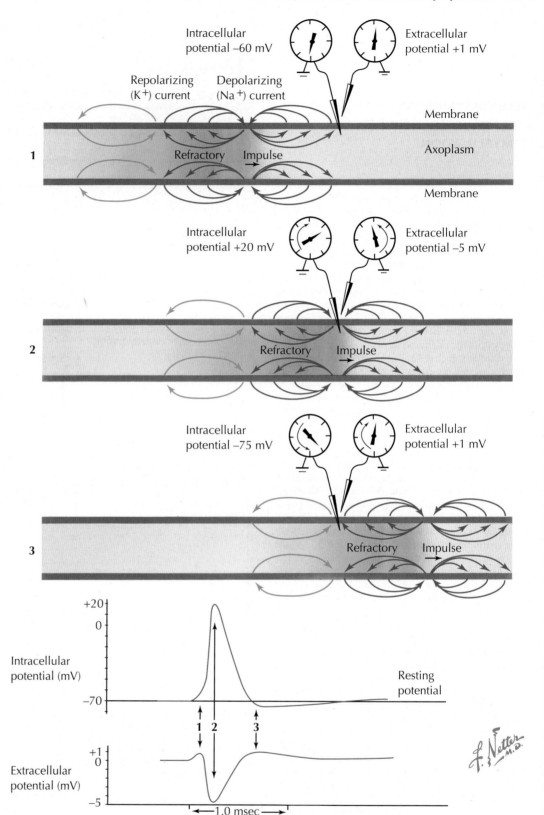

IMPULSE PROPAGATION

Propagation of nerve impulses occurs when current spreads from a small, active area of the axonal membrane to adjacent inactive areas.

ACTION POTENTIAL PROPAGATION

The propagation of an action potential can be divided into three stages when measured at a single point on an axon at which microelectrodes have been positioned to record intracellular and extracellular potentials, each with respect to a "ground" (the bath fluid). The intracellular electrode records the transmembrane potential, and the extracellular electrode records small voltage changes produced by the flow of current through the extracellular fluid.

Stage 1. The nerve impulse approaches the recording point from the left but is distant to the recording sites. The inward flow of sodium ions [Na$^+$] at the active region creates a current that must be balanced by the outward flow of other ionic currents at adjacent regions. This outward flow of current is passive, that is, not initiated by a change in membrane permeability. The passive flow of outward current through the membrane resistance is measured as positive voltage shift at the extracellular membrane. The intracellular electrode begins to record depolarization of the axonal membrane as the active region approaches.

Stage 2. As the activity approaches, the transmembrane depolarization at the intracellular recording point becomes greater, until it reaches the threshold for action potential initiation. At this point, the membrane becomes active. The passive outward current flow shifts to an active inward flow of Na$^+$ current. In accordance with this reversal in the direction of current flow, the voltage recorded by the extracellular electrode shifts from positive to negative. The intracellular potential further depolarizes because the inward current flow is caused by a change in [Na$^+$] membrane permeability, shifting the membrane potential toward E_{Na} (+50 to 65 mV).

The strong flow of inward current at the recording point gives rise to a passive flow of outward current through the axonal membrane at adjacent regions. An action potential is thus triggered to the right. It does not occur on the left immediately because the membrane is temporarily refractory.

Stage 3. After the intracellular potential reaches peak depolarization, [Na$^+$] channel inactivation occurs, and [Na$^+$] permeability is again reduced to a low level while potassium ion [K$^+$] permeability increases, moving the potential toward E_K^+ (−90 mV). The increase in [K$^+$] permeability and outward current flow related to the adjacent active region leads to a final transient positivity of extracellular voltage. Because of the repolarizing [K$^+$] current and inactivation of [Na$^+$] channels during the refractory period, this outward current gives rise to another action potential.

Plate 6.8

Peripheral Neuropathies

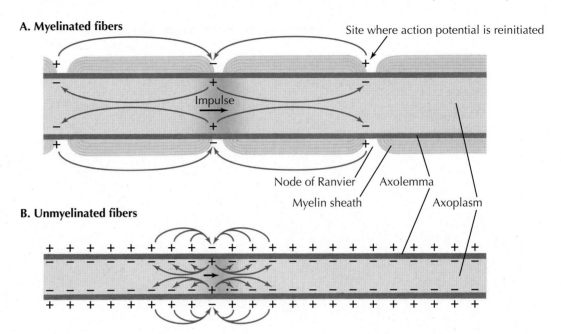

A. Myelinated fibers

Site where action potential is reinitiated

Impulse

Node of Ranvier   Axolemma

Myelin sheath   Axoplasm

B. Unmyelinated fibers

Conduction Velocity

The velocity of action potential propagation along an axon depends on the distance that suprathreshold depolarization spreads in front of the active zone. The conduction velocity can be increased either by increasing the axonal diameter (longitudinal resistance of the axoplasm is inversely proportionate to the diameter squared) or by decreasing the transverse capacitance between the inner and outer axon. A single, unmyelinated giant squid axon of 500-μm diameter achieves approximately 25 m/sec conduction velocity. However, in fibers where the transverse membrane resistance is increased by the addition of a myelin sheath, conduction velocities in excess of 100 m/sec are achieved with axonal diameters of less than 20 μm.

In a myelinated nerve fiber, a lamellated Schwann cell membrane envelops 1- to 2-mm segments of axon sequentially. Between these segments are short lengths of axon with little or no covering, called *nodes of Ranvier;* the covered regions are called *internodes.* According to the saltatory conduction theory, myelin increases the transverse resistance of the internodes, while the resistance at the nodes remains normal. As a result, when the axonal membrane at a node becomes active (Plate 6.8 *A*), the passive outward currents produced by this activity are prevented from flowing through the membrane of the adjacent internode; instead, they flow through the membrane of the next node.

The resulting depolarization triggers an action potential at this node. Thus unlike impulse propagation in an unmyelinated axon (Plate 6.8, *B*), which proceeds continuously in very small steps, the impulse in a myelinated axon jumps from node to node and results in a much faster conduction velocity.

As shown in Plate 6.8, *C,* mammalian peripheral nerves contain myelinated fibers with diameters of 0.5 to 20 μm and conduction velocities of 3 to 120 m/sec, and unmyelinated fibers with diameters of less than 2 μm and conduction velocities of 0.5 to 2.0 m/sec. In 1930 Erlanger and Gasser published a classification of peripheral nerve fibers, based on conduction velocity. Three groups of fibers were defined according to descending conduction velocity, designated A (with subgroups α, β, and γ), B, and C. A further subgroup, Aδ, was added later. This classification refers to both afferent (sensory) and efferent (motor) fibers, whereas a more recent classification of nerve fibers into groups I, II, III, and IV refers only to afferent fibers.

C. Classification of nerve fibers by size and conduction velocity

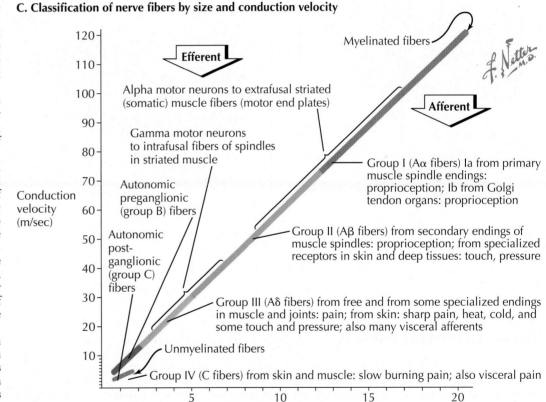

Efferent

Myelinated fibers

Afferent

Alpha motor neurons to extrafusal striated (somatic) muscle fibers (motor end plates)

Gamma motor neurons to intrafusal fibers of spindles in striated muscle

Autonomic preganglionic (group B) fibers

Autonomic post-ganglionic (group C) fibers

Conduction velocity (m/sec)

Unmyelinated fibers

Group I (Aα fibers) Ia from primary muscle spindle endings: proprioception; Ib from Golgi tendon organs: proprioception

Group II (Aβ fibers) from secondary endings of muscle spindles: proprioception; from specialized receptors in skin and deep tissues: touch, pressure

Group III (Aδ fibers) from free and from some specialized endings in muscle and joints: pain; from skin: sharp pain, heat, cold, and some touch and pressure; also many visceral afferents

Group IV (C fibers) from skin and muscle: slow burning pain; also visceral pain

Fiber diameter (microns)

The properties and functions of the different classes of nerve fibers are summarized in Plate 6.8, *C.* In the somatic efferent system, fibers supplying skeletal muscle fibers (alpha motor) have conduction velocities ranging from 50 to 100 m/sec (Aα and Aβ ranges), and fibers supplying the intrafusal muscle fibers of muscle spindles (gamma motor) have conduction velocities ranging from 10 to 40 m/sec (Aγ and Aδ ranges). Autonomic efferent fibers fall either into group B (preganglionic fibers) or group C (postganglionic fibers). In the afferent system, the larger myelinated fibers carry information from specialized receptors that respond to only one type of stimulus, whereas many smaller myelinated fibers carry information about noxious stimuli that give rise to the sensation of prickling pain. The function of unmyelinated sensory fibers (group IV, or C, fibers) is not entirely clear. Stimulation of these fibers as a group evokes only the sensation of burning pain, but experiments have shown that many of these fibers carry information about a specific type of stimulus (touch, pressure, temperature), and only a restricted group is specifically sensitive to noxious stimuli.

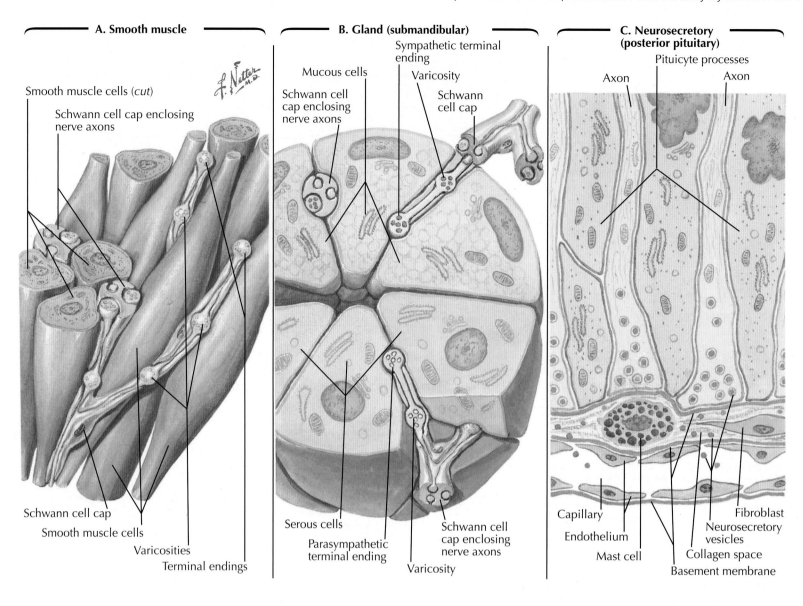

A. Smooth muscle

Smooth muscle cells (*cut*)

Schwann cell cap enclosing
nerve axons

Schwann cell cap

Smooth muscle cells

Varicosities

Terminal endings

B. Gland (submandibular)

Sympathetic terminal
ending

Mucous cells

Varicosity

Schwann cell
cap enclosing
nerve axons

Schwann
cell cap

Serous cells

Parasympathetic
terminal ending

Schwann cell
cap enclosing
nerve axons

Varicosity

**C. Neurosecretory
(posterior pituitary)**

Pituicyte processes

Axon

Axon

Capillary

Endothelium

Mast cell

Fibroblast

Neurosecretory
vesicles

Collagen space

Basement membrane

VISCERAL EFFERENT ENDINGS

Efferent endings involved in the control of smooth muscle, glandular activity, and neurosecretion differ from central and neuromuscular synapses because they do not exhibit the discrete one-to-one relationship between presynaptic endings and postsynaptic cells and may have synapses as wide as 2000 Å. Neurotransmitters released by efferent endings reach the interstitium or bloodstream, where they influence the activity of near or distant effector cells.

Autonomic neuromuscular endings control diverse functions like heart rate, intestinal and urogenital activity, pupillary size, and blood pressure. The morphologic features of this type of ending are shown in Plate 6.9, *A,* which illustrates a three-dimensional reconstruction of the smooth muscle lining the colon. Bundles of the unmyelinated postganglionic fibers that innervate intestinal muscle are enveloped by individual Schwann cells.

As these bundles run between smooth muscle cells, each axon exhibits bead-like swellings filled with synaptic vesicles at various points along its length. At these *varicosities* ("boutons en passant"), the surrounding Schwann cell membranes are drawn back so that the released transmitter can diffuse into the interstitial space and act on nearby smooth muscle cells. After forming numerous varicosities, an individual axon loses its Schwann cell sheath, forming a final terminal ending with similar structure to the other varicosities.

Autonomic nerve endings in exocrine glands are structurally similar to autonomic neuromuscular endings. In the case of the submandibular gland (Plate 6.9, *B*), bundles of unmyelinated postganglionic fibers sheathed by Schwann cells form varicosities and terminal endings in the spaces between secretory cells. In this gland, as in many structures innervated by autonomic fibers, two types of endings are seen. *Sympathetic endings,* which in this gland excite mucous cells to produce mucous saliva, are filled with densely staining vesicles indicating the

presence of norepinephrine. *Parasympathetic endings,* which act on serous cells to produce watery saliva, are filled with clear vesicles that contain acetylcholine.

The endings in the posterior pituitary gland (Plate 6.9, *C*) and adrenal medulla are uniquely capable of releasing neurosecretory vesicles into the bloodstream in response to action potentials conducted into the nerve terminal. In the posterior pituitary, axons of neurons in the supra-optic and paraventricular nuclei of the hypothalamus run between supporting cells called pituicytes, to terminate directly on the basement membrane that separates the collagen space around a capillary. Vesicles within the terminals contain one of the two posterior pituitary hormones, oxytocin or vasopressin (antidiuretic hormone). The morphology of the endings suggests that a hormone released by the arrival of action potentials in the nerve terminal diffuses through the collagen space, entering the capillary via pores between endothelial cells. This diffusion process may be aided by mast cells, which are known to play a role in capillary permeability.

Plate 6.10

Peripheral Neuropathies

Glabrous skin

Epidermis Dermal papilla Sweat gland

Krause's end bulb

Free nerve ending

Meissner's corpuscle

Pacinian corpuscle Merkel's disk Free nerve ending

Hairy skin

Hair Hair follicle

Merkel's disk
Free nerve ending

Sebaceous gland

Nerve plexus around hair follicle

Ruffini terminals Pacinian corpuscle

Detail of Merkel's disk

Lobulated nucleus Desmosomes Merkel cell

Basil epithelial cells

Cytoplasmic protrusion

Mitochondria

Expanded axon terminal Granulated vesicles Schwann cell

Basement membrane
Axon terminal
Mitochondrion
Schwann cell

Cross section

Axon
Schwann cells

Detail of free nerve ending

Skin biopsy section immunostained with protein gene product 9.5 showing epidermal nerve fibers (*arrows*).

CUTANEOUS RECEPTORS

Glabrous and hairy skin both contain a wide variety of receptors for the purpose of detecting mechanical, thermal, or painful stimuli applied to the body surface. Because of the difficulties in visualizing these receptors and in stimulating an individual receptor in isolation, some uncertainties still exist in regard to precise identification of the functions of each receptor type. Functional classification is further complicated because a receptor may respond to different stimuli with different intensity. How "crosstalk" of this kind is resolved by the CNS is still unknown.

Three types of receptors are common to glabrous and hairy skin: pacinian (lamellated) corpuscles, *Merkel disks,* and free nerve endings. The *pacinian corpuscle* has been identified as a quickly adapting mechanoreceptor, and its mechanical transduction process has been extensively studied. The primary role of pacinian corpuscles appears to be the sensing of brief touch or vibration.

Merkel disks are slowly adapting mechanoreceptors structured to respond to deformation of the skin surface. Typically, one afferent fiber of large-to-medium diameter branches to form a cluster of Merkel disks situated at the base of a thickened region of epidermis. Each nerve terminal branch ends in a disk enclosed by a specialized accessory cell (Merkel cell). The distal surface of the Merkel cell holds to nearby epidermal cells with cytoplasmic protrusions and desmosomes, while the base of the cell anchors in the underlying dermis. Thus movement of the epidermis relative to the dermis will exert a stretching or shearing force on the two ends of the Merkel cell. Numerous granulated vesicles within each Merkel cell suggest the capability of chemical synaptic transmission, though attempts to demonstrate this have failed. Direct mechanical transduction by the nerve ending has not been ruled out as a possibility. However, whatever the transduction mechanism, the Merkel cell/Merkel disk ending appears to play a role in the sensing of both touch and pressure.

The "free nerve ending" is made up of a branching nerve axon, which is entirely or partially surrounded by Schwann cells. The axon/Schwann cell complex is further surrounded by a basement membrane. Free nerve endings originate from thinly myelinated or unmyelinated fibers that branch extensively in the

dermis and extend into the epidermis. These endings respond to strong mechanical and thermal stimuli, and they are particularly activated by painful stimuli.

The other receptors found in glabrous skin are *Meissner corpuscles* (tactile corpuscles), in which the terminal branches of a myelinated axon intertwine in a basketlike array of accessory cells, and *Krause end bulbs,* in which a thinly myelinated fiber forms a club-shaped ending. Meissner corpuscles have been tentatively identified as quickly adapting mechanoreceptors subserving

the sense of touch, whereas Krause end bulbs may be thermoreceptors.

The most important receptors in hairy skin are the *hair follicle endings,* in which axon terminals of sensory nerve fibers wrap themselves around a hair follicle. These endings are quickly adapting mechanoreceptors that provide information about any force applied to the hair and thus to the skin. Hairy skin also contains the splayed *Ruffini terminals,* which may be involved in the sensing of steady pressure applied to hairy skin.

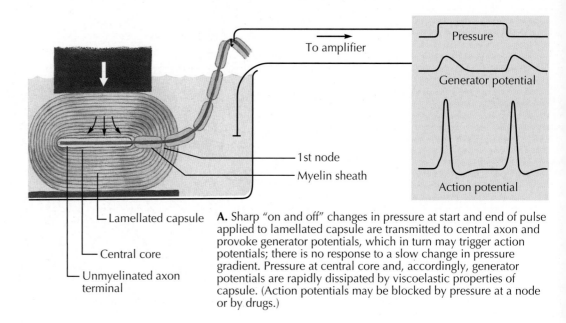

A. Sharp "on and off" changes in pressure at start and end of pulse applied to lamellated capsule are transmitted to central axon and provoke generator potentials, which in turn may trigger action potentials; there is no response to a slow change in pressure gradient. Pressure at central core and, accordingly, generator potentials are rapidly dissipated by viscoelastic properties of capsule. (Action potentials may be blocked by pressure at a node or by drugs.)

B. In absence of capsule, axon responds to slow as well as to rapid changes in pressure. Generator potential dissipates slowly, and there is no "off" response.

PACINIAN CORPUSCLE

The pacinian corpuscle is one of the mechanoreceptors that transform mechanical force or displacement into action potentials. In a simple mechanoreceptor, such as the pacinian corpuscle, transduction of the mechanical stimulus into action potentials occurs in three stages. First, the mechanical stimulus is modified by the viscoelastic properties of the receptor and the accessory cells surrounding it. Then, the modified mechanical stimulus acts on the mechanically sensitive membrane of the receptor cell to produce a change—a generator potential—in the transmembrane potential of the receptor cell. Finally, the generator potential acts to produce action potentials in the afferent nerve fiber linked to the mechanoreceptor.

The pacinian corpuscle consists of the unmyelinated terminal part of an afferent nerve fiber that is surrounded by concentric lamellae formed by the membranes of numerous supporting cells. This specialized axon terminal membrane demonstrates increased ionic permeability when deformed by applied pressure. Although the permeability change appears to be nonspecific, the principal ion flux that occurs is an inflow of sodium ions (Na^+) because of the great difference in the electrochemical potential of this ion on the two sides of the membrane. The Na^+ influx causes a depolarizing current to flow through the axon terminal and the nearby nodes of Ranvier of the afferent fiber. The depolarization caused by this current comprises the generator potential. If the depolarization is great enough, it will produce an action potential at the point of lowest threshold, in this case, at the first node. This action potential then propagates along the afferent fiber to the CNS.

The pacinian corpuscle is specifically adapted to respond to rapidly changing mechanical stimulation. Experiments on isolated pacinian corpuscles have shown that this adaptation involves both the physical

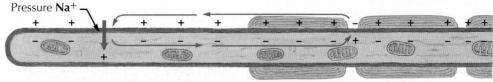

Pressure applied to axon terminal directly or via capsule causes increased permeability of membrane to Na^+, thus setting up ionic generator current through the first node.

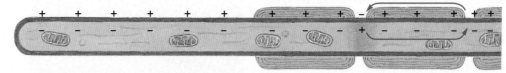

If resultant depolarization at first node is great enough to reach threshold, an action potential appears, which is propagated along the nerve fiber.

structure of the receptor and the properties of the action potential–generating mechanism.

When pressure is applied to an intact pacinian corpuscle, single action potentials are evoked at the beginning and end of the pressure pulse. If action potentials are blocked by a drug such as tetrodotoxin, the generator potentials evoked by the pressure pulse can still be recorded. In the intact pacinian corpuscle, these potentials consist of rapidly decaying depolarizations that occur at the beginning and end of the pulse.

If all the lamellae of the sheath, except the innermost, are dissected away, the response of the pacinian corpuscle to the pressure pulse is modified. The generator potential now decays slowly throughout the period of applied pressure, and no additional depolarization appears at the termination of the pulse. This finding indicates that the viscoelastic properties of the intact capsule dissipate applied pressure, which means that only sudden pressure changes can reach the membrane of the nerve terminal and produce a generator potential.

Plate 6.12

Peripheral Neuropathies

MUSCLE AND JOINT RECEPTORS

Several types of mechanoreceptors located in the joints and muscles provide the CNS with vital proprioceptive information about the position of the parts of the body and the length and tension of various muscles.

JOINT RECEPTORS

Four types of receptors have been described in the joint capsule and ligaments. The parts played by these four receptor types in signaling joint position are not completely understood. *Golgi-type* endings (Wyke type III) reside in ligaments but not in joint capsules and are innervated by large, myelinated (Aα) fibers. These are slowly adapting mechanoreceptors that respond to movements at the extreme joint position with changes in their tonic discharge rates to protect joints. *Ruffini terminals* and *paciniform corpuscles* (Wyke types I and II), which resemble pacinian corpuscles but are smaller, are found in the joint capsule and are innervated by medium-diameter (Aβ) fibers. Ruffini terminals respond to both movement and position, whereas paciniform corpuscles respond primarily to movement. *Free nerve endings,* supplied by thinly myelinated (Aδ) fibers and unmyelinated C fibers (Wyke type IV), are found in both ligaments and joint capsules and are thought to respond to extreme, painful movement of the joint.

MUSCLE RECEPTORS

Muscles also contain four types of receptors, two of which—Golgi tendon organs and muscle spindles—are specific to muscle and contribute to the proprioceptive control of reflexes.

Golgi tendon organs are encapsulated receptors located in a tendon, close to the junction of the tendon and the corresponding muscle. The tendon organ capsule surrounds a bundle of tendon fascicles, which are connected to 3 to 25 muscle fibers. Each tendon organ is innervated by a single group Ib (Aα) fiber that enters the capsule and forms "flower spray" (secondary) endings in contact with the tendon fascicles. Because it is connected in series with the muscle fibers, the tendon organ is stretched and thereby excited when muscle tension increases. Tension produced by active muscle contraction has been shown to be more effective in exciting tendon organs than tension produced by passive muscle stretch.

The *muscle spindle* is a complex receptor consisting of *intrafusal fibers,* a bundle of small muscle fibers encased in a sheath. The fibers typically do not run the entire length of the muscle; instead, they insert into one or both ends of the sheath of a large extrafusal muscle fiber. The intrafusal fibers are of two types: smaller *nuclear chain fibers,* in which the cell nuclei lie in a line along the middle portion of the fiber, and larger *nuclear bag fibers,* in which the nuclei are more clustered. Both nuclear bag and nuclear chain fibers are innervated by small-diameter gamma motor fibers, which increase the sensitivity of the spindle by causing a contraction of the intrafusal muscle fibers. Each spindle receives afferent innervation from a single, large group Ia (Aα) fiber, which forms large *annulospiral* (primary) endings around both nuclear chain and nuclear bag fibers, and from one to five medium group II (Aα) fibers, which form flower spray endings chiefly on nuclear chain

fibers. Because these spindles lie parallel to the extrafusal muscle fibers, they are stretched when the muscle lengthens. The range of muscle stretch encountered during normal movement excites both kinds of afferent fibers but in somewhat different fashions. The group II fibers respond to lengthening with an increase in their tonic discharge rate, which remains constant as long as the muscle is stretched, whereas the group Ia fibers respond especially vigorously to the dynamic phase of

muscle lengthening and, more weakly, to maintained stretch.

The remaining two classes of muscle receptors include *pacinian corpuscles,* which are innervated by group II (Aβ) fibers and respond to vibratory stimuli, and *free nerve endings,* which are innervated by group III (Aδ) or IV (C) fibers and respond to strong, noxious stimuli. Thus they resemble corresponding types of receptors found in other tissues.

Alpha motor neurons to extrafusal striated muscle end plates

Gamma motor neurons to intrafusal striated muscle end plates

Ia (Aα) fibers from annulospiral endings (proprioception)

II (Aβ) fibers from flower spray endings (proprioception); from paciniform corpuscles (pressure) and pacinian corpuscles (pressure)

III (Aδ) fibers from free nerve endings and from some specialized endings (pain and some pressure)

IV (unmyelinated) fibers from free nerve endings (pain)

Ib (Aα) fibers from Golgi tendon organs (proprioception)

Aα fibers from Golgi-type endings

Aβ fibers from paciniform corpuscles and Ruffini terminals

Aδ and C fibers from free nerve endings

Alpha motor neuron to extrafusal muscle fiber end plates

Gamma motor neuron to intrafusal muscle fiber end plates

II (Aβ) fiber from flower spray endings

Ia (Aα) fiber from annulospiral endings

Extrafusal muscle fiber

Intrafusal muscle fibers

γ1 plate endings

γ2 trail endings

Sheath

Lymph space

Nuclear chain fiber

Nuclear bag fiber

Detail of muscle spindle

—— **Efferent fibers**
—— **Afferent fibers**

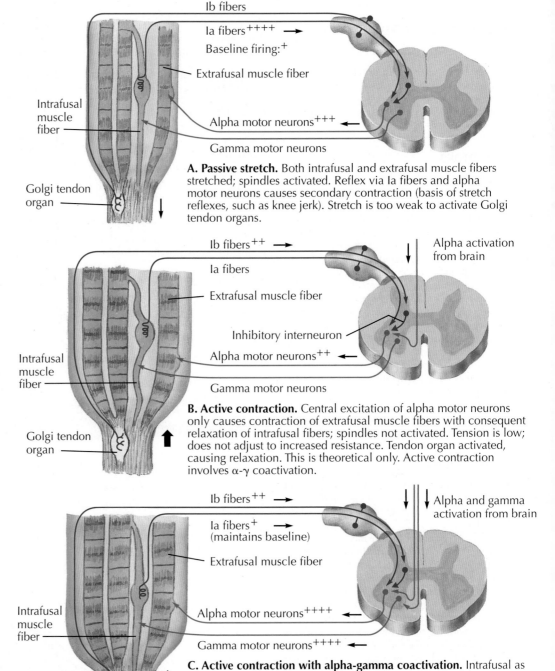

A. Passive stretch. Both intrafusal and extrafusal muscle fibers stretched; spindles activated. Reflex via Ia fibers and alpha motor neurons causes secondary contraction (basis of stretch reflexes, such as knee jerk). Stretch is too weak to activate Golgi tendon organs.

B. Active contraction. Central excitation of alpha motor neurons only causes contraction of extrafusal muscle fibers with consequent relaxation of intrafusal fibers; spindles not activated. Tension is low; does not adjust to increased resistance. Tendon organ activated, causing relaxation. This is theoretical only. Active contraction involves α-γ coactivation.

C. Active contraction with alpha-gamma coactivation. Intrafusal as well as extrafusal fibers contract; spindles activated, reinforcing contraction stimulus via Ia fibers in accord with resistance. Tendon organ activated, causing relaxation if load is too great.

PROPRIOCEPTIVE REFLEX CONTROL OF MUSCLE TENSION

The higher motor control centers of the brain receive information from *muscle spindles* and *Golgi tendon organs* via group I fibers from dorsal spinal roots. The central processing of this proprioceptive information helps to coordinate and smooth movements and other muscle activity. However, abrupt changes in body position and orientation require a faster method of compensation because the relay to and from the brain requires time and may be too slow. Muscle spindles and tendon organs work quickly and directly at the spinal level via collateral fibers creating monosynaptic or oligosynaptic reflex arcs. This spinal segmental processing functions effectively even when there is a loss of connection with the brain centers, such as spinal cord transection or other disease states.

When muscle spindles in a muscle respond to stretching, they transmit activity via afferent Ia fibers to directly stimulate the alpha motor neurons supplying that particular muscle. The same Ia fibers also inhibit antagonist muscles through interneuron connections. By contrast, Golgi tendon organ activity transmitted by Ib afferent fibers stimulate spinal interneurons to inhibit the alpha motor neurons supplying a particular muscle, relaxing that muscle in response to high muscle tension.

PASSIVE STRETCH

When the muscle is passively lengthened, both extrafusal and intrafusal fibers are stretched (Plate 6.13, *A*). The stretch activates *muscle spindles,* sending a volley of activity through group Ia and group II (not shown) fibers; this provokes reflex excitation of alpha motor neurons, leading to extrafusal muscle fiber contraction opposing the applied lengthening force. Golgi tendon organs, which respond poorly to passive stretch, do not discharge under these circumstances. More rapid or intense initial stretching stimuli produce proportionately more rapid or intense reflex contraction; for example, the knee jerk. If either the afferent or the efferent arc of the reflex is damaged, there will be a change of the expected jerk response, which makes this reflex a useful clinical test.

ACTIVE CONTRACTION

The role of spinal reflexes during active contraction of a muscle is shown in Plate 6.13, *B* and *C*. A situation in which there is higher stimulation of alpha motor neurons only (Plate 6.13, *B*), brings about the contraction of the extrafusal fibers, which leads to a shortening of the muscle overall and a slackening of the intrafusal fibers. This results in a termination of activity in the muscle spindles and Ia fibers. The increase in muscle tension, however, is sufficient to activate the Golgi tendon organs and the Ib afferent fibers that attempt to inhibit the alpha motor neurons via interneurons. Sufficient Ib inhibition will lead to relaxation or cessation of muscle contraction.

In a normal situation during voluntary contraction of a muscle (Plate 6.13, *C*), commands from the brain excite both alpha and gamma motor neurons, resulting in the stimulation and shortening of both extrafusal and intrafusal fibers. The muscle spindles are activated and produce a discharge of Ia fibers, which thus reinforce the higher stimulation of the alpha motor neurons. This reinforced motor neuron activity increases the spring-like tension of the contracting muscle and helps it adjust to changes in the load. The activated Ib afferent fibers from the Golgi tendon organs oppose the alpha motor neurons through a feedback mechanism that reduces tension and causes relaxation if the load becomes too great. The role of this "force feedback" mechanism is not well understood.

Plate 6.14

Peripheral Neuropathies

CHARCOT-MARIE-TOOTH DISEASE OVERVIEW (HEREDITARY MOTOR AND SENSORY NEUROPATHY)

Inherited neuropathies affecting motor and large sensory fibers have been named Charcot-Marie-Tooth disease (CMT) or, synonymously, hereditary motor and sensory neuropathy (HMSN). CMT is a very common genetic disorder, affecting approximately 1 in 2500 people.

Symptom onset of inherited polyneuropathies tends to be very slow or insidious. High arches of the feet (pes cavus), curling of the toes (hammertoes), gradually progressive weakness of the feet and ankles, and mild gait problems are often the initial manifestations. These may first be identified by the patient or a family member, but in many cases it is a healthcare provider such as a school nurse who first notices. Examination reveals symmetric ankle dorsiflexion weakness and reduced vibration sensation at the toes because distal motor and sensory fibers are first and most severely affected. For most patients, negative (e.g., sensory loss) sensory symptoms predominate over positive (e.g., pain, prickling, tingling) sensory symptoms, although these can occur as well. Autonomic features are uncommon. These disorders are chronic, lifelong, and slowly progressive.

Approximately 30% to 40% of all chronic polyneuropathies may be associated with a specific genetic mutation. In some cases of hereditary polyneuropathy, there is a clear pattern of familial inheritance, but in others, a careful inquiry of neuropathic symptoms may reveal a family history even without a previous formal diagnosis. Autosomal dominant transmission is the most commonly recognized mode of inheritance, but X-linked recessive, mitochondrial, and autosomal recessive types also occur.

The classifications of the different types of hereditary polyneuropathy were initially based on clinical and electrophysiologic features. More recently, however, advances in genetics have led to identification of many specific genetic mutations known to produce polyneuropathy, and the classification of hereditary polyneuropathies has been modified. In 2018 the naming scheme for CMT was updated to include the mode of inheritance, the types of nerve fibers affected (CMT if large motor and sensory fibers; hereditary sensory and autonomic neuropathy [HSAN] if autonomic and sensory), the primary nature (demyelinating, axonal, indeterminate), and the gene in question if known. This updated nomenclature differs from the previous classifications that assigned number and letter combinations.

The most commonly recognized primarily demyelinating CMT is AD-CMT-De-PMP22 (formerly CMT1A), an autosomal dominant deletion of the *PMP22* gene associated with conduction velocities below 35 m/s. Rarer recessive forms of demyelinating CMT such as AR-CMT-De-GDAP1 (formerly HMSN4A) also occur, typically from birth or infancy, and are generally more severe with other associated abnormalities (e.g., deafness, vocal cord or diaphragm paralysis) depending on

the associated gene. AD-CMT-Ax-MFN2 (formerly CMT2A) is the most diagnosed primarily axonal form of CMT, but many patients with axonal forms of CMT do not have an identifiable gene mutation. Déjerine-Sottas syndrome (DSS, formerly CMT3) is a severe inherited demyelinating neuropathy that manifests by age 2 years and may be inherited as autosomal dominant, autosomal recessive, or noninherited sporadic (de novo) mutations in the *MPZ* gene or associated with other gene mutations. XD-CMT-In-GJB1 (formerly CMTX) is an

X-linked inherited neuropathy, usually with more severe clinical manifestations in males, with conduction velocities ranging between primarily demyelinating or axonal ranges (30–40 m/s). Refsum disease (previously CMT4) is a very rare disorder that causes a relative block in the degradation of phytanic acid and clinically mimics infantile CMT in many respects but is now thought to be a separate, non-CMT multisystem disorder. The classification of inherited neuropathies continues to change as new mutations are recognized.

Swelling of great auricular nerve or other individual nerves, particularly the ulnar or the peroneal nerves, may be visible or palpable.

Thin (stork-like) legs with very high arches (pes cavus) and claw foot or hammertoes due to atrophy of peroneal, anterior tibial, and long extensor muscles of toes

Loss of ankle jerk

Patient walks gingerly due to loss of position sense and/or painful dysesthesia

Footdrop

Graduated glove-and-stocking hypesthesia

Impaired vibration sense

CHARCOT-MARIE-TOOTH DISEASE: COMMON TYPES

Common autosomal dominant demyelinating and axonal forms of CMT disease cause motor and sensory dysfunction. Symptoms may not be evident early in life because the progression is often very slow, and patients are able to compensate for their physical limitations. Symptoms of inherited neuropathy are typically not reported until the second or third decade of life or even later. Early symptoms include clumsiness when walking, difficulty running, a history of "weak ankles," with difficulty doing activities such as ice skating or roller skating; frequent tripping or ankle sprains are often reported. These symptoms are sometimes so well-compensated that some patients achieve impressive athletic skills despite their neuropathy. On examination, some degree of distal lower extremity weakness and atrophy is usually present. High arched feet and hammertoes are common. Hand weakness can also occur but usually later in the course of the disease. Sensory findings are present on examination but are more often large-fiber sensory loss; pain, prickling, and tingling are less common and usually not major features of the disease.

NCS distinguishes predominantly demyelinating from axonal neuropathies. In demyelinating neuropathies, conduction velocities are generally less than 60% of normal and may be as low as 15% of normal. Slowing of nerve conduction can be used to identify affected family members before they are symptomatic. The degree of conduction slowing is uniform across all nerves. Distal latencies may be significantly prolonged, consistent with slowing along the entire course of nerves. Temporal dispersion and conduction block are usually not present.

In contrast to demyelinating CMT, NCS in axonal CMT reveals low-amplitude motor and sensory responses, with relatively preserved conduction velocities (0.40 m/s by definition) and distal latencies. Needle EMG shows a greater degree of active motor axon loss (fibrillation potentials) and motor unit potential remodeling (long-duration motor units).

Nerve biopsy is not necessary for diagnosis if a causative CMT gene is found but may be useful when genetic testing is negative and other causes of neuropathy need to be excluded. In demyelinating CMT, nerve biopsy demonstrates a reduced number of large, myelinated nerve fibers and "onion bulbs" (circumferentially arranged Schwann cell processes) due to repeated demyelination and attempted remyelination. Thinly myelinated and "naked" axons with very thin or no layers of myelin surrounding axons may be seen. Teased fiber preparations on nerve biopsy show areas of segmental demyelination and remyelination. Although both inherited and acquired forms of demyelinating polyradiculoneuropathy may have similar findings of demyelination and remyelination, acquired forms are more likely to show inflammatory changes and a pattern of onion bulb formations intermixed with normal myelinated fibers. Nerve biopsies of primarily axonal forms of CMT show diffuse loss of axons, with degenerating profiles best seen with teased fiber preparations in longitudinal view of axonal degeneration at varying temporal stages that suggest an indolent and ongoing process.

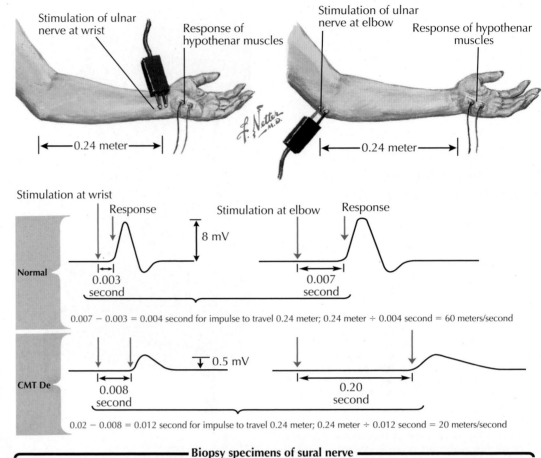

0.007 − 0.003 = 0.004 second for impulse to travel 0.24 meter; 0.24 meter ÷ 0.004 second = 60 meters/second

0.02 − 0.008 = 0.012 second for impulse to travel 0.24 meter; 0.24 meter ÷ 0.012 second = 20 meters/second

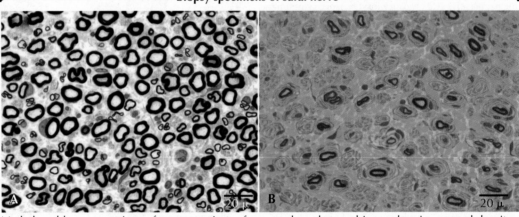

Biopsy specimens of sural nerve

Methylene blue preparations of epoxy sections of a normal sural nerve biopsy showing normal density and size distribution of small and large myelinated fibers (**A**) and a sural nerve biopsy of a patient with CMT disease (**B**) showing slight decrease in density with fewer large myelinated fibers and essentially all fibers surrounded by onion bulbs.

Genetic testing has an increasing role in the diagnosis of inherited neuropathies. Duplication of the *PMP22* gene was found to be a common cause of demyelinating CMT early on, but subsequently other genetic mutations have been found to produce similar demyelinating CMT phenotypes, including defects in the genes myelin protein zero *(MPZ), EGR2,* and *GJB1.* Similarly, several gene abnormalities have been found to cause axonal CMT, including *MFN2, MPZ, EGR2, PRX, NFL, LITAF, MME,* and *GJB1.* Identification of a specific genetic abnormality is important, both for genetic counseling of the patient and family members and for implicating potential targets for future therapeutics.

There is currently no curative genetic therapy available for CMT, and no treatment has been found to be effective in slowing the progression of neuropathy. Because there are many causative gene mutations and new genes continue to be identified, it is unlikely a single treatment strategy will be effective for all types of CMT. Disability caused by CMT varies dramatically; some patients eventually require a wheelchair, whereas others are minimally affected. In many cases, CMT is only identified in preceding ancestors after a younger, more affected family member is diagnosed. Patients with severe footdrop may benefit from ankle-foot orthoses to avoid muscle fatigue and falls. Painless injury to the feet or other areas with hypesthesia is a risk for patients with CMT. Foot care is important to prevent ulceration and amputations. In extreme cases, patients may develop a joint deformity of the ankle called a Charcot joint. Use of a cane, hiking stick, trekking pole, or other gait aid can markedly improve quality of life.

Plate 6.16

Peripheral Neuropathies

EARLY ONSET AND OTHER RARE FORMS OF CHARCOT-MARIE-TOOTH DISEASE AND INHERITED NEUROPATHIES

Déjerine-Sottas syndrome (DSS) is a rare form of inherited or sporadic genetic demyelinating neuropathy presenting in infancy or early childhood. The syndrome may be caused by several genetic mutations, including the *MPZ, PMP22, PRX, GJB1,* and *EGR2* genes. Motor developmental milestones are delayed in affected children. They walk later than their unaffected siblings, some not until 4 years of age. Most acquire other motor skills slowly. The course may be insidiously progressive. Many cases of DSS occur on the basis of a de novo mutation and are not inherited. Weakness of the distal musculature is noted mainly in the feet and legs early in the disease, later becoming evident in the upper extremities, manifesting as difficulty with performing fine tasks and manipulating small objects. Deep tendon reflexes are absent. Large fiber sensation is impaired but may be difficult to reliably assess at a young age. Miotic pupils unresponsive to light stimuli are seen in some patients. Skeletal abnormalities such as pes cavus and kyphoscoliosis develop in many patients, as in other inherited or long-standing peripheral neuropathies. Careful examination may reveal thickened peripheral nerves as are seen in some patients with later-onset demyelinating CMT. These hypertrophic nerves are usually easier to palpate than see. The course of this illness is progressive, and by adolescence most patients require assistance to walk, including need for a wheelchair.

The cerebrospinal fluid (CSF) protein is often increased. NCS may show absent sensory potentials and marked slowing of motor conduction velocity, with values in the range of 5 to 20 m/sec, characteristic of a severe demyelinating process. Temporal dispersion and conduction block are not typically present. Nerve biopsy, usually not necessary for diagnosis, demonstrates a characteristic histologic picture of large onion bulbs (redundant Schwann cell processes resulting from repetitive demyelination and attempts at remyelination) and very little intact myelin so that almost all of the axons are "naked." Nerve biopsies typically do not have inflammatory changes. Genetic testing may show mutations in known associated genes.

AR-CMT-De-GDAP1 is a rare autosomal recessive demyelinating polyneuropathy. The clinical course is severe and generally diagnosed in infancy or early life because of marked weakness. NCS typically shows a demyelinating pattern. In addition to length-dependent neuropathy, there may be vocal cord paralysis or deafness. Several other genes cause similar findings with autosomal recessive inheritance, including *MTMR2, SBF2, SBF1, SH3TC2, NDRG1, EGR2, PRX, FGD4,* and *SURF1.*

XLD-CMT-In-GJB1 is an X-linked dominant inherited neuropathy that accounts for 10% to 15% of all CMT cases. HMSN X is usually more severe in males owing to the X-linked dominant inheritance. It usually becomes symptomatic in early adulthood. NCS shows varying degrees of conduction slowing, with intermediate velocity

Difficulty in locomotion is often a presenting symptom. Child walks late.

Loss of pupillary reflex

Loss of deep tendon reflexes

Glove-and-stocking hypesthesia

Electron micrograph of an onion bulb with a myelinated fiber in center surrounded by attenuated Schwann cell processes

Refsum Disease

Retinitis pigmentosa is a characteristic feature of Refsum disease, which may clinically resemble Déjerine-Sottas disease or Friedreich ataxia.

slowing intermediate between demyelinating and axonal ranges. Nerve biopsy shows predominantly axonal loss. Genetic testing for *GJB1,* the gene producing connexin-32, may be helpful diagnostically.

Refsum disease is a very rare autosomal recessive disorder characterized by abnormal fatty acid oxidation, leading to elevated levels of phytanic acid in the blood. Refsum disease usually begins in adolescence with a slowly evolving peripheral neuropathy, although it has a remitting-relapsing course in some patients. Most subjects have retinitis pigmentosa characterized

by night blindness. Associated pupillary changes, nerve deafness, ataxia, cardiomyopathy, and ichthyosis may also be seen. In some patients, ataxia mimicking Friedreich ataxia is the initial sign. CSF findings and results of nerve conduction velocity studies are similar to those of DSS. Although phytanic acid is a relatively ubiquitous compound found in many foods, a carefully controlled diet that excludes whole milk, all vegetables except potatoes, fatty meats, chocolate, and nuts can prevent further relapses and may improve the clinical condition.

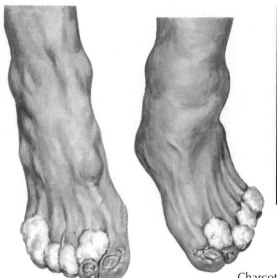

X-ray film showing dissolution of ankle joints

Charcot joints of both ankles, resulting from lack of pain sensation. Cotton pledgets protect ulcerated toes.

Testing of sensory (sural) nerve conduction (antidromic)

} Recording leads

Sural nerve

Lateral sural nerve

Medial sural nerve

Ground

Stimulus

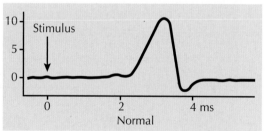

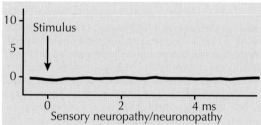

Normal

Sensory neuropathy/neuronopathy

HEREDITARY SENSORY AND AUTONOMIC NEUROPATHY

Hereditary sensory and autonomic neuropathy (HSAN) is a rare condition characterized primarily by loss of small-fiber sensory modalities and pain. In many cases, inheritance is autosomal dominant. The clinical presentation generally reflects the damage to small unmyelinated or thinly myelinated sensory nerve fibers and autonomic fibers. As such, strength is mostly spared, as are large-fiber sensory modalities (e.g., vibration, touch, and proprioception). Small-fiber sensation of pain and temperature is disturbed. A main complication is development of painless injuries, which can occur with repetitive trauma. Local ulcerations may not be detected unless there is visible blood or infection develops, risking the health of the limb. The development of a Charcot joint can occur, and sometimes amputations are necessary when tissue damage is severe. A typical presentation of HSAN in middle and old age is the development of burning feet. A family history of polyneuropathy is frequently not appreciated unless family members are directly questioned.

A careful history and neurologic examination are crucial in these patients. Family history is very important, particularly a history of painful feet or amputations. Neurologic examination should include testing of small-fiber sensory modalities (pinprick sensations and temperature sensation). Although these clinical findings may mimic the dissociated sensory loss seen in syringomyelia, in that disorder there is primary involvement at the level of the central part of the spinal cord. In contrast, with HSAN the small neurons at the level of the dorsal root ganglia appear to be involved.

NCS and EMG are useful for assessing large-fiber sensory and motor nerve fibers and are a mainstay of diagnosis for CMT but are usually not as revealing in HSAN. Dedicated small nerve fiber testing can help clarify the diagnosis, including quantitative sensory testing, autonomic function testing, and thermoregulatory sweat test, which can show focal areas of sweat loss in this disorder. Skin biopsy to evaluate epidermal nerve fiber density can be a useful diagnostic tool. Nerve biopsies are not standard diagnostic tools in these cases, but if performed, they may show a relative reduction in small nerve fibers. A randomized controlled trial of L-serine in patients with HSAN1 was associated with clinical improvement in neuropathy severity and decreased blood levels of toxic sphingolipids. Routine and intensive foot care and properly fitted footwear help avoid ulcers and amputations.

Plate 6.18

Peripheral Neuropathies

GUILLAIN-BARRÉ SYNDROME

Guillain-Barré syndrome (GBS) is the name given to acute immune polyneuropathies that vary in severity and distribution but typically manifest in the United States as a sudden demyelinating polyradiculoneuropathy causing ascending flaccid paralysis. The most common form of GBS in the United States is demyelinating, also described as acute inflammatory demyelinating polyradiculopathy (AIDP). The disease results from an attack on the myelin sheath by inflammatory cells, causing myelin breakdown and, in severe cases, secondary axonal damage. AIDP affects peripheral nerves in all segments between the spinal nerve root and the distal ending of the nerve. In about 60% of patients, an antecedent infection (e.g., virus or bacteria) precedes the syndrome by a few weeks, but this is not a requirement for diagnosis. In the past there was concern for an association between GBS and influenza vaccination; however, this association has not been verified in recent large-scale epidemiologic studies. In many of these instances, preceding vaccination was likely a coincidental event during the season when GBS is most common.

Mild cases of AIDP may never come to medical attention, but the typical presentation is acute ascending paralysis, reaching worst severity within 4 weeks. Paresthesias (tingling, prickling) are the earliest symptoms in about 50% of patients, but motor findings are the most characteristic. Symptoms worsen over the span of hours to days, most often spreading from the toes upward. In severe cases, respiratory involvement can occur, requiring intubation. Autonomic dysfunction may coexist, manifesting as hemodynamic instability with labile blood pressure, heart rate, and cardiac arrhythmias, requiring hemodynamic support. In this clinical setting neurocritical care may be required.

Other forms of GBS present differently. Acute motor axonal neuropathy (AMAN), an axonal variant of GBS with a worse long-term prognosis, is more common in Asia and in other areas of the world. These forms include acute autonomic ganglioneuropathy with predominantly autonomic manifestations such as orthostatic hypotension; cranio-pharyngeal-brachial variant, which causes sudden demyelination involving the face, bulbar muscles, neck, and arms with relative sparing of the legs; and Miller-Fisher syndrome (MFS) characterized by ataxia, areflexia, and ophthalmoplegia.

Nearly all patients with AIDP require hospitalization, even in mild cases, because progression of weakness is expected. The standard of care treatment is intravenous immunoglobulin (IVIg) or plasmapheresis. Supportive measures are necessary. Monitoring and management of respiratory and autonomic dysfunction have significantly reduced mortality. Other complications that should be prevented or treated include deep vein thrombosis, pulmonary emboli, pressure sores, and hyponatremia. Early involvement with physical therapy is important. AIDP is self-limiting and monophasic for

— **Pathogenesis** —

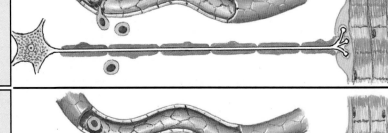

Stage I. Lymphocytes migrate through endoneurial vessels and surround nerve fiber, but myelin sheath and axon not yet damaged.

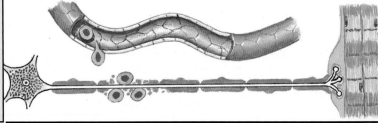

Stage II. More lymphocytes extruded and macrophages appear. Segmental demyelination begins; however, axon not yet affected.

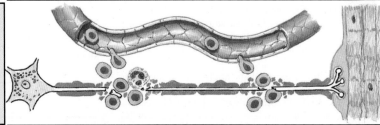

Stage III. Multifocal myelin sheath and axonal damage. Central chromatolysis of nerve cell body occurs and muscle begins to develop denervation atrophy.

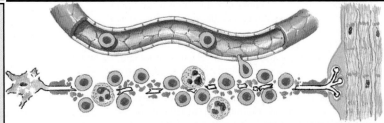

Stage IV. Extensive axonal destruction. Some nerve cell bodies irreversibly damaged, but function may be preserved because of adjacent less-affected nerve fibers.

From Asbury, Arnson, and Adams

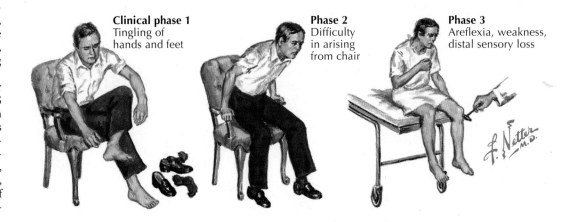

Clinical phase 1
Tingling of hands and feet

Phase 2
Difficulty in arising from chair

Phase 3
Areflexia, weakness, distal sensory loss

the majority of patients. The maximum deficit is seen in 2 to 4 weeks, and after that improvement follows. The course of recovery can be predicted by the severity at onset and the degree of axonal damage identified. If axonal damage is severe, maximum recovery may take more than a year, and there may be significant residual weakness. Most patients eventually recover from AIDP, but the course is variable, and approximately 20% are left with some permanent disability.

DIAGNOSIS OF AIDP

EDX studies can be useful for evaluating patients with severe weakness for the diagnosis of AIDP, but much of the most characteristic electrophysiologic features may be absent on studies done in the very early stages of the disease process. Loss or prolongation of F-wave latencies or H reflexes are the earliest EDX findings in AIDP and may be the only electrophysiologic abnormality in

GUILLAIN-BARRÉ SYNDROME (Continued)

the first few days after onset of symptoms. Over time, other features of demyelination, such as prolonged distal latencies, slowed conduction velocity, and temporal dispersion, may emerge. EMG is performed to detect neurogenic changes in muscles from axonal injury, which is secondary to the inciting inflammatory demyelinating process, or can be primary in the case of AMAN or some other GBS variants. The findings on EDX studies mirror the degree of underlying pathologic changes in the four stages of the AIDP, as shown in Plate 6.18.

There are no classic serologic findings associated with AIDP. CSF classically demonstrates cyto-albuminologic dissociation, which means there is high CSF protein with few or no cells present. This finding may not be detectable until 24 to 72 hours after the illness begins, so its absence in the early stages of the disease does not exclude GBS.

The differential diagnosis for AIDP needs to be carefully considered because the classic electrophysiologic features are often not present early in the disease process. Acute spinal cord lesions may be confused with AIDP. Spinal cord lesions may cause rapidly progressive paralysis, but sensory examination usually demonstrates a spinal cord level. In a process involving only anterior horn cells, flaccid paralysis can occur, but with more extensive spinal cord injury, hyperreflexia and spasticity develop after the acute phase. These upper motor neuron signs are often very helpful in distinguishing a spinal cord lesion from AIDP. However, in the acute state, these other features (e.g., hyperreflexia) may not be present. Spinal cord lesions also typically cause early bowel and bladder dysfunction. Back pain may be a feature of either disorder. If there is high clinical suspicion for a primary spinal cord injury, magnetic resonance imaging (MRI) can be diagnostically helpful. Clinical findings in a number of toxic, metabolic, or infectious processes, including arsenic poisoning, acute intermittent porphyria (AIP), or *botulism*, may resemble those of AIDP but can be differentiated by history of exposures and other associated features.

A carefully documented history and appropriate laboratory studies usually point to the specific mechanism. Infectious diseases that should be considered include poliomyelitis, diphtheria, Lyme disease, West Nile infection, and human immunodeficiency virus (HIV). CSF pleocytosis should be a strong clue that the underlying process is infectious. A bull's-eye rash or presence in an endemic area should prompt evaluation for Lyme disease; Lyme serology and spinal fluid evaluation can be performed. West Nile exposure can be evaluated in blood or spinal fluid. As is the case with Lyme disease, markers for acute infection should be sought. Acute ascending paralysis mimicking AIDP can also be associated with HIV infection. Pupillary abnormality points

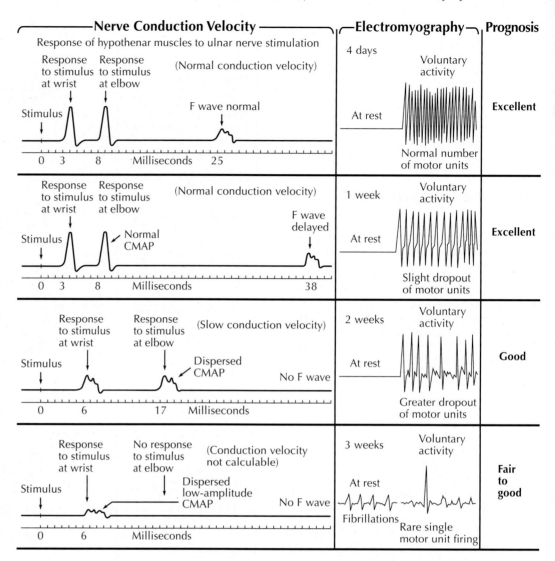

Nerve Conduction Velocity	Electromyography	Prognosis

Nerve Conduction Velocity — Response of hypothenar muscles to ulnar nerve stimulation

Response to stimulus at wrist / Response to stimulus at elbow / (Normal conduction velocity)
Stimulus — F wave normal
0 3 8 Milliseconds 25

Electromyography: 4 days — Voluntary activity; At rest — Normal number of motor units — **Excellent**

Response to stimulus at wrist / Response to stimulus at elbow / (Normal conduction velocity)
Stimulus — Normal CMAP — F wave delayed
0 3 8 Milliseconds 38

Electromyography: 1 week — Voluntary activity; At rest — Slight dropout of motor units — **Excellent**

Response to stimulus at wrist / Response to stimulus at elbow / (Slow conduction velocity)
Stimulus — Dispersed CMAP — No F wave
0 6 17 Milliseconds

Electromyography: 2 weeks — Voluntary activity; At rest — Greater dropout of motor units — **Good**

Response to stimulus at wrist / No response to stimulus at elbow / (Conduction velocity not calculable)
Stimulus — Dispersed low-amplitude CMAP — No F wave
0 6 Milliseconds

Electromyography: 3 weeks — Voluntary activity; At rest — Fibrillations / Rare single motor unit firing — **Fair to good**

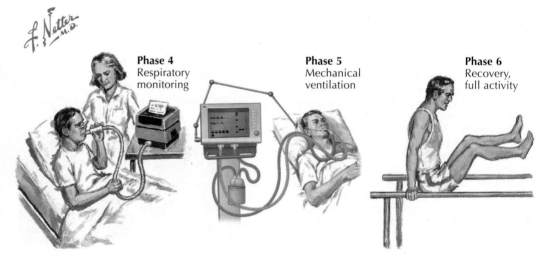

Phase 4 Respiratory monitoring

Phase 5 Mechanical ventilation

Phase 6 Recovery, full activity

to either diphtheria or *botulism*, both of which also have predominant bulbar symptoms. AIP may mimic classic AIDP with or without accompanying psychosis, and the patient should be questioned about use of any medication that could precipitate a porphyric crisis. Clues to an attack of AIP include a personal or family history of similar events, coexisting acute neuropsychiatric symptoms, and severe abdominal pain. Severe weakness can occur as part of a porphyric attack. The

pathology is primarily axonal rather than demyelinating, although this distinction is difficult to establish in the acute setting; urine porphyrins can be tested if the clinical suspicion is high. The scalp and skin should be carefully examined to exclude the presence of a tick that could produce tick paralysis. Associated facial palsy may suggest sarcoidosis, whereas bulbar symptoms may also be seen with myasthenia gravis, which rarely mimics AIDP.

Plate 6.20

Peripheral Neuropathies

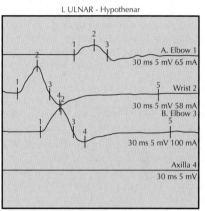

Principal manifestation of CIDP is four-extremity weakness; paresthesias in the feet and hands are also noted. On examination, patient is weak (shoulder abduction testing) and areflexic and demonstrates sensory loss in the feet and hands. NCS/EMG demonstrate a predominantly demyelinating sensorimotor polyradiculoneuropathy.

CHRONIC INFLAMMATORY DEMYELINATING POLYRADICULONEUROPATHY

Chronic inflammatory demyelinating polyradiculoneuropathy (CIDP) is sometimes thought of as a long-term form of AIDP because of the similar electrophysiologic similarities and immune-mediated etiology. Similar to AIDP, CIDP tends to be motor predominant, with significant weakness causing disability, although the weakness of CIDP is usually not as severe as it is with AIDP. Sensory symptoms such as "dead" numbness or lack of feeling are more specific, whereas sensory symptoms such as paresthesias and pain are unusual early in CIDP. Imbalance caused by sensory loss (sensory ataxia) is often present. Large myelinated fibers have the greatest amount of myelin and are therefore most susceptible to demyelination in CIDP. Damage to large, myelinated fibers causes weakness and loss of joint position sense and vibration sense. The symptoms of CIDP tend to be slowly progressive with maximum deficit occurring greater than 8 weeks after symptom onset. The course of disease can either be relapsing-remitting or chronic progressive. Respiratory and severe bulbar involvement rarely occur. Clinically evident autonomic dysfunction is rare in CIDP.

The diagnosis of CIDP can be challenging. Patients generally have both proximal and distal weakness on examination. Deep tendon reflexes are markedly reduced or absent. Distal sensory loss is often found on clinical examination. EDX studies are required for accurate diagnosis. They demonstrate signs of acquired demyelination including conduction block and temporal dispersion of compound muscle action potentials, with prolonged distal and F-wave latencies and slowed conduction velocities. CSF examination usually reveals elevated spinal fluid protein without an increased white blood cell count. Nerve biopsy is not usually necessary for diagnosis but typically demonstrates segmental demyelination, onion bulb formations, and inflammation within the endoneurium and epineurium. Teased nerve fiber preparation reveals demyelination and remyelination along individual nerve strands.

The differential diagnosis of CIDP includes other acquired or hereditary polyradiculoneuropathies. The diagnosis of CIDP becomes more complex in cases in which there are mixed features of demyelination and axonal loss, leading to uncertainty about which process was first. Diabetic polyneuropathy often shows mixed

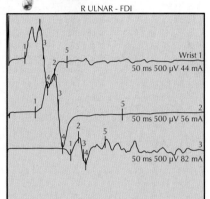

R ULNAR - FDI

Wrist 1
50 ms 500 µV 44 mA

50 ms 500 µV 56 mA

50 ms 500 µV 82 mA

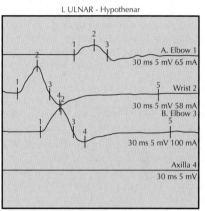

L ULNAR - Hypothenar

A. Elbow 1
30 ms 5 mV 65 mA

Wrist 2
30 ms 5 mV 58 mA
B. Elbow 3
30 ms 5 mV 100 mA

Axilla 4
30 ms 5 mV

Motor nerve conduction study of the ulnar motor nerve in a patient with CIDP. The waveform tracings *(left)* illustrate temporal dispersion. On proximal stimulation above the elbow *(lower tracing)*, there is a marked increase in the duration of the CMAP, as well as a significant drop in the amplitude, which is called temporal dispersion. The waveform tracings *(right)* illustrate conduction block. On proximal stimulation above the elbow *(top tracing)*, there is a significant drop in the amplitude compared with CMAPs elicited with more distal stimulation. Temporal dispersion and conduction block are both indicative of acquired demyelination, occurring somewhere in the nerve between the above-elbow and below-elbow stimulation sites.

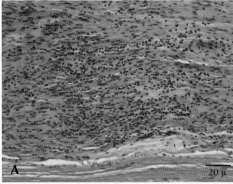

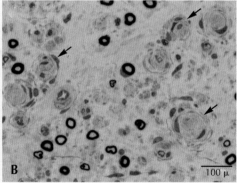

Biopsies of nerves from CIDP. Longitudinal paraffin hematoxylin and eosin preparation of a sciatic nerve biopsy showing endoneurial inflammation (**A**). Methylene blue–stained epoxy section of a sural nerve biopsy showing some fibers with large onion bulbs without myelinated fibers at their centers (**B**, *arrows*), whereas other myelinated fibers do not have onion bulbs (a pattern typical of CIDP).

axonal and demyelinating EDX features and can become severe enough to cause disability. Other conditions may also cause a mixed axonal and demyelinating polyradiculopathy, such as POEMS syndrome (polyneuropathy, organomegaly, endocrinopathy, monoclonal protein, skin changes). POEMS syndrome is an underrecognized condition and may be suggested when patients who have been suspected to have CIDP do not have a response to immunotherapy. Lymphoma can invade nerve roots and cause a polyradiculoneuropathy; CSF cytology and nerve biopsy can be helpful diagnostically when this is suspected.

Variants of CIDP include focal and multifocal forms, including chronic inflammatory demyelinating mononeuropathy, multifocal acquired demyelinating sensory and motor neuropathy, and chronic inflammatory

sensory polyradiculopathy. In these variants, diagnosis is more difficult, and sometimes MRI and fascicular nerve biopsy can be helpful.

The treatment of CIDP differs from patient to patient. In general, CIDP is treated with immunomodulatory agents, including IVIg, corticosteroids, and plasma exchange (PLEX). Controlled trials have shown these agents to be effective. When necessary, oral steroid-sparing immunomodulatory agents are used, but comparative data for their relative efficacy are lacking. CIDP treatment is usually successful in reducing disability, but without treatment, many patients require assistive devices or a wheelchair. With treatment, many can lead essentially typical lives. Long-term immune therapy treatment is commonplace because of the chronic nature of the condition.

DIABETIC NEUROPATHIES

Diabetic peripheral nerve damage takes many forms, including diabetic sensory and motor polyneuropathy, autonomic neuropathy, small-fiber sensory polyneuropathy, compression mononeuropathy, and microvasculitic radiculoplexus neuropathy. Most types of diabetic neuropathy occur in patients with long-standing diabetes, but some forms may occur soon after onset of diabetes.

CLINICAL MANIFESTATIONS

Diabetic polyneuropathy (DPN) is one of the most common neuropathies recognized in clinical practice. It is classically length dependent with prominent sensory symptoms including sensory loss and painful paresthesias. Autonomic neuropathy can occur along with DPN and other forms of diabetic neuropathy or independently. Features of autonomic neuropathy include orthostatic hypotension and supine hypertension, sweating loss, gastrointestinal dysmotility, erectile dysfunction, and urge urinary incontinence and neurogenic bladder. Patients with diabetes have a greater risk of compression mononeuropathies than the general population, including median mononeuropathy at the wrist (carpal tunnel syndrome) and ulnar mononeuropathy at the elbow. Diabetic radiculoplexus neuropathy (DRPN) usually manifests as severe unilateral thigh or upper arm pain, with associated weight loss, followed by weakness and sensory loss. Months after the initial attack, the contralateral side may become involved. DRPN is usually a monophasic illness but can sometimes recur. It can present segmentally in the lower limb (lumbosacral), the trunk (thoracic), or the upper limb (cervical) segment; the lower limb presentation is most common.

DPN generally occurs in long-standing diabetes mellitus, usually in patients who already have nephropathy and retinopathy associated with their diabetes. NCS and EMG can be helpful to establish the diagnosis, distribution, and severity of neuropathy. In DPN, NCS usually shows distally decreased compound muscle action potential and sensory neve action potential amplitudes with mildly prolonged distal latencies and slowed conduction velocities. In lumbosacral DRPN, there is evidence of patchy and asymmetric involvement of proximal and distal segments, including the nerve root, plexus, and distal nerve. Electrophysiologic studies are also useful for evaluating focal neuropathies, including mononeuropathies at the common sites of compression. An autonomic reflex screen and thermoregulatory sweat test can be helpful to assess suspected autonomic neuropathy. Other testing, such as gastrointestinal motility and urodynamic studies, can be useful in some cases. Nerve biopsies are rarely performed in diabetic neuropathies but show axonal loss. In cases of DRPN, pathologic changes of microvasculitis have been found.

Overall, the best treatment strategy for diabetic neuropathies is to manage the diabetes, which prevents worsening and may allow for healing over time. Foot care is important to prevent injuries and ulcerations due to pressure and lack of pain sensation. Neuropathic pain management is very important to improve the quality of life in patients with painful diabetic neuropathies. Supportive treatments for autonomic neuropathy can be considered depending on the symptoms (e.g., for orthostatic hypotension, compressive garments, management of fluid and salt intake, and pharmacologic approaches). In DPN, the cause of the neuropathy is related to the length and severity of the exposure to hyperglycemia. Consequently, treatment is centered on optimizing diabetic control. In DRPN, in contrast, the putative mechanism is ischemic injury from microvasculitis. A controlled trial with intravenous methylprednisolone did show some efficacy, and immunomodulatory therapy can be considered. Usually, the treatment should be a short course because the disease is most frequently monophasic.

Paresthesia, hyperalgesia, or hypesthesia

Loss of vibration sense

Pupillary abnormalities

Orthostatic hypotension and nocturnal hypertension

Polyradiculopathy
Nocturnal diarrhea
Neurogenic bladder
Impotence

Autonomic neuropathy

Serial skip paraffin section of a microvessel above (**A**) and at (**B**) regions of microvasculitis in the superficial radial nerve of a patient with diabetic radiculoplexus neuropathy. Sections are stained with hematoxylin and eosin.

5μ

A   B

Patients with diabetic polyneuropathy are prone to the development of superimposed mononeuropathies at common sites of entrapment, including the ulnar nerve at the elbow segment, median nerve at the carpal tunnel in the wrist, and peroneal nerve at the fibular head.

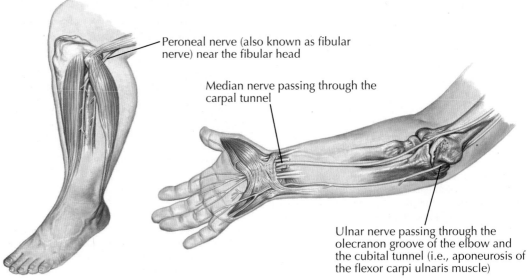

Peroneal nerve (also known as fibular nerve) near the fibular head

Median nerve passing through the carpal tunnel

Ulnar nerve passing through the olecranon groove of the elbow and the cubital tunnel (i.e., aponeurosis of the flexor carpi ulnaris muscle)

Plate 6.22

Peripheral Neuropathies

MONOCLONAL PROTEIN–ASSOCIATED NEUROPATHIES

Many neuropathies can occur in patients with monoclonal proteins, also called paraproteinemia. However, in many cases these may not be causative. Neuropathies are more common in older patients, as is the presence of a monoclonal protein, so the presence of a monoclonal protein should not always be interpreted as the cause of neuropathy. Neuropathies have been reported with monoclonal gammopathy of undetermined significance (MGUS), with amyloidosis, and with malignancies such as osteosclerotic myeloma (POEMS syndrome), lymphoma, Waldenström macroglobulinemia, and immunoglobulin M (IgM) monoclonal gammopathy. The matter is further complicated by toxic neuropathies that sometimes occur as adverse effects of some agents used to treat these monoclonal gammopathies and associated lymphoproliferative disorders.

IGM MGUS NEUROPATHY

Several types of neuropathy have been associated with IgM MGUS. Distal acquired demyelinating symmetric (DADS) neuropathy is the most common IgM MGUS neuropathy and presents with sensory-predominant polyneuropathy of insidious onset, particularly in men older than 50 years. Because of profound sensory involvement, gait unsteadiness (sensory ataxia) is a common symptom. When motor signs are present, they are usually confined to the distal (toes, ankles, fingers, wrists) muscles. Tremor is also a frequent finding. These patients are often found to have associated myelin-associated glycoprotein (MAG) autoantibodies. Motor NCS demonstrates widespread symmetric slowing. In many cases, distal latencies are dramatically prolonged, resulting in a short terminal latency index. This finding implies that the motor conduction velocity slowing is more pronounced in distal nerve segments and is considered an EDX hallmark of DADS neuropathy. In neuropathies felt to have a clear association with anti-MAG antibodies or with other monoclonal proteins in the absence of a more severe hematologic disorder, some immunomodulatory treatments (e.g., rituximab) have been tried with varying degrees of success.

Waldenström macroglobulinemia may cause an IgM neuropathy presenting with sensory or sensorimotor polyneuropathy or polyradiculoneuropathy.

AMYLOID NEUROPATHY

Amyloid is an amorphous protein material that can deposit in nerves, causing neuropathy, but also in many other tissues, including fat, gastrointestinal, kidney, and heart, leading to multisystem damage and, in some cases, death. Amyloidosis causing neuropathy can be divided into primary amyloidosis (associated with a bone marrow disorder) and inherited forms. Primary

AMYLOID NEUROPATHY

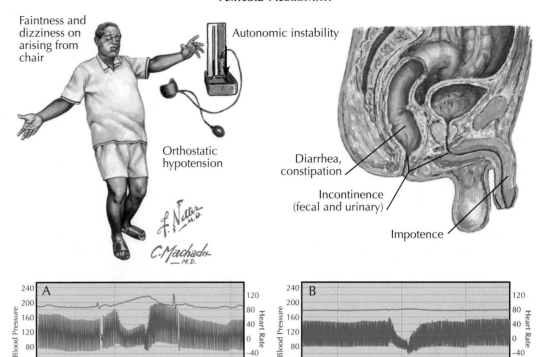

Blood pressure (BP) and heart rate (HR) responses to the Valsalva maneuver showing a normal response in a male aged 80 years (**A**) and a patient with amyloid autonomic neuropathy (female aged 68 years) (**B**). In the normal recording (**A**), the maneuver-induced fall in BP results in an increase in heart rate (vagal baroreflex response), followed by a BP rise (late phase II), followed by a transient fall (phase III, resulting from cessation of the maneuver), a rapid BP recovery, and a BP overshoot (phase IV). All the BP increments are the result of an increase in total peripheral resistance. In the amyloid recording (**B**), baroreflex failure is manifest as a failure of HR to rise and a loss of late phases II and IV and delayed BP recovery after phase III.

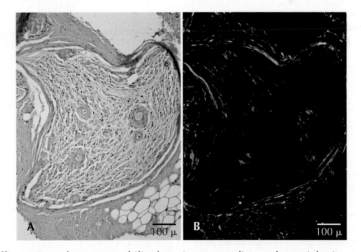

Sural nerve paraffin sections show congophilic deposits surrounding endoneurial microvessels (Congo red stain, **A**) and apple green birefringence under polarized light (**B**). These changes are diagnostic of amyloidosis.

amyloidosis occurs in patients with an abnormal serum monoclonal protein with elevated free light chains that deposit into tissues. Inherited forms of ayloidosis include those caused by various mutations of the transthyretin (TTR) protein largely made by the liver and other rare subtypes of misfolded proteins. Approximately 15% of patients with primary amyloidosis develop neuropathy. These neuropathies are usually severe, lower limb predominant, and symmetric. The distribution may begin in a length-dependent fashion but continue to progress beyond the thighs and elbows for some patients. Typically, small nerve fibers are more involved than large nerve fibers, causing prominent pain, sensory loss, orthostasis, and lack of sweating. Diagnosis can be challenging and requires a high clinical suspicion. In cases of primary amyloidosis, the presence of a monoclonal protein with high free light chains in the blood prompts further evaluations, including assessment of kappa and lambda light chains in the blood, urine, and tissue biopsy.

DISTAL ACQUIRED DEMYELINATING SYMMETRIC (DADS) NEUROPATHY

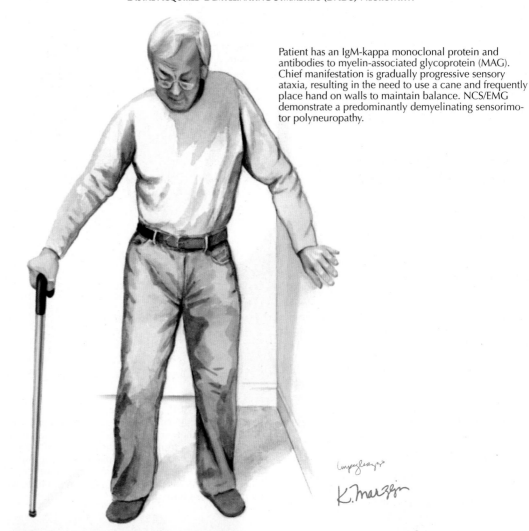

Patient has an IgM-kappa monoclonal protein and antibodies to myelin-associated glycoprotein (MAG). Chief manifestation is gradually progressive sensory ataxia, resulting in the need to use a cane and frequently place hand on walls to maintain balance. NCS/EMG demonstrate a predominantly demyelinating sensorimotor polyneuropathy.

MONOCLONAL PROTEIN–ASSOCIATED NEUROPATHIES (Continued)

Familial amyloid polyneuropathy associated with TTR mutations is suspected when patients describe a prominent family history of bilateral carpal tunnel syndrome, polyneuropathy, early cardiomyopathy, lumbosacral spine stenosis, and early disability or death (before age 60 years) in affected family members. Genetic testing for TTR mutations has become widely available.

Tissue biopsy can be helpful for both hereditary and primary amyloidosis. Potential sites of biopsy include subcutaneous fat, rectum, epidermis, and peripheral nerve. Other tissues suspected to be affected can be biopsied as well. A negative biopsy does not exclude the diagnosis because deposition is not necessarily uniform among organs.

Treatment of amyloidosis depends on the type of amyloid demonstrated. Treatments for primary amyloidosis include melphalan, peripheral blood stem cell transplant, and other advanced chemotherapeutic options. Hereditary TTR amyloidosis can be treated effectively with genetic therapies that silence the production of the abnormal TTR protein within the liver, preventing further deposition and allowing some nerve recovery. These medications are often given in combination with TTR stabilizers that prevent the large, misfolded TTR tetramers from breaking into individual pieces that tend to deposit in tissues. Trials to demonstrate efficacy of gene-silencing therapies in amyloid cardiomyopathy are ongoing at the time of this publication.

POEMS SYNDROME

POEMS syndrome (polyneuropathy, organomegaly, endocrinopathy, monoclonal gammopathy, and skin changes) is an uncommon systemic paraneoplastic disorder causing a predominantly demyelinating polyradiculoneuropathy. POEMS syndrome arises as a consequence of an osteosclerotic myeloma or Castleman disease. Neurologic manifestations of POEMS syndrome include progressive proximal and distal weakness, hypo- or areflexia, sensory loss, and neuropathic pain that progresses to severe disability over the span of months to years. Patients with POEMS syndrome are often initially diagnosed with CIDP but do not respond well to immunotherapies, leading to delay in diagnosis.

Aside from the neurologic manifestations, there are other critical systemic features of POEMS syndrome. Organomegaly (hepatosplenomegaly) can be detected by a medical examination, directed abdominal ultrasound, or computed tomography (CT) but may be discovered incidentally during imaging performed for other reasons. Endocrinopathies include hypogonadism with elevated follicle-stimulating hormone, hypothyroidism, and adrenal insufficiency. A monoclonal protein can generally be demonstrated by serum and urine protein

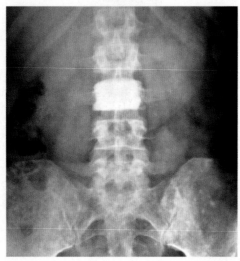

X-ray film showing osteosclerotic myeloma affecting isolated vertebra as seen in POEMS syndrome

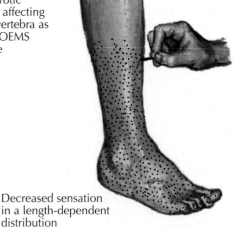

Decreased sensation in a length-dependent distribution

electrophoresis and immunofixation, but the total quantity of protein is often very low, so 24-hour urine collection or advanced serum mass spectrometry techniques such as MALDI-TOF may be required to detect it. Skin changes may include discoloration, nail changes, or hypertrichosis, among others. Thrombocytosis is a common laboratory finding. The presence of elevated levels of vascular endothelial growth factor (VEGF) in the blood is an important support for the diagnosis, although treatment with corticosteroids may cause a

false-negative VEGF response. Screening for osteosclerotic myeloma can be performed with skeletal radiographs, and Castleman disease can be identified with CT imaging of the body and sometimes positron emission tomography. Early referral to a hematologist is crucial for effective management of this disorder. Treatment strategies are dependent on the underlying etiology. If a single osteosclerotic myeloma is found, local irradiation can be effective. If the disease process is more diffuse, peripheral blood stem cell transplantation can be beneficial.

Plate 6.24

Peripheral Neuropathies

FIBRINOID NECROSIS

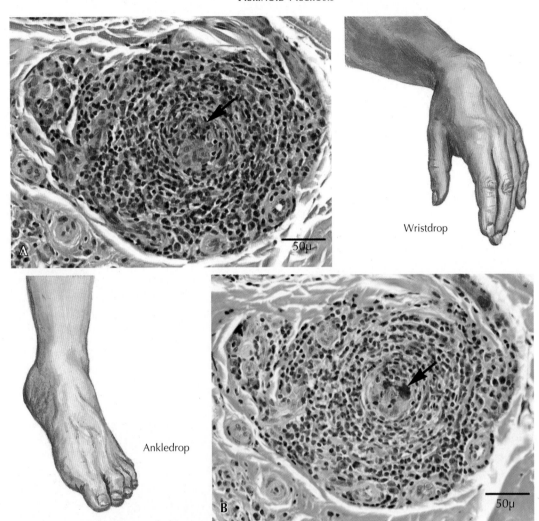

Wristdrop

Ankledrop

VASCULITIC NEUROPATHY AND OTHER CONNECTIVE TISSUE DISORDERS ASSOCIATED WITH NEUROPATHY

Vasculitic neuropathies can occur in an isolated fashion affecting only peripheral nerves, or they can occur as part of a systemic vasculitic process, such as polyarteritis nodosa, eosinophilic granulomatosis with polyangiitis (Churg-Strauss syndrome), microscopic polyangiitis, and granulomatosis with polyangiitis. Vasculitic neuropathy can also be seen in other primary connective tissue diseases, such as rheumatoid arthritis. Nerves receive blood flow via small arteries and microvessels (large and small arterioles), not large or medium-sized arteries. Vasculitides associated with connective tissue disorders attack these small vessels and microvessels, involving all the arterial vessels within the nerves (small arteries and large arterioles) and often producing fibrinoid necrosis of vessel walls. By contrast, nonsystemic vasculitis of nerves, including diabetic and nondiabetic radiculoplexus neuropathies, involve only the microvessels (small arterioles) and can be pathologically described as a microvasculitis of nerves (see Plate 6.21).

Vasculitic neuropathies typically produce a syndrome of asymmetric, painful weakness and sensory loss progressing in a stepwise fashion. In long-standing cases and in about 20% of new cases, patients appear to have a length-dependent symmetric peripheral neuropathy resulting from confluent and overlapping individual nerve trunk injuries in the affected areas. In systemic vasculitis, fever, weight loss, and other systemic features often accompany the neurologic symptoms. In polyarteritis nodosa the skin, heart, kidneys, and other organ systems may be involved. Asthma, especially with adult onset, can be a clue to the diagnosis of eosinophilic granulomatosis with polyangiitis. Renal involvement is common in microscopic polyangiitis and granulomatosis with polyangiitis.

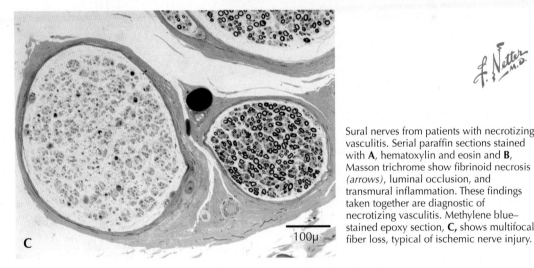

The asymmetry and non–length-dependent distribution of neuropathic findings are major clues to this diagnosis, as is a clinical history of stepwise progression to involve different peripheral nerves, particularly when accompanied by pain. In diabetic lumbosacral radiculoplexus neuropathy, there is typically lower limb pain and weakness with associated weight loss. Electrophysiologic studies are consistent with asymmetric or "patchy" axonal loss in most cases, although the pattern may be confluent and symmetric in some patients. Diagnosis of systemic vasculitis depends on serologies, including connective tissue markers, sedimentation rate, and C-reactive protein, and evidence of clinical involvement of other organ systems. In these cases, biopsy of an affected nerve and surrounding epineurial blood vessels is often diagnostic. Pathologic findings include axonal degeneration with prominent chronic inflammation (lymphocytic) involving and disrupting the layers of

Sural nerves from patients with necrotizing vasculitis. Serial paraffin sections stained with **A**, hematoxylin and eosin and **B**, Masson trichrome show fibrinoid necrosis *(arrows)*, luminal occlusion, and transmural inflammation. These findings taken together are diagnostic of necrotizing vasculitis. Methylene blue–stained epoxy section, **C**, shows multifocal fiber loss, typical of ischemic nerve injury.

SJÖGREN SYNDROME

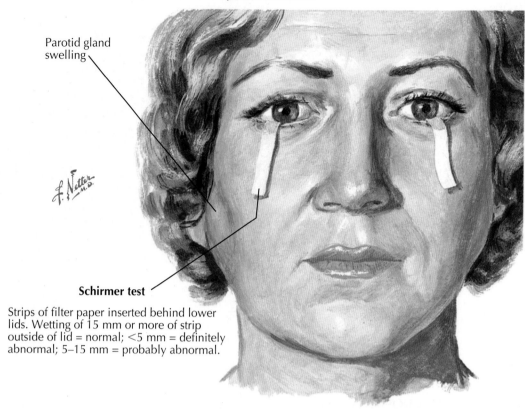

Parotid gland swelling

Schirmer test
Strips of filter paper inserted behind lower lids. Wetting of 15 mm or more of strip outside of lid = normal; <5 mm = definitely abnormal; 5–15 mm = probably abnormal.

VASCULITIC NEUROPATHY AND OTHER CONNECTIVE TISSUE DISORDERS ASSOCIATED WITH NEUROPATHY (Continued)

vessel walls. In some cases, inflammation leads to blood vessel wall fibrinoid necrosis, also called necrotizing vasculitis. Treatment of vasculitides requires immunosuppressive agents. Some patients with nonsystemic microvasculitis of peripheral nerves are managed with corticosteroids. Patients with evidence of systemic necrotizing vasculitis with or without associated connective tissue disorder often need higher potency immunosuppression and long-term management.

SYSTEMIC LUPUS ERYTHEMATOSUS

Systemic lupus erythematosus (SLE) is a multisystem disorder that can manifest with variable combinations of fever, rash, alopecia, arthritis, pleuritis, pericarditis, nephritis, anemia, leukopenia, thrombocytopenia, and nervous system disease. Neuropathy is reported in approximately 20% of patients with SLE. The most common neuropathy phenotype in SLE is mild, gradually progressive, length-dependent, sensory, or sensorimotor neuropathy. Patients often note positive (prickling, tingling, pain) and negative (dead-type numbness) sensory symptoms. In less than 5% of patients with SLE, the pattern is of multiple mononeuropathies, likely secondary to vasculitis. Less commonly, patients have pure small-fiber neuropathy.

SJÖGREN SYNDROME

Sjögren syndrome (SS) is a systemic autoimmune disease that primarily affects middle-aged women. The criteria for diagnosis include sicca symptoms (dry eyes, dry mouth), objective evidence of keratoconjunctivitis, evidence of chronic lymphocytic sialoadenitis, and the

Lymphocytic infiltration in salivary gland

Xerophthalmia
Sicca syndrome
Rheumatoid disease
Xerostomia
Clinical triad

Serology
1. Rheumatoid factor (high titer)
2. Antinuclear antibodies
3. Antibodies to salivary duct epithelium demonstrated by immunofluorescence (in 50% of cases)
4. Agar gel precipitins to lymphoid extracts

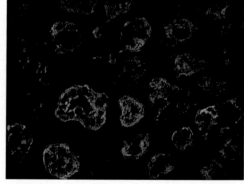

presence of either anti–SS-A or anti–SS-B antibodies. Rash, arthralgias, and Raynaud phenomenon are also common. Peripheral neuropathy is reported to occur in 10% to 30% of patients with SS. The neuropathy of SS is secondary to vasculitis in some cases and secondary to mononuclear cell infiltration without vasculitis (e.g., ganglionitis) in other cases. There may also be other mechanisms of neuropathy in patients. For example, the etiology of the small-fiber neuropathy seen in some

cases of SS may be different. Several patterns of neuropathy are seen in association with SS: sensory ataxic neuropathy, painful sensory neuropathy without ataxia, multiple mononeuropathies, multiple cranial neuropathies, trigeminal sensory neuropathy, autonomic neuropathy with anhidrosis, and radiculoneuropathy. Abnormal pupils and orthostatic hypotension are relatively common accompaniments to many of these neuropathies and should be sought on examination.

Plate 6.26

Peripheral Neuropathies

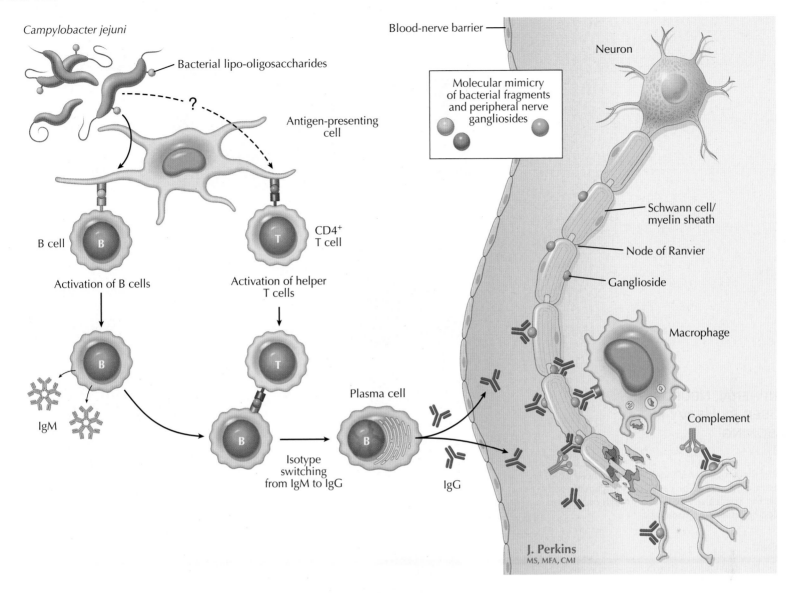

Campylobacter jejuni

Bacterial lipo-oligosaccharides

Blood-nerve barrier

Neuron

Antigen-presenting cell

Molecular mimicry of bacterial fragments and peripheral nerve gangliosides

B cell

CD4+ T cell

Schwann cell/ myelin sheath

Activation of B cells

Activation of helper T cells

Node of Ranvier

Ganglioside

IgM

Macrophage

Plasma cell

Complement

Isotype switching from IgM to IgG

IgG

J. Perkins
MS, MFA, CMI

IMMUNOPATHOGENESIS OF GUILLAIN-BARRÉ SYNDROME

Although much of the pathophysiology of GBS is yet unknown, there is overwhelming clinical, therapeutic, serologic, pathologic, and animal model evidence supporting the hypothesis that it is an immune-mediated or autoimmune disorder. Multiple mechanisms, including humoral (B-cell or autoantibody-mediated) and cellular (T-cell–mediated) immunologic processes, cytokines secretion, blood-nerve barrier breakdown, neutrophil and macrophage activation, and complement activation contribute to cellular infiltration into nerves and roots, inflammation, myelin breakdown, and nerve fiber damage in GBS. The sequence and relative importance of these processes, however, are not precisely known. The proven efficacy of antibody-clearing treatments such as PLEX and IVIg indicates a role of autoantibodies in causation. Although neural autoantibodies are demonstrated with passive transfer experiments, precise epitopes such autoantibodies are directed against are unknown in the majority of GBS cases.

GBS has multiple subtypes. AIDP is the most common subtype in most regions of the world. AIDP is characterized by acute development of distal as well as proximal weakness of extremities, sensory changes, and loss of deep tendon reflexes. AIDP is often associated with weakness of facial and other cranial muscles. In severe cases, respiratory muscle weakness may ensue. Symptoms progress over days to a few weeks. Elevated protein in CSF is a sign of nerve root inflammation. EDX testing usually shows physiologic evidence of demyelination (loss of Schwann cells and consequent slowing and conduction block) with relative preservation of nerve fiber (axon) function. Most patients with GBS recover well over weeks to months with treatment. Many patients with AIDP report an infection days to a few weeks preceding symptom onset. Multiple pathogens such as *Campylobacter jejuni*, cytomegalovirus (CMV), Epstein-Barr virus, HIV, mycoplasma, Zika virus, and, most recently, SARS-CoV-2 (COVID-19) have been implicated as GBS triggers. Molecular mimicry between microbe antigen and peripheral nerve or Schwann cell epitopes is hypothesized.

Molecular mimicry is demonstrated especially with a variant of GBS called acute motor axonal neuropathy (AMAN), frequently a seasonal illness in Asian countries. AMAN is often triggered by preceding *C. jejuni* infection, which is a diarrheal illness. The microbe shares epitope similarity with neural gangliosides, notably GM1. It is hypothesized that infection triggers anti-GM1 immunoglobulin G (IgG) antibodies, which cause blockage of sodium channels, followed by complement-mediated axolemmal injury to motor fibers at the nodes of Ranvier, resulting in an axon loss (rather than demyelinating) motor neuropathy. AMAN may have a worse prognosis than AIDP because recovery from axonal damage is typically slower and less complete than from demyelinating (Schwann cell damage) nerve injury. Another variant of GBS called Miller Fisher syndrome (MFS) is characterized by prominent extraocular muscle weakness. MFS is associated with another antiganglioside antibody (anti-GQ1b).

Closely related to self-limited GBS is CIDP, which has a relapsing or progressive course. Although there are several parallels between GBS and CIDP, there are notable differences. CIDP is rarely preceded by an infection and only rarely affects cranial and respiratory muscles. PLEX and IVIg treat GBS as well as CIDP; corticosteroids, however, can improve CIDP but do not improve GBS. Lymphocytic and macrophagic infiltrates and Schwann cell proliferation (onion bulbs) are more typical of CIDP. Neural autoantibodies probably have a role in the causation of CIDP, but specific epitopes they are directed against are not known in most cases. Notable exceptions are anti-GM1 IgM antibodies (causing a motor variant of CIDP called multifocal motor neuropathy), anti-MAG IgM antibodies (causing a distally predominant demyelinating neuropathy), and IgG4 antibodies directed against specific paranodal proteins (causing atypical CIDP requiring B-cell–depleting treatments).

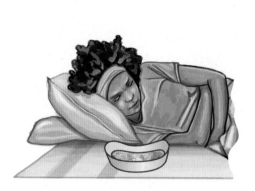

History of nausea and vomiting may suggest arsenic poisoning in patient with peripheral neuropathy.

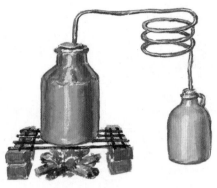

Antique copper utensils (e.g., still used for bootleg liquor) and runoff waste from copper smelting plant may be sources of arsenic poisoning.

PERIPHERAL NEUROPATHY CAUSED BY HEAVY METAL POISONING

Peripheral neuropathy secondary to heavy metal exposure is rare but should be considered in patients with risk factors, particularly exposure through occupation, hobbies, or deliberate poisoning.

ARSENIC

Arsenic has a ubiquitous distribution in the environment, particularly as an impurity in copper ores. Although arsenic poisoning represents a notorious method of homicide, the presence of excessive levels of arsenic in a patient should not immediately indicate a possible criminal cause. Arsenic contamination may be due to agricultural industrial exposure, such as copper smelting. Other sources have included drinking tainted well water and in the production of stained glass. The clinical manifestations of arsenic poisoning vary. Usually, the initial symptoms are gastrointestinal rather than neuropathic, and vomiting, diarrhea, and abdominal pain are common early signs of poisoning. The peripheral nerve manifestations ultimately follow, usually as painful, length-dependent sensory symptoms followed by weakness. These symptoms may continue to progress even after the source of exposure is gone, as with many other toxic neuropathies. CNS findings are often present, such as confusion and psychiatric symptoms. Skin changes may eventually occur, with erythema or abnormal areas of pigmentation. Occasionally, if the amount ingested is sufficiently large, growth-arrest lines (*Mees lines*) may be seen in the fingernails. The diagnosis is confirmed by analysis of a 24-hour urine sample, a more sensitive indicator than serum values that can decrease rapidly after exposure has ceased. Differentiation between inorganic and organic arsenic is important because some dietary sources (e.g., seafood) can result in elevations of urinary arsenic in a nontoxic form. Samples of hair and nails may provide supporting evidence of arsenic

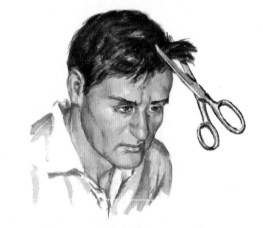

Although 24-hour urinalysis is the best diagnostic test for arsenic, hair and nail analysis may also be helpful.

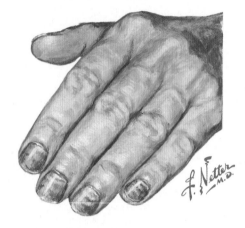

Mees lines on fingernails are characteristic of arsenic poisoning.

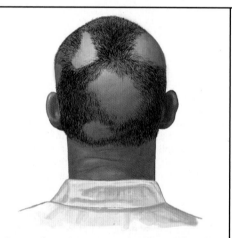

Spotty alopecia associated with peripheral neuropathy characterizes thallium poisoning.

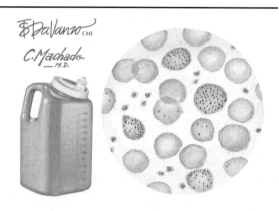

Lead poisoning, now relatively rare, causes basophilic stippling of red blood cells; 24-hour urinalysis is a diagnostic test.

exposure and may be useful to analyze long after the exposure has ceased. If electrophysiologic tests are performed, they will generally be consistent with axonal peripheral neuropathy. The most important treatment components are removal of the source of the arsenic and use of chelating agents.

NEUROPATHIES CAUSED BY OTHER METALS

Gold salts, formerly used in treating rheumatoid arthritis, have sometimes produced a distal sensorimotor peripheral neuropathy, although sometimes this can be difficult to separate clinically from neuropathy secondary to rheumatoid arthritis itself. Improvement in neuropathic symptoms after discontinuation of gold salts usually confirms an underlying toxic mechanism. Ingestion of thallium salts, occasionally used in rodenticides and insecticides, causes a potentially severe sensorimotor neuropathy associated with development of alopecia 10 to 30 days after ingestion. Exposure to lead, now seen infrequently, can cause a predominantly motor neuropathy, often initially involving wrist and finger extensors.

Plate 6.28

Peripheral Neuropathies

METABOLIC, TOXIC, AND NUTRITIONAL PERIPHERAL NEUROPATHIES

There are many metabolic, toxic, and nutritional causes of peripheral neuropathy, with alcohol abuse being the most common etiology in this category.

ALCOHOL

The prevalence of neuropathy in alcohol use is uncertain but has been estimated to exist in approximately 50% of those with alcohol use disorder. The incidence of neuropathy correlates with the age of the patient and the duration of alcohol use. The pathophysiology is uncertain, but the direct toxic effect of alcohol on peripheral nerves seems to be the most important etiology. Alcoholic neuropathy has a phenotype similar to other metabolic neuropathies. The neuropathy is often distal, symmetric, sensory predominant, and slowly progressive. There are often positive neuropathic sensory symptoms, such as tingling and/or burning, as well as loss of nociceptive sensation on examination. Other vitamin and nutritional deficiencies may coexist, such as thiamine and vitamin B_{12}.

THIAMINE (VITAMIN B₁)

Thiamine (vitamin B_1) deficiency most commonly occurs in chronic alcohol use disorder, chronic gastrointestinal disorders associated with recurrent vomiting, malignancy, and after weight reduction (bariatric) surgery. Severe vitamin B_1 deficiency causes congestive heart failure (wet beriberi), peripheral neuropathy (dry beriberi), Wernicke encephalopathy, and Korsakoff syndrome. Neuropathy associated with thiamine deficiency may present with acute onset or insidiously with distal, symmetric, sensory, or sensorimotor neuropathy with positive neuropathic sensory symptoms (e.g., tingling). Thiamine-deficient patients may develop weakness, numbness, and loss of balance (ataxia). Evaluation for thiamine deficiency should include measurement of whole-blood thiamine.

VITAMIN B₁₂ DEFICIENCY

Multiple nutritional deficiencies can result in peripheral neuropathy. Vitamin B_{12} deficiency can lead to both peripheral neuropathy and myelopathy, pathologically described as subacute combined degeneration. Vitamin B_{12} deficiency can result from deficient diet and various causes of malabsorption, including pernicious anemia, inflammatory bowel disease, and bowel resection surgery (including gastric bypass surgeries). Vitamin B_{12} deficiency usually presents with distal numbness (large-fiber sensory modalities) and paresthesias associated with progressive gait unsteadiness. It can also give rise to cognitive dysfunction. Diagnosis begins with serologic testing for vitamin B_{12} and methylmalonic acid. EDX studies show findings of axonal sensorimotor peripheral neuropathy. Somatosensory evoked potentials may show central conduction slowing, reflecting spinal cord involvement. MRI of the spinal cord may at times show abnormal T2 signal in the posterior columns of the spinal cord. Treatment with vitamin B_{12} supplementation may be oral or intramuscular, depending on whether the etiology of the deficiency is poor dietary intake or malabsorption. Follow-up serologic studies should be done to ensure adequate supplementation. The neurologic symptoms may take months to years to improve, even after normalization of vitamin B_{12} levels.

HYPOTHYROIDISM

Hypothyroidism is a common disorder that affects women more than men. The diagnosis should be considered in patients with symptoms such as fatigue, weight gain, cold intolerance, coarse dry hair and skin, constipation, depression, and abnormal menstrual cycles. Neuropathic symptoms often include paresthesias, numbness, and pain. Patients often describe subjective weakness without clear weakness on examination.

UREMIA

Peripheral neuropathy due to uremia occurs in patients with chronic kidney failure who are on dialysis, but it has become less frequent with the advent of kidney transplantation. The neuropathy in uremia is similar to other neuropathies due to a metabolic cause, often being distal, symmetric, sensory predominant, and slowly progressive. Patients have symptoms of numbness, paresthesias, burning, and imbalance. Other symptoms include restless legs, cramps, and weakness. The diagnosis should be considered in patients with end-stage renal disease with a creatinine level of 5 mg/dL or higher or creatinine clearance less than 12 mL/min.

Etiology

Diabetic

Alcoholic

Uremic

Drug-related
Isoniazid
Disulfiram
Vincristine
Hydralazine
Other medications

Thiamine deficiency (beriberi)

Common early manifestations

Loss of tendon reflexes

Paresthesia

Numbness of feet

Painful, tender muscles (pain on compressing calf)

Dry beriberi. Emaciation, great weakness, aphonia may appear (poor prognosis; vagus nerve involved), wristdrop, footdrop

Wristdrop

Ankledrop

Hypothyroidism

Dry, brittle hair

Edema of face and eyelids

Cold intolerance

Diminished perspiration

Coarse (follicular keratosis), cool, dry, yellowish (carotenemia) skin

Lethargy, memory impairment, slow cerebration (psychoses may occur)

Thick tongue, slow speech

Deep, coarse voice

Enlarged heart, poor heart sounds

Diastolic hypertension (frequently)

Slow pulse

Ascites

Menorrhagia (amenorrhea may occur late in disease)

Weakness

Reflexes, prolonged recovery

LEPROSY AND OTHER INFECTIONS SOMETIMES CAUSING PERIPHERAL NEUROPATHY

LEPROSY

Leprosy (Hansen disease) is a common global cause of peripheral neuropathy due to infection with *Mycobacterium leprae*. This organism tends to affect nerves close to the skin where body temperature is cooler. Most people are not susceptible to infection. Leprosy has been eliminated from parts of the world as a result of improved standards of living. The host's individual response to the infection dictates whether leprosy takes on a tuberculoid, lepromatous, or borderline form. In tuberculoid leprosy, the spread of the bacilli is limited, and focal, asymmetric disease results. The skin is often hypopigmented. In lepromatous leprosy, spread of the bacilli is widespread and the clinical manifestations reflect extensive involvement of regions with cooler body temperature. The hallmark clinical feature of leprosy is sensory loss, often first recognized when a traumatic injury produces limited or no pain. Involved nerves may become enlarged and hardened. Treatment stops ongoing nerve damage and helps existing nerves to heal. However, leprosy is a chronic disease requiring long-term treatment.

LYME DISEASE

Lyme disease in the United States is caused by *Borrelia burgdorferi* infection transmitted by the *Ixodes* tick. In the majority of infected individuals, Lyme disease manifests first with erythema migrans, a painless and nonpruritic skin lesion that evolves over days to weeks. Patients typically have flu-like symptoms and may have infection of large joints, meninges, heart, or peripheral nerve. Approximately 15% of patients develop neurologic complications days to weeks after untreated infection. The typical neurologic manifestations are one or more elements of a triad of polyradiculoneuritis, lymphocytic meningitis, and cranial neuritis. Polyradiculopathy or polyradiculoneuropathy is typically sensorimotor, painful, asymmetric, and not length dependent (involvement of nerve roots). Approximately 5% of untreated patients develop chronic axonal neuropathy, with symptoms of relatively symmetric, distal paresthesias. Serologic testing may be negative early in the course and should be repeated if the clinical suspicion is high. Positive serologies should be confirmed by Western blot analysis. CSF in acute disease typically shows modest lymphocytic pleocytosis and mild increase in protein. In chronic infection, the IgG synthesis rate is increased, and oligoclonal bands may be present. CSF Lyme polymerase chain reaction (PCR) has 40% to 50% sensitivity and 97% specificity.

HUMAN IMMUNODEFICIENCY VIRUS

Symptomatic neuropathies occur in approximately 10% to 15% of HIV-1–infected patients, and the incidence increases as the immunodeficiency worsens. Distal symmetric sensory polyneuropathy is the most common manifestation, with distal pain, paresthesias, and numbness in a symmetric length-dependent manner. It involves sensory or sensory and motor nerve fibers and is gradually progressive. The neuropathy is similar to that associated with nucleoside analog reverse-transcriptase

inhibitors (dideoxyinosine, dideoxycytidine, 29-39-didehydro-29-39-dideoxythymidine [Stavudine]) used in the treatment of HIV. Polyradiculopathy is a much less common manifestation. AIDP can rarely occur at the time of seroconversion (CD4 counts ≥500). Polyradiculopathy can also be seen in moderately advanced HIV (CD4 counts 200–500), presenting with a CIDP pattern. In both cases, CSF examination typically demonstrates lymphocytosis of 10 to 50 cells/mm^3. Mononeuritis multiplex is an infrequent complication of HIV (0.1%–3% of patients). In advanced HIV (CD4 counts < 50), coinfection with CMV can cause painful mononeuritis multiplex, polyradiculoneuropathy, or polyradiculopathy. In these cases, CSF demonstrates polymorphonuclear pleocytosis in 5%, and CMV PCR in CSF is positive in 90% of cases.

HEPATITIS C VIRUS

Hepatitis C virus (HCV) is the most common chronic blood-borne viral infection in the United States. Neuropathy associated with HCV may affect approximately 10% of patients, with a higher prevalence (up to 30%) in those with serologic evidence of type II or type III cryoglobulinemia. Different pathophysiologic mechanisms have been suggested, including virus-triggered nerve microvasculitis and intravascular deposits of cryoglobulins, leading to disruption of the vasa nervorum microcirculation. Peripheral neuropathy may present as a distal, asymmetric sensory or sensorimotor polyneuropathy or as multiple mononeuropathies. Patients often have prominent symptoms of prickling, burning, or pain. Palpable purpura on the ankles is common and should be sought during the examination.

LEPROSY (HANSEN DISEASE)

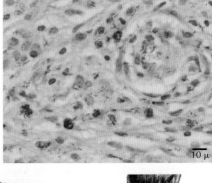
Sural nerve paraffin sections stained with Fite showing many acid-fast bacilli of a patient with leprosy

10 μ

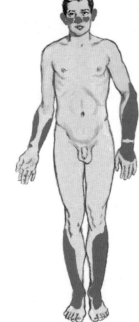
Typical early pattern of sensory loss in Hansen disease tends to affect cooler skin areas not following either segmental or nerve distribution; the area kept warm by a watchband is not affected.

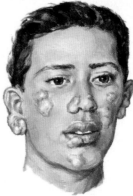
Patches and plaques on face and ears

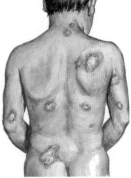
Multiple patches seen in lepromatous leprosy; central healed areas tend to be hypesthetic or anesthetic (dimorphous leprosy)

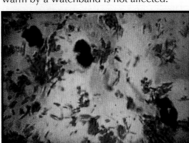
Biopsy specimen of nerve reveals abundant acid-fast bacilli (*M. leprae*).

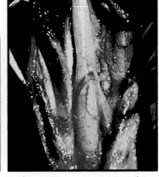
Median nerve appears normal when deep *(top)*, grossly thickened and hyperemic when superficial *(bottom)*.

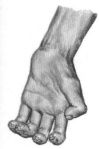
Late-stage finger contractures with ulcerations due to sensory loss

AUTONOMIC NERVOUS SYSTEM AND ITS DISORDERS

AUTONOMIC NERVOUS SYSTEM: GENERAL TOPOGRAPHY

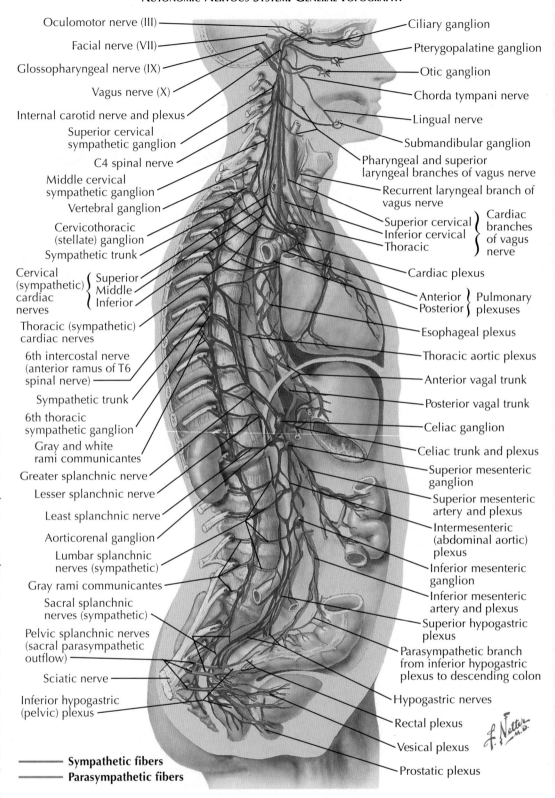

Oculomotor nerve (III)

Facial nerve (VII)

Glossopharyngeal nerve (IX)

Vagus nerve (X)

Internal carotid nerve and plexus

Superior cervical sympathetic ganglion

C4 spinal nerve

Middle cervical sympathetic ganglion

Vertebral ganglion

Cervicothoracic (stellate) ganglion

Sympathetic trunk

Cervical (sympathetic) cardiac nerves { Superior Middle Inferior }

Thoracic (sympathetic) cardiac nerves

6th intercostal nerve (anterior ramus of T6 spinal nerve)

Sympathetic trunk

6th thoracic sympathetic ganglion

Gray and white rami communicantes

Greater splanchnic nerve

Lesser splanchnic nerve

Least splanchnic nerve

Aorticorenal ganglion

Lumbar splanchnic nerves (sympathetic)

Gray rami communicantes

Sacral splanchnic nerves (sympathetic)

Pelvic splanchnic nerves (sacral parasympathetic outflow)

Sciatic nerve

Inferior hypogastric (pelvic) plexus

Ciliary ganglion

Pterygopalatine ganglion

Otic ganglion

Chorda tympani nerve

Lingual nerve

Submandibular ganglion

Pharyngeal and superior laryngeal branches of vagus nerve

Recurrent laryngeal branch of vagus nerve

Superior cervical / Inferior cervical / Thoracic } Cardiac branches of vagus nerve

Cardiac plexus

Anterior / Posterior } Pulmonary plexuses

Esophageal plexus

Thoracic aortic plexus

Anterior vagal trunk

Posterior vagal trunk

Celiac ganglion

Celiac trunk and plexus

Superior mesenteric ganglion

Superior mesenteric artery and plexus

Intermesenteric (abdominal aortic) plexus

Inferior mesenteric ganglion

Inferior mesenteric artery and plexus

Superior hypogastric plexus

Parasympathetic branch from inferior hypogastric plexus to descending colon

Hypogastric nerves

Rectal plexus

Vesical plexus

Prostatic plexus

——— **Sympathetic fibers**
——— **Parasympathetic fibers**

GENERAL TOPOGRAPHY OF AUTONOMIC NERVOUS SYSTEM

The nervous system is divided into somatic and autonomic divisions: the somatic division controls predominantly voluntary activities, whereas the autonomic system regulates involuntary functions. The two divisions develop from the same primordial cells; they comprise closely associated central and peripheral components and are both built up from afferent, efferent, and interneurons linked to produce ascending and descending nerve pathways and reflex arcs.

The *central autonomic components* include regions of the cerebral cortex, diencephalon, and brainstem. In the cerebral cortex, autonomic areas include the frontal premotor areas, telencephalic cortex in the hippocampus, insular cortex, anterior cingulate gyrus, and anteromedial prefrontal cortex. The central nucleus of the amygdala and the bed nucleus of the stria terminalis are known as the extended amygdala and modulate the autonomic responses to emotions.

The hypothalamus integrates autonomic and endocrine responses and includes nuclei in three functional zones: periventricular, lateral, and medial. Nuclei in the periventricular region control biologic rhythms; the suprachiasmatic nucleus, the pacemaker for the circadian rhythms, and the paraventricular nuclei are involved in endocrine responses by modulating the anterior pituitary. The lateral hypothalamic nuclei are involved in arousal and behavior, whereas the medial hypothalamic area, including the medial preoptic region, is involved in homeostatic functions such as thermoregulation. The periaqueductal gray nuclei of the midbrain integrate autonomic and behavioral response to nociceptive environmental stimuli. The parabrachial nucleus of the pons and the nucleus of tractus solitarius in the medulla are the principal relay nuclei in the control of cardiovascular, respiratory, and visceral function in response to environmental stimuli. The reticular formation of the anterolateral medulla contains the primary premotor neurons that control the respiratory motor neurons of the brainstem and cervical spinal cord as well as the sympathetic neurons in the intermediolateral column of the thoracic spinal cord.

These higher and lower levels of representation are interconnected by ascending and descending tracts, or pathways. For example, efferent autonomic inputs originating in the frontal premotor cortical areas descend through fasciculi, usually via synaptic relays in the thalamus, hypothalamus, and reticular formation, and end in certain cranial nerve nuclei and thus influence involuntary muscles, blood vessels, and exocrine and endocrine glands supplied by them. Other fibers descend still farther and form synapses with neurons in the intermediolateral columns in the thoracic and upper two lumbar spinal cord segments and with neurons in the gray matter of the second to fourth sacral cord segments.

Afferents to the central autonomic area are conveyed by cranial and spinal pathways. Afferent innervation from baroreceptors, chemoreceptors, and pulmonary and gastrointestinal autonomic receptors is conveyed

Plate 7.2

Autonomic Nervous System and Its Disorders

AUTONOMIC NERVOUS SYSTEM

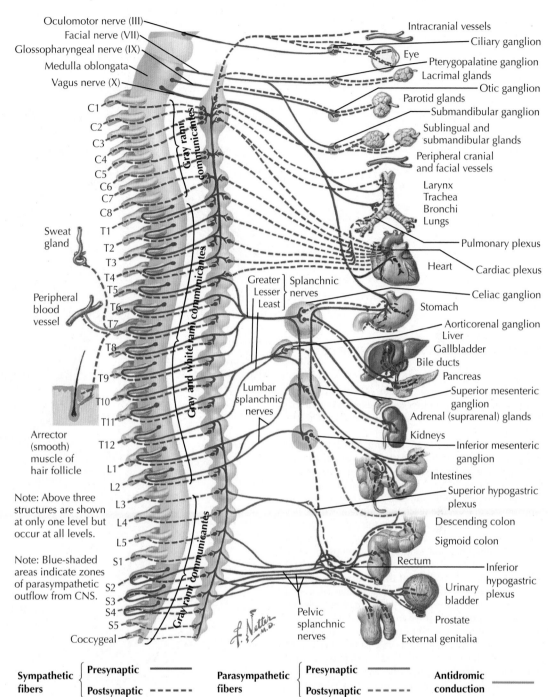

Oculomotor nerve (III)
Facial nerve (VII)
Glossopharyngeal nerve (IX)
Medulla oblongata
Vagus nerve (X)

Intracranial vessels
Ciliary ganglion
Eye
Pterygopalatine ganglion
Lacrimal glands
Otic ganglion
Parotid glands
Submandibular ganglion
Sublingual and submandibular glands
Peripheral cranial and facial vessels
Larynx
Trachea
Bronchi
Lungs
Pulmonary plexus
Heart
Cardiac plexus
Celiac ganglion
Stomach
Aorticorenal ganglion
Liver
Gallbladder
Bile ducts
Pancreas
Superior mesenteric ganglion
Adrenal (suprarenal) glands
Kidneys
Inferior mesenteric ganglion
Intestines
Superior hypogastric plexus
Descending colon
Sigmoid colon
Rectum
Inferior hypogastric plexus
Urinary bladder
Prostate
External genitalia

Gray rami communicantes
Gray and white rami communicantes
Gray rami communicantes

C1, C2, C3, C4, C5, C6, C7, C8
T1, T2, T3, T4, T5, T6, T7, T8, T9, T10, T11, T12
L1, L2, L3, L4, L5
S1, S2, S3, S4, S5
Coccygeal

Sweat gland
Peripheral blood vessel
Arrector (smooth) muscle of hair follicle

Greater / Lesser / Least Splanchnic nerves
Lumbar splanchnic nerves
Pelvic splanchnic nerves

Note: Above three structures are shown at only one level but occur at all levels.

Note: Blue-shaded areas indicate zones of parasympathetic outflow from CNS.

Sympathetic fibers { Presynaptic ——— | Postsynaptic – – – –
Parasympathetic fibers { Presynaptic ——— | Postsynaptic – – – –
Antidromic conduction ———

GENERAL TOPOGRAPHY OF AUTONOMIC NERVOUS SYSTEM (Continued)

by the vagus and glossopharyngeal nerves to the nucleus of the tractus solitarius. The information is relayed from this nucleus to the more rostral autonomic centers; visceral input and taste are relayed to the anteromedial nucleus of thalamus and then to the insular cortex. Humoral signals are relayed to the central autonomic areas by the circumventricular organs that lack a blood-brain barrier, such as the subfornical organ, the lamina terminalis in the third ventricle, and the area postrema.

The *peripheral components* of the autonomic nervous system include sympathetic ganglia and the paravertebral sympathetic trunks, which extend from the cranial base to the coccyx. Other sympathetic and parasympathetic ganglia include the ciliary, pterygopalatine, otic, submandibular, and carotid in the cranial region; prevertebral plexuses and ganglia, such as the cardiac, celiac, mesenteric, aortic, and hypogastric; plexuses located on or in the walls of viscera and vessels; and ganglia associated with the liver and adrenal gland.

The axons of autonomic neurons in the cranial nerve nuclei and sacral spinal segments usually produce effects opposite to those produced by the axons of neurons in the thoracolumbar intermediolateral cell columns. The cranial and sacral groups comprise the *parasympathetic system,* and the more numerous thoracolumbar groups comprise the *sympathetic system.* The neurons of sympathetic and parasympathetic systems are morphologically similar; they are smallish, ovoid, multipolar cells with myelinated axons and variable number of dendrites.

The axons of the autonomic nerve cells in the nuclei of the cranial nerves, in the thoracolumbar intermediolateral columns, and in the gray matter of the sacral spinal segments are termed preganglionic fibers and form synapses in peripheral ganglia. The axons of the ganglion cells are called postganglionic fibers; these unmyelinated axons convey efferent output to the viscera, vessels, and other structures.

The *cranial parasympathetic preganglionic fibers* form synapses in the ciliary, pterygopalatine, otic, submandibular, cardiac, and celiac ganglia and in much smaller ganglia in the walls of the trachea, bronchi, and gastrointestinal

tract. The corresponding sacral fibers form synapses in the inferior hypogastric (pelvic) plexuses, within the enteric plexuses of the distal colon and rectum, and in the walls of the urinary bladder and other pelvic viscera. Most of the *thoracolumbar sympathetic preganglionic fibers* synapse in sympathetic trunk ganglia, but some fibers pass through the sympathetic trunk ganglia to form synapses in other ganglia, such as the celiac, mesenteric, and renal.

Parasympathetic relay ganglia are located near the structures innervated or within the walls of hollow organs or solid viscera; therefore parasympathetic postganglionic fibers are relatively short. Sympathetic relay ganglia are generally more distant from the structures they innervate, so sympathetic postganglionic fibers are often much longer than their parasympathetic

counterparts. Plate 7.2 illustrates the arrangement of the preganglionic and postganglionic fibers to all the important viscera, the positions of the ganglia in which the synaptic relays occur, and the consequent disparities in the lengths of the postganglionic fibers. For example, in the heart, sympathetic preganglionic fibers synapse with the neurons in the superior cervical to the fifth thoracic sympathetic ganglia; the relatively long postganglionic fibers are conveyed to the heart in the cervical and thoracic sympathetic cardiac nerves. The parasympathetic preganglionic fibers reach the heart in the cardiac branches of the vagus nerves and relay in ganglia of the cardiac plexus or in small subendocardial ganglia; their postganglionic fibers are relatively short.

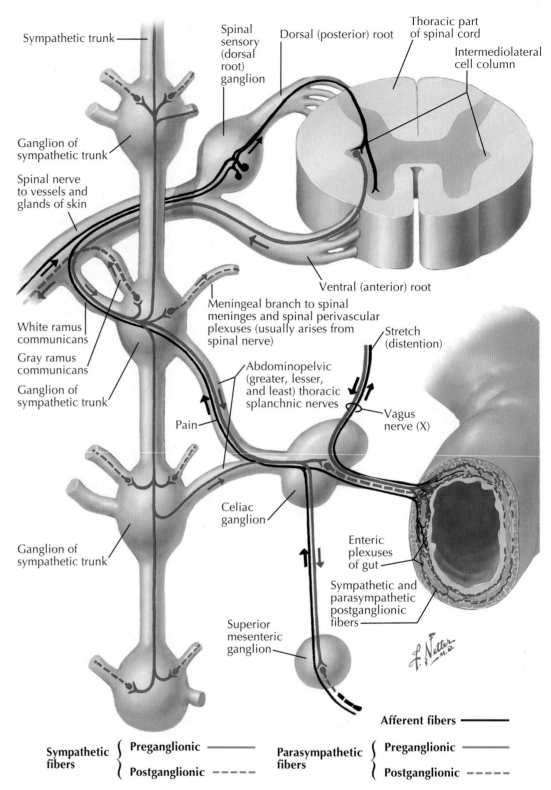

Sympathetic trunk

Spinal sensory (dorsal root) ganglion

Dorsal (posterior) root

Thoracic part of spinal cord

Intermediolateral cell column

Ganglion of sympathetic trunk

Spinal nerve to vessels and glands of skin

White ramus communicans

Gray ramus communicans

Ganglion of sympathetic trunk

Ganglion of sympathetic trunk

Ventral (anterior) root

Meningeal branch to spinal meninges and spinal perivascular plexuses (usually arises from spinal nerve)

Abdominopelvic (greater, lesser, and least) thoracic splanchnic nerves

Pain

Stretch (distention)

Vagus nerve (X)

Celiac ganglion

Enteric plexuses of gut

Sympathetic and parasympathetic postganglionic fibers

Superior mesenteric ganglion

f. Netter

Afferent fibers ——————

Sympathetic fibers { Preganglionic —————— Postganglionic - - - - -

Parasympathetic fibers { Preganglionic —————— Postganglionic - - - - -

AUTONOMIC REFLEX PATHWAYS

Plate 7.3 shows the arrangement of a typical spinal autonomic reflex arc, in this example involving the enteric plexus in the gut. Similar reflex arcs exist in the brainstem.

The autonomic reflex arc is similar to the somatic reflex arc, although in the somatic arcs the interneurons and their connections are entirely within the central nervous system (CNS). In the autonomic arcs, the interneurons are within the CNS, but their axons synapse outside the CNS to reach the ganglia in which they terminate. Initially, the autonomic and somatic components of the nervous system develop together, but during the embryonic and fetal phases, groups of nerve cells migrate outward along the spinal nerve roots and form ganglia, such as those of the sympathetic trunks, and more peripheral ganglia, such as the celiac and mesenteric (see Plate 7.13). These migrant cells are efferent autonomic neurons, and to maintain their synaptic relationships, the axons of the interneurons must follow them to reach the autonomic ganglion cells with which they form synapses. These axons are termed *preganglionic fibers,* whereas the axons of ganglionic neurons lie beyond the ganglia and are called *postganglionic fibers.*

The preganglionic fibers are myelinated, and when seen together, as in the large groups of sympathetic preganglionic fibers passing from all the thoracic and the upper two lumbar spinal nerves to nearby sympathetic trunk ganglia, they are almost white in color and constitute the *white rami communicantes.* Afferent myelinated fibers pass through these rami to the spinal nerves and contribute to their whitish appearance. The postganglionic fibers are unmyelinated and appear grayish pink in color when seen in mass. They form the *gray rami communicantes* connecting each sympathetic trunk ganglion to the adjoining spinal nerves.

One part of a *parasympathetic arc* (vagal) is illustrated; the efferent preganglionic fibers arise from the dorsal vagal nucleus and reach the walls of the intestine by vagal branches that are part of, and synapse with, cells in the ganglia forming the enteric plexus; postganglionic fibers innervate the intestines. The cell bodies of the afferent pseudounipolar neurons are also located in afferent ganglia of the enteric plexus, and their central axonal processes travel to the brainstem in the vagal nerve to synapse with the neurons in the dorsal vagal nuclei.

Plate 7.3 also shows that sympathetic preganglionic fibers emerge through the anterior root of the thoracic or upper lumbar spinal nerves. They all pass through white rami communicantes to the adjacent sympathetic trunk ganglia. Many of these preganglionic fibers synapse with the cells of the ganglia; others pass upward or downward in the sympathetic trunks to form synapses with neurons in other cervical, lumbar, and sacral ganglia. Still other preganglionic fibers pass through the sympathetic trunk ganglia without relaying and run in splanchnic nerves to end in ganglia, such as the celiac and mesenteric or the adrenal medulla. The postganglionic axons all pass to adjacent spinal nerves as gray rami communicantes; this explains why all spinal nerves have gray rami communicantes, whereas white rami communicantes are limited to the thoracolumbar region. Also shown is the recurrent meningeal sympathetic branch carrying postganglionic fibers to the spinal meninges and the spinal perivascular plexuses.

Plate 7.4

Autonomic Nervous System and Its Disorders

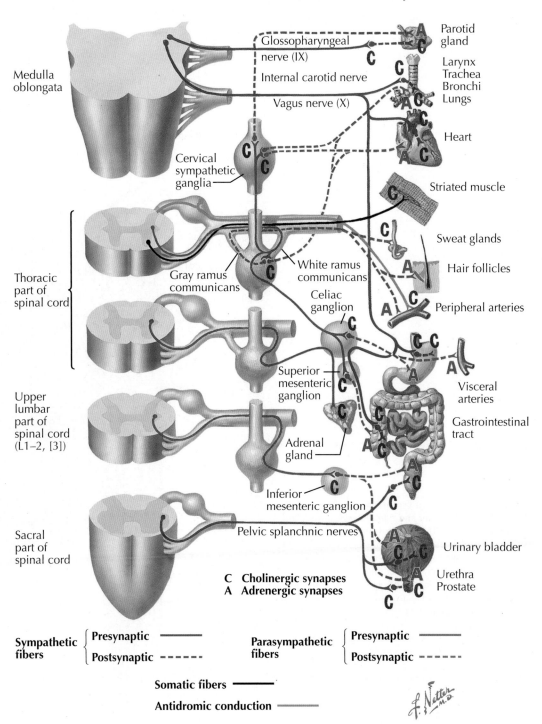

Medulla oblongata

Glossopharyngeal nerve (IX)

Internal carotid nerve

Vagus nerve (X)

Parotid gland

Larynx
Trachea
Bronchi
Lungs

Heart

Cervical sympathetic ganglia

Striated muscle

Thoracic part of spinal cord

Gray ramus communicans

White ramus communicans

Sweat glands

Hair follicles

Celiac ganglion

Peripheral arteries

Superior mesenteric ganglion

Visceral arteries

Upper lumbar part of spinal cord (L1–2, [3])

Gastrointestinal tract

Adrenal gland

Inferior mesenteric ganglion

Sacral part of spinal cord

Pelvic splanchnic nerves

Urinary bladder

Urethra
Prostate

C Cholinergic synapses
A Adrenergic synapses

Sympathetic fibers { Presynaptic ——— Postsynaptic - - - - - }

Parasympathetic fibers { Presynaptic ——— Postsynaptic - - - - - }

Somatic fibers ———

Antidromic conduction ———

CHOLINERGIC AND ADRENERGIC NERVES

The terms *adrenergic* and *cholinergic,* introduced by Dale in 1933, are based on the concept that synaptic transmission between autonomic nerve fibers, and between the postganglionic axon and the structures they innervate, is effected by adrenergic or cholinergic chemicals.

Epinephrine (adrenaline) and the closely related *norepinephrine* (noradrenaline) are the chief neurotransmitters at peripheral sympathetic or *adrenergic* terminations, whereas *acetylcholine* is generally associated with parasympathetic, or *cholinergic,* effects. However, in reality, acetylcholine is an important neurotransmitter at synapses in both sympathetic and parasympathetic pathways. Dale's terms were initially applied only to *postganglionic fibers;* acetylcholine, in fact, is the chief neurotransmitter at synapses between *preganglionic fibers* and ganglionic neurons of both the sympathetic and parasympathetic systems.

Plate 7.4 shows the sites at which acetylcholine (C) and norepinephrine (A) are the chief neurotransmitters. Other chemical substances, such as adenosine

triphosphate, gamma-aminobutyric acid, a polypeptide called substance P, histamine, glutamic acid, and prostaglandins, have also been implicated as neurotransmitters.

Sympathetic, or adrenergic, efferent nerve fibers usually elicit active reactions in effector structures, such as smooth (unstriated) muscle or glands, which are the reverse of the diminished activity produced by parasympathetic, or cholinergic, fibers. Thus stimulation of the sympathetic and parasympathetic cardiac nerves produces cardiac acceleration and deceleration. However, these effects are not universal. For example, activity of the alimentary adrenergic nerves produces slowing of gastrointestinal motility; conversely, activity in the cholinergic supply results in acceleration of gastric and

intestinal movements. Similar reactions occur in other structures. Thus in the urinary tract, the sympathetic nerves produce relaxation of the bladder wall, and the parasympathetic nerves cause contraction, so the former have been aptly described as "filling" and the latter as "emptying" nerves.

Sweat glands are classified as apocrine or eccrine glands. The apocrine glands open into the lumen of the sweat glands in the axilla, perineum, and periareolar region and are innervated by adrenergic fibers and probably respond to humoral epinephrine. The eccrine sweat glands open directly into the skin and are innervated by sympathetic postganglionic fibers that are cholinergic. Eccrine glands are one of the most important skin appendages and play a vital role in temperature regulation.

AUTONOMIC NERVES IN HEAD

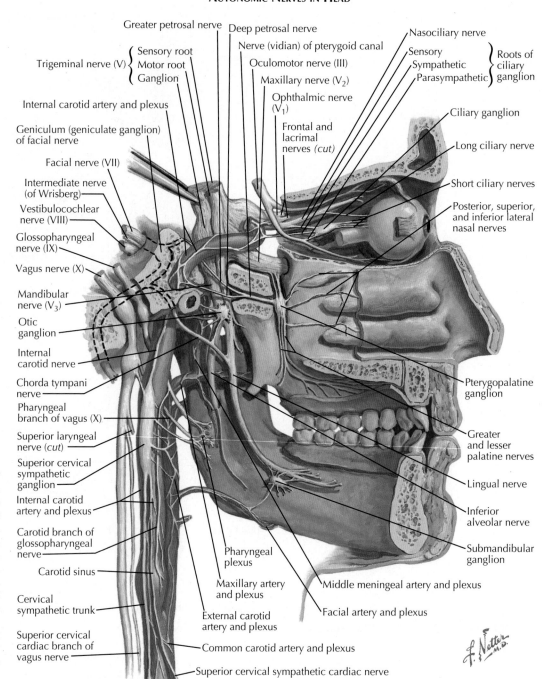

Greater petrosal nerve

Deep petrosal nerve

Nerve (vidian) of pterygoid canal

Nasociliary nerve

Trigeminal nerve (V) { Sensory root, Motor root, Ganglion

Oculomotor nerve (III)

Sensory, Sympathetic, Parasympathetic } Roots of ciliary ganglion

Internal carotid artery and plexus

Maxillary nerve (V₂)

Ophthalmic nerve (V₁)

Ciliary ganglion

Geniculum (geniculate ganglion) of facial nerve

Frontal and lacrimal nerves (cut)

Long ciliary nerve

Facial nerve (VII)

Short ciliary nerves

Intermediate nerve (of Wrisberg)

Posterior, superior, and inferior lateral nasal nerves

Vestibulocochlear nerve (VIII)

Glossopharyngeal nerve (IX)

Vagus nerve (X)

Mandibular nerve (V₃)

Otic ganglion

Internal carotid nerve

Chorda tympani nerve

Pterygopalatine ganglion

Pharyngeal branch of vagus (X)

Superior laryngeal nerve (cut)

Greater and lesser palatine nerves

Superior cervical sympathetic ganglion

Lingual nerve

Internal carotid artery and plexus

Inferior alveolar nerve

Carotid branch of glossopharyngeal nerve

Submandibular ganglion

Carotid sinus

Pharyngeal plexus

Cervical sympathetic trunk

Maxillary artery and plexus

Middle meningeal artery and plexus

Superior cervical cardiac branch of vagus nerve

External carotid artery and plexus

Facial artery and plexus

Common carotid artery and plexus

Superior cervical sympathetic cardiac nerve

AUTONOMIC NERVES IN HEAD AND NECK

The cervical part of each sympathetic trunk generally has four ganglia: *superior* and *middle cervical, vertebral,* and *cervicothoracic.* The superior and middle cervical ganglia are usually connected by a single cord, but the middle cervical, vertebral, and cervicothoracic ganglia are connected by several cords, one or more of which form a loop, the ansa subclavia, around the subclavian artery and sometimes also around the vertebral artery. A true inferior cervical ganglion is present only in about 20% of individuals; in the majority, the lowest cervical and uppermost thoracic ganglia are fused to form the cervicothoracic (stellate) ganglion.

The *superior cervical ganglion* is fusiform in shape. It is produced by the coalescence of the upper three or four cervical ganglia. The preganglionic fibers emerge through the uppermost thoracic spinal nerves and ascend as the cervical sympathetic trunk; a relatively small number of these fibers are from adjacent cervical nerve roots. A small proportion of the preganglionic fibers pass through it without interruption and relay at higher levels in the internal carotid ganglia.

The superior cervical ganglion receives and supplies communicating, visceral, vascular, muscular, osseous, and articular rami. It communicates with the last four cranial nerves or their branches, with the vertebral arterial plexus and, occasionally, with the phrenic nerve. It supplies gray rami to the upper three or four cervical spinal nerves, and the contained postganglionic fibers are distributed with the branches of the cervical nerves. *Visceral fibers* pass to the larynx, pharynx, and heart, and other fibers are carried in vascular plexuses to the salivary, lacrimal, pituitary, pineal, thyroid, and other glands. *Vascular fibers* are supplied to the internal and external carotid arteries and form plexuses around them; nerve continuations from these plexuses form subsidiary plexuses around all their branches. From the

internal carotid plexus, minute caroticotympanic offshoots join the tympanic branch of the glossopharyngeal nerve and thus reach the tympanic plexus. A deep petrosal branch unites with the greater petrosal nerve to form the *nerve of the pterygoid canal,* which constitutes the *sympathetic root of the pterygopalatine ganglion.* The sympathetic fibers are postganglionic and run through the ganglion without relaying, to be distributed to vessels and glands in the nose, palate, nasopharynx, and orbit. The *sympathetic root of the ciliary ganglion* arises from the cranial end of the ipsilateral internal carotid nerves or plexus; its fibers are postganglionic, having relayed in the superior cervical or internal carotid ganglia; they pass through the ganglion and run onward in the ciliary nerves to supply the ocular vessels and the dilator pupillae. In addition to postganglionic efferent

fibers, many *visceral efferent* and *afferent fibers* are present in the vascular plexuses. They convey sympathetic efferent output to the pituitary, lacrimal, salivary, thyroid, and other smaller glands in the territories supplied by the carotid arteries, and they also transmit sensory information from the same structures. In a similar fashion, sympathetic fibers are carried to adjacent *osseous, articular,* and *muscular* structures.

The *middle cervical ganglion* is much smaller than the superior ganglion and usually represents fused fifth and sixth cervical ganglia. It contributes gray rami communicantes to the fifth and sixth cervical nerves and sends fibers to the vertebral periarterial plexus. Inconstant strands form interconnections with the vagus, phrenic, and recurrent laryngeal nerves, and *visceral branches* are supplied to the thyroid and parathyroid glands. The

Plate 7.6

Autonomic Nervous System and Its Disorders

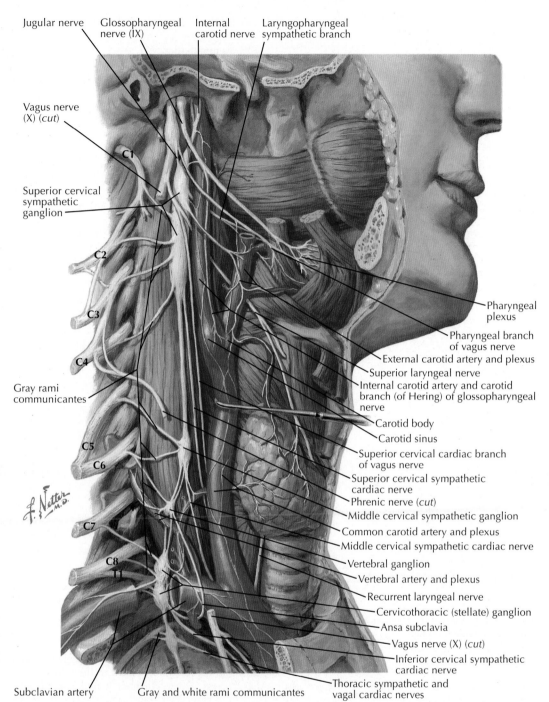

AUTONOMIC NERVES IN NECK

Jugular nerve
Glossopharyngeal nerve (IX)
Internal carotid nerve
Laryngopharyngeal sympathetic branch
Vagus nerve (X) (cut)
C1
Superior cervical sympathetic ganglion
C2
C3
C4
Gray rami communicantes
C5
C6
C7
C8
T1
Subclavian artery
Gray and white rami communicantes

Pharyngeal plexus
Pharyngeal branch of vagus nerve
External carotid artery and plexus
Superior laryngeal nerve
Internal carotid artery and carotid branch (of Hering) of glossopharyngeal nerve
Carotid body
Carotid sinus
Superior cervical cardiac branch of vagus nerve
Superior cervical sympathetic cardiac nerve
Phrenic nerve (cut)
Middle cervical sympathetic ganglion
Common carotid artery and plexus
Middle cervical sympathetic cardiac nerve
Vertebral ganglion
Vertebral artery and plexus
Recurrent laryngeal nerve
Cervicothoracic (stellate) ganglion
Ansa subclavia
Vagus nerve (X) (cut)
Inferior cervical sympathetic cardiac nerve
Thoracic sympathetic and vagal cardiac nerves

AUTONOMIC NERVES IN HEAD AND NECK (Continued)

ganglion may give off the middle cervical sympathetic cardiac nerve and contributes several twigs to the esophagus and trachea. *Vascular branches* help in the innervation of the common carotid, inferior thyroid, and vertebral arteries and the jugular veins. Fibers pass to adjacent muscular, osseous, and articular structures, usually alongside the arteries supplying them.

The *vertebral ganglion* is small and is located anterior to the vertebral artery, near its point of entry into the transverse foramen of the sixth cervical vertebra. It may receive gray rami communicantes from the sixth and/ or seventh cervical nerves and thus may represent a detached element of the middle cervical ganglion or the cervicothoracic ganglion. It gives off *vascular branches* that accompany the vertebral artery; it may be connected by fibers to the vagus and phrenic nerves, and it supplies tiny *visceral branches* to the thyroid gland, trachea, and esophagus.

The *cervicothoracic (stellate) ganglion* is formed by the fusion of the seventh and eighth cervical ganglia with the first and/or second thoracic ganglia. It is an irregularly fusiform structure with many radiating branches. The cervicothoracic ganglion is situated posterior to the first part of the subclavian artery, the origin of the vertebral artery, the vertebral vein, and the apex of the lung. It lies anterior to the last cervical transverse process, the neck of the first rib, and the anterior primary ramus of the eighth cervical nerve as it passes outward to unite with the corresponding ramus of the first thoracic nerve to form the inferior trunk of the brachial plexus. The vertebral vessels run over the upper pole of the ganglion, and the superior intercostal vessels run lateral to it at the level of the neck of the first rib. An aponeurotic slip from the scalene muscles spreads out to become attached to the suprapleural membrane and may veil the ganglion

during the anterior operative approach. If a scalenus minimus is present, it may also obscure the ganglion.

The cervicothoracic ganglion receives white rami communicantes from the first and second thoracic nerves and sends gray rami communicantes to the eighth cervical and first thoracic nerves and, occasionally, to the seventh cervical and second thoracic nerves. These rami carry efferent and afferent sympathetic fibers to and from the brachial plexus and the uppermost intercostal nerves, thus helping to innervate *vessels, sweat glands, arrectores pilorum, bones,* and *joints* in the upper limbs and superior parts of the chest wall. The ganglion or the ansa subclavia invariably communicates with the ipsilateral phrenic nerve and almost constantly with the vagus or the recurrent laryngeal nerve. Fibers are supplied to the heart, esophagus,

trachea, and thymus. Some vascular fibers from the ganglion pass directly to the large vessels in the cervicothoracic inlet, but most of the sympathetic fibers for the upper limb structures enter the inferior trunk of the brachial plexus. They pass mainly into the medial cord of the plexus and then into the median and ulnar nerves and, to a lesser extent, into the axillary, radial, musculocutaneous, and other branches of the plexus. Vasomotor and sudomotor disturbances, or causalgia, are therefore most likely to follow irritation or injury to the inferior trunk of the brachial plexus or to the ulnar or median nerves.

Most of the preganglionic fibers for the upper limbs emerge through the anterior rami of the second to sixth or seventh thoracic nerves, and the second and third nerves probably contain the majority of the fibers.

AUTONOMIC DISTRIBUTION TO THE HEAD AND THE NECK

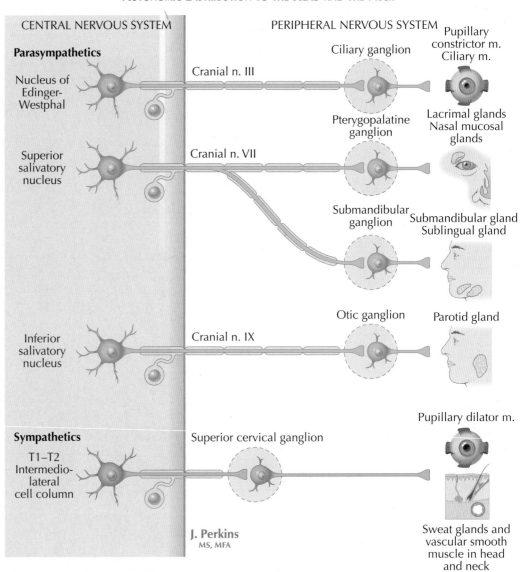

CENTRAL NERVOUS SYSTEM   PERIPHERAL NERVOUS SYSTEM

Parasympathetics

Nucleus of Edinger-Westphal — Cranial n. III — Ciliary ganglion → Pupillary constrictor m. Ciliary m.

Superior salivatory nucleus — Cranial n. VII — Pterygopalatine ganglion → Lacrimal glands Nasal mucosal glands

Submandibular ganglion → Submandibular gland Sublingual gland

Inferior salivatory nucleus — Cranial n. IX — Otic ganglion → Parotid gland

Sympathetics

T1–T2 Intermedio-lateral cell column — Superior cervical ganglion → Pupillary dilator m.

Sweat glands and vascular smooth muscle in head and neck

J. Perkins
MS, MFA

AUTONOMIC INNERVATION OF EYE

The eye receives a rich innervation by the sympathetic and parasympathetic systems.

SYMPATHETIC FIBERS

The sympathetic *preganglionic fibers* for the eye arise from the intermediolateral column of the thoracic cord and travel in the ipsilateral first, second, and occasionally third thoracic spinal nerves. They pass through white rami communicantes to the sympathetic trunks; the fibers ascend to the superior cervical ganglion where they relay, although a few synapse higher in the internal carotid ganglia. The *postganglionic fibers* run either in the internal carotid plexus and enter the orbit through its superior fissure, or else they run alongside the ophthalmic artery in its periarterial plexus. Some of the ocular sympathetic fibers may make a detour through the caroticotympanic nerves and tympanic plexus before rejoining the cavernous part of the internal carotid plexus by means of a branch that emerges from the anterior surface of the petrous part of the temporal bone near the greater petrosal nerve; thereafter, they accompany the other ocular fibers.

Some of the branches passing through the superior orbital fissure form the *sympathetic root of the ciliary ganglion;* their contained fibers pass through it without relaying to become incorporated in the 8 to 10 *short ciliary nerves.* Other branches join the ophthalmic nerve or its nasociliary branch and reach the eye in the two to three *long ciliary nerves* that supply the radial musculature in the iris (dilator pupillae). Both long and short ciliary nerves also contain afferent fibers from the cornea, iris, and choroid. Fibers conveyed in the short ciliary nerves pass through a communicating ramus from the ciliary ganglion to the nasociliary nerve; this ramus is called the *sensory root of the ciliary ganglion.* The parent cells of these sensory fibers are located in the trigeminal (semilunar) ganglion, and their central processes end in the *sensory trigeminal nuclei* in the brainstem. The sensory trigeminal nuclei have multiple interconnections with other somatic and autonomic centers and thus influence many reflex reactions. Other sympathetic fibers from the internal carotid plexus reach the eye through the ophthalmic periarterial plexus and its subsidiary plexuses around the central retinal, ciliary, scleral, and conjunctival arteries (see Plate 7.5).

PARASYMPATHETIC FIBERS

The parasympathetic preganglionic fibers for the eye are the axons of cells in the *autonomic, (Edinger-Westphal) oculomotor nucleus.* They run in the third cranial nerve and exit in the *motor root of the ciliary ganglion,* where they relay. The axons of these ganglionic cells are postganglionic parasympathetic fibers, which reach the eye in the *short ciliary nerves* and are distributed to the constrictor fibers of the iris (sphincter pupillae), to the ciliary muscle, and to the blood vessels in the eyeball.

VISUAL CENTERS

The visual reflex centers are located in the tectal and pretectal areas of the mesencephalon. They are connected to the lateral geniculate bodies (lower visual centers) and to the superior colliculi in which the *tectospinal tracts* originate; these connections provide the anatomic basis for the reflex movements of the head and eyes in response to visual stimuli. The light and accommodation reflexes are affected through pretectal

Plate 7.8

Autonomic Nervous System and Its Disorders

CILIARY GANGLION

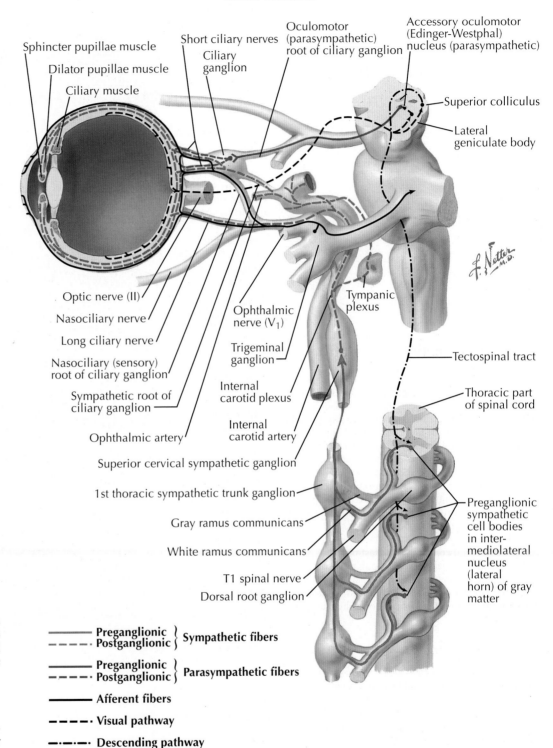

Sphincter pupillae muscle
Dilator pupillae muscle
Ciliary muscle
Short ciliary nerves
Ciliary ganglion
Oculomotor (parasympathetic) root of ciliary ganglion
Accessory oculomotor (Edinger-Westphal) nucleus (parasympathetic)
Superior colliculus
Lateral geniculate body
Optic nerve (II)
Nasociliary nerve
Long ciliary nerve
Nasociliary (sensory) root of ciliary ganglion
Sympathetic root of ciliary ganglion
Ophthalmic artery
Ophthalmic nerve (V₁)
Trigeminal ganglion
Internal carotid plexus
Internal carotid artery
Tympanic plexus
Tectospinal tract
Thoracic part of spinal cord
Superior cervical sympathetic ganglion
1st thoracic sympathetic trunk ganglion
Gray ramus communicans
White ramus communicans
T1 spinal nerve
Dorsal root ganglion
Preganglionic sympathetic cell bodies in inter-mediolateral nucleus (lateral horn) of gray matter

Preganglionic / Postganglionic } Sympathetic fibers
Preganglionic / Postganglionic } Parasympathetic fibers
Afferent fibers
Visual pathway
Descending pathway

AUTONOMIC INNERVATION OF EYE (Continued)

connections. Fibers from the lateral geniculate bodies are connected through synapses in pretectal nuclei to the accessory oculomotor nucleus (Edinger-Westphal nuclei), which controls the sphincter pupillae and the ciliary muscle.

PUPILLARY LIGHT REFLEX

Light causes pupillary constriction (miosis). The impulse generated by the light travels from the retina by the optic nerve and optic tract to bilateral pretectal nuclei in the midbrain, decussating in the posterior commissure. The axons from the pretectal nuclei terminate in the accessory oculomotor nuclei. Preganglionic parasympathetic information travels via the oculomotor nerve to the ciliary ganglion. Postganglionic fibers from the ciliary ganglion traverse the short ciliary nerves to innervate the sphincter pupillae muscle of the iris. If one eye is stimulated by light, both pupils will react; ipsilateral (direct response) and contralateral (consensual response) pupils both respond because of the termination of the fibers of the optic tract in the pretectal nuclei bilaterally.

Dilation of the pupil (mydriasis) occurs from postganglionic sympathetic innervation from the superior cervical ganglion. Preganglionic fibers arise from the neurons first and second thoracic intermediolateral column and by the upper thoracic spinal nerves, and white rami communicantes reach the superior cervical ganglion. From there, they traverse the long ciliary nerves to the dilator pupillae. Pupils also dilate in response to pain, presumably due to fibers from the sensory system reaching the preganglionic neurons (pupillary skin reflex).

ACCOMMODATION REFLEX

In viewing objects that are near, the pupils constrict, the eyes move medially, and the lens changes shape to become more convex. The reflex for this begins in the retina and then involves the optic nerve, optic tract, lateral geniculate bodies, optic radiations, and visual cortical centers. From there, the impulse is thought to reach the "near response neurons" in the pretectal nuclei by corticotectal fibers. From the pretectal nuclei, the information reaches the oculomotor nuclei. The parasympathetic fibers reach the sphincter pupillae via the ciliary ganglion and short ciliary nerves. The parasympathetic fibers cause stimulation of the ciliary muscles, which causes relaxation of the zonule, and the lens becomes more spheric; the medial recti are activated by the ventral oculomotor nuclei, causing the eyes to converge.

THORACIC SYMPATHETIC CHAIN AND SPLANCHNIC NERVES

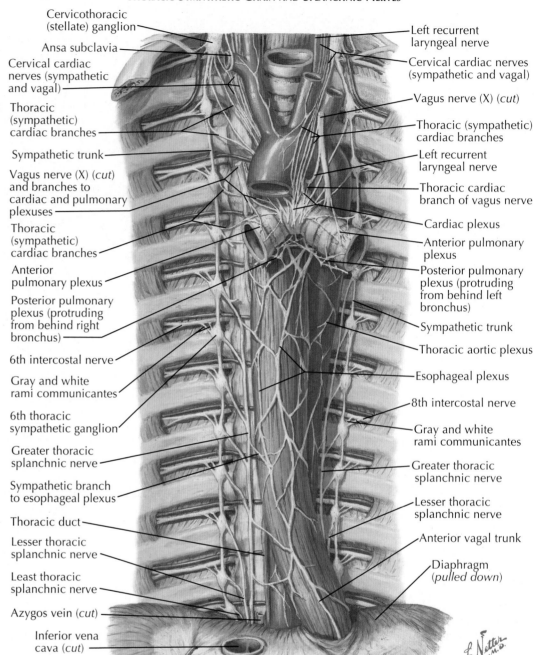

Cervicothoracic (stellate) ganglion

Ansa subclavia

Cervical cardiac nerves (sympathetic and vagal)

Thoracic (sympathetic) cardiac branches

Sympathetic trunk

Vagus nerve (X) (cut) and branches to cardiac and pulmonary plexuses

Thoracic (sympathetic) cardiac branches

Anterior pulmonary plexus

Posterior pulmonary plexus (protruding from behind right bronchus)

6th intercostal nerve

Gray and white rami communicantes

6th thoracic sympathetic ganglion

Greater thoracic splanchnic nerve

Sympathetic branch to esophageal plexus

Thoracic duct

Lesser thoracic splanchnic nerve

Least thoracic splanchnic nerve

Azygos vein (cut)

Inferior vena cava (cut)

Left recurrent laryngeal nerve

Cervical cardiac nerves (sympathetic and vagal)

Vagus nerve (X) (cut)

Thoracic (sympathetic) cardiac branches

Left recurrent laryngeal nerve

Thoracic cardiac branch of vagus nerve

Cardiac plexus

Anterior pulmonary plexus

Posterior pulmonary plexus (protruding from behind left bronchus)

Sympathetic trunk

Thoracic aortic plexus

Esophageal plexus

8th intercostal nerve

Gray and white rami communicantes

Greater thoracic splanchnic nerve

Lesser thoracic splanchnic nerve

Anterior vagal trunk

Diaphragm (pulled down)

AUTONOMIC NERVES IN THORAX

The thoracic parts of the sympathetic trunks lie anterior to the junctions between the heads and necks of the ribs and posterior to the pleura. There are usually 10 or 11 ganglia on each side; the first is often incorporated into the cervicothoracic (stellate) ganglion (see Plate 7.6), and the last thoracic and first lumbar ganglia may also be united. The interganglionic cords are usually single, but double or triple cords between some adjacent ganglia are not uncommon. The thoracic trunks supply or receive communicating, visceral, vascular, muscular, osseous, and articular branches.

Each ganglion receives at least one white ramus communicans and contributes at least one gray ramus to the adjacent spinal nerve, although several white and gray rami communicantes may be attached to each ganglion. Visceral branches are supplied to the heart and pericardium, lungs, trachea and bronchi, esophagus, and thymus.

SYMPATHETIC CARDIAC NERVES

Three pairs of sympathetic cardiac nerves arise from the cervical trunk ganglia, and the others emerge from the upper thoracic ganglia.

The *superior cervical sympathetic cardiac nerves* originate from the corresponding trunk ganglia. On the right, the nerve passes posterolateral to the brachiocephalic artery and aortic arch; on the left, it curves downward over the left side of the aortic arch to reach the cardiac plexus.

The *middle cervical sympathetic cardiac nerves* are usually larger than the corresponding superior and inferior nerves. They arise from the middle cervical and vertebral ganglia of the sympathetic trunks and usually run independently to the cardiac plexus.

The *inferior cervical sympathetic cardiac nerves* consist of fibers arising from the cervicothoracic ganglia and subclavian ansae.

The *thoracic sympathetic cardiac nerves* are four or five slender branches that run forward and medially from the thoracic trunk ganglia to the cardiac plexus.

PARASYMPATHETIC CARDIAC NERVES

Three pairs of parasympathetic (vagal) cardiac nerves are usually present. The *superior cervical vagal cardiac branches* leave the vagus nerves in the upper part of the neck. The *inferior cervical vagal cardiac branches* arise in the lower third of the neck and descend posterolateral to the brachiocephalic artery and aortic arch on the right side; on the left side, they descend lateral to the left common carotid artery and aortic arch. The *thoracic vagal cardiac branches* arise at or below the level of the thoracic inlet.

Multiple interconnections exist between all the sympathetic and parasympathetic cardiac nerves and between the cardiac and other visceral branches of the sympathetic trunks.

Other *thoracic sympathetic branches* supply the thoracic viscera from the paired greater, lesser, and lowest thoracic splanchnic nerves, although these are mainly destined to supply abdominal structures and contain a mixture of preganglionic, postganglionic, and afferent fibers. The *greater (major) splanchnic nerve* lies medial to the ipsilateral sympathetic trunk and enters the abdomen by piercing the crus of the diaphragm. The *lesser (minor) splanchnic nerve* lies slightly lateral to the greater splanchnic nerve and also usually pierces the diaphragmatic crus. The *lowest (imus) splanchnic nerve* is inconstant.

Minute twigs from the sympathetic trunks join and innervate the intercostal arteries. Other sympathetic postganglionic fibers reach these vessels in fascicles from adjacent intercostal nerves or their branches, and these also carry sudomotor and pilomotor fibers.

The muscular, osseous, and articular fibers from the thoracic sympathetic trunks and their branches supply the adjacent structures concerned; their exact functions are uncertain.

Plate 7.10

Autonomic Nervous System and Its Disorders

AUTONOMIC NERVES IN THORAX (Continued)

INNERVATION OF HEART

The heart is supplied by sympathetic nerves arising mainly in the neck because the heart develops initially in the cervical region and later migrates into the thorax, taking its nerves down with it. The parasympathetic supply is conveyed in cardiac branches of the vagus nerves.

The *sympathetic preganglionic cardiac fibers* leave the spinal cord in the anterior roots of the upper four to five thoracic spinal nerves and enter the white or mixed rami communicantes passing to adjacent thoracic sympathetic trunk ganglia. Some of the fibers relay here; others ascend in the trunks to form synapses in the cervical ganglia, giving rise to the *cardiac nerves* (see earlier discussion). Most cardiac fibers are postganglionic and pass through the cardiac plexus without relaying, to be distributed to the heart wall and its vessels via the *coronary plexuses.*

The *parasympathetic preganglionic (vagal) fibers* are the axons of cells in the dorsal vagal nucleus. From the vagal cardiac nerves, they relay in ganglia of the *cardiac plexus* or in *intrinsic cardiac ganglia,* which are located mainly in the atrial subepicardial tissue along the coronary sulcus and around the roots of the great vessels. The sinoatrial node and the atrioventricular node and bundle have a rich supply of parasympathetic innervation. Ventricular ganglia are scanty, but enough of them exist to cast doubts on the hypothesis that ventricular innervation is purely sympathetic.

The more important afferent and efferent pathways in cardiac innervation are shown in the illustration. The peripheral processes of the afferent pseudounipolar neurons in the posterior root ganglia transmit input from cardiac receptors of various types and from terminal nerve networks in reflexogenic zones, such as those in and around the large cardiac venous openings, the interatrial septum, and the ascending aorta. Some of their central processes are implicated in spinal reflex arcs, whereas others ascend to the dorsal vagal nuclei in the medulla oblongata, the nearby reticular formation, or the hypothalamus and frontal cortex.

The thoracic sympathetic cardiac nerves carry many *afferent pain fibers* from the heart and great vessels, and this endows them with a clinical interest disproportionate to their small size, because their surgical destruction produces alleviation of angina pectoris. Other cardiac pain afferents run in the middle and inferior cervical sympathetic cardiac nerves; however, after entering the corresponding cervical ganglia, they descend within the sympathetic trunks to the thoracic region before passing through rami communicantes to the upper four or five thoracic spinal nerves.

Afferent vagal fibers from the heart and vessels play an important role in modifying efferent output that adjusts the rate and strength of the heartbeat; usually, they depress cardiac activity. In humans, the afferent vagal information pass through cardiac branches of the recurrent laryngeal nerves to the main vagus nerves and thus to the brainstem.

Afferent pericardial fibers from the fibrous and parietal serous pericardium are carried mainly in the phrenic nerves, but those from the visceral serous pericardium join the coronary arterial plexuses.

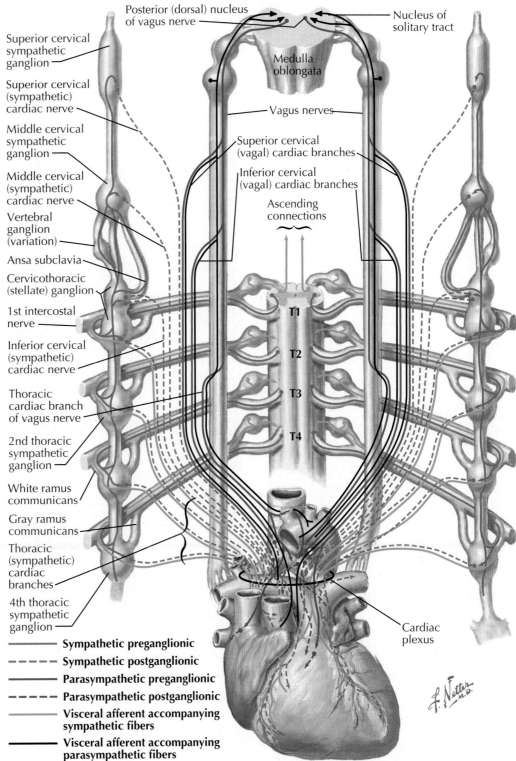

INNERVATION OF HEART

Posterior (dorsal) nucleus of vagus nerve
Nucleus of solitary tract
Medulla oblongata
Vagus nerves
Superior cervical (vagal) cardiac branches
Inferior cervical (vagal) cardiac branches
Ascending connections

Superior cervical sympathetic ganglion
Superior cervical (sympathetic) cardiac nerve
Middle cervical sympathetic ganglion
Middle cervical (sympathetic) cardiac nerve
Vertebral ganglion (variation)
Ansa subclavia
Cervicothoracic (stellate) ganglion
1st intercostal nerve
Inferior cervical (sympathetic) cardiac nerve
Thoracic cardiac branch of vagus nerve
2nd thoracic sympathetic ganglion
White ramus communicans
Gray ramus communicans
Thoracic (sympathetic) cardiac branches
4th thoracic sympathetic ganglion

Cardiac plexus

T1
T2
T3
T4

——— **Sympathetic preganglionic**
- - - - **Sympathetic postganglionic**
——— **Parasympathetic preganglionic**
- - - - **Parasympathetic postganglionic**
——— **Visceral afferent accompanying sympathetic fibers**
——— **Visceral afferent accompanying parasympathetic fibers**

INNERVATION OF BLOOD VESSELS

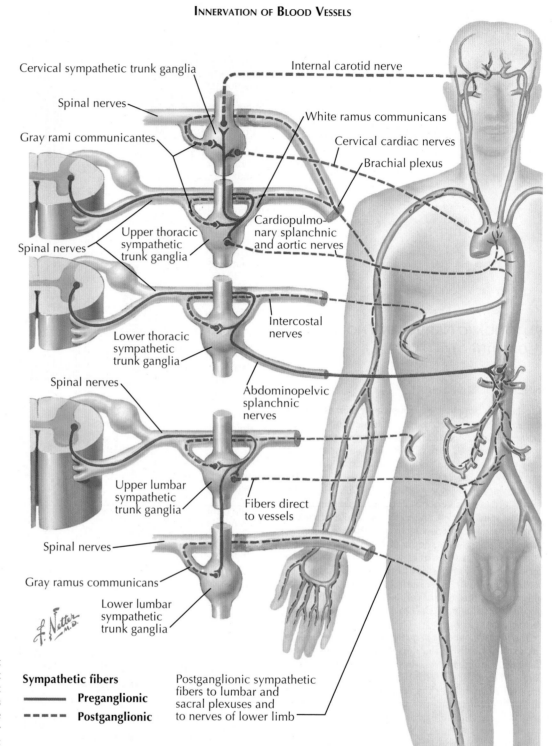

Cervical sympathetic trunk ganglia

Spinal nerves

Gray rami communicantes

Internal carotid nerve

White ramus communicans

Cervical cardiac nerves

Brachial plexus

Upper thoracic sympathetic trunk ganglia

Spinal nerves

Cardiopulmonary splanchnic and aortic nerves

Intercostal nerves

Lower thoracic sympathetic trunk ganglia

Spinal nerves

Abdominopelvic splanchnic nerves

Upper lumbar sympathetic trunk ganglia

Fibers direct to vessels

Spinal nerves

Gray ramus communicans

Lower lumbar sympathetic trunk ganglia

Sympathetic fibers

——— **Preganglionic**

- - - - **Postganglionic**

Postganglionic sympathetic fibers to lumbar and sacral plexuses and to nerves of lower limb

INNERVATION OF BLOOD VESSELS

Blood vessels are innervated by afferent and efferent autonomic nerves. All receive sympathetic fibers, but some may not have a parasympathetic supply. The great vessels near the midline in the neck and body cavities receive direct innervation from adjacent parts of the sympathetic trunks. Some of these vessels and their branches also obtain supplies from nearby autonomic plexuses, which contain both sympathetic and parasympathetic elements. Thus the ascending aorta, the aortic arch and its branches, and the superior vena cava receive offshoots from the cardiac plexus; the pulmonary vessels receive offshoots from the pulmonary plexuses; the celiac, hepatic, gastric, splenic, superior mesenteric, renal, and adrenal vessels and the portal and inferior caval veins receive offshoots from the celiac and superior mesenteric plexuses; the inferior mesenteric vessels receive offshoots from the corresponding plexus; and the pelvic vessels receive offshoots from the superior and inferior hypogastric plexuses.

The chief outflow of sympathetic preganglionic fibers is through the anterior roots of spinal nerves T1 to L2. The fibers pass in white rami communicantes to adjacent sympathetic trunk ganglia, where many relay. The

axons of these ganglionic cells (postganglionic fibers) may pass in nerves to nearby structures, such as midline vessels and prevertebral plexuses (cardiac, celiac, mesenteric), or they may join the lowest cervical, thoracic, and upper lumbar spinal nerves through gray rami communicantes, to be distributed with them to vessels and glands in the thoracic and abdominal cavities and limbs.

Other preganglionic fibers, however, do not relay in adjacent trunk ganglia but ascend or descend in the sympathetic trunks to form synapses in the cervical or

lower lumbar and sacral ganglia. The axons (postganglionic fibers) of the cervical ganglionic cells supply the vessels and glands in the head and neck, whereas others contribute to the sympathetic cervical cardiac nerves. Some of the postganglionic fibers arising in the lumbar and sacral ganglia run in lumbar and sacral splanchnic nerves to the mesenteric and hypogastric plexuses, but others pass through gray rami communicantes to the lumbar, sacral, and coccygeal spinal nerves to be distributed with them and their branches to vessels, sweat glands, and arrectores pilorum muscles in the loin,

Plate 7.12

Autonomic Nervous System and Its Disorders

CAROTID BODY AND CAROTID SINUS

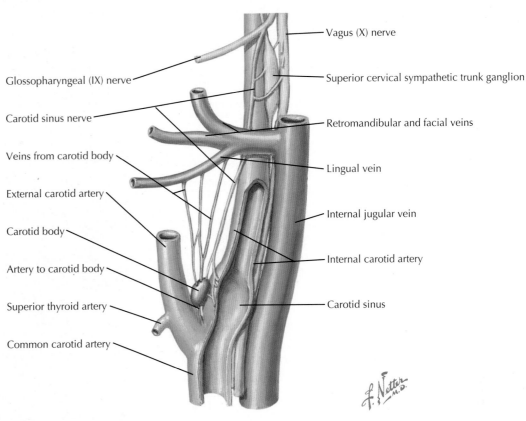

Vagus (X) nerve

Glossopharyngeal (IX) nerve

Superior cervical sympathetic trunk ganglion

Carotid sinus nerve

Retromandibular and facial veins

Veins from carotid body

Lingual vein

External carotid artery

Internal jugular vein

Carotid body

Internal carotid artery

Artery to carotid body

Superior thyroid artery

Carotid sinus

Common carotid artery

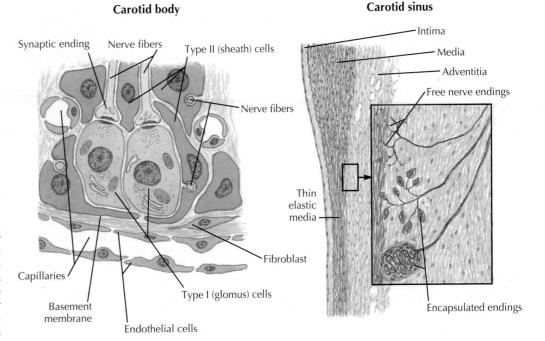

Carotid body

Synaptic ending   Nerve fibers   Type II (sheath) cells

Nerve fibers

Fibroblast

Capillaries

Type I (glomus) cells

Basement membrane

Endothelial cells

Carotid sinus

Intima

Media

Adventitia

Free nerve endings

Thin elastic media

Encapsulated endings

INNERVATION OF BLOOD VESSELS (Continued)

lower abdominal wall, buttocks, perineum, and lower limbs.

The vascular nerves from the diverse sources unite around individual vessels in wide-meshed *perivascular adventitial plexuses*. Fascicles arising from these sink inward to form more delicate plexuses between the adventitial and medial coats, from which nerve fibers originate to ramify in the media and in the zone between the media and intima. Subsidiary perivascular plexuses extend along the vessel branches and are augmented at intervals by branchlets from nearby cranial or spinal nerves, which contain autonomic fibers. Thus innervation is segmental rather than longitudinal, and only relatively short lengths of arteries can be denervated by the removal of adventitial cuffs.

Most cranial and spinal nerves contain efferent and afferent vascular fibers. The oculomotor (III), trigeminal (V), facial (VII), vagus (X), glossopharyngeal (IX), phrenic, ulnar, median, pudendal, and tibial nerves contain relatively large numbers of vascular fibers. Accordingly, lesions involving these nerves are more likely to produce vasomotor and other autonomic disturbances. Vascular disorders are usually more evident

in peripheral arteries and arterioles (like those in the fingers and toes) and in arteriovenous anastomoses because they have thicker muscular layers and a richer innervation than larger arteries, which have more elastic tissue in their walls. Arteries supplying erectile tissues and the skin are also richly innervated, whereas the nerve supply to veins and venules is comparatively sparse. Nerve fibers are often associated with capillaries, but their functions are unknown.

CAROTID SINUS AND CAROTID BODY

The carotid sinus is a dilation at the beginning of the internal carotid artery; the tunica media is thin, and adventitia are thicker with multiple terminations of the glossopharyngeal nerve. The carotid sinus contains baroreceptors, which play an important role in the control of intracranial blood pressure. The carotid body is a small reddish-brown structure behind the bifurcation of the common carotid artery and is a chemoreceptor.

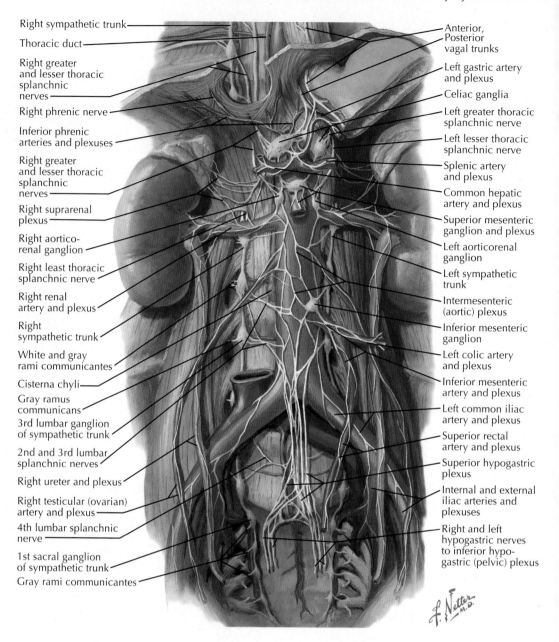

Right sympathetic trunk

Thoracic duct

Right greater and lesser thoracic splanchnic nerves

Right phrenic nerve

Inferior phrenic arteries and plexuses

Right greater and lesser thoracic splanchnic nerves

Right suprarenal plexus

Right aortico-renal ganglion

Right least thoracic splanchnic nerve

Right renal artery and plexus

Right sympathetic trunk

White and gray rami communicantes

Cisterna chyli

Gray ramus communicans

3rd lumbar ganglion of sympathetic trunk

2nd and 3rd lumbar splanchnic nerves

Right ureter and plexus

Right testicular (ovarian) artery and plexus

4th lumbar splanchnic nerve

1st sacral ganglion of sympathetic trunk

Gray rami communicantes

Anterior, Posterior vagal trunks

Left gastric artery and plexus

Celiac ganglia

Left greater thoracic splanchnic nerve

Left lesser thoracic splanchnic nerve

Splenic artery and plexus

Common hepatic artery and plexus

Superior mesenteric ganglion and plexus

Left aorticorenal ganglion

Left sympathetic trunk

Intermesenteric (aortic) plexus

Inferior mesenteric ganglion

Left colic artery and plexus

Inferior mesenteric artery and plexus

Left common iliac artery and plexus

Superior rectal artery and plexus

Superior hypogastric plexus

Internal and external iliac arteries and plexuses

Right and left hypogastric nerves to inferior hypogastric (pelvic) plexus

AUTONOMIC NERVES AND GANGLIA IN ABDOMEN

There are more sympathetic nerves in the abdomen and pelvis than anywhere else because these cavities contain the major parts of the digestive and urogenital systems, the adrenal glands, and the extensive peritoneum.

The abdominal sympathetic nerves include the lumbar parts of the sympathetic trunks and their branches and contribute to the celiac, mesenteric, intermesenteric (abdominal aortic), hepatic, renal, adrenal, superior hypogastric, and other plexuses, including all subsidiary plexuses. Apart from the lumbar sympathetic trunks and branches, however, all the autonomic plexuses mentioned contain both sympathetic and parasympathetic elements.

The lumbar parts of the sympathetic trunks are directly continuous above with their thoracic counterparts behind the medial arcuate ligaments, whereas below they pass over the pelvic brim and behind the common iliac vessels to become the sacral parts of the sympathetic trunks. The trunks lie in the retroperitoneal connective tissue on the anterolateral aspect of the lumbar vertebrae, along the medial margins of the psoas muscles; the right trunk is partly overlapped by the inferior vena cava and the cisterna chyli, and the left trunk is just lateral to the abdominal aorta. There are usually four lumbar ganglia on each side; the intervening cords may be single or split into two or even three strands. Each trunk supplies or receives communicating, visceral, vascular, muscular, osseous, and articular branches.

Only the upper two or, occasionally, three lumbar spinal nerves contribute white rami communicantes to the adjacent lumbar trunk ganglia, but every lumbar

spinal nerve receives one or more gray communicating rami from adjacent trunk ganglia. White rami contain preganglionic and visceral afferent fibers, whereas gray rami contain vasomotor, sudomotor, and pilomotor fibers, which are distributed with the lumbar spinal nerves.

Three or four lumbar splanchnic nerves arise on each side and are seldom arranged symmetrically. The *first lumbar splanchnic nerve* arises from the first lumbar ganglion and ends in the renal, celiac, and/or intermesenteric plexuses, but some fibers may end directly in the duodenum, pancreas, and gastroesophageal junction. The *second lumbar splanchnic nerve* arises from the second lumbar ganglion and ends mainly in the intermesenteric plexus, although it may give direct contributions to the renal plexus, duodenum, and pancreas. The *third lumbar splanchnic nerve* usually originates from the third and fourth ganglia and ends in the upper part of the superior hypogastric plexus. The *fourth lumbar splanchnic nerve*, when present, arises from the fourth and/or the inconstant fifth lumbar ganglion and joins the lower part of the

superior hypogastric plexus or the homolateral hypogastric nerve; it communicates with the ureteric and testicular plexuses.

Vascular fibers from the lumbar sympathetic trunks and their lumbar splanchnic branches pass to the abdominal aorta and the inferior vena cava, where they form the delicate intermesenteric and caval plexuses. All the aortic branches and vena caval tributaries are surrounded by subsidiary plexuses continuous with those around the parent vessels. Twigs from the right sympathetic trunk also supply the cisterna chyli and the commencement of the thoracic duct. Nerve fibers from the renal plexus, sometimes reinforced by fascicles from the second and third lumbar splanchnic nerves, usually join the plexus around the common or external iliac arteries.

Muscular, osseous, and articular fibers supply the adjacent muscles, vertebrae, and joints in the lumbar region. They contain postganglionic (efferent) fibers, which are possibly vasomotor, and afferent fibers conveying impulses from meningeal, bony, and articular structures.

Plate 7.14

Autonomic Nervous System and Its Disorders

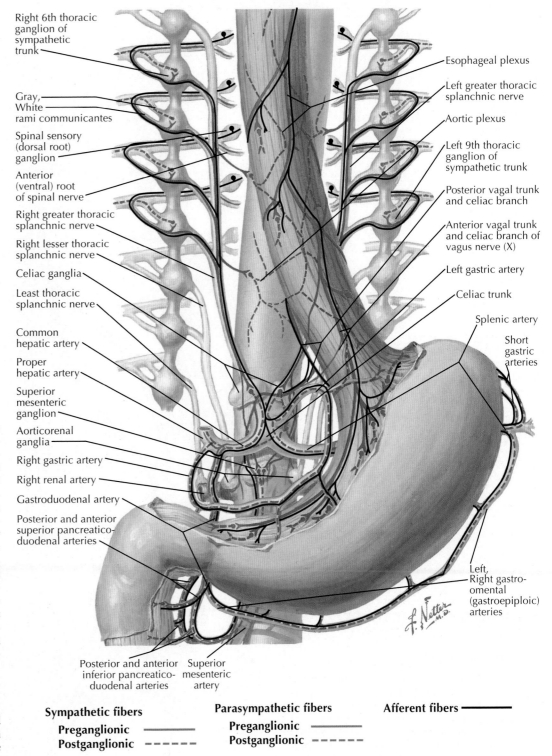

Right 6th thoracic ganglion of sympathetic trunk

Gray, White rami communicantes

Spinal sensory (dorsal root) ganglion

Anterior (ventral) root of spinal nerve

Right greater thoracic splanchnic nerve

Right lesser thoracic splanchnic nerve

Celiac ganglia

Least thoracic splanchnic nerve

Common hepatic artery

Proper hepatic artery

Superior mesenteric ganglion

Aorticorenal ganglia

Right gastric artery

Right renal artery

Gastroduodenal artery

Posterior and anterior superior pancreatico-duodenal arteries

Esophageal plexus

Left greater thoracic splanchnic nerve

Aortic plexus

Left 9th thoracic ganglion of sympathetic trunk

Posterior vagal trunk and celiac branch

Anterior vagal trunk and celiac branch of vagus nerve (X)

Left gastric artery

Celiac trunk

Splenic artery

Short gastric arteries

Left, Right gastro-omental (gastroepiploic) arteries

Posterior and anterior inferior pancreatico-duodenal arteries

Superior mesenteric artery

Sympathetic fibers
Preganglionic ———
Postganglionic - - - - -

Parasympathetic fibers
Preganglionic ———
Postganglionic - - - - -

Afferent fibers ———

INNERVATION OF STOMACH AND PROXIMAL DUODENUM

SYMPATHETIC FIBERS

The gastric sympathetic preganglionic fibers are the axons of cells located in the intermediolateral cell columns of the sixth to ninth or tenth thoracic spinal segments. They reach the celiac plexus via the *sympathetic trunk ganglia* and the *greater (major)* and *lesser (minor) thoracic splanchnic nerves*. Some of the fibers form synapses in trunk ganglia, but most continue through them to end in synapses within the *celiac* and *superior mesenteric ganglia*. The resulting postganglionic fibers may run in fascicles ending directly in the stomach and duodenum, but the majority are conveyed to their destinations in the *perivascular plexuses* along the various branches of the celiac trunk. These plexuses are composed mainly of sympathetic fibers, but they also contain parasympathetic fibers derived from the celiac branches of the vagal trunks. The sympathetic postganglionic fibers traverse the intramural enteric ganglia without relaying and are distributed mainly to the gastric musculature and blood vessels.

PARASYMPATHETIC FIBERS

The two *vagus nerves* form an *esophageal plexus* around the lower esophagus, which is reinforced by twigs from the *thoracic parts* of the *sympathetic trunks* and from the *greater (major)* and *lesser (minor) thoracic splanchnic nerves*. Before reaching the diaphragm, the meshes of the esophageal plexus are reconstituted to form *anterior* and *posterior vagal trunks*. In general, more fibers from the left vagus enter the anterior trunk, whereas the posterior trunk contains more fibers from the right vagus, although the anatomic relationships are highly variable. The vagal trunks give off gastric, pyloric, hepatic, and celiac branches.

Anterior and *posterior gastric branches* supply the corresponding surfaces of the stomach. They run between the layers of the lesser omentum and give off branches that radiate over the surfaces of the stomach and can be traced for some distance in the subperitoneal tissue before they sink into muscle coats; no definite anterior or posterior gastric plexuses exist. Often, one branch on both the anterior and posterior aspects is larger than the others—the *greater anterior* and *greater posterior gastric nerves*. *Pyloric branches* arise from the anterior vagal trunk or its greater anterior gastric branch and supply the pyloric antrum, pylorus, and superior (first) part of the duodenum. *Hepatic branches* are provided by both vagal trunks; that from the anterior trunk arises near the gastric cardiac ostium and is called the *hepatogastric nerve* because it supplies offshoots to the hepatic plexus and stomach (there may be more than one hepatogastric nerve). The hepatic contribution from the posterior vagal trunk usually reaches the hepatic plexus through its celiac branch. Both vagal trunks give off *celiac branches,* and the posterior branch is larger than the anterior. All efferent (preganglionic) vagal fibers ending in the stomach make synaptic contacts with ganglionic neurons in the gastric parts of the *myenteric* and *submucous plexuses;* the resulting postganglionic fibers are distributed to the gastric musculature, glands, and vessels, where they exert both motor and secretory effects (see Plate 7.17).

AFFERENT FIBERS

Afferent parasympathetic and sympathetic fibers pursue reverse routes to those described for vagal and sympathetic efferent fibers.

INNERVATION OF THE INTESTINE

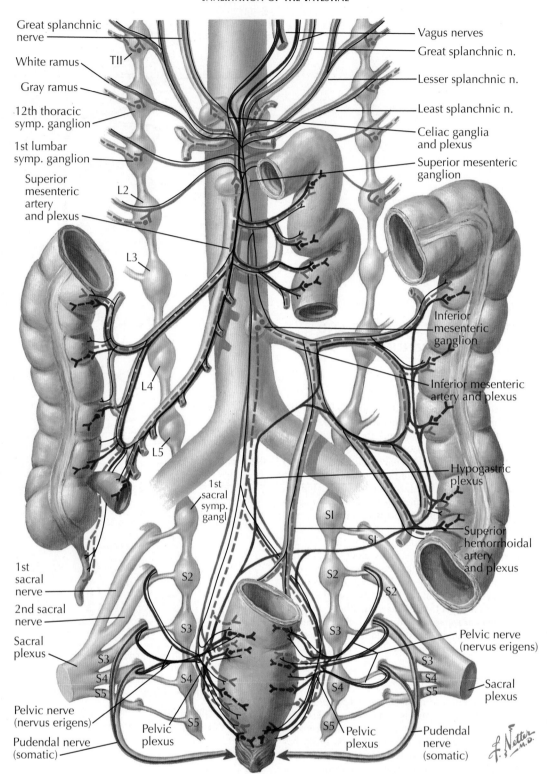

Great splanchnic nerve
White ramus
Gray ramus
12th thoracic symp. ganglion
1st lumbar symp. ganglion
Superior mesenteric artery and plexus
TII
L2
L3
L4
L5
1st sacral symp. gangl
1st sacral nerve
2nd sacral nerve
Sacral plexus
Pelvic nerve (nervus erigens)
Pudendal nerve (somatic)
S3
S4
S5
Pelvic plexus
S5

Vagus nerves
Great splanchnic n.
Lesser splanchnic n.
Least splanchnic n.
Celiac ganglia and plexus
Superior mesenteric ganglion
Inferior mesenteric ganglion
Inferior mesenteric artery and plexus
Hypogastric plexus
Superior hemorrhoidal artery and plexus
SI
SI
S2
S2
S3
S4
S5
Pelvic nerve (nervus erigens)
Sacral plexus
Pudendal nerve (somatic)
Pelvic plexus

INNERVATION OF INTESTINES

SYMPATHETIC FIBERS

The preganglionic sympathetic fibers to the intestines are the axons of intermediolateral cells located in the lowest four or five thoracic and upper two lumbar spinal segments. Some form synapses in the *sympathetic trunk ganglia,* but most are conveyed in the *thoracic, lumbar,* and *sacral splanchnic nerves* to the celiac, mesenteric, and hypogastric plexuses, where they relay. From the celiac and superior mesenteric plexuses, an unknown proportion of fibers descend in the *intermesenteric* and *hypogastric nerves* to the inferior mesenteric and hypogastric plexuses. Postganglionic fibers from ganglionic synapses, along with afferent and preganglionic parasympathetic fibers, are carried to the intestines in branches of the various plexuses.

The *parasympathetic supply* to the intestines is derived from the vagus and pelvic splanchnic nerves. The *vagal* contributions pass to the celiac plexus in the *larger* and *smaller celiac branches* arising, respectively, from the *posterior* and *anterior vagal trunks.* Some fibers are distributed with branches of the *celiac plexus* to the stomach and duodenum (see Plate 7.14), but others descend to the *superior mesenteric plexus.* They comprise efferent

(preganglionic) and afferent fibers and innervate the small intestines and the colon almost to the left colic flexure. Parasympathetic fibers follow the same routes to the intestines as sympathetic postganglionic fibers but are still preganglionic and end by forming synapses in the enteric plexuses (see Plate 7.17).

The *pelvic splanchnic nerves* arise from the second, third, and fourth sacral nerves. They contain parasympathetic preganglionic and afferent fibers, which

include those supplying the distal end of the transverse colon and left colic flexure, the descending and sigmoid colons, and the rectum. They join the *inferior hypogastric (pelvic) plexuses* and are distributed with their branches. The preganglionic intestinal fibers pass through the ganglia in these plexuses without relaying; like their vagal counterparts, they end by making synaptic contacts in the *enteric plexuses.* Some branches pass directly to the rectum and lower end of the

Plate 7.16

Autonomic Nervous System and Its Disorders

AUTONOMIC INNERVATION OF SMALL INTESTINE

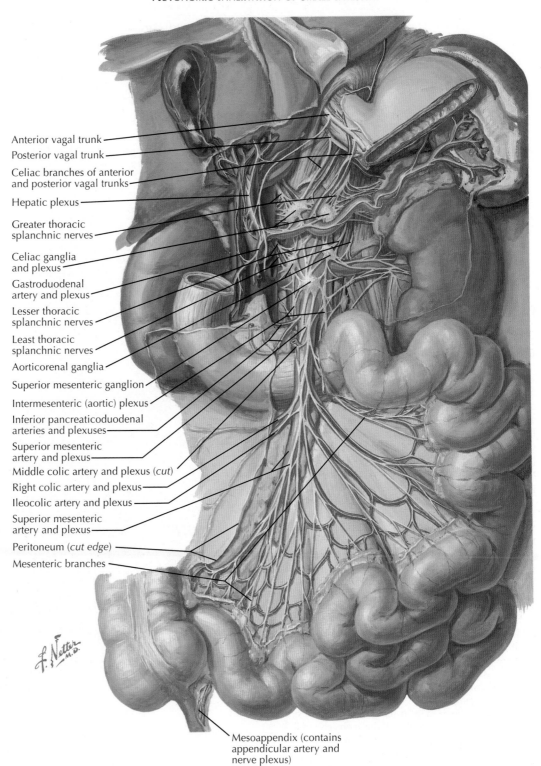

Anterior vagal trunk

Posterior vagal trunk

Celiac branches of anterior and posterior vagal trunks

Hepatic plexus

Greater thoracic splanchnic nerves

Celiac ganglia and plexus

Gastroduodenal artery and plexus

Lesser thoracic splanchnic nerves

Least thoracic splanchnic nerves

Aorticorenal ganglia

Superior mesenteric ganglion

Intermesenteric (aortic) plexus

Inferior pancreaticoduodenal arteries and plexuses

Superior mesenteric artery and plexus

Middle colic artery and plexus (cut)

Right colic artery and plexus

Ileocolic artery and plexus

Superior mesenteric artery and plexus

Peritoneum (cut edge)

Mesenteric branches

Mesoappendix (contains appendicular artery and nerve plexus)

INNERVATION OF INTESTINES (Continued)

sigmoid colon, others accompany rectal and colic vessels, and still others may ascend in the *hypogastric nerves* to the *superior hypogastric plexus* and then to the *inferior mesenteric plexus,* to be distributed with its branches to the distal parts of the colon. However, the majority of the parasympathetic fibers for these parts of the colon pursue a different course: they arise by several filaments from the *pelvic splanchnic nerves* or the *inferior hypogastric plexuses* and run upward across the sigmoid and left colic vessels. They can be traced as far as the left colic flexure, and they supply offshoots to the adjacent parts of the sigmoid and descending colons and communicate with branches of the inferior mesenteric plexus.

Afferent pathways, in general, follow (in reverse direction) both the sympathetic and the parasympathetic supplies to the small and large bowel. The afferent components of the vagus and pelvic nerves and of the sympathetic pathways subserve reflex activity, but most localized sensations referable to the gastrointestinal tract appear to be mediated through the sympathetic afferents.

At the anorectal junction, the autonomic innervation gives way to somatic innervation.

AUTONOMIC NERVOUS SYSTEM ROLE IN GUT MOTILITY

The enteric nervous system (ENS) is a complex network of neurons and nerve fibers located within the gut wall that consists of the two ganglionic strata: the myenteric (Auerbach) plexus, between the two layers of the external muscle, and the submucosal (Meissner) plexus, which extends from the esophagus to the anal canal and is responsible for peristaltic activity, secretion of mucosal glands, vasoconstriction and vasodilation, water absorption, and electrolyte balance. The parasympathetic and sympathetic fibers exert external regulatory influences on the ENS. The cholinergic terminals of the parasympathetic system, acting on the smooth muscles of the small and large intestine and also via the enteric plexuses, cause increased motility of the intestine and increased secretory activity of the glands. Postganglionic fibers of the sympathetic nervous system release norepinephrine, causing decreased motility.

ENTERIC PLEXUSES

Enteric plexuses exist within the walls of the alimentary tract, from the esophagus to the rectum. They form microscopic networks and consist of bundles of nerve fibers (axons) and dendrites, which link ganglia located chiefly at nodal points in the meshes. These networks are most evident between the layers of the muscle coats (myenteric, or Auerbach, plexus) and in the submucosa (submucosal, or Meissner, plexus). Tenuous subserous plexuses with sparsely disposed nerve cells are present in those parts of the gastrointestinal tract that possess peritoneal coverings.

The *myenteric (Auerbach) plexus* is relatively coarse, with thicker meshes and larger ganglia. The main, or primary, meshes give off fascicles that form secondary networks in the interstices of the primary networks. These, in turn, split into minute bundles of fibers that ramify between the muscle tunics and supply them. The *submucosal (Meissner) plexus* is more delicate, and its meshes are more irregular. Its delicate offshoots mostly end in relation to cells forming the muscularis mucosae or form rarefied periglandular plexuses, whereas other offshoots end in almost invisible subepithelial plexuses.

The patterns and densities of these plexuses vary in different parts of the alimentary tract. They are less well defined in the upper part of the esophagus but are well developed from the stomach to the lower end of the rectum. The ganglia are not uniformly distributed. The density of ganglionic cells in the plexuses is lowest in the esophagus, rises steeply in the stomach until it reaches a peak at the pylorus, falls to an intermediate level throughout the small intestines, and gradually increases along the colon to reach another, lesser peak in the rectum.

The extrinsic nerves involved contain *efferent* and *afferent sympathetic* and *parasympathetic fibers* derived from thoracic, lumbar, and sacral branches of the sympathetic trunks and from the vagus and pelvic splanchnic nerves. Most of the sympathetic efferent fibers entering the enteric plexuses are postganglionic, whereas parasympathetic efferent fibers are still preganglionic. The vagal fibers form synapses with ganglion cells located in the enteric plexuses, from the esophagus to the distal third of the transverse colon; below this level, the preganglionic parasympathetic fibers are carried in branches of the pelvic splanchnic

nerves. Thus in this as in other situations, the parasympathetic postganglionic fibers are very much shorter than their sympathetic counterparts.

Many interconnections exist between the myenteric and submucosal plexuses. In general, the former are mainly concerned with the innervation of the muscle layers in the visceral walls, whereas the latter are chiefly involved with supplying the glands and muscularis mucosae and in forming delicate subepithelial plexuses. The enteric plexuses and their subdivisions are also

responsible for supplying adjacent vessels and transmitting sensory impulses. The sympathetic innervation is primarily inhibitory to peristalsis and stimulatory to the sphincters, whereas the parasympathetic innervation is the opposite.

Afferent fibers from the alimentary tract are conveyed to the CNS through the same sympathetic and parasympathetic nerves that carry the corresponding efferent fibers. There is also evidence that local reflex arcs exist.

Peritoneal layers of mesentery

Branch of straight artery (arteriae rectae) to intestine and accompanying nerves

Subserous plexus

Longitudinal intramuscular plexus

Myenteric (Auerbach) plexus

Circular intramuscular plexus

Submucosal (Meissner) plexus

Periglandular plexus

Visceral peritoneum (serosa)

Subserous connective tissue

Longitudinal muscle

Intermuscular stroma

Circular muscle

Submucosa

Submucosal glands

Muscularis mucosae

Mucosa and intestinal glands

Lumen

Note: Intestinal wall is shown much thicker than in actuality.

Myenteric (Auerbach) plexus lying on longitudinal muscle coat. Fine tertiary bundles crossing meshes (duodenum of guinea pig, Champy-Coujard, osmic stain, ×20).

Submucous plexus (Meissner) (ascending colon of guinea pig. Stained by gold impregnation, ×20).

Group of multipolar neurons, type II, in ganglion of myenteric (Auerbach) plexus (ileum of cat; Bielschowsky silver stain, ×200)

Pseudounipolar neuron within ganglion of myenteric plexus (ileum of cat; Bielschowsky silver stain ×375)

Plate 7.18

Autonomic Nervous System and Its Disorders

INNERVATION OF LIVER AND BILIARY TRACT

The liver, biliary tract, and gallbladder receive their nerve supplies from sympathetic and parasympathetic sources. The *preganglionic sympathetic fibers* originate mainly in the seventh to tenth thoracic segments and pass to the celiac plexus via the sympathetic trunk ganglia and the greater and lesser thoracic splanchnic nerves (see Plates 7.13 and 7.14). Most of the fibers form synapses in the celiac ganglia, although some may relay in small ganglia located in the porta hepatis. The *postganglionic sympathetic fibers* reach the liver in the hepatic plexuses, which also contain parasympathetic and afferent fibers. The *parasympathetic supply* is provided by branches of the vagal trunks.

Afferent fibers from the liver and biliary tract are conveyed through the hepatic and celiac plexuses to the *thoracic splanchnic nerves* or to branches of the *vagus nerves.* The sympathetic afferents reach the seventh to twelfth thoracic spinal cord segments through the corresponding posterior spinal nerve roots, whereas the vagal afferents are carried upward to the brainstem. The right, and possibly the left, phrenic nerve also conveys afferents from receptors in the peritoneal lining over the liver and biliary tract, which can be stimulated by stretching, such as by acute hepatic enlargement or distention of the gallbladder. The resultant pain in the right shoulder region associated with liver and biliary tract disorders is an example of referred pain.

LIVER

The *hepatic plexuses* lie in the right free margin of the lesser omentum anterior to the epiploic (omental) foramen. They are formed mainly by offshoots from the *celiac plexus,* which contain sympathetic and parasympathetic efferent and afferent fibers, supplemented by direct contributions from the *anterior vagal trunk* and by indirect contributions from the *right phrenic nerve.* They are arranged in two interconnected groups, one of which lies along the anterior and lateral sides of the hepatic artery and the other posterior to the common bile duct and portal vein.

Subsidiary plexuses surround and accompany the branches of the hepatic artery, portal vein, and right and left hepatic ducts as they enter and ramify within the liver; their offshoots penetrate between the cells of the liver lobules to form a widespread *parenchymal plexus.* Histochemical studies reveal that the nerve fibers in relation to the hepatocytes and sinusoids are parasympathetic, whereas sympathetic fibers remain mainly or entirely associated with vessels in the interlobular spaces. Direct contacts between the terminations of nerve fibers and liver cells have been observed in electron micrographs.

GALLBLADDER

The gallbladder is supplied by perivascular nerve fibers accompanying the right hepatic and cystic arteries from

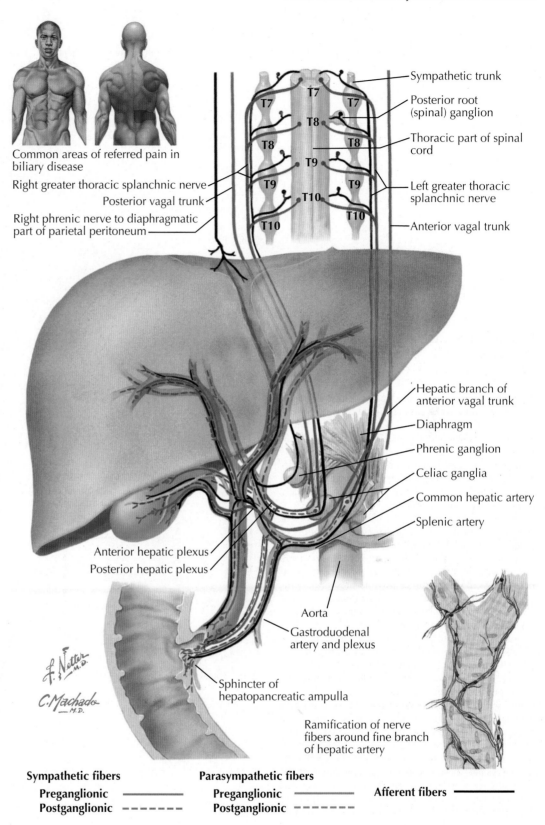

Common areas of referred pain in biliary disease

Right greater thoracic splanchnic nerve
Posterior vagal trunk
Right phrenic nerve to diaphragmatic part of parietal peritoneum

Sympathetic trunk
Posterior root (spinal) ganglion
Thoracic part of spinal cord
Left greater thoracic splanchnic nerve
Anterior vagal trunk

T7 T7 T7
T8 T8
T8 T8
T9 T9
T9 T10 T9
T10 T10

Hepatic branch of anterior vagal trunk
Diaphragm
Phrenic ganglion
Celiac ganglia
Common hepatic artery
Splenic artery

Anterior hepatic plexus
Posterior hepatic plexus

Aorta
Gastroduodenal artery and plexus

Sphincter of hepatopancreatic ampulla

Ramification of nerve fibers around fine branch of hepatic artery

Sympathetic fibers
Preganglionic ————
Postganglionic --------

Parasympathetic fibers
Preganglionic ————
Postganglionic --------

Afferent fibers ————

the *anterior hepatic plexus* and by other nerve fibers extending along the cystic duct from the *posterior hepatic plexus.* The common bile duct (choledochal duct) is supplied by twigs from both anterior and posterior hepatic plexuses and by offshoots from the plexus around the gastroduodenal artery and its retroduodenal branches. The arrangement of the nerves within the walls of these structures resembles that in the enteric plexuses.

Both the sphincter ampullae and the sphincter of the choledochal duct are supplied by sympathetic and parasympathetic fibers. The former normally cause contraction of the sphincters and dilation of the gallbladder, whereas the latter produce the opposite effects.

Anterior vagal trunk / Celiac plexus and ganglia
Right greater thoracic splanchnic nerve / Posterior vagal trunk / Left greater thoracic splanchnic nerve
Right phrenic nerve / Left phrenic nerve
Right inferior phrenic artery and plexus / Left inferior phrenic artery and plexus
Right adrenal (suprarenal) gland / Left adrenal (suprarenal) gland
Right lesser thoracic splanchnic nerve / Left lesser thoracic splanchnic nerve
Right least thoracic splanchnic nerve / Aorticorenal ganglia
Right renal ganglion and plexus / Left least thoracic splanchnic nerve
Left renal ganglion and plexus
Left sympathetic trunk
Right sympathetic trunk / Left 1st lumbar splanchnic nerve
Right 1st lumbar splanchnic nerve / Superior mesenteric ganglion

Intermediolateral cell column (lateral horn of gray matter)
T10 / T11 / T12 / L1
Greater thoracic splanchnic nerve (preganglionic fibers) / Celiac ganglion
Postganglionic fibers supply blood vessels / Medulla / Cortex
Spinal cord / Sympathetic trunk
Preganglionic fibers ramify around cells of medulla
Adrenal (suprarenal) gland

INNERVATION OF ADRENAL GLANDS

The adrenal (suprarenal) glands show a high degree of species variation, which also applies to their nerve supplies. The cortex and medulla differ in their development. The *medullary (chromaffin) cells* are modified migrant neuroblasts from the neural crest and are homologous with ganglion cells in the sympathetic trunks. Accordingly, they are innervated directly by preganglionic fibers. Relative to their size, the adrenal medullae are more richly innervated than any other viscus.

The *preganglionic sympathetic fibers* are the axons of cells located in the intermediolateral gray columns of mainly the lower three or four thoracic and upper one or two lumbar segments of the spinal cord. They emerge in the anterior rootlets of the corresponding spinal nerves, pass in white rami communicantes to the sympathetic trunks, and leave them in the thoracic and first lumbar splanchnic nerves that run to the celiac, aorticorenal, and renal ganglia. Some of the fibers conveying impulses for the adrenal vessels may relay in these ganglia, but the majority continue onward to enter the adrenal branches of the celiac plexus.

Some of the *parasympathetic fibers* reaching the celiac plexus through the vagal trunks may be concerned with adrenal innervation and may relay in small ganglia near or in the glands, but as yet no definite proof of this hypothesis exists. The adrenal parasympathetic supply may well emerge via posterior spinal nerve root efferents, which enter the thoracic splanchnic nerves and thereafter follow the same routes as the sympathetic preganglionic fibers; however, the existence of such posterior root efferents is still unproven. A proportion of the fibers in the adrenal nerves may be afferent and enter the spinal cord through the ninth to eleventh thoracic spinal nerves.

ADRENAL NERVES

Numerous fine nerves pass outward to each gland from the *celiac plexus* and *ganglia*. They are joined by contributions from the terminations of the *greater* and *lesser thoracic splanchnic nerves,* and they communicate with the ipsilateral *phrenic nerve* and *renal plexus*.

Many nerve fibers from the adrenal nerves enter the gland through its hilus and medial margin. Other nerve fibers spread out over the gland to form a delicate *subcapsular plexus* from which fascicles penetrate the cortex to run alongside arterioles in the trabeculae to the medulla. The majority of nerve fibers entering the gland end in the medulla, where they ramify profusely and give off fibers that mostly terminate in synaptic-type contacts with the chromaffin cells. As already stated, these are the homologues of ganglion cells in the sympathetic trunks. Some fibers invaginate the cell membranes deeply but do not penetrate them. A minority of fibers innervate the medullary arterioles and the central vein, which has an unusually thick muscle coat.

Multipolar or bipolar neurons, singly or in small groups, have been noted within the adrenal medullae. Their significance and the destinations of their axons have not yet been determined, although it is assumed that the cells are the final relay stations in the parasympathetic pathways.

Plate 7.20

Autonomic Nervous System and Its Disorders

AUTONOMIC NERVES AND GANGLIA IN PELVIS

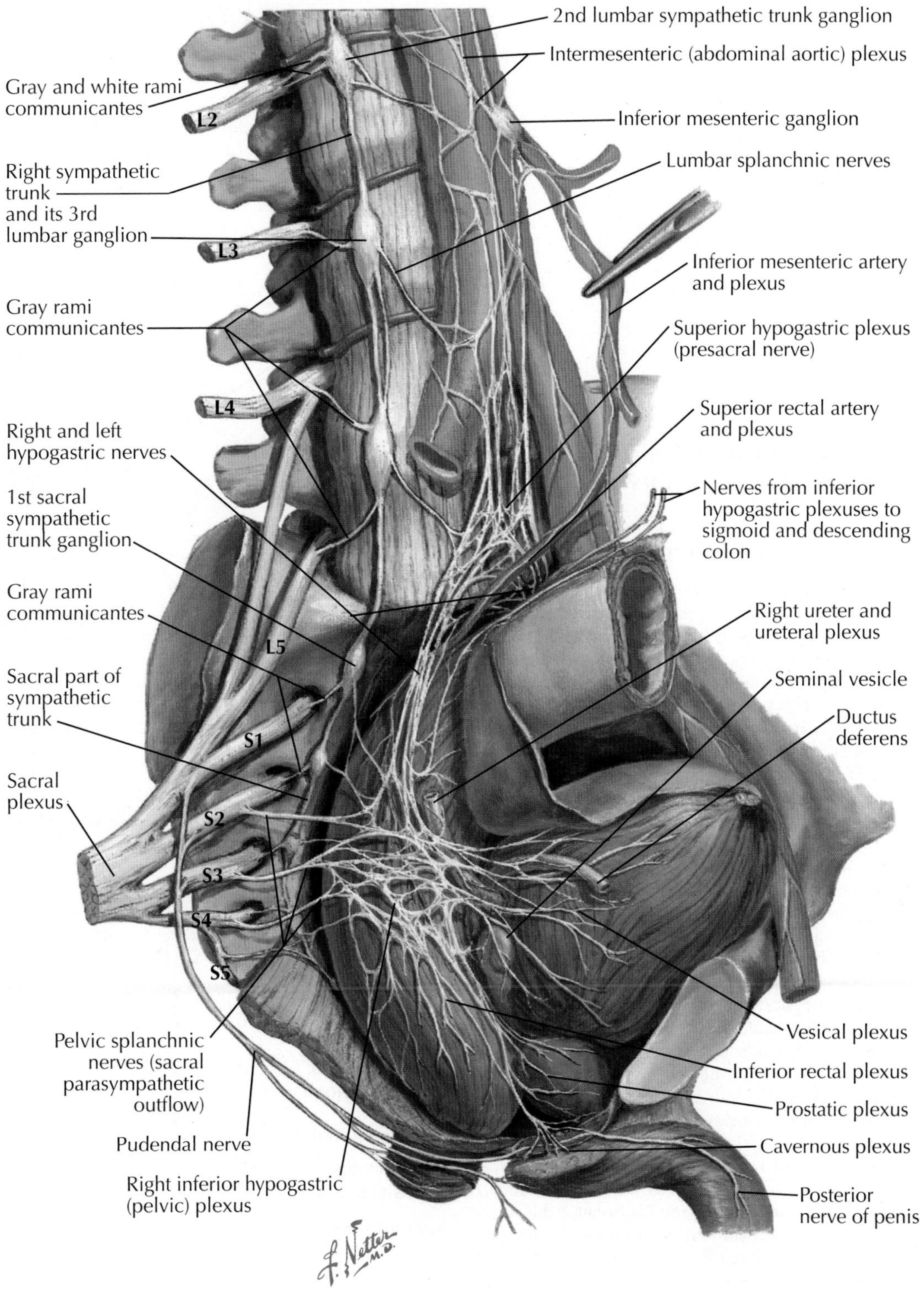

Sympathetic fibers reach the pelvis through the sympathetic trunks and the superior hypogastric plexus and in visceral and vascular nerves accompanying and supplying such structures as the colon, ureters, and the inferior mesenteric and common iliac vessels. *Parasympathetic fibers* emerge in the anterior roots of the second, third, and sometimes fourth sacral spinal nerves and leave them in the slender bilateral pelvic splanchnic nerves (nervi erigentes) that join the corresponding inferior hypogastric (pelvic) plexuses and are distributed with their branches.

SYMPATHETIC FIBERS

The lumbar and sacral parts of the sympathetic trunks are directly continuous at the level of the pelvic brim. The sacral trunks lie in the pelvic fascia behind the parietal peritoneum and rectum and on the anterior surface of the sacrum, just medial to its anterior foramina and the nerves and vessels passing through them. Below, they converge and unite in a single tiny "ganglion impar" anterior to the coccyx. In general, four, or sometimes three, sacral trunk ganglia exist on each side. No white rami communicantes are present in this region, but each ganglion supplies one or more gray rami communicantes containing postganglionic sympathetic fibers to the adjoining sacral and coccygeal spinal nerves; these fibers are conveyed in branches of the sacral and coccygeal plexuses to vessels, sweat glands, arrectores pilorum muscles, striated muscles, bones, and joints.

The pelvic sympathetic trunk ganglia also supply slender rami, the *sacral splanchnic nerves*, which pass to the inferior hypogastric plexuses. The majority of sympathetic fibers, however, reach these plexuses through the *right* and *left hypogastric nerves*, formed just below the level of the lumbosacral junction by the splitting of the median superior hypogastric plexus (often misleadingly referred to as the "presacral nerve"; a single nerve is very rare). Similarly, the right and left hypogastric nerves are more often elongated plexuses consisting of several nerves interconnected by oblique strands, which incline downward on each side, behind the peritoneum and lateral to the sigmoid colon and rectosigmoid junction, to end in the upper parts of the homolateral inferior hypogastric plexus.

The *inferior hypogastric plexuses* are situated on each side of the rectum and the lower part of the bladder, prostate, and seminal vesicles. In females, the cervix of the uterus and vaginal fornices replace the prostate gland and seminal vesicles as medial relations. The

plexuses supply branches to the pelvic viscera and genitalia and often form subsidiary plexuses (such as the rectal, prostatic, and vesical). The branches contain visceral, glandular, vascular, and afferent fibers, often combined in the nerve fascicles supplying the various structures concerned (see Plates 7.21 to 7.24). The *sympathetic efferent fibers* in these branches, like those in the gray rami communicantes connecting the ganglia of the pelvic sympathetic trunks to the sacral and coccygeal spinal nerves, are almost entirely postganglionic because most or all of the sympathetic preganglionic fibers involved in the supply of pelvic, perineal, gluteal,

and lower limb structures relay in lumbar and sacral trunk ganglia; a minority may form synapses in ganglia within the inferior hypogastric plexuses.

The *parasympathetic fibers* in the *pelvic splanchnic nerves*, which arise from the sacral nerves and end in the *inferior hypogastric plexuses*, are preganglionic. Some relay in ganglia within the plexuses, but many more form synapses in ganglia located near or within the walls of the viscera and vessels innervated.

Other branches from the inferior hypogastric plexuses ascend to assist in the innervation of the distal colon and the renal pelvises.

Gray and white rami communicantes

Right sympathetic trunk and its 3rd lumbar ganglion

Gray rami communicantes

Right and left hypogastric nerves

1st sacral sympathetic trunk ganglion

Gray rami communicantes

Sacral part of sympathetic trunk

Sacral plexus

Pelvic splanchnic nerves (sacral parasympathetic outflow)

Pudendal nerve

Right inferior hypogastric (pelvic) plexus

2nd lumbar sympathetic trunk ganglion

Intermesenteric (abdominal aortic) plexus

Inferior mesenteric ganglion

Lumbar splanchnic nerves

Inferior mesenteric artery and plexus

Superior hypogastric plexus (presacral nerve)

Superior rectal artery and plexus

Nerves from inferior hypogastric plexuses to sigmoid and descending colon

Right ureter and ureteral plexus

Seminal vesicle

Ductus deferens

Vesical plexus

Inferior rectal plexus

Prostatic plexus

Cavernous plexus

Posterior nerve of penis

f. Netter m.d.

L2 · L3 · L4 · L5 · S1 · S2 · S3 · S4 · S5

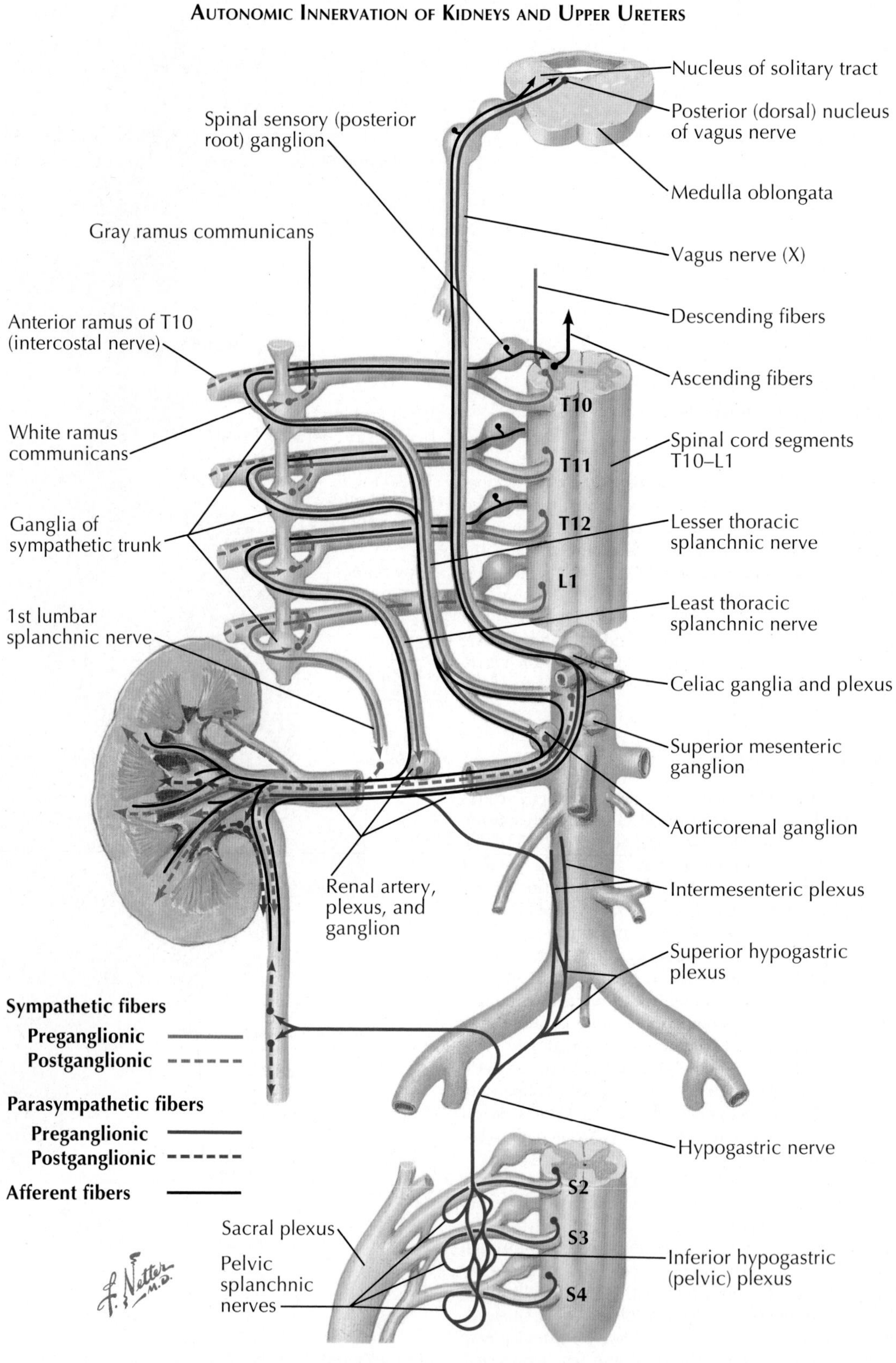

AUTONOMIC INNERVATION OF KIDNEYS AND UPPER URETERS

Labels on illustration:
- Nucleus of solitary tract
- Posterior (dorsal) nucleus of vagus nerve
- Medulla oblongata
- Vagus nerve (X)
- Descending fibers
- Ascending fibers
- Spinal cord segments T10–L1
- Lesser thoracic splanchnic nerve
- Least thoracic splanchnic nerve
- Celiac ganglia and plexus
- Superior mesenteric ganglion
- Aorticorenal ganglion
- Intermesenteric plexus
- Superior hypogastric plexus
- Hypogastric nerve
- Inferior hypogastric (pelvic) plexus
- Spinal sensory (posterior root) ganglion
- Gray ramus communicans
- Anterior ramus of T10 (intercostal nerve)
- White ramus communicans
- Ganglia of sympathetic trunk
- 1st lumbar splanchnic nerve
- Renal artery, plexus, and ganglion
- Sacral plexus
- Pelvic splanchnic nerves
- T10, T11, T12, L1, S2, S3, S4

Sympathetic fibers
Preganglionic ———
Postganglionic - - - -

Parasympathetic fibers
Preganglionic ———
Postganglionic - - - -

Afferent fibers ———

INNERVATION OF KIDNEYS, URETERS, AND URINARY BLADDER

KIDNEY AND UPPER URETER

The *preganglionic sympathetic fibers* for the kidneys and upper ureters emerge from the spinal cord through the anterior nerve roots of the eleventh and twelfth thoracic spinal nerves and, often, the tenth thoracic and first lumbar spinal nerves as well. The fibers then pass in white rami communicantes to adjacent ganglia in the sympathetic trunks. They leave the ganglia in the splanchnic nerves: the lesser, lowest thoracic, first lumbar, and second lumbar. The lesser thoracic splanchnic nerve usually ends in the ipsilateral celiac or aorticorenal ganglia, and the other nerves mentioned may do the same, although they usually end directly in the renal plexus or in the small renal ganglion lying posterior or posterosuperior to the renal artery. Most of the preganglionic fibers form synaptic relays in the aorticorenal or posterior renal ganglia or in smaller ganglia incorporated into the renal plexuses. The *postganglionic sympathetic fibers* form fascicles that surround and accompany the upper ureteric, renal, pelvic, calyceal, and segmental branches of the renal vessels.

Some *parasympathetic fibers* are carried through the vagal contributions to the celiac plexus and are conveyed onward to the kidneys in the renal branches of this plexus; others emerge through the pelvic splanchnic nerves and may reach the renal collecting tubules, renal calyces and renal pelvis, and upper ureter by a more indirect route. Such an arrangement is understandable on embryologic grounds because the structures mentioned are all derived from buds developed from the cloacal ends of the mesonephric (wolffian) ducts. These pelvic parasympathetic fibers join the inferior hypogastric plexuses, ascend in the hypogastric nerves to the superior hypogastric plexus, and exit in fine branches that ascend retroperitoneally to enter the inferolateral parts of the homolateral renal plexus.

Afferent fibers from the kidneys and upper ureter follow similar routes in the reverse direction, but they do not form relays in peripheral ganglia; their cell bodies are located in posterior spinal nerve root ganglia. The central processes of these ganglion cells enter the spinal cord mainly through the posterior nerve roots of the tenth to twelfth thoracic spinal nerves and then ascend in or alongside the spinothalamic tracts and also in the posterior white columns of the cord.

Within the renal hilus and sinus, the *renal plexus* supplies nerve fibers to the renal pelvis, calyces, and upper ureter. Other nerve fibers form rich plexuses around the renal vessels and their branches and accompany them into the kidney. They contain mostly unmyelinated fibers and relatively few of the myelinated type. The *sympathetic fibers* are distributed to the smooth muscle in the renal pelvis and calyces, to the vascular musculature, and possibly to the juxtaglomerular cells and glomeruli. The *parasympathetic fibers* supply the muscle in the pelvis, calyces, and upper ureter, but it is uncertain whether they supply the vessels and tubules. *Sensory nerve endings* have reputedly been detected in the pelvis and ureter, in the adventitia of the larger vessels, and near the glomeruli.

URINARY BLADDER AND LOWER URETER

The *preganglionic sympathetic cells* concerned with vesical innervation are located in the upper two lumbar segments and perhaps also in the lowest thoracic segment of the spinal cord. The sites where the preganglionic fibers form synapses with the ganglionic neurons

Plate 7.22

Autonomic Nervous System and Its Disorders

INNERVATION OF URINARY BLADDER AND LOWER URETER

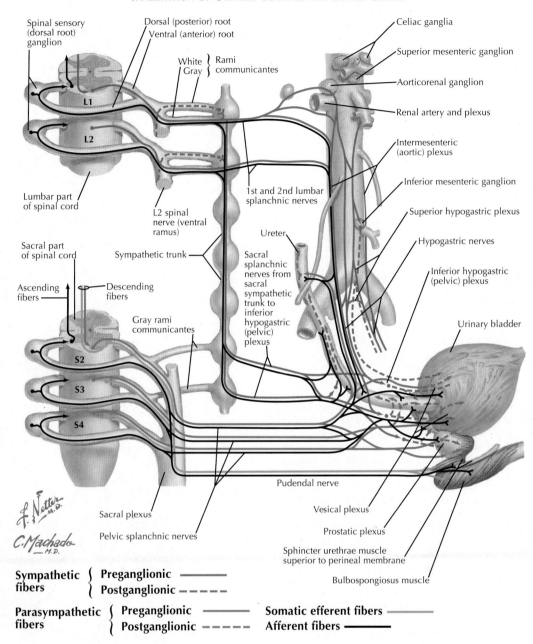

Spinal sensory (dorsal root) ganglion

Dorsal (posterior) root

Ventral (anterior) root

Celiac ganglia

Superior mesenteric ganglion

Aorticorenal ganglion

White } Rami
Gray } communicantes

L1

L2

Renal artery and plexus

Lumbar part of spinal cord

1st and 2nd lumbar splanchnic nerves

Intermesenteric (aortic) plexus

Inferior mesenteric ganglion

L2 spinal nerve (ventral ramus)

Sacral part of spinal cord

Sympathetic trunk

Ureter

Sacral splanchnic nerves from sacral sympathetic trunk to inferior hypogastric (pelvic) plexus

Superior hypogastric plexus

Hypogastric nerves

Inferior hypogastric (pelvic) plexus

Ascending fibers

Descending fibers

Gray rami communicantes

Urinary bladder

S2

S3

S4

Pudendal nerve

Vesical plexus

Prostatic plexus

Sacral plexus

Pelvic splanchnic nerves

Sphincter urethrae muscle superior to perineal membrane

Bulbospongiosus muscle

Sympathetic fibers { Preganglionic ——— / Postganglionic - - - - -

Parasympathetic fibers { Preganglionic ——— / Postganglionic - - - - -

Somatic efferent fibers ———

Afferent fibers ▬▬▬

INNERVATION OF KIDNEYS, URETERS, AND URINARY BLADDER (Continued)

that give off the postganglionic fibers have not been determined accurately. The *preganglionic parasympathetic cells* are located in the second to fourth sacral segments of the spinal cord, and their axons (nervi erigentes) relay in ganglia close to or within the wall of the urinary bladder. The neurons in the anterior gray matter of the sacral spinal cord S1 to S3, the *Onuf nucleus,* provide the motor supply to the external urethral sphincter through the motor branches of the pudendal nerve. *Afferent fibers* pursue similar pathways but in the reverse direction; thus some vesical sensory impulses enter the cord through the upper lumbar and last thoracic posterior nerve roots, whereas others from the neck of the bladder and the lowest parts of the ureters reach the cord via the pelvic splanchnic nerves and the posterior nerve roots of the second to fourth sacral nerve segments.

Many fascicles from the *extrinsic vesical plexuses* enter the bladder wall, mainly alongside its blood vessels. They divide and subdivide and are ultimately carried to all parts, forming a widespread *intramural,* or *intrinsic, vesical plexus.* The nerve fasciculi are most conspicuous in the trigonal and neighboring regions, becoming more scattered and attenuated toward the fundus. Many small ganglia are present on the surface or are buried more deeply between the muscular bundles, and these are more numerous in the trigonal region. Many fibers enter the submucosa and penetrate between the mucosal cells, where they apparently end in small boutons.

Most of the nerve fasciculi in the urinary bladder wall contain unmyelinated or finely myelinated fibers. A small proportion of larger myelinated and, presumably, sensory fibers are connected with terminal arborizations regarded as stretch receptors. Many other putative sensory endings have been described in the submucosa and mucous membrane. The parasympathetic nerves may transmit many or most of the afferent fibers from the trigonal area of the urinary bladder and from the lowest parts of the ureters, including those conveying painful impulses. However, some afferents from the neck of the bladder and prostatic urethra may reach the spinal cord via the pudendal nerves.

Sensations associated with vesical distention may be mediated through sympathetic pathways because vague discomfort may still be experienced by patients with transverse lesions of the cord below the level of the uppermost lumbar segments. This suggests that there is an afferent inflow from the bladder through the upper lumbar or lowest thoracic posterior spinal nerve roots. Alternatively, such sensations may be produced by the stimulation of nerve endings in the peritoneum over a distended bladder. However, presacral neurectomy

(removal of the superior hypogastric plexus) rarely completely alleviates discomfort in patients with painful and intractable cystitis because only a proportion of the vesical afferent fibers traverse the hypogastric nerves and superior hypogastric plexus. Other afferent fibers traveling in the perivascular plexuses of the vesical and iliac arteries may also reach the superior hypogastric plexus. Beyond the plexus, the fibers run in lumbar splanchnic nerves to the sympathetic trunks, pass through rami communicantes to the upper lumbar and lowest thoracic spinal nerves, and enter the spinal cord through the posterior roots of these nerves.

The parasympathetic supply to the bladder produces contraction of the walls and relaxation of the sphincteric mechanism and is thus actively involved in micturition. Many credit the sympathetic supply with opposing effects, such as relaxation of the detrusor muscles of the vesical wall by activation of β-adrenergic receptors and contraction of the internal sphincter by activation of α-adrenergic receptors. However, the

sympathetic nervous system may play a minor role in bladder function, and the preponderance of evidence suggests that human bladder function depends on the integrity of the parasympathetic and somatic motor innervation of the bladder.

There are multiple interactive reflex arcs that are important in the volitional control of the bladder. The first is a connection between the posteromedial frontal lobe to the pontine nuclei via the basal ganglia. Lesions of this loop result in detrusor hyperreflexia and failure of volitional suppression of the detrusor reflex. The second reflex arc extends from the pontine nuclei to the motor neurons of the sacral region that innervate the bladder; again, interruption results in detrusor hyperreflexia. The third reflex arc includes afferents from the detrusor muscle to the motor neurons of the bladder, and the fourth involves afferents from the external urethral sphincter to the motor nuclei; loss of these reflex arcs results in distention of the bladder with failure to empty.

MALE REPRODUCTIVE ORGANS

Sympathetic trunk and ganglia
Greater splanchnic nerve (T5–9)
T10
Gray ramus communicans
T11
White ramus communicans
T12
Lesser splanchnic nerve
Least splanchnic nerve
L1
Upper lumbar splanchnic nerves
L2
L3
Gray ramus communicans
L4
Testicular artery and plexus
Ductus deferens and plexus
Inferior extent of peritoneum
Pelvic splanchnic nerves
Sacral plexus
Pudendal nerve
Inferior hypogastric (pelvic) plexus
Vesical plexus
Prostatic plexus
(Greater and lesser) cavernous nerves of penis

Celiac ganglia
Superior mesenteric ganglion
Left aorticorenal ganglion
Renal ganglion
Intermesenteric (aortic) plexus
Inferior mesenteric ganglion
Testicular artery and plexus
Superior hypogastric plexus
Hypogastric nerves
Ductus deferens and plexus
Pelvic splanchnic nerves
Sacral plexus
Pudendal nerve
Posterior nerves of penis
Epididymis
Testis

S1, S2, S3, S4, S5 (left and right)

| Sympathetic fibers | Presynaptic ——— Postsynaptic – – – – | Parasympathetic fibers | Presynaptic ——— Postsynaptic – – – – | Afferent fibers ——— |

INNERVATION OF REPRODUCTIVE ORGANS

The nerves supplying the male and female genital organs contain sympathetic and parasympathetic efferent and afferent fibers; their origins are similar in both sexes.

Sympathetic preganglionic fibers are the axons of intermediolateral column cells located in the lowest two or three thoracic and upper one or two lumbar segments of the spinal cord. They emerge in the anterior nerve roots of the corresponding spinal nerves and leave them in white rami communicantes passing to adjacent sympathetic trunk ganglia. They course via the thoracic and the upper lumbar splanchnic nerve, the celiac, intermesenteric (aortic) and superior hypogastric plexuses, and the hypogastric nerves to the *inferior hypogastric (pelvic) plexuses.* Many of these fibers relay in the lowest thoracic and upper lumbar sympathetic trunk ganglia or within the celiac plexus, but others do not relay until they reach ganglia in the inferior hypogastric plexuses. Consequently, the postganglionic fibers to the pelvic organs may be either long or relatively short. A minority of the sympathetic fibers for the pelvic viscera descend in the sympathetic trunks to emerge in the tiny *sacral splanchnic nerves* and thus join the inferior hypogastric plexuses.

Preganglionic parasympathetic fibers reach the inferior hypogastric plexuses in *pelvic splanchnic nerves* arising from the second, third, and fourth sacral spinal nerves. Nerve fibers from the *inferior hypogastric plexuses* supply the genital organs, and most of them relay in ganglia close to the prostate gland, neck of the bladder, cervix of the uterus, and upper vagina. Others relay in microscopic ganglia in or near the walls of seminal vesicles, deferent ducts, epididymis, and uterine tubes. There are no ganglia within the substance of the testes and ovaries. Inconclusive evidence suggests that parasympathetic fibers reach the outer parts of the uterine tubes by passing through the celiac plexus into the superior ovarian nerves that help supply the oviducts. Histochemical studies indicate that parasympathetic innervation of the genital systems in both sexes is less abundant than sympathetic innervation.

Afferent fibers exist in both the sympathetic and parasympathetic pathways and follow the same routes as the efferent fibers but in the reverse direction. Their parent pseudounipolar cells are situated in the posterior root ganglia of the lower thoracic, upper lumbar, and midsacral spinal nerves. The peripheral processes of these cells transmit impulses from the genital organs, ducts, and vessels. Their central processes carry the impulses into the cord, where many are carried to the brain in ascending pathways in the lateral and posterior white columns, whereas others form synapses with lateral cornual cells in the related cord segments and are thus involved in spinal reflex arcs.

MALE REPRODUCTIVE ORGANS

The nerves supplying the testis, epididymis, and ductus (vas) deferens are derived from three bilateral sources.

A *superior group* arises by rootlets from the *renal* and *intermesenteric plexuses,* with inconstant contributions from the *lumbar splanchnic nerves* and the origin of the *superior mesenteric plexus.* One or two small ganglia are associated with these rootlets. They communicate with

Plate 7.24

Autonomic Nervous System and Its Disorders

INNERVATION OF REPRODUCTIVE ORGANS (Continued)

the superior ureteric nerves and, on the right side, with branches supplying the duodenum and pancreas. The rootlets coalesce to form two or three slender nerves, which descend on the testicular artery to the *testis*.

A *middle group* arises by rootlets from the *superior hypogastric plexus* and from the ipsilateral *hypogastric nerve* and often communicates with the *middle ureteric* and *genitofemoral nerves*. The resultant nerves are mostly or entirely distributed to the *epididymis* and the *ampulla* of the *ductus deferens*.

An *inferior group* of a few small nerves arises from the *inferior hypogastric plexus* and from the nerve loops around the *lower end of the ureter*. This third group is closely associated with small nerves given off from the anterior part of the inferior hypogastric plexus to the seminal vesicles, prostate gland, ejaculatory ducts, and the base of the urinary bladder. The *prostatic* and *urethral nerve fibers* communicate with branchlets of the *pudendal nerves,* and offshoots from these united nervelets innervate the corpora cavernosa, the corpus spongiosum and the part of the urethra within it, and the bulbourethral glands. The nerve fibers supplying the cavernous structures and their vessels are termed the *penile cavernous nerves,* whereas their ramifications are often called the *cavernous plexuses.*

FEMALE REPRODUCTIVE ORGANS

The autonomic nerves supplying the female genital organs have similar origins to those supplying the male genital organs.

The *superior group* coalesces to form two or three slender nerves, which accompany the ovarian artery and supply nerve fibers to it and to the *ovary* and outer parts of the *uterine tube*. Their terminal fibers communicate with *uterine fibers* innervating the inner end of the uterine tube. Most of the afferent fibers in these nerves enter the spinal cord through the posterior roots of the tenth and the eleventh thoracic nerves, although a number may enter through the ninth or twelfth nerves.

The *middle group* helps to supply the *ovaries* and the *uterine tube* and vessels and gives off fascicles to the common and external iliac arteries.

The *inferior group* consists of nerves that enter the *cervix* of the *uterus* and the *vagina* directly, often alongside branches of the uterine and vaginal vessels, and

other nerves that ascend with or near the uterine artery, supplying nerve fibers to the *body* and *fundus* of the *uterus,* as well as to the artery and its branches. The terminal nerve fibers supply the uterine end and isthmus of the *uterine tube,* where they communicate with corresponding nerve fibers from the superior and middle groups of nerves.

The *uterine nerves* ramify throughout the myometrium. The fibers, which are predominantly unmyelinated and adrenergic in type, are most plentiful around

the uterine end of the uterine tube, in the cervix, and near the arterial branches.

The nerves entering the upper part of the *vagina* contain tiny ganglia. They break up into nerve fibers that supply the vaginal arteries and give off fascicles to the muscular and mucous coats of the vagina and urethra, the erectile tissue of the vestibular bulb and corpora cavernosa clitoridis, and the greater and lesser vestibular glands. These nerves contain a mixture of sympathetic and parasympathetic efferent and afferent fibers.

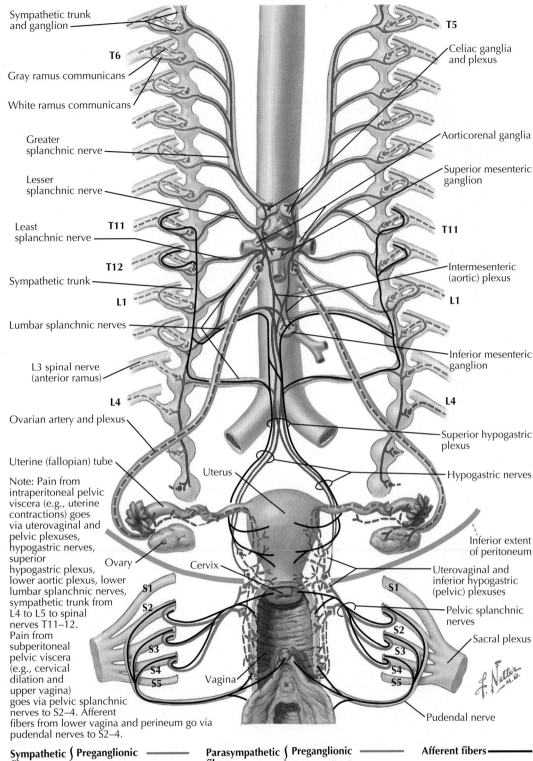

FEMALE REPRODUCTIVE ORGANS

SUDOMOTOR TESTING

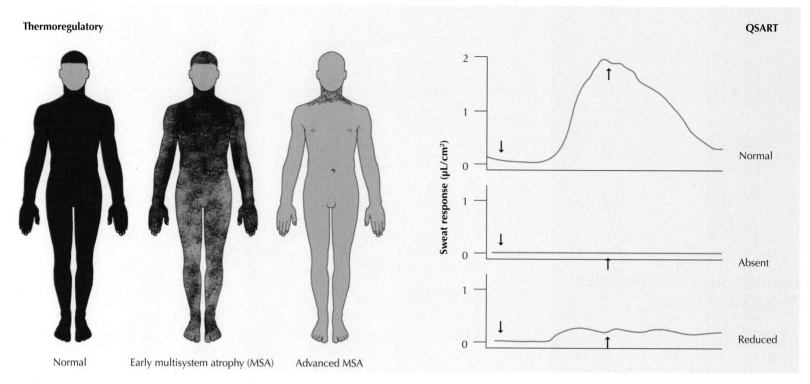

Thermoregulatory

Normal   Early multisystem atrophy (MSA)   Advanced MSA

QSART

Sweat response (μL/cm²)

Normal

Absent

Reduced

AUTONOMIC TESTING

Autonomic testing suggests the extent and pattern of autonomic involvement and can aid in the precise diagnosis and subsequent management of patients with dysautonomias. Tests are performed to assess both the sympathetic and parasympathetic systems. The autonomic battery usually consists of tests of sudomotor sympathetic function (sweat tests), cardiovagal function (heart rate response to deep breathing and Valsalva maneuver [VM]), and adrenergic cardiovascular function (tilt table test). The slope of the blood pressure responses during VM is an additional tool to assess both cardiovagal and adrenergic cardiovascular responses.

SWEAT TESTING

The thermoregulatory sweat test consists of the visual detection of skin humidity in response to warm external temperature. A dye that changes color when moist is applied to the patient's skin, and the ambient temperature is raised by 1°C by a heat cradle over the torso.

As the patient starts to sweat, the dye changes to a dark purple color. This test measures abnormalities in the sweat pathways at all levels (afferent, central, and efferent). The quantitative sudomotor axon reflex test (QSART) evaluates postganglionic sudomotor cholinergic fibers more objectively. It involves the iontophoresis of acetylcholine, resulting in an axon reflex. An impulse travels antidromically to reach a branch point and then orthodromically to the sweat gland, stimulating the release of acetylcholine from the nerve terminal to evoke the sweat response. A multicompartment sweat capsule is attached to the skin to measure the sweat response at standardized sites. Abnormality indicates that postganglionic sudomotor sympathetic axons are dysfunctional. QSART is usually normal in preganglionic lesions. The sympathetic skin response (a voltage change at the skin surface after an electric stimulus) also reflects postganglionic sudomotor function, with results correlating with those of other sweat tests.

CARDIOVAGAL TESTING

Cardiovagal function is assessed by measuring the heart rate response to deep breathing, the VM, and

standing. For the heart rate response to deep breathing, the patient inspires and expires deeply at six breaths per minute, and the difference between the maximum and minimum heart rate response is calculated. For VM, the subject makes a forced expiration to maintain a column of mercury at 30 to 40 mm for 15 seconds, and the ratio of the maximum heart rate during the maneuver to the lowest rate occurring within 30 seconds of its conclusion is determined. Concurrent measurement of beat-to-beat blood pressure (BP) enables quantification of baroreflex sensitivity. There are four main phases to the response to the VM; during phase I, there is a transient rise in BP due to increased intrathoracic and intraabdominal pressure. In early phase II (II_e), the reduced venous return results in a fall in BP followed by a compensatory increase in heart rate and peripheral resistance, resulting in an increase in BP in the late phase II (II_L). During phase III, there is a transient decline in BP from a reduction in intrathoracic pressure as the forced expiration is released, and in phase IV, the BP overshoots due to normalized venous return and cardiac output in the presence of persistently increased peripheral resistance. Late-phase II (II_L) is a function of α-adrenergic and phase IV of β-adrenergic responses;

Plate 7.26   Autonomic Nervous System and Its Disorders

CARDIOVAGAL TESTING AND HEAD-UP TILTING

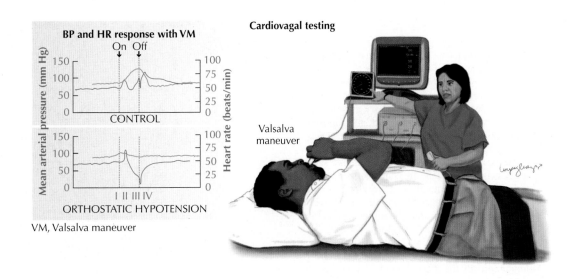

BP and HR response with VM

CONTROL

ORTHOSTATIC HYPOTENSION

I II III IV

VM, Valsalva maneuver

Cardiovagal testing

Valsalva
maneuver

AUTONOMIC TESTING
(Continued)

they can be used to assess sympathetic adrenergic integrity. Abnormality may lead to an excessive decline in blood pressure in phase II, with no BP overshoot in phase IV.

On standing, the heart rate increases, peaking at about the 15th beat after standing, and then declines to reach a stable state at about the 30th beat. The ratio of the R-R interval at the 15th and 30th beats after standing provides a test of parasympathetic (vagal) function. It is age dependent, but in young adults a ratio of less than 1.04 is abnormal. The biphasic response that occurs on standing is not present with passive tilt.

HEAD-UP TILTING

Patients with sympathetic dysfunction have a progressive decline in blood pressure during head-up tilt to 70 degrees. The heart rate response is also usually attenuated and does not compensate fully for the fall in blood pressure. If the patient is being evaluated for neurocardiogenic syncope or delayed orthostatic hypotension, prolonged tilting beyond 10 minutes, often for about 45 minutes, is needed.

ISOMETRIC HANDGRIP

During sustained handgrip, sympathetic outflow increases due to muscle contraction, increasing the BP. For testing purposes, a 30% maximal contraction for 3 to 5 minutes is required; diastolic BP usually increases by more than 15 mm Hg.

NEUROCHEMICAL TESTING

Measurement of supine and upright plasma norepinephrine levels provides a measure of postganglionic release of norepinephrine; levels usually double on

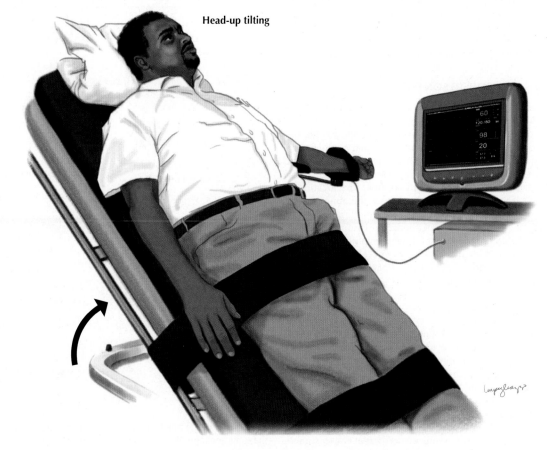

Head-up tilting

standing. With preganglionic lesions, supine levels are normal, but there is a limited rise or no change in the standing level. In postganglionic lesions of the sympathetic system, both supine and standing values are low.

[131]I-labeled metaiodobenzylguanidine (MIBG) scintigraphy is useful in evaluating cardiac sympathetic innervation.

OTHER TESTS

Other tests of value include skin biopsy to detect cutaneous nerve pathology. Special stains of the dermal nerves may be worthwhile. These include use of Congo red (viewed under polarized light) for amyloid neuropathies and alpha-synuclein stains for synucleinopathies such as pure autonomic failure.

ABNORMAL PUPILLARY CONDITIONS

ADIE'S TONIC PUPIL

The tonic pupil, or Adie's pupil, results from parasympathetic denervation. The tonically dilated pupil does not usually respond to light but responds to accommodation with slow constriction and then remains constricted for longer than normal (light-near dissociation). There is degeneration of the ciliary ganglion and the short ciliary nerves, sometimes with aberrant reinnervation. Most cases are idiopathic, but other causes include inflammation, ischemia, tumor, trauma, and paraneoplastic and autonomic neuropathies. When idiopathic, it is seen usually in young females, but it may occur in males and manifest at any age. It is commonly associated with reduced or absent muscle stretch reflexes in the lower limbs and sometimes with abnormalities of thermoregulatory sweating. The pupillary abnormality is commonly unilateral but may become bilateral.

Although initially the affected pupil is larger than the contralateral pupil, with time it can become smaller. The pupil is very sensitive to acetylcholine (probably due to denervation supersensitivity), with strong, tonic constriction; this can be demonstrated by the vigorous miotic response to methacholine chloride and 0.1% pilocarpine. The intact sympathetic innervation is demonstrated by the normal response to cocaine.

ARGYLL ROBERTSON PUPIL

This was initially described in neurosyphilis or tabes dorsalis. The classic findings include a normal near or convergence reflex with normal pupillary responses to accommodation and an abnormal pupillary response to light. In addition, the pupils are small and irregular and constrict with physostigmine and dilate variably with atropine and cocaine. The location of the lesion in the brain that causes the abnormal response is thought to be the rostral midbrain, near the periaqueductal gray. Although previously thought to be pathognomonic of neurosyphilis, it is now recognized in diabetes, viral encephalitis, multiple sclerosis, and other inflammatory and degenerative diseases of the brain.

HORNER SYNDROME

Horner syndrome results from loss of sympathetic innervation to the eye and is characterized by ptosis (droopy eyelid), miosis (constricted pupil), and facial anhidrosis (impaired facial sweating). Additional findings may include pigmentary changes in the iris. Pupillary reactions to light and accommodation are normal. The anisocoria (inequality in pupil size) is accentuated in dim light. The ptosis is due to paralysis of the Muller muscle; this is the sympathetically innervated smooth muscle of the upper eye lid. Acquired Horner syndrome may be central, preganglionic, or postganglionic. A central lesion may involve the first-order neuron at any point from the cell origin in the hypothalamus to its termination in the intermediolateral column of the spinal cord. Causes include brainstem infarction, tumor, and syringomyelia (cavitation in the spinal cord). Preganglionic Horner syndrome is due to involvement of the second-order neuron from its origin in the intermediolateral column to its termination in the superior cervical ganglion; causes include trauma or tumor of the cervical or upper thoracic spinal cord and lesion of the

lower trunk of the brachial plexus, such as by tumors of the lung apex, jugular vein puncture, and thyroid surgery. Postganglionic Horner syndrome results from lesions of the third-order neuron in the sympathetic ganglion and the pathway leading to its termination in the face and eye, such as by extracranial carotid artery dissection, intracranial lesion in the carotid canal, or cavernous sinus pathology. Use of cocaine eye drops (which block the reuptake of norepinephrine) will help distinguish true Horner syndrome from physiologic anisocoria; 1 hour after instillation of 4% to 10% cocaine drops, a normal pupil will have dilated more than a pupil with sympathetic dysfunction (irrespective of site of lesion), increasing the baseline anisocoria. Apraclonidine,

an α-adrenergic receptor agonist will cause the affected pupil to dilate (because of α-adrenergic supersensitivity), whereas the normal pupil will constrict. Pharmacologic testing will also differentiate between central, preganglionic, and postganglionic lesions. Hydroxyamphetamine (1%) drops instilled into the eye do not affect the pupil of patients with Horner syndrome resulting from a lesion of the third-order postganglionic neuron, whereas dilation occurs in normal pupils and in patients with Horner syndrome with an intact third-order neuron because of release of norepinephrine. Similarly, 1% solution of phenylephrine hydrochloride will dilate the pupil in postganglionic lesions (third-order neurons) but not normal pupils.

Pupillary light reflex

Light

Optic nerves

Short ciliary nerves

Ciliary ganglion

Optic chiasm

CN III

Optic tract

Red nucleus

Edinger-Westphal nucleus

Pretectal nucleus

Adie's tonic pupil

Affected pupil unreactive to light — Normal pupil

Methacholine drops

Constriction — No effect

Pilocarpine drops

Constriction — No effect

Argyll Robertson pupil
Usually bilateral; normal left pupil shown for comparison

Ptosis

Miosis

Affected pupil unreactive to light — Normal pupil

Atropine drops

No effect — Dilation

Horner syndrome

Right-sided Horner syndrome — Normal left eye

Ptosis

Miosis

Central or Preganglionic lesion

Cocaine drops

No effect — Dilation

Hydroxyamphetamine drops

Dilation — Dilation

Phenylephrine drops

No effect — No effect

Postganglionic lesion

Cocaine drops

No effect — Dilation

Hydroxyamphetamine drops

No effect — Dilation

Phenylephrine drops

Dilation — No effect

Hypothalamus (origin)

Central pathway

Postganglionic pathway

Superior cervical ganglion

Preganglionic pathway

Plate 7.28

Autonomic Nervous System and Its Disorders

CLINICAL PRESENTATION OF AUTONOMIC DISORDERS

Patients usually have symptoms due to both parasympathetic and sympathetic dysfunction. The former is characterized by dry mucous membranes, particularly the eyes and mouth, with gastrointestinal and urogenital symptoms: early satiety, nausea, vomiting, constipation, diarrhea, urinary bladder dysmotility, and erectile dysfunction. Feelings of light-headedness or syncope when assuming an upright posture and alteration of sweating are symptoms of impaired sympathetic function. Sexual dysfunction is due to combined parasympathetic and sympathetic disorders. Signs of autonomic dysfunction include fixed heart rates, orthostatic hypotension, and tonic pupils, with normal strength and sensation unless somatic nerves are also affected.

Autonomic disorders may be classified as peripheral (central) and acute (chronic) disorders.

ACUTE PERIPHERAL AUTONOMIC DISORDERS

Acute and subacute autonomic neuropathies are usually due to toxic, metabolic, autoimmune, or paraneoplastic causes. Primary autonomic polyneuropathies represent an uncommon subgroup. However, many length-dependent polyneuropathies have associated autonomic fiber involvement. Impotence is such an example in diabetic polyneuropathies.

Antecedent viral infections may occur in patients with *autoimmune autonomic neuropathy,* suggesting that it may be a variant of Guillain-Barré syndrome. This is usually a severe generalized disorder, but restricted milder forms also occur. Orthostatic intolerance, anhidrosis, mydriasis, hypotonic bladder, and gastrointestinal dysmotility are common presentations. Autonomic tests are abnormal. Recovery is slow and incomplete. High titers of ganglionic nicotinic acetylcholine receptor antibodies are reported, supporting an autoimmune basis. Immunotherapy with intravenous immunoglobulin may help; in some instances, a trial of long-term immunosuppression (with mycophenolate, azathioprine, or rituximab) may be indicated.

Guillain-Barré syndrome preferentially involves somatic fibers but causes dysautonomia in two-thirds of cases, especially affecting the cardiovascular (labile blood pressure, cardiac arrhythmias) and gastrointestinal systems (hypomotility presenting as ileus or gastroparesis). Bladder dysfunction is less common. Autonomic complications may be life-threatening; patients must therefore be monitored in the intensive care unit.

CAUSES OF DYSAUTONOMIA

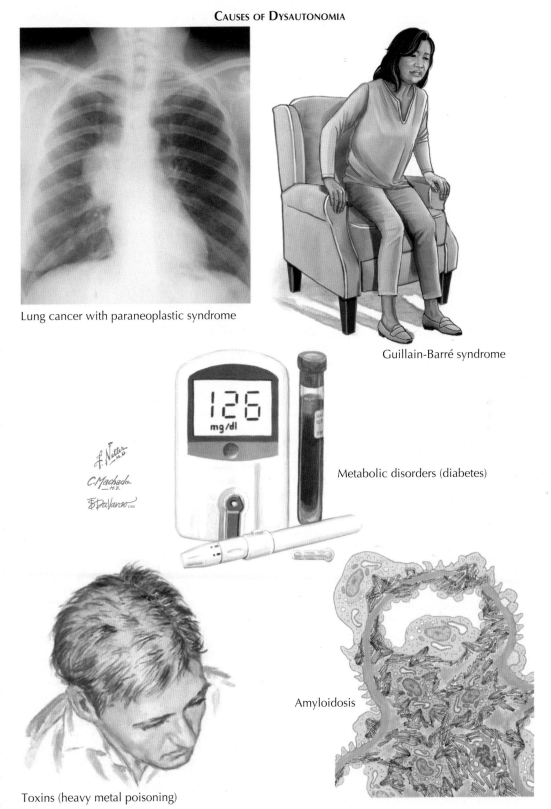

Lung cancer with paraneoplastic syndrome

Guillain-Barré syndrome

Metabolic disorders (diabetes)

Amyloidosis

Toxins (heavy metal poisoning)

Paraneoplastic autonomic neuropathy is indistinguishable from autoimmune autonomic neuropathy and often follows a subacute course. Gastrointestinal dysmotility is a common manifestation. Associated symptoms and signs due to more widespread involvement of the nervous system may occur, such as encephalitis, myelitis, or neuropathy. Antineuronal nuclear antibody type 1 and CRMP-5 are associated with small cell lung cancer. The presence of other antibodies should also be sought. Computed tomography (CT) scans of the chest, abdomen, and pelvis as well as positron emission tomography–CT may be indicated. In Lambert-Eaton myasthenic syndrome, which is associated with presynaptic voltage-gated calcium channel antibody (P/Q type), significant dysautonomia may occur, with symptoms usually consisting of dry mouth, constipation, and erectile dysfunction. Therapy involves treatment of the underlying cancer and immunotherapy; 3,4 diaminopyridine may also be of benefit.

MULTIPLE SYSTEM ATROPHY

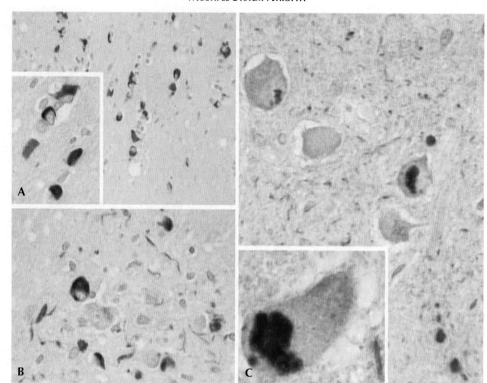

Synuclein positive neural and glial inclusions in multiple system atrophy

CLINICAL PRESENTATION OF AUTONOMIC DISORDERS (Continued)

Sensory neuronopathy–associated *Sjögren syndrome* may have autonomic manifestations, primarily orthostatic hypotension.

Hereditary porphyria manifests with acute attacks of dysautonomic symptoms (abdominal pain, vomiting, constipation, hypertension, and tachycardia) in addition to psychiatric symptoms and motor polyneuropathies. Diagnosis requires demonstration of increased urinary excretion of porphobilinogen. Prompt hemin administration may lead to rapid resolution of an attack. Givosiran is a small interfering RNA (siRNA) directed against the hepatic *ALAS1* gene and may be used to reduce the frequency of attacks. Liver transplantation may be effective in severely affected patients.

Toxins, including medications (particularly cisplatin and vinca alkaloids), may cause peripheral neuropathies with autonomic features. Other autonomic nerve toxins include organophosphates, thallium, arsenic, hexacarbons, and acrylamide.

CHRONIC PERIPHERAL AUTONOMIC DISORDERS

Autonomic neuropathies are common accompaniments of diabetic peripheral neuropathies and correlate with duration and control of diabetes. Autonomic testing reveals evidence of cardiovagal dysfunction manifested by impairment of heart rate response to VM or deep breathing.

Postural orthostatic tachycardia syndrome (POTS) is a subacute disorder seen predominantly in young females. It is characterized by orthostatic symptoms associated with significant rise in heart rate on standing, without orthostatic hypotension or other clinical or laboratory evidence of autonomic neuropathy, except for occasional mild distal loss of sweating. Diagnosis is made in adults by symptoms of orthostatic intolerance, along with an increase in heart rate of greater than 30 beats/min or heart rate exceeding 120 beats/min on standing or head-up tilt.

Amyloidosis is a multisystem disorder that may be sporadic or familial. Amyloidosis results from extracellular deposition of fibrils that exhibit apple green birefringence with Congo red staining when viewed with a polarizing microscope. Amyloid may be due to a plasma cell dyscrasia (AL amyloid). Heritable amyloidosis is due to mutations in genes coding for transthyretin (TTR), gelsolin, or apolipoprotein. Amyloidosis compli-

cating systemic diseases (AA amyloid) is less common. TTR amyloidosis can present with peripheral neuropathy, autonomic neuropathy, and/or cardiomyopathy. Wild-type TTR amyloidosis is not associated with genetic mutations in the TTR gene; it commonly presents with cardiomyopathy. Autonomic neuropathy often occurs and presents with symptoms of somatic small fiber dysfunction, orthostatic intolerance, and constipation alternating with diarrhea. AL amyloidosis is treated by chemotherapy, often followed by autologous hematopoietic transplantation. TTR amyloidosis treatment includes RNA-targeted therapies and includes patisiran, an siRNA that reduces the hepatic production of the inherited and wild-type TTR protein. Inotersen is an antisense oligonucleotide that also inhibits TTR production. Tafamidis and diflunisal also reduce the formation of TTR amyloid. Finally, liver transplantation is also used in inherited TTR amyloidosis. Studies are ongoing on the role of gene editing using CRISPR (clustered regularly interspersed short palindromic repeats) and CRISPR-associated protein 9 endonuclease.

Pure autonomic failure is also known as idiopathic autonomic failure, with orthostatic hypotension as the primary symptom. It is an insidious process with typical signs of disordered autonomic function. The absence of parkinsonian features helps differentiate this disorder from multiple systems atrophy. It results from postganglionic sympathetic neuron degeneration. Patients may progress to develop Parkinson disease, multiple systems atrophy, or dementia with Lewy bodies.

Hereditary autonomic neuropathies are rare disorders. Hereditary sensory and autonomic neuropathy type III, also known as Riley-Day syndrome, is an autosomal recessive disorder with defective control of blood pressure, sweating, temperature, and lacrimation in children. It is seen primarily in children of Ashkenazi Jewish descent; the causative gene is located on chromosome 9q31 and encodes for 1 kappa B kinase complex–associated

protein; treatment is supportive. Dysautonomic manifestations are less pronounced in other hereditary sensory and autonomic neuropathies.

CENTRAL DISORDERS

Parkinson disease is associated with significant autonomic dysfunction, particularly in long-standing disease. There is loss of pigmented dopaminergic cells in substantia nigra; other pigmented nuclei, including locus coeruleus and dorsal vagal nucleus, are affected; this may explain the dysautonomia. Symptoms include constipation, sialorrhea, rhinorrhea, erectile dysfunction, and orthostatic hypotension. Peripheral sympathetic denervation of the heart is common, contributing to the symptoms of orthostatic hypotension. Treatment consists of symptomatic management.

Multiple systems atrophy, a degenerative disorder, is characterized by parkinsonian features with autonomic, cerebellar, and corticospinal involvement. When autonomic symptoms predominate, the disorder is sometimes called *Shy-Drager syndrome.* Dysautonomia presents as orthostatic hypotension; urinary symptoms of urgency, frequency, retention, and incontinence; and decreased sweating. Erectile dysfunction is common in males. Sleep and breathing abnormalities are also common. Fludrocortisone is the medication of choice for the treatment of orthostatic hypotension. Other agents that are useful include the α-adrenergic agonist midodrine and norepinephrine precursor droxidopa.

Spinal cord disorders may also cause autonomic symptoms. Common disorders include trauma, syringomyelia, and multiple sclerosis. They usually manifest with arrhythmias, blood pressure lability, and bladder atony. Treatment is of the underlying disorder and also involves managing the prominent autonomic symptoms.

PAIN

NEUROANATOMY OF THE ASCENDING PAIN PATHWAYS

Pain propagation is initiated with activation of nociceptors that are distributed within skin, muscle, joints, and viscera. These receptors include small-diameter $A\delta$- and C-fiber free nerve endings representing distal primary afferent neurons. Cutaneous $A\delta$ fibers (myelinated) mediate sharp sensation of first-phase or acute pain known to trigger withdrawal responses. These include two fiber groups: (1) high-threshold *mechanoreceptors fibers,* which respond to mechanical stimuli of high intensity and, after sensitization, to noxious heat, and (2) *mechanothermal receptors* for extreme (i.e., noxious) heat and cold sensation. Once sensitized, these receptors are activated by mechanical stimuli even at nonnoxious thresholds.

C-type fibers (unmyelinated) slowly propagate dull, burning (secondary) pain sensation information. Some C fibers are modality specific and respond only to thermal, mechanical, or chemical noxious stimuli. However, the majority of C fibers are polymodal, which means that they respond to both thermal and mechanical noxious stimuli as well as to chemical substances (e.g., potassium ions, prostaglandins, substance P, and histamine). A unique C-fiber subtype responds to high-intensity thermal stimuli and also mediates flare responses after tissue damage. Some C-type nociceptors, designated *silent receptors,* are primarily activated by inflammation.

The cell bodies of sensory neurons are located primarily in the dorsal root ganglia (DRG) or trigeminal ganglia in addition to satellite cells that modulate neuron-immune interactions. The diversity of primary afferent nociceptors may be broadly characterized as either peptidergic or nonpeptidergic. Ion channels play an essential role in the regulation of neuronal excitability. Key channel proteins for the generation of inward membrane currents on nociceptors include voltage-gated sodium (Na_v) and calcium (Ca_v) channels. The peptidergic subpopulation expresses calcitonin gene-related peptide (CGRP) and/or substance P. In contrast, the nonpeptidergic subpopulation binds isolectin B4 or expresses P2X3 receptor. Most human nociceptors have a peptidergic phenotype, and DRG neurons express transient receptor potential vanilloid receptor 1 (TRPV1) and TrkA, the high-affinity nerve growth factor receptor.

The primary afferent fibers travel through dorsal nerve roots and enter the dorsal horn of the spinal cord, where they divide in a "T" pattern. They travel two to three spinal segments within the Lissauer tract in both rostral and caudal directions and send collateral projections to the gray matter along the entire four- to six-segment length, thus transmitting pain signals over a broad spinal cord area.

Both myelinated and unmyelinated primary afferent fibers project predominantly to the superficial laminae of the dorsal horn. Although there is considerable overlap in the projection of fibers, signaling innocuous and noxious stimuli, there exists some degree of functional segregation at the postsynaptic level in the superficial laminae. Dorsal horn neurons are classified into three distinct groups. The specific nociceptive neurons that respond exclusively to noxious stimuli are found in Rexed laminae I, II, V, and VI. Their receptive fields in lamina I are punctiform and display somatotopic organization.

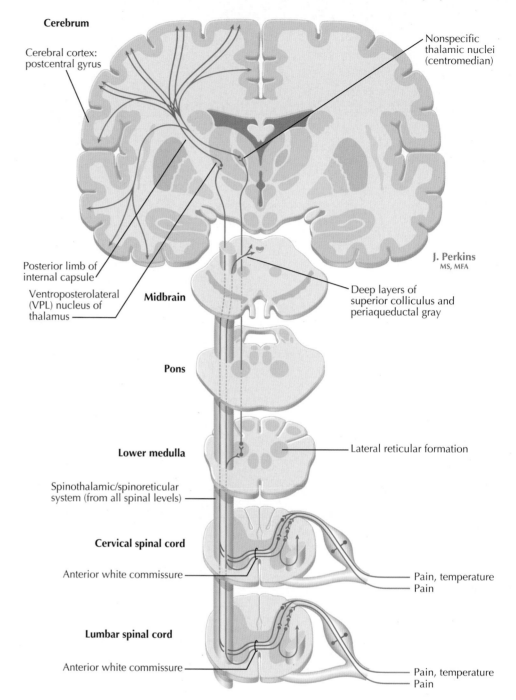

J. Perkins
MS, MFA

Lamina I neurons are classified into several modality-selective classes, relaying information from particular subsets of small-diameter fibers and relating the current physiologic status of body tissues. The two nociceptive cell types, *nociceptive-specific* (NS) and *polymodal nociceptive* (HPC, for heat, pinch, and cold) have different characteristics. NS neurons receive mainly $A\delta$ inputs associated with first pain and relay information about noxious stimuli localization and physical quality. HPC cells receive polymodal C-nociceptor information and are associated with second pain. Lamina I cells relate current physiologic conditions of all body tissues and regulate spinal cord excitability, and therefore pain behavior, through the activation of descending inhibitory and excitatory pathways from the brainstem.

Lamina V neurons are large cells with dendrites extending across the dorsal horn, receiving myelinated primary afferent input from $A\beta$, $A\delta$, and C fibers. According to *gate control theory,* this fiber group is important for segmental suppression of pain; however, their inhibitory role is not yet confirmed. Almost all of lamina V consists of *wide dynamic range* (WDR) cells, which have large receptive fields and high-frequency ongoing discharges. WDR neurons demonstrate graded responses to pressure and noxious stimuli, including heat, cold, and deep and visceral stimulation. Their activity represents integration of all dorsal horn afferent inputs. In contrast to lamina I neurons, WDR cells are not somatotopically organized; their complex excitatory and inhibitory receptive fields are musculotopically organized. Their main characteristic is to code stimulus intensity; they demonstrate increasing frequencies of response from innocuous to noxious stimulation.

Intrinsic dorsal horn neurons promote interaction of afferent and efferent nociceptive stimuli and are also responsible for their transfer to supraspinal structures. These are classified as (1) *projection neurons* directly transmitting information to supraspinal centers, (2)

Plate 8.2

Pain

NEUROANATOMY OF THE ASCENDING PAIN PATHWAYS (Continued)

intersegmental propriospinal neurons integrating several spinal levels, and (3) interneurons having inhibitory or excitatory features. Nociceptive projection neurons relay information to various brainstem and diencephalon regions, including the thalamus, periaqueductal gray, bulbar reticular formation, and limbic structures within the hypothalamus, amygdala, and other sites. There is also a visceral nociceptive pathway within the postsynaptic posterior column pathway.

The spinothalamic tract (STT) mediates sensations of pain, cold, warmth, and touch. This pathway originates from WDR, NS, and nonnociceptive dorsal horn neurons in laminae I, II, and deeper lamina V. Most STT axons decussate transversely through the anterior white commissure of the spinal cord and ascend through the contralateral anterolateral funiculus. Passing through the brainstem, the STT sends collateral projections to the medullary, pontine, and midbrain reticular formation, including gigantocellularis and paragigantocellularis nuclei and periaqueductal gray matter. These are probably responsible for descending suppressor system activation, as well as behavioral and neurovegetative responses to pain. Three STT afferent forms are recognized, including a monosynaptic neospinothalamic pathway (anterior STT) that directly projects to lateral complex thalamic nuclei involved in sensory-discriminative pain components. Another is a multisynaptic paleospinothalamic pathway (dorsal STT) projecting to posterior medial and intralaminar complex thalamic nuclei involved in the motivational-affective aspects of pain. Lastly, there is a monosynaptic spinothalamic pathway projecting directly to thalamic medial central nucleus that is related to affective components of pain sensation.

The thalamus is the main relay structure for sensory information destined for the cortex; it is involved in reception, integration, and transfer of nociceptive potentials. NS and WDR neurons project to the ventroposterolateral (VPL), ventroposteromedial (VPM), and ventroposteroinferior (VPI) nuclei, collectively the main somatosensory relay. It receives both noxious and innocuous information of cutaneous, muscular, and articular origin. These nuclei have numerous interconnections with the somatosensory (SI) cortex. The VPI nucleus participates in the processing of visceral pain, occurring through the postsynaptic dorsal column pathway with nucleus gracilis projections.

The VPM nucleus is likewise involved in sensory-discriminative aspects of thermal, mechanical, and tactile information. Owing to its projections to the prefrontal cortex, the convergence of fibers arising from the parabrachial region within the lateral pons at the locus coeruleus level, as well as to amygdala, hypothalamic, and periaqueductal gray interconnections, the VPM nucleus is likely involved with emotional pain, as well as psychomotor and autonomic reactions to painful stimuli. Posterior division of the ventromedial nucleus and posterior nucleus are essential parts of the medial nociceptive system, establishing insular and cingulate cortex connections involved in affective-cognitive aspects of pain. Specific STT projections, originating from lamina I, suggest that these nuclei are noxious information integration centers, especially for cases of freezing and visceral sensations.

The thalamus medial complex receives afferent input from laminae I and V of the STT, interconnecting with the striatum and the cerebellum. This is responsible for the control of attention and motor responses, suggesting that this area may be involved in escape behavior in the presence of harmful stimuli.

Ultimately the nociceptive signal is relayed from the thalamus to a variety of cortical regions. Two systems of nociceptive cortical projection are commonly distinguished: the lateral and medial systems. There are three important cortical regions: SI cortex, secondary somatosensory (SII) cortex, and the anterior cingulate cortex (ACC). The lateral nociceptive system participates directly in the sensory-discriminative ascription of nociception involving specific thalamic nuclei, projecting to NS and WDR neurons of the SI and SII cortices. NS neurons are associated with topographic localization of peripheral stimuli, whereas WDR neurons code the intensity of these stimuli. Nociceptive neurons in the SII

cortex code the painful stimulus in temporal terms. Both SI and SII cortices have connections with the posteroparietal area and the insula, responsible for somatosensory input association with learning and memory. This pathway is crucial to assessment of the stimuli features and behavioral decisions in relation to the prefrontal cortex functions. Conversely, the medial nociceptive system has more diffuse projections from the medial thalamus to SI and SII and limbic structures, such as the insula and the ACC. Accordingly, it is predominantly responsible for the motivational-affective component of pain.

The insula relays information from the lateral nociceptive system to the limbic system, mainly via the amygdala and prefrontal cortex associated with the emotional and affective component and with memory integral to the painful experience. The ACC coordinates inputs from parietal areas with frontal cortical regions, integrating the perception of threat with the appropriate pain behavior.

Somatosensory afferents to the spinal cord

Principal fiber tracts of spinal cord

J. Perkins
MS, MFA

- Ascending pathways
- Descending pathways
- Fibers passing in both directions

F. Netter
M.D.

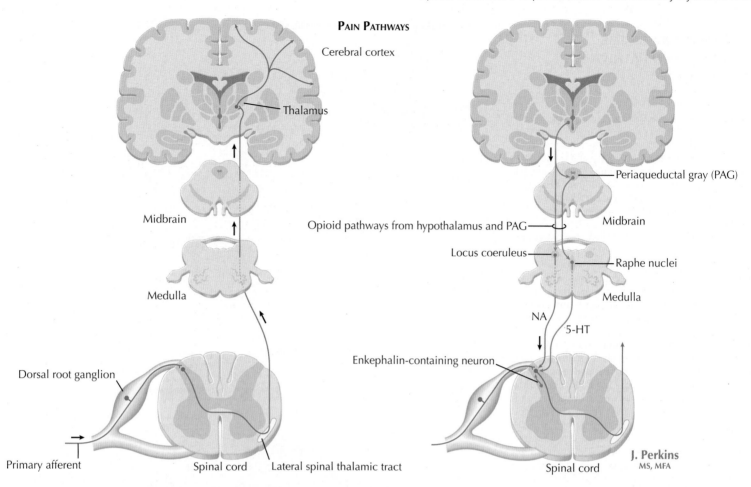

PAIN PATHWAYS

Cerebral cortex

Thalamus

Midbrain

Medulla

Dorsal root ganglion

Primary afferent

Spinal cord

Lateral spinal thalamic tract

Periaqueductal gray (PAG)

Opioid pathways from hypothalamus and PAG

Midbrain

Locus coeruleus

Raphe nuclei

Medulla

NA

5-HT

Enkephalin-containing neuron

Spinal cord

J. Perkins
MS, MFA

DESCENDING NOCICEPTIVE PATHWAYS AND NEUROCHEMICAL FOUNDATIONS OF DESCENDING PAIN MODULATION

DESCENDING NOCICEPTIVE PATHWAYS

Descending control of spinal nociception arises from various brain areas and is pivotal in determining the experience of pain, both acute and chronic. Several central nervous system (CNS) areas exert a top-down modulation of nociceptive processing. Projections from prefrontal, anterior cingulate, and insular cortices, as well as hypothalamus and amygdala to the brainstem pain modulatory system, support the notion of emotional and affective regulation of pain transmission. Attention, anticipation, control over pain, and religious beliefs affect pain perception, supporting the importance of the ACC and frontal lobes in modulation of nociceptive processing.

The current model of descending pain modulation involves both inhibitory and facilitatory influences on spinal nociceptive transmission. The balance between inhibition and facilitation is dependent on different behavioral, emotional, and pathologic conditions. Intense stress or fear is associated with decreased response to pain, whereas inflammation, nerve injury, or sickness is associated with hyperalgesia that partially can be ascribed to descending facilitatory mechanisms. Several studies suggest that descending facilitatory systems are also activated by safety signals that follow an aversive event. In addition, descending facilitation of spinal nociception contributes to central sensitization and

development of secondary hyperalgesia. Finally, hyperalgesia encountered during acute opioid abstinence also entails descending nociceptive facilitation from the rostral ventromedial medulla.

A number of supraspinal sites activated by nociceptive input contribute to central modulation of pain. The most prominent ones include *periaqueductal gray* (PAG) and rostral ventromedial medulla (RVM). The effects of descending modulation are exerted in the spinal dorsal horn on the synapse between the primary afferent and projection neurons or on interneurons that synapse with projection neurons, by inhibiting the release of neurotransmitter from primary afferent fibers or by inhibiting the function of neurotransmitter receptors on the postsynaptic neuron.

In awake, behaving animals, *anterolateral* PAG stimulation leads to immobility, sympathoinhibition, and analgesia, as well as inhibition of nociceptive dorsal horn neurons, including STT cells. The PAG contains a large number of neurons. Local injection of opioids, nonspecific *enkephalin, substance P,* and *gamma-aminobutyric acid (GABA)ergic* excitants or neuropeptides into the PAG produces analgesia in animals. Excitatory pathways projecting from the PAG to the brainstem are subject to inhibitory control by GABAergic inhibitory neurons within the PAG. Analgesic opioids and cannabinoids relieve GABAergic control and thus induce analgesia. The PAG is significantly interconnected with the hypothalamus and limbic forebrain structures, including the amygdala. This suggests that cognitive and emotional aspects influence ascending nociceptive input, further modulating the resultant experience of pain. Major brainstem inputs to the PAG originate from the *nucleus cuneiformis, the locus coeruleus, the pontomedullary reticular*

formation and parabrachial area, and other *catecholaminergic nuclei.*

Major descending projections from the anterolateral PAG are to the rostral ventromedial medulla, including the *nucleus raphe magnus* and adjacent *reticular formation.* The PAG pain-modulating action is relayed almost exclusively through the RVM, which, in turn, sends bilateral descending projections through posterolateral spinal funiculi terminating within the spinal dorsal horn. The *RVM* is a functional term describing the *midline pontomedullary area* in which opioid injection or electrical stimulation produces *antinociception,* that is, analgesia. It includes the *nucleus raphe magnus* and *adjacent reticular formation* and projects diffusely to dorsal horn laminae important in nociceptive processing, including superficial layers and deep dorsal horn.

With increasing understanding of RVM neuronal physiology, it is recognized that this area is central to the mediation of the bidirectional control of nociception. It receives projections from serotonin-containing neurons of the dorsal raphe, neurotensinergic neurons of the PAG, and limbic and prelimbic cortex, including the anterior insula. Nonselective stimulation or inactivation of RVM neurons can either suppress or facilitate nociception, depending on the functional background. This suggests that there are parallel inhibitory and facilitatory output pathways from the RVM to the spinal cord. Adjacent neurons are simultaneously under facilitatory and inhibitory control from supraspinal structures. The equilibrium between inhibition and facilitation determines the net effect of descending modulation on nociceptive transmission.

The RVM includes three distinct types of neurons: (1) neurons that begin discharging just before the

Plate 8.4

Pain

DESCENDING NOCICEPTIVE PATHWAYS AND NEUROCHEMICAL FOUNDATIONS OF DESCENDING PAIN MODULATION (Continued)

withdrawal from noxious heat, entering a period of activity ("ON cells"); (2) neurons that stop discharging before the withdrawal reflex, entering a period of silence ("OFF cells"); and (3) neurons that do not demonstrate consistent changes in activity when withdrawal reflex occurs ("neutral cells"). ON and OFF cells send projections specifically to laminae I, II, and V of the dorsal horn. Activation of OFF cells produces behavioral antinociception and is required for the analgesic opioid effect. In contrast, direct, selective activation of ON cells produces hyperalgesia; their discharge is associated with enhanced nociception. Thus OFF cells exert a net inhibitory effect on nociception, whereas the ON cells play a facilitatory role in the descending modulation of pain.

The role of *neutral cells* in pain modulation is unexplained. One theory is that neutral cells are recruited to become ON or OFF cells during development of chronic pain states, which is supported by wide variations of ON and OFF cell excitability under basal conditions. At least some neutral cells are *serotonergic*. Considering the importance of serotonin in nociceptive modulation, this suggests that neutral cells may be involved in the descending control of pain transmission.

The *locus coeruleus* and the *A5 and A7 noradrenergic cell groups* of the *posterolateral pons* are the main source of noradrenergic input to the dorsal horn. These regions send bilateral projections that primarily descend to contralateral laminae I, II, and V of the spinal dorsal horn, exerting an antinociceptive effect. The PAG sends input to the locus coeruleus and the A7 region. RVM neurons containing substance P or enkephalin also send input to A7. Consequently, the *posterolateral pontine tegmentum* provides a corresponding pathway for the PAG and RVM to provide descending nociception control over the spinal dorsal horn. *Posterolateral pontine systems* may also provide cortical control of spinal pain transmission. The anterior insular cortex has locus coeruleus and RVM connections, suggesting that inhibition of the insular outflow disinhibits noradrenergic neurons of the locus coeruleus.

NEUROCHEMICAL FOUNDATIONS OF DESCENDING PAIN MODULATION

Opioids have long been considered the archetypical analgesics, with endogenous opioids ("enkephalins") believed to play a pivotal role in the modulation of pain transmission. Recently, however, monoaminergic pathways have been shown to mediate modulation of nociceptive processing. Monoaminergic systems include *serotonergic, noradrenergic,* and *dopaminergic neurons* that elicit either *antinociceptive* or *pronociceptive* effects, depending on the type of receptor involved and its location. Monoaminergic modulation entails complex interplay between primary nociceptive afferents, dorsal horn projection neurons, local interneurons, and glial cells.

The RVM is the major source of *serotonergic input* to the dorsal horn; it is the final common output for descending influences from rostral brain regions projecting to the superficial and deep dorsal horn. The *PAG-RVM serotonergic pathway* is considered to be the major endogenous pain modulatory system and the main target of supraspinal opioid analgesia. *Serotonergic*

neurons can exert *antinociceptive action* (in response to chemical stimuli and neurogenic inflammation) as well as *pronociceptive action* (in response to mechanical stimuli), depending on the activation of different serotonergic receptors.

Noradrenergic neurons originating from locus coeruleus and A5 and A7 pontine tegmentum groups provide inhibition of nociceptive input via *presynaptic alpha-2 receptors*. In this case noradrenergic modulation relies upon volume transmission, in contrast to the serotonergic system mediating punctate synaptic transmission. The effect of this noradrenergic system is essentially an extrasynaptic spread of neuroactive substances that may be involved in late and long-lasting changes of a group of neurons. The analgesic effects mediated through presynaptic alpha-2 receptors

involve presynaptic inhibition in primary afferents, postsynaptic inhibition of projection neurons, as well as a complex interplay with opioid and adenosine antinociceptive systems.

Dopaminergic pathways originate mainly from A11 neurons of the *periventricular posterior thalamus*. Their activation results in diminished response to noxious stimuli mediated by *D2 receptors*, with concomitant inhibition of neurotransmitter release from primary afferents. Conversely, *D1 receptor* activation engenders facilitated nociception transmission, both directly and by opioid antagonism. The possible mechanism of action for dopamine may rely on local dopamine concentration; low levels activate antinociceptive D2 receptors, and high levels elicit pronociceptive effects via D1 receptor.

ENDORPHIN SYSTEM

Stimuli from higher centers (psychologic, placebo effect, etc.)
Periaqueductal gray matter
Cerebral aqueduct
Enkephalin-containing neuron
Morphine
Mesencephalon
Indirect pathways
Morphine
Raphe magnus nucleus
Medullary reticular neuron
Afferent pain fibers in trigeminal nerve
Spinal trigeminal tract and nucleus
Enkephalin-containing neuron
Medulla oblongata
Serotonin pathway
Spinoreticula pathway
Posterolateral funiculus
Lamina I pain interneuron
Lamina V interneuron
Afferent pain neuron of dorsal root ganglion
Anterolateral funiculus
Spinal cord
Enkephalin-containing neuron in substantia gelatinosa (lamina II)
Spinoreticular neuron

NOCICEPTIVE PROCESSING AND CENTRAL NERVOUS SYSTEM CORRELATES OF PAIN

NEUROPATHIC PAIN

The International Association for the Study of Pain defines neuropathic pain as pain caused by a lesion or disease of the somatosensory nervous system. Peripheral neuropathic pain results from a diverse array of insults to the peripheral nervous system (PNS) variously caused by mechanical trauma, metabolic diseases (e.g., diabetes mellitus), infection (e.g., herpes zoster), tumor invasion, or neurotoxic chemicals. Associated risk factors include sex, age, anatomic site of the injury, and even the severity of acute postoperative pain. Epidemiologic studies identify the prevalence of neuropathic pain to be as high as 5%.

Neural injury triggers a range of processes affecting primary afferent receptors and their axons and cell bodies and unleashes a complex immune response in central neurons and glial cells. Some of these processes facilitate healing and normative repair, such as removal of cell and myelin debris, recruitment of antiapoptotic strategies, induction of axonal growth and sprouting, synaptic remodeling, and remyelination. In contrast, animal neurophysiologic studies demonstrate that some of these secondary effects have a maladaptive effect. Other well-characterized effects leading to chronic pain include central sensitization, ectopic impulse generation, reduced central inhibition, neuronal loss, and glial scarring.

PERIPHERAL SENSITIZATION

Various signaling molecules, including cytokines, chemokines, neurotransmitters, neurotrophic factors, and excess protons released as a result of tissue injury and inflammation, directly activate or sensitize nociceptors. Increased expression of ion channels involved in pain transmission is an important mechanism leading to development of peripheral sensitization. Peripheral nerve injury leads to increased expression of specific *voltage-gated sodium* (Na_v) channels and TRPV1 cation channels in the primary afferent terminals, axonal sprouts at the lesion site, demyelinated areas, and adjacent unharmed nociceptors in the site of injury. These channel changes are significant for the expression of neuropathic pain.

Peripheral sensitization has several important ramifications. It reduces the threshold for nociceptor activation, causes primary hyperalgesia (augmentation of normally noxious stimuli), and elicits spontaneous depolarization in primary afferent fibers (ectopic activity). Concomitantly, the peripheral injury enables these neurotrophic factors to migrate in a retrograde direction, thus affecting DRG and dorsal horn cells.

ECTOPIC IMPULSE GENERATION

The persistence of an unpleasant sensory and emotional experience in the absence of an identifiable ongoing stimulus is a characteristic feature of neuropathic pain. This spontaneous pain can occur as a result of ectopic action potential generation in primary afferent neurons. It may originate both from ectopic activity in nociceptors and from low-threshold large myelinated afferents due to central sensitization and altered connectivity in the spinal cord. Ectopic discharges originating in the cell body of injured primary afferents may cause antidromic stimulation, the release of mediators,

and neurogenic inflammation at the periphery. Ectopic impulses can also generate along neuromas and from the sprouting of sympathetic efferents, forming "baskets" around DRG cells. Sympathetic sensory coupling is believed to play an important role in the pathophysiology of inflammatory pain, complex regional pain syndrome (CRPS), diabetic neuropathy, postherpetic neuralgia (PHN), phantom limb sensations, and other conditions. Also, deafferentation (loss of normal afferent input) can lead to sensitization and ectopic discharges in spinal cord or thalamic neurons.

Voltage-gated sodium channels are important influences on the generation of ectopic activity; their role in the pathogenesis of neuropathic pain is supported by the reversal of nociceptive effects by nonselective sodium channel blockers such as local anesthetics. DRG neurons express several types of sodium channels that are either sensitive or resistant to tetrodotoxin.

CENTRAL SENSITIZATION

This is a form of *activity-dependent synaptic plasticity* that also has a pivotal role in the pathophysiology of neuropathic pain. It is responsible for *secondary hyperalgesia,* characterized as increased pain intensity to noxious stimuli experienced beyond the distribution of the inciting area of injury, and *tactile allodynia,* defined as pain due to a normally innocuous stimulus. *Central sensitization* represents amplification in the functional status of neurons and nociceptive circuits, caused by reduced inhibition, increased membrane excitability, and enhanced synaptic efficacy. Because these changes appear in the CNS neurons, the perceived pain does not reflect the presence, intensity, or duration of peripheral stimuli. On the contrary, it corresponds to a pathologic state of responsiveness or increased activity of the nociceptive system.

SPINOTHALAMIC AND SPINORETICULAR NOCICEPTIVE PROCESSING IN THE SPINAL CORD

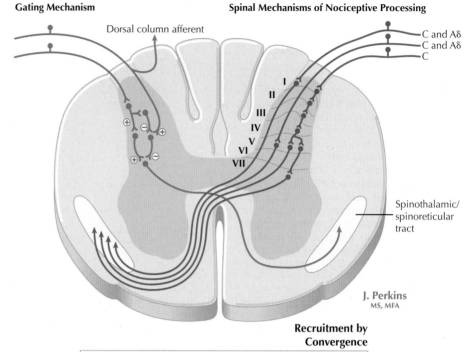

Gating Mechanism   **Spinal Mechanisms of Nociceptive Processing**

Dorsal column afferent

C and Aδ
C and Aδ
C

Spinothalamic/ spinoreticular tract

J. Perkins
MS, MFA

Recruitment by Convergence

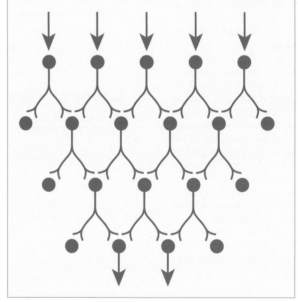

Plate 8.6

Pain

Nociceptive Processing and Central Nervous System Correlates of Pain (Continued)

The development of central sensitization often requires high-intensity, repetitive, and continuous noxious input. Induction and maintenance of central sensitization are dependent on *N*-methyl-D-aspartate receptors (NMDARs) that are ubiquitous within the superficial laminae synapses of the dorsal horn. Normally, the voltage-dependent NMDAR pore is blocked by a magnesium ion (Mg^{2+}). Continuous release of glutamate, substance P, and CGRP leads to sufficient membrane depolarization to force Mg^{2+} to leave the NMDAR channel, allowing glutamate to bind to the receptor and generate an inward current. This allows entry of calcium ion (Ca^{2+}) into the neuron, activating various intracellular pathways that contribute to the maintenance of central sensitization. This early, acute phase of central sensitization results in activation of intracellular kinases that phosphorylate NMDA subunits and other receptors, enhancing their activity and density and leading to *postsynaptic hyperexcitability*. Alterations in transcription in the dorsal horn contribute to the delayed or late phase of central sensitization. Increased synthesis of transmitters and neuromodulators, such as glutamate, substance P, CGRP, brain-derived neurotrophic factor (BDNF), or nitric oxide (NO), results in presynaptic functional changes in the dorsal horn. All of these processes can increase membrane excitability, facilitate synaptic strength, and decrease inhibitory influences on dorsal horn neurons. Of note, these alterations are not necessarily restricted to the activated synapse (*homosynaptic facilitation*) but can easily spread to adjacent synapses (*hetero-synaptic facilitation*). Consequently, these modulatory processes lead to enhanced responsiveness of nociceptive neurons, which lasts longer than the initiating stimuli, or results in activation of nociceptive networks by stimuli that are subthreshold compared with the preinjury baseline.

DISINHIBITION

Several local inhibitory circuits and descending inhibitory pathways serve to modulate the perception of pain. However, after peripheral nerve injury, primary afferents, dorsal horn neurons, and GABAergic inhibitory neurons undergo a number of maladaptive changes. Primary afferents express fewer opioid receptors, and dorsal horn neurons are less susceptible to inhibition by mu opioid agonists. Activation of GABAergic receptors may provoke paradoxic excitation and spontaneous activity. This loss of local inhibition promotes pain transmission, especially the Aβ fiber–mediated pain.

LOW-THRESHOLD Aβ FIBER–MEDIATED PAIN

These fibers mediate not only touch, pressure, vibratory, and joint movement sensation but also, and very importantly, the suppression of nociceptive pain caused by rubbing the affected area. However, after neural lesions, Aβ fibers begin to activate superficial dorsal horn nociceptive projection neurons. Peripheral injury induces regenerative responses to help damaged neurons in reconnecting with their targets. These gene-activated growth stimuli may cause sprouting of Aβ fibers into the superficial layers of dorsal horn. Regenerative

Central Nervous System Neurotransmitters, Receptors, and Drug Targets

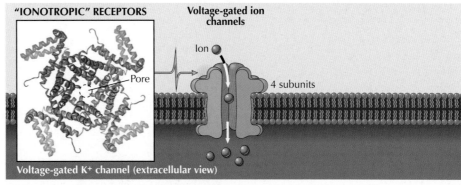

"IONOTROPIC" RECEPTORS

Voltage-gated ion channels

Ion

Pore

4 subunits

Voltage-gated K+ channel (extracellular view)

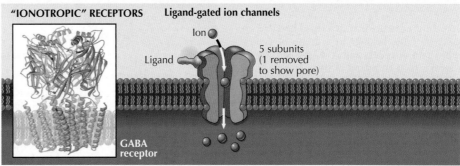

"IONOTROPIC" RECEPTORS

Ligand-gated ion channels

Ion

Ligand

5 subunits (1 removed to show pore)

GABA receptor

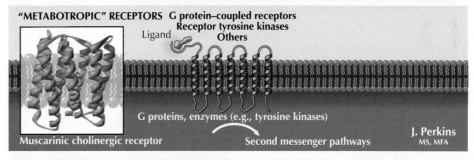

"METABOTROPIC" RECEPTORS

G protein–coupled receptors
Receptor tyrosine kinases
Others

Ligand

G proteins, enzymes (e.g., tyrosine kinases)

Muscarinic cholinergic receptor

Second messenger pathways

J. Perkins
MS, MFA

Select CNS Neurotransmitters and Neuromodulators

Acetylcholine	Dopamine	Glycine	Oxytocin
Adenosine	Eicosanoids	Histamine	Somatostatin
AMP, ADP, ATP	Endothelins	Neuropeptide Y	Substance P
Anandamide	Epinephrine	Neurosteroids	(tachykinins)
Aspartate	FMRF-amide-related	Neurotensin	Taurine
Bombesin	peptides	NO (nitric oxide)	Vasoactive intestinal
Bradykinin	GABA	Norepinephrine	polypeptide (VIP)
Calcitonin gene-related	Galanin	Opioid peptides	Vasopressin
peptide (CGRP)	Gastrin	(endorphins,	
Cholecystokinin	Glutamate	enkephalins,	
Cytokines	Glutamine	dynorphins)	

sprouts may demonstrate ectopic activity or be activated by otherwise subthreshold stimuli. Along with central sensitization, these changes *manifest clinically as the ability to generate pain in areas outside of injured nerve territories* and are usually coupled with a loss of C-fiber terminals.

NEUROIMMUNE INTERACTIONS

Macrophages have a central role in the immune surveillance of the PNS. They clear cellular debris and serve as antigen-presenting cells to activate T lymphocytes. Both macrophages and T cells use cytokines and chemokines as means of communication with neurons, oligodendrocytes, Schwann cells, and spinal microglia. Peripheral nerve injury unleashes *microglial activation* in the dorsal horn; this occurs in close proximity to the injured afferent. The activated spinal microglia *express chemokine receptors* and *release immune mediators* (interleukin [IL]-1B, IL6, tumor necrosis factor-α [TNF-α], BDNF), inducing and maintaining maladaptive pain conditions. Mediators released by microglia and astrocytes, as well as cytokines/chemokines produced by DRG cells, directly activate nociceptors, cause peripheral sensitization by increasing the excitability of primary afferents, and stimulate adjacent chemokine-expressing neurons. Changes in the expression and function of the transient receptor potential channels and increases in sodium and calcium currents contribute to induction of action potentials. TNF-α also has been shown to stimulate DRG neurons and enhance the expression of chemokines, and its antagonists abolish neuropathic pain behavior in animal models.

Plate 8.7

THALAMUS

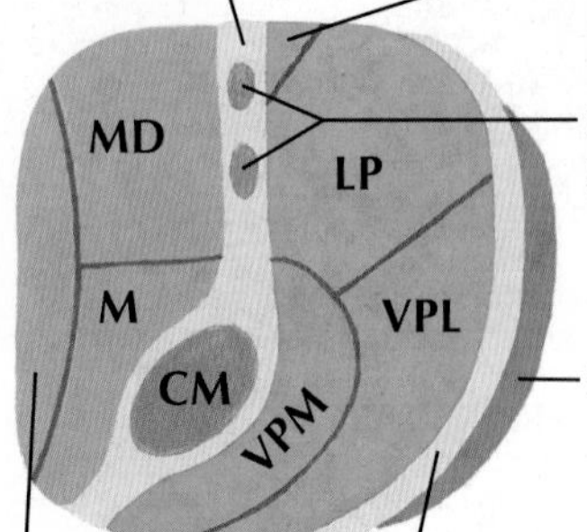

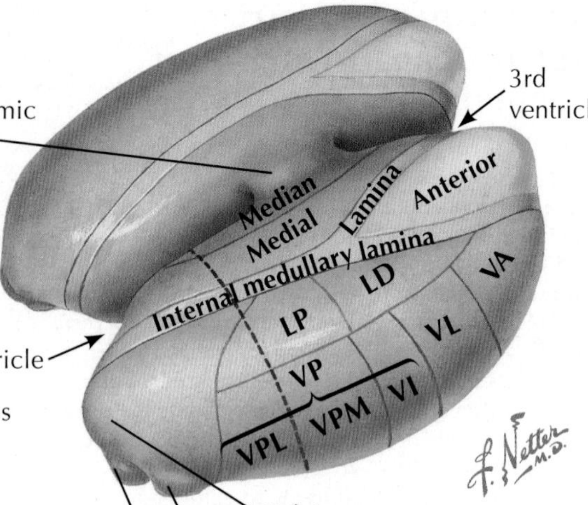

Thalamic nuclei

CM	Centromedian
LD	Lateral dorsal
LP	Lateral posterior
M	Medial
MD	Medial dorsal
VA	Ventral anterior
VI	Ventral intermedial
VL	Ventral lateral
VP	Ventral posterior
VPL	Ventroposterolateral
VPM	Ventroposteromedial

Schematic section through thalamus (at level of broken line shown in figure at right)

Schematic representation of thalamus (external medullary lamina and reticular nuclei removed)

Lateral nuclei
Medial nuclei
Anterior nuclei

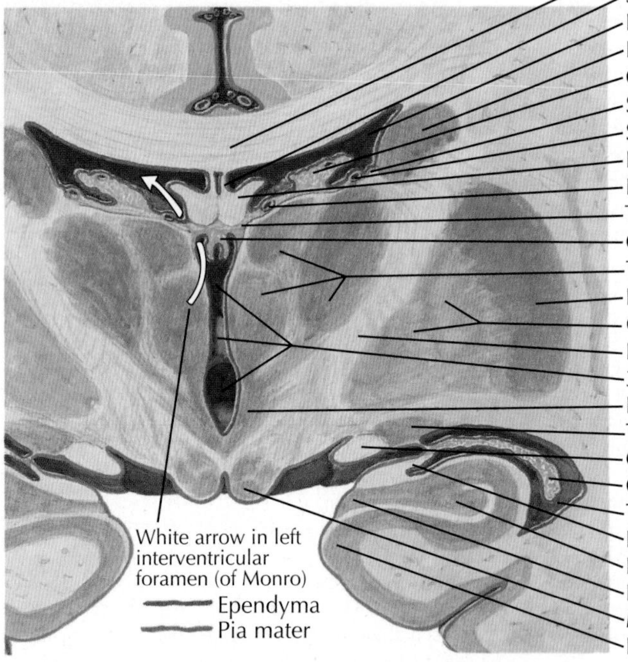

THALAMIC PAIN SYNDROME

Thalamic pain syndrome, first described by Dejerine and Roussy in 1906, belongs to a group of central neuropathic pain disorders and is most often the result of a stroke, be it an infarct or hemorrhage. However, recognition that noncerebrovascular etiologies and lesions to CNS structures other than the thalamus may give rise to this pattern of symptoms has led to a broadening of the eponymous terminology to include central poststroke pain (CPSP) or central pain syndrome. The defining clinical features of this syndrome include persistent allodynia, hypersensitivity to mechanical or thermal stimuli, and muscle weakness and sensory impairment affecting the side contralateral to the lesion. CPSP can develop weeks to years after the inciting stroke, with incidence of 8% within the first year after a stroke. CPSP has a spectrum of severity from mild numbness to a debilitating condition that severely affects quality of life, undercuts rehabilitation efforts, and leads to psychological disturbances. At the time of its earliest description and for many years thereafter, this condition was considered relatively rare, and treatment options typically offered minimal analgesic benefit.

Pathophysiology. The thalamus plays a central role in modulation of sensory information between the periphery and cerebral cortex. Various hypothesized mechanisms underlie the pathophysiology of CPSP, three of which are central imbalance, central disinhibition, and central sensitization. Central imbalance is associated with the exam finding of dissociated sensory loss. This is characterized by hypersensitivity to thermal and noxious stimuli and intact sensory perception to touch and vibration. It is speculated that this symptom pattern is attributable to an imbalance of inputs among STTs and spared dorsal column/medial lemniscus activity. Central disinhibition is thought to account for the abnormal thermal sensation, burning pain, and cold allodynia at the level of the medial thalamus and ACC. The concept of central sensitization postulates that changes in electrophysiologic properties of nociceptive neurons lead to hyperexcitability through multiple mechanisms. From a clinical, practical standpoint there is currently no way to correlate these symptom features with an underlying mechanism or localization. As such, therapy based on the underlying pain mechanism or localization is not possible based on our current understanding of the pathophysiology of these syndromes.

Clinical Manifestations. Thalamic pain syndrome or CPSP is primarily diagnosed by its onset after stroke, location of lesion, and presentation and pattern of symptoms. CPSP appears in patients at variable

Coronal section of brain: posterior view

times after the initial ischemic event, ranging from weeks to months or even years later. The pain qualities most commonly associated with this syndrome are described as burning, stinging, stabbing, or shooting; hyperalgesia to temperature and touch are often noted. The primary features of CPSP include sensory

and motor deficits contralateral to the ischemic lesion. Pain may travel from the extremities and may be accompanied by facial paresthesia; anesthesia may also occur in regions affected by the stroke. CPSP is more common in right-sided strokes. The majority of pain is classified as a persistent constant pain, daily

Plate 8.8

Pain

CLINICAL MANIFESTATIONS RELATED TO THALAMUS SITE IN INTRACEREBRAL HEMORRHAGE

Pathology	CT scan	Pupils	Eye movements	Motor and sensory deficits	Other
Thalamus		Constricted, poorly reactive to light bilaterally	Both lids retracted; eyes positioned downward and medially; cannot look upward	Slight contralateral hemiparesis, but greater hemisensory loss	Aphasia (if lesion on left side)

THALAMIC PAIN SYNDROME (Continued)

intermittent pain lasting seconds to minutes with relief limited to a few hours, or hypersensitivity, hyperpathia, or allodynia in response to various stimuli. The latter classification has been reported in 65% of patients with CPSP, although any or all of the pain characteristics may be present.

Treatment. Management of CPSP remains a major therapeutic challenge. Due to the severity and quality of the pain, many patients have both associated motor deficits (e.g., spasticity) and psychological distress that need to be addressed in addition to the need for analgesic treatment. So far, there are few class I randomized controlled trials (RCTs) on CPSP treatment. Lately, however, new pharmacologic treatments have emerged and have been evaluated in various clinical trials. A recent RCT study on duloxetine demonstrated that despite some advantageous biologic effects, duloxetine is no more effective in controlling neuropathic pain than placebo. One RCT of pregabalin demonstrated significant reduction in pain intensity as well as improvements in sleep and global patient status. There is evidence for the dose-dependent analgesic benefit of opioids in these syndromes. Inhaled cannabis has been shown to improve spasticity in patients not receiving relief from traditional treatment options. Smoked cannabis causes a reduction in both spasticity and pain in patients with treatment-resistant spasticity.

Currently, a multimodal pharmacologic approach is endorsed by some experts specializing in the treatment of patients with CPSP, although no trials have been published so far on polypharmacy for CPSP. Part of the rationale for this approach is to improve the tolerability of analgesics that exert their pharmacologic effect and have side effects mediated centrally. These experts advocate tricyclic antidepressants and gabapentinoids as first-line treatment. In CPSP, fluvoxamine is the only selective serotonin reuptake inhibitor that has been tested, and it reduces the pain if started within 1 year of the stroke. If improvement in pain intensity is not seen and the pain has a shooting characteristic, anticonvulsants such as carbamazepine are added to the medication regimen. The timing of incorporation of opioids should be tailored to individual patient risk factors for aberrant drug-taking behavior with this class of therapy. Some clinical reports show that transdermal buprenorphine can show promising results for central neuropathic pain, which can also improve patient compliance and quality of life. In addition, tapentadol has shown some promising results in patients with neuropathic pain.

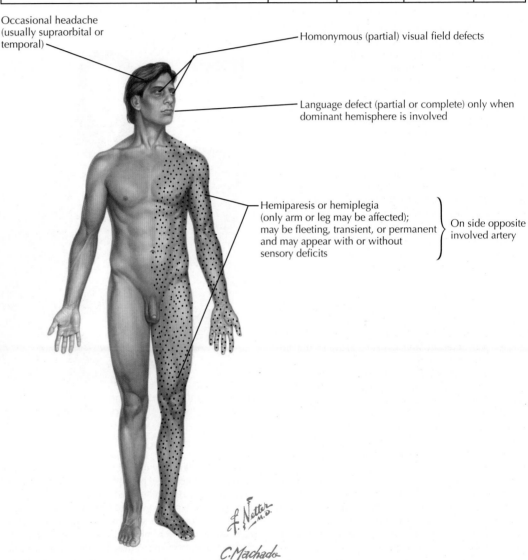

Occasional headache (usually supraorbital or temporal)

Homonymous (partial) visual field defects

Language defect (partial or complete) only when dominant hemisphere is involved

Hemiparesis or hemiplegia (only arm or leg may be affected); may be fleeting, transient, or permanent and may appear with or without sensory deficits } On side opposite involved artery

Invasive procedures include deep brain, spinal cord, and motor cortex stimulation, and various ablative approaches have been presented in small series with modest and often short-lived therapeutic benefit. Repetitive transcranial magnetic stimulation has shown benefit with reductions in visual analog scale for pain, but data are preliminary.

Some patients with CPSP might also benefit from psychological treatment addressing chronic pain behaviors, and poststroke rehabilitation seems to be of utmost importance in this group of patients. In a case report, mirror therapy typically used for CRPS was beneficial for central poststroke pain.

COMPLEX REGIONAL PAIN

Complex regional pain syndrome (CRPS), previously known as reflex sympathetic dystrophy, is an important chronic neuropathic pain syndrome with a distinctive clinical presentation that often implicates the autonomic nervous system. The epidemiology of CRPS is difficult to estimate because of the spectrum of symptom severity and paucity of clinical signs in many cases, but in studies maximizing diagnostic sensitivity, incidence rates as high as the 30% range in postsurgical series and 20% to 25% in extremity fractures have been ventured. Chronic CRPS rated as "severe" occurs in less than 2% of cases.

Pathophysiology. The precise pathophysiology of CRPS remains unclear, but the emerging consensus from recent studies indicates that CRPS involves more than one underlying mechanism. One of the proposed explanations involves altered cutaneous innervation after injury. Other studies underline the roles of central and peripheral sensitization in the development of CRPS. Hyperalgesia and allodynia encountered after initial tissue trauma are attributed to local release of several pronociceptive neuropeptides that leads to enhanced responsiveness of nociceptors and lowered thresholds for innocuous thermal and mechanical stimuli.

Excessive function of sympathetic nervous system (SNS) has been long believed to be responsible for common autonomic features of CRPS. Reduced SNS function in the early phase of CRPS may also help explain the common phenomenon of a warm, red extremity in acute CRPS. Furthermore, increased sympathetic activity may contribute to nociceptive excitation through adrenergic receptors that are expressed on nociceptive fibers after nerve trauma.

Finally, there is also evidence pointing to an important role of the CNS in the pathophysiology of CRPS. Several studies have shown that the region of somatosensory cortex representing the affected limb is considerably reduced. Such brain plasticity is reportedly associated with greater pain intensity and hyperalgesia, and impaired tactile discrimination.

Clinical Findings. Although CRPS has been documented in visceral trauma, it occurs predominantly in fractures and surgical trauma to the extremities, including distal radial fractures, carpal tunnel release, and numerous arthroscopic procedures. The major clinical features of CRPS are spontaneous pain, allodynia, hyperalgesia, edema, vasomotor instability, autonomic dysfunction, and progressive trophic changes. Pain is typically experienced in a distribution beyond the initially affected nerve(s) and may spread to involve the entire affected limb and, rarely, the contralateral limb as well. Weakness, tremor, and other motor anomalies may occur in the affected extremity, resulting in profound loss of function. CRPS occurs as two subtypes, with the presence of an identifiable noxious stimulating event delineating between the two. Type I CRPS develops in the absence of an identifiable focal nerve lesion and can develop after a minor fracture or trauma, whereas type II CRPS occurs in the presence of identifiable nerve damage.

Various diagnostic tools, including thermography, sweat testing, radiographic testing, and sympathetic blocks, have their advocates, but the diagnosis remains clinical. Abnormal sweat production may be measured in the affected extremity to provide quantitative description of symptom report.

Treatment. Treatment of CRPS requires a multidisciplinary approach to manage symptoms and preserve

Acute reflex sympathetic dystrophy. Hand swollen, red, and painful.

Associated severe disuse osteoporosis

Chronic reflex sympathetic dystrophy. Hand atrophic, cold, and painful, with slight clawing of fingers.

In chronic reflex sympathetic dystrophy, right upper limb atrophic, stiffened. Arm held at rest protectively to avoid pain.

function. The outcome of CRPS may be more favorable with early diagnosis and prompt treatment. Management of symptoms is typically based on severity of pain and may include interventional and pharmacologic therapy.

One first-line treatment for the functional consequences of CRPS is physiotherapy, which includes range-of-motion exercise, desensitization, and isometric strengthening. A number of interventional therapeutic approaches blocking the SNS to reduce CRPS symptoms demonstrate symptomatic relief in addition to improvements in function and reduced analgesic medication use. Regional anesthetic blocks, such as sympathetic blockade, sympathectomy, and somatic blockade, are used in patients with moderate to severe pain and are often used in combination with nonpharmacologic approaches. Neuromodulation technologies, such as spinal cord stimulation (SCS), have also shown promise in the treatment of CRPS; a subpopulation of patients may experience a durable robust response, but treatment matching remains a challenge. DRG stimulation has demonstrated efficacy in clinical

trials in CRPS populations. These data suggest that DRG stimulation may have better outcomes than SCS in patients with CRPS.

Pharmacotherapy for symptom-oriented treatments includes antidepressants such as tricyclics, adjuvants such as gabapentinoids, corticosteroids, topical analgesics, opioids, bisphosphonates, and free radical scavengers. Tricyclic antidepressants (TCAs) and antiepileptics, such as gabapentin, are effective in treating neuropathic pain, yet their effectiveness has not been studied specifically in patients with CRPS. Controlled studies of bisphosphonates for the indication of CRPS have not provided rigorous evidence to support their use in this indication. Small, uncontrolled studies may support the use of the NMDAR modulator ketamine for symptomatic relief in patients with CRPS. Opioids may be used when tolerated because this class of analgesic has demonstrated efficacy in neuropathic pain. However, the development of tolerance may be problematic, and the potential for abuse and misuse requires judicious use and close monitoring.

Plate 8.10

Pain

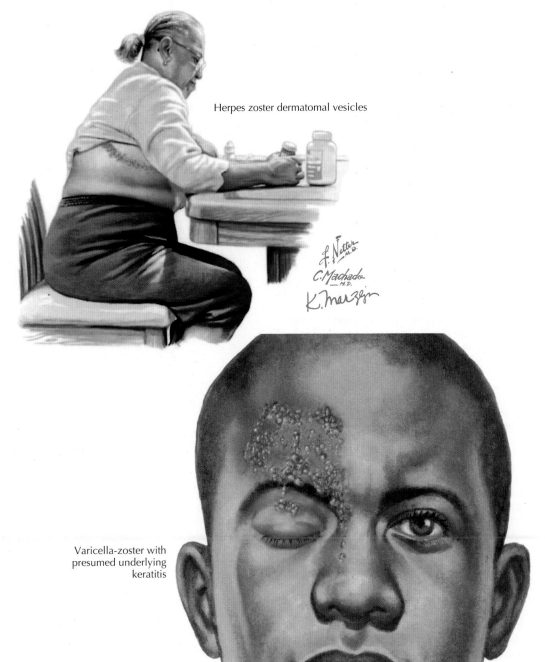

Herpes zoster dermatomal vesicles

Varicella-zoster with presumed underlying keratitis

HERPES ZOSTER

Known to the layman as "shingles," herpes zoster is an acute neuralgia typically confined to the distribution of a specific spinal nerve root or cranial nerve. It is the most common infection of the PNS in industrialized nations. After causing primary infection, known as "chicken pox," the varicella-zoster virus (VZV) becomes latent in trigeminal, autonomic, and dorsal root ganglia as a result of acquired cell-mediated immunity. Since the introduction of live-attenuated vaccine in 1996, a greater than 97% decline in varicella cases has been observed. The virus can reactivate after a variable period of time, causing an extremely painful vesicular skin rash. Pain is often the most debilitating symptom associated with herpes zoster. Age and immunosuppression are the most important factors in the reactivation of the virus; however, stress, trauma, surgery, and a family history of herpes zoster can also reactivate VZV.

Herpes zoster causes complications in as many as 10% of patients treated for non-Hodgkin lymphoma. Other significant subpopulations at increased risk of acute herpes zoster include those on corticosteroid therapy or patients who are therapeutically immunosuppressed, such as transplant recipients.

A serious chronic complication of herpes zoster is postherpetic neuralgia (PHN), characterized by severe and persistent pain more than 90 days after resolution of the vesicular rash; in its most severe forms, this syndrome is highly refractory to treatment. Several risk factors for the development of PHN have been identified, such as age over 50 years, female sex, a severe disseminated rash, severe pain at onset, the presence of a prodrome, and polymerase chain reaction–detectable viremia.

Pathophysiology. The DRG is the primary site of infection. The VZV, a DNA-type virus, is the same virus that causes chickenpox in children. Current theories suggest that the virus, which is also similar to herpes simplex virus, migrates up the peripheral nerve to the DRG subsequent to an attack of chickenpox in childhood. The virus then lies dormant for many years until the decrement in immunologic surveillance occurs and the virus reactivates. When this occurs, the DRG may be destroyed by an acute inflammatory reaction. Concomitantly, the virus spreads down the nerve root and peripheral nerve to the skin, producing the characteristic rash.

Clinical Findings. The rash is reminiscent of chickenpox but confined to a radicular or cranial nerve distribution. Its onset is often heralded by a few days of either severe localized pain or nonspecific discomfort in the affected area. The vesicles appear 72 to 96 hours later.

As with varicella, more than half of patients are affected in the thoracic region, as well as the ophthalmic branch of the trigeminal nerve.

A serious primary complication of VZV is PHN, or chronic neuropathic pain in the affected nerve territory that persists after the skin eruptions and acute inflammatory response have subsided. Although PHN may improve over time, the incidence and severity of symptoms directly correlate with advanced age at rash onset and the degree of rash severity. The pain may be characterized either as persistent burning or lancinating pain precipitated by friction of the skin; intense itching and formication can be present as well.

Treatment. Recombinant zoster vaccine (RZV; Shingrix) has surpassed the live-attenuated vaccine (Zostavax, Merck & Co.) as the first-line vaccine for the prevention of herpes zoster in patients aged 50 years and older. Immunocompetent adults should get two doses of RZV 2 to 6 months apart, whether or not they have already received the live-attenuated vaccine or had herpes zoster. It should not, however, be used for the treatment of herpes zoster or PHN. Antivirals such as acyclovir, valacyclovir, and famciclovir reduce the acute and symptomatic period if taken within 3 days of rash appearance. The latter two drugs also decrease the incidence and severity of PHN but do not prevent its occurrence. TCAs, adjuvants such as gabapentin and pregabalin, topical lidocaine (5%), topical high-dose (8%) capsaicin, and opioid medication have all proved efficacious in relieving pain related to PHN. Opioid analgesics, including oxycodone, have demonstrated analgesic benefit in the acute and subacute phase after acute herpes zoster reactivation and are commonly used in combination with nonopioid therapies.

OCCIPITAL NEURALGIA

Occipital neuralgia, as defined by the International Headache Society, is paroxysmal shooting pain within the distribution of the greater, lesser, and third occipital nerves. The pain involves occipital and periauricular areas and may radiate to the lateral scalp and periorbital area. Occipital neuralgia episodes may be provoked with palpation of the occipital nerves, especially at the anatomic landmark of the occipital notch. Increased muscle tone modulated by psychosocial factors may modulate pain intensity in the distribution of the occipital nerve. In one prospective registry from a subspecialty headache clinic population evaluating 5515 patients, only 1.2% were diagnosed with occipital headache; the vast majority of diagnosed cases were in females (79%). Although there is no definitive localizing test to characterize the epidemiology of occipital neuralgia, multiple studies indicate that the greater occipital nerve accounts for the majority of cases. One study found that in roughly 8.7% of cases both the greater and lesser nerves were involved.

Pathophysiology. Occipital neuralgia may have various etiologies, mostly categorized as neurogenic, vascular, muscular, or osteogenic. Trauma to the C2 root due to traction injury (e.g., whiplash injury) and arthritic changes of the atlantoaxial joint are possible mechanical causes of occipital neuralgia. Other postulated mechanisms include entrapment with sustained contraction or spasm of the posterior neck muscles as they pass through the inferior oblique, semispinalis, and the aponeurosis of the superior trapezius. Osteogenic origins include osteoarthritis and arthritic degeneration of the spine, which lead to nerve impingement by hypertrophied atlantoaxial ligaments. Instances of vascular etiology include irritation of C1/C2 nerve roots by diverging branches of the posterior inferior cerebellar artery and dural arteriovenous fistulas in the cervical regions. Tumors of the second and third cervical dorsal roots account for more uncommon, neurogenic causes. Some cases can occur after Arnold-Chiari malformation surgery or other craniocervical surgeries. It has also been reported after radiofrequency ablation and cryoablation. Most often, however, the inciting factor is not disclosed with clinical evaluation, and the neuropathic changes in the greater or lesser occipital nerve are considered idiopathic. Perhaps these pathophysiologic mechanisms will be more easily identified with the increased availability of 3-T magnetic resonance imaging (MRI), providing more accurate detail.

Clinical Findings. The differential diagnosis for occipital neuralgia includes primary headache syndromes such as migraine, cluster headache, and trigeminal autonomic cephalgia, in addition to referred myofascial pain, cervicogenic headache localizing to articular structures such as the facet joint, and tension-type headache. Occipital neuralgia is typically described as stabbing pain with periods of aching pain between the paroxysmal episodes. Retroorbital pain may be explained by the convergence of nociceptive pathways in the dorsal root of C2 and the pars caudalis division of the spinal trigeminal nucleus. Additionally, visual deficits, ringing in the ears, dizziness, and nasal congestion may accompany painful periods because of the involvement of cranial nerves VIII, IX, and X and the cervical sympathetic trunk. Upon physical examination, dysesthesia is elicited along the greater and lesser occipital nerve as well as tenderness to palpation. Diagnosis is confirmed via diagnostic nerve block of the occipital nerve, along with imaging scans to identify any suspected lesions.

Third occipital nerve (dorsal ramus of C3 spinal nerve)

Epicranial aponeurosis (galea aponeurotica)

Greater occipital nerve (dorsal ramus of C2 spinal nerve)

Occipital belly (occipitalis) of occipitofrontalis muscle

Occipital artery

Posterior auricular artery

Semispinalis capitis and splenius capitis muscles in posterior triangle of neck

Great auricular nerve (cervical plexus C2, 3)

Sternocleidomastoid muscle

Lesser occipital nerve (cervical plexus C2)

Trapezius muscle

Posterior cutaneous branches of dorsal rami of C4, 5, 6 spinal nerves

Rectus capitis posterior minor muscle

Rectus capitis posterior major muscle

Semispinalis capitis muscle (cut and reflected)

Vertebral artery (extradural part)

Obliquus capitis superior muscle

Suboccipital nerve (dorsal ramus of C1 spinal nerve)

Posterior arch of atlas (C1 vertebra)

Obliquus capitis inferior muscle

Occipital artery

Greater occipital nerve (dorsal ramus of C2 spinal nerve)

Splenius capitis muscle (cut and reflected)

Third occipital nerve (dorsal ramus of C3 spinal nerve)

Longissimus capitis muscle

Splenius cervicis muscle

Semispinalis cervicis muscle

Semispinalis capitis muscle (cut)

Splenius capitis muscle (cut)

Treatment. Treatment depends on whether an identifiable lesion or compression is present. Occipital nerve blocks are often effective at attenuating pain intensity in this region. Ultrasound-guided greater occipital nerve blocks provide better pain reduction at 4 weeks than landmark-based greater occipital nerve blocks for patients with occipital neuralgia or cervicogenic headache. Patients with multiple sclerosis in whom the pain may localize to demyelinating lesions of CNS structures are far less likely to respond to occipital nerve blocks compared with other phenotypes with peripheral localizations. Most treatments, however, are aimed at symptom reduction and relief of any accompanying muscle tension. Empiric use of drugs based on efficacy data from other neuropathic syndromes is common. These agents include adjuvants such as TCAs and anticonvulsants such as oxcarbazepine and gabapentin. Botulinum toxin type A injections have been studied in a preliminary fashion. Pulsed radio frequency of the C2 or C3 DRG has also been evaluated in small preliminary studies if injection of local anesthetics and corticosteroids of the greater occipital nerve is only transiently beneficial. An emerging body of evidence may support the use of subcutaneous peripheral nerve stimulation in intractable, severe cases of occipital neuralgia; however, sham-controlled studies are needed to support this practice.

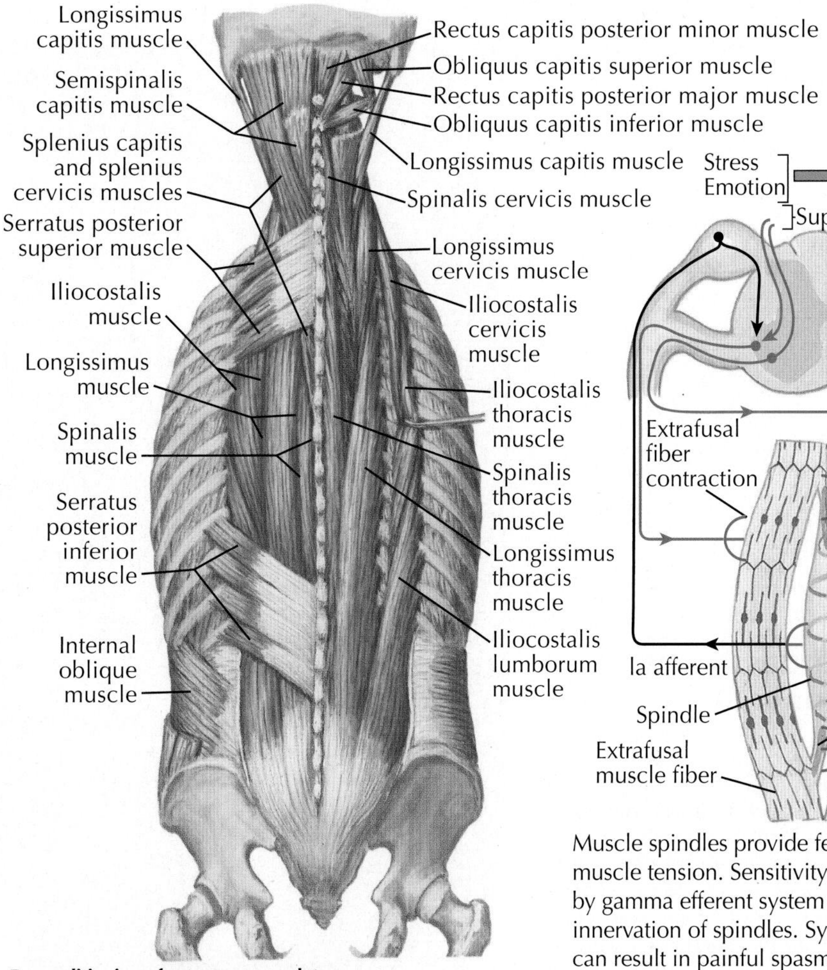

Plate 8.12

Pain

Longissimus capitis muscle
Semispinalis capitis muscle
Splenius capitis and splenius cervicis muscles
Serratus posterior superior muscle
Iliocostalis muscle
Longissimus muscle
Spinalis muscle
Serratus posterior inferior muscle
Internal oblique muscle

Rectus capitis posterior minor muscle
Obliquus capitis superior muscle
Rectus capitis posterior major muscle
Obliquus capitis inferior muscle
Longissimus capitis muscle
Spinalis cervicis muscle
Longissimus cervicis muscle
Iliocostalis cervicis muscle
Iliocostalis thoracis muscle
Spinalis thoracis muscle
Longissimus thoracis muscle
Iliocostalis lumborum muscle

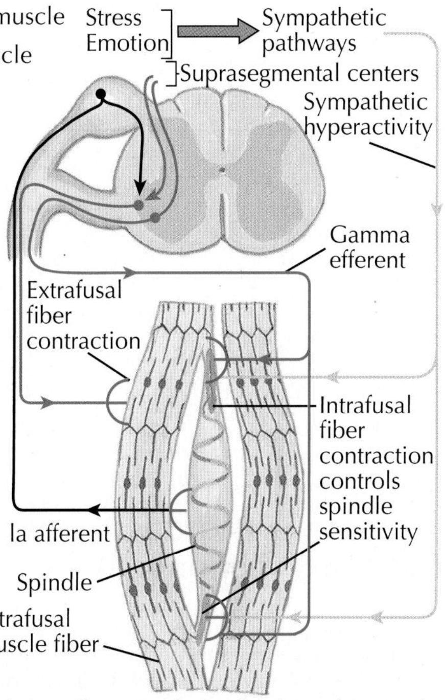

Stress Emotion
Sympathetic pathways
Suprasegmental centers
Sympathetic hyperactivity
Gamma efferent
Extrafusal fiber contraction
Intrafusal fiber contraction controls spindle sensitivity
Ia afferent
Spindle
Extrafusal muscle fiber

Muscle spindles provide feedback mechanism for muscle tension. Sensitivity of spindles modulated by gamma efferent system and by sympathetic innervation of spindles. Sympathetic hyperactivity can result in painful spasm of spindles.

Deconditioning of extensor musculature

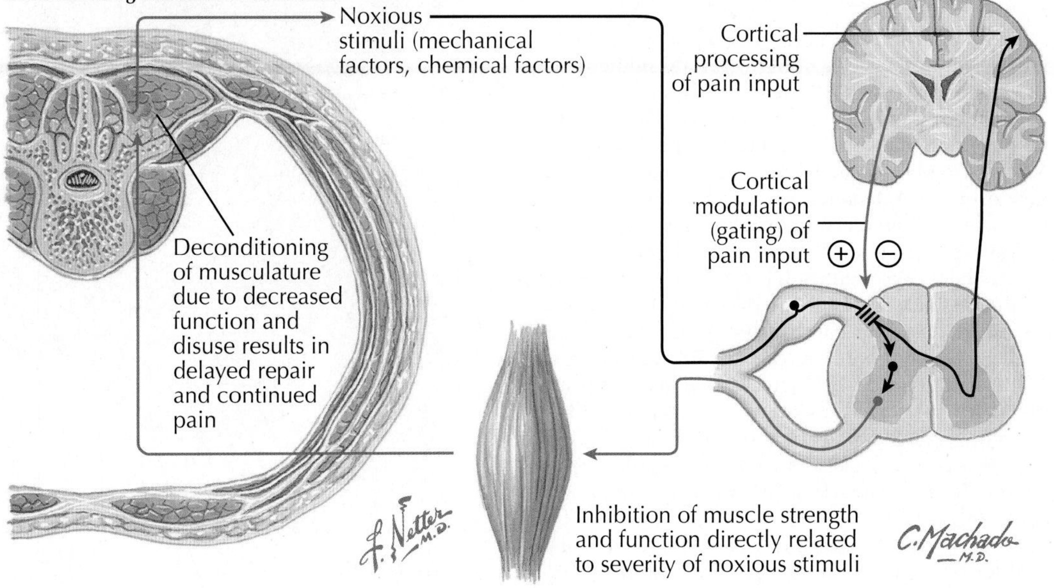

Noxious stimuli (mechanical factors, chemical factors)
Deconditioning of musculature due to decreased function and disuse results in delayed repair and continued pain
Cortical processing of pain input
Cortical modulation (gating) of pain input
Inhibition of muscle strength and function directly related to severity of noxious stimuli

Myofascial Factors in Low Back Pain

Myofascial structures are implicated in virtually all acute and chronic low back pain (CLBP) syndromes. Myofascial pain syndrome (MPS) is strictly defined by the presence of local and referred pain that originates from a myofascial trigger point (MTrP). This symptom pattern overlaps clinically with pain referred from diverse somatic structures such as ligaments, articular surfaces, periosteum, scar tissue, skin, and tendons. Trigger points, defined as a zone of intense pain associated with a hardened muscle band, may be identified on physical examination; however, it is not uncommon that syndromes with a myofascial component lack a discrete TrP when somatic pain is referred pain from deeper muscles such as the psoas into the inguinal region.

Clinical studies suggest that MPS is the most common cause of CLBP, with 60% to 97% patients examined exhibiting myofascial abnormalities. Less clear is the extent to which centralized mechanisms of pain manifest as myofascial symptoms due to either increases in muscle tone associated with psychosocial factors (e.g., anxiety) or dysregulation of nociceptive processing that localizes to the CNS. The prevalence varies from 30% of general medical clinic patients with regional pain to as high as 85% to 93% of patients presenting to specialty pain management centers. Women are even three times more likely to experience from MTrPs compared with men. MPS is more commonly identified in those aged 27 to 50 years.

Pathophysiology. The development of MPS is often associated with postural derangements such as muscle overload, dystonia, and fatigue. Postural abnormality (e.g., scoliosis) may reflect asymmetric extensor or flexor tone in a group of paraspinal muscles. Secondary causes of myofascial pain are extremely common as well and include distinct presentations such as painful spasm in the context of spondylolisthesis or increases in tone in the setting of emotional stress. The most common cause of MTrP formation is repetitive stress on one or more muscles or muscle groups. In the low back, MPS may also develop because of structural inadequacies, such as small hemipelvis or short leg or arm. An MTrP is defined by Simons and Travell as a hyperirritable spot in skeletal muscle that is associated with a hypersensitive palpable nodule in a taut band. The key pathoanatomic abnormalities associated with MTrPs appear to be principally located at the center of a muscle in its motor endplate zone. Precipitating factors may cause the facilitated release of acetylcholine at motor end plates, sustained muscle fiber contractions and local ischemia with release of vascular and neuroactive substances, and muscle pain. More acetylcholine may then be released, thus perpetuating the muscle spasm. The abundance of the nociceptors in muscle, joints, skin, and blood vessels may explain the severity of pain and exquisite tenderness in the muscle upon palpation.

Some experts speculate that chronicity in myofascial pain syndromes is attributable to altered sensory processing as characterized by central sensitization with alteration in supraspinal inhibitory descending pain control pathways.

POSTERIOR ABDOMINAL WALL: INTERNAL VIEW

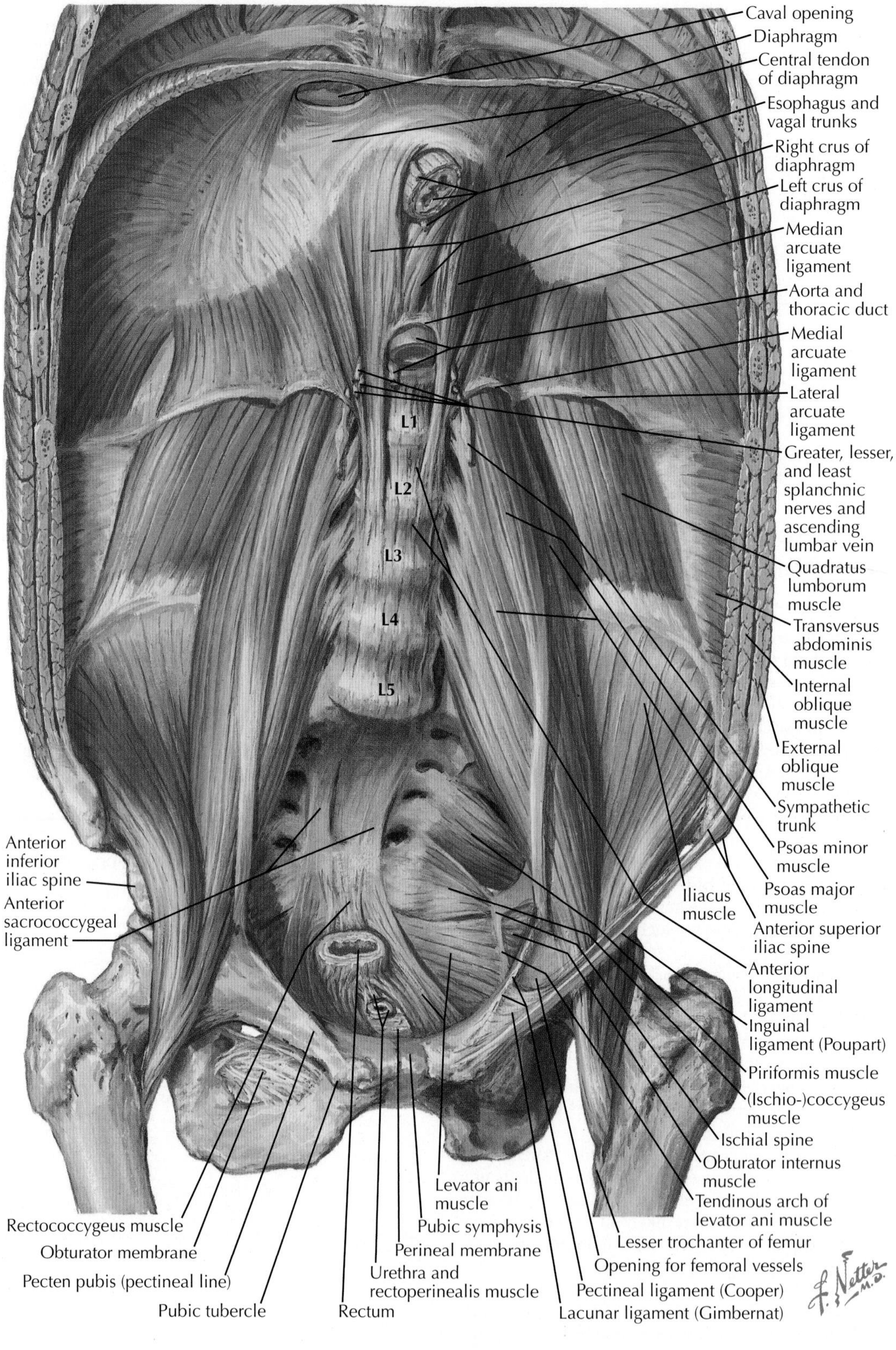

Labels (clockwise from top right):
Caval opening
Diaphragm
Central tendon of diaphragm
Esophagus and vagal trunks
Right crus of diaphragm
Left crus of diaphragm
Median arcuate ligament
Aorta and thoracic duct
Medial arcuate ligament
Lateral arcuate ligament
Greater, lesser, and least splanchnic nerves and ascending lumbar vein
Quadratus lumborum muscle
Transversus abdominis muscle
Internal oblique muscle
External oblique muscle
Sympathetic trunk
Psoas minor muscle
Psoas major muscle
Anterior superior iliac spine
Anterior longitudinal ligament
Inguinal ligament (Poupart)
Piriformis muscle
(Ischio-)coccygeus muscle
Ischial spine
Obturator internus muscle
Tendinous arch of levator ani muscle
Lesser trochanter of femur
Opening for femoral vessels
Pectineal ligament (Cooper)
Lacunar ligament (Gimbernat)
Iliacus muscle
Levator ani muscle
Pubic symphysis
Perineal membrane
Urethra and rectoperinealis muscle
Rectum
Pubic tubercle
Pecten pubis (pectineal line)
Obturator membrane
Rectococcygeus muscle
Anterior sacrococcygeal ligament
Anterior inferior iliac spine

L1, L2, L3, L4, L5

f. Netter M.D.

MYOFASCIAL FACTORS IN LOW BACK PAIN (Continued)

Clinical Findings. The characteristic symptoms of myofascial pain may begin after a discrete trauma or may be of insidious onset. Patients note regional deep aching sensations, varying in intensity from mild to severe. Functional complaints include decreased work tolerance, impaired muscle coordination, stiff joints, fatigue, and weakness. Patients experiencing chronic myofascial pain may report sleep disturbances, mood changes, and stress.

The physical examination is conducted to ascertain the clinical criteria of MPS. Several studies have suggested that the most reliable physical signs of trigger points are pain recognition, taut band, tender point, referred pain, and local twitch response. MTrPs usually appear in muscular structures used for posture maintenance, such as quadratus lumborum, gluteus maximus, gluteus medius, iliocostalis, iliopsoas, levator ani, longissimus thoracis, lower rectus abdominis, multifidi, piriformis, and rotators. In the instance of low back pain (LBP), quadratus lumborum, used for trunk stabilization and posture, is the most common source of MTrP. Palpation of MTrP will produce or increase regional pain and may elicit a referred, radiating pain pattern. Additionally, snapping palpation or needling of MTrP may provoke a local twitch response (detectable contraction) or a reaction known as a "jump sign" (involuntary jerk).

Patients with chronic MTrPs should also be evaluated for perpetuating factors, such as postural abnormalities, ergonomic factors, and hypothyroidism.

Treatment. Treatment of chronic myofascial pain syndromes often requires a comprehensive approach that combines rehabilitation therapies, oral analgesics, and even local interventions. The primary aim is reduction in pain intensity associated with MTrP. In the long term, flexibility has to be restored to the muscle, and any associated precipitating factors have to be removed. Psychosocial factors may play a significant role. Maladaptive pain-coping behaviors, such as fear avoidance and catastrophizing, have been shown to significantly increase the risk of chronic pain in general and LBP in particular.

Medication is a useful supplementary treatment. Acetaminophen, nonsteroidal antiinflammatory drugs (NSAIDs), or cyclooxygenase (COX)-2 selective inhibitors may be used, particularly if there is a local inflammatory component.

Rehabilitation approaches, such as neuromuscular relaxation techniques, heat therapy, and electrical therapy, may also help control muscle pain and spasm.

Needling of MTrPs is one of the most common treatments for MPS. A number of relevant studies have been published demonstrating possible effectiveness; however, none of them established a causal relationship between direct needling of MTrPs and improvement in symptoms. The value of the precision afforded by ultrasound guidance for treatment of myofascial pain syndrome remains unclear regardless of technique and injectate.

Plate 8.14

Pain

LUMBAR ZYGAPOPHYSEAL JOINT BACK PAIN

Lumbar zygapophyseal (facet) joint degeneration is a leading cause of axial predominant CLBP. Facet-mediated pain results from a multifactorial process that is intimately tied to degeneration of the intervertebral disks. Facet syndromes are defined as pain originating from any structure integral to both the function and configuration of the lumbar zygapophyseal (l-z) joints, including the fibrous capsule, synovial membrane, hyaline cartilage surfaces, and bony articulations.

Pathophysiology. In rare instances the development of l-z joint arthropathy can be traced to a specific inciting event; however, the overwhelming majority of cases of l-z joint pain are the result of repetitive strain accumulated with load bearing over the course of a lifetime. The mechanical consequences of disk degeneration are not only reduced disk height but also segmental microinstability. Such changes lead to an increase in the load on the facets and provoke subluxation of the joints as well as cartilage alteration.

Several other conditions, such as rheumatoid arthritis, ankylosing spondylitis, synovial impingement, chondromalacia facetae, pseudogout, meniscoid entrapment, and capsular and synovial inflammation, may also predispose patients to chronic facet joint strain.

Lumbar facet joints are richly innervated with encapsulated, unencapsulated, and free nerve endings, containing substance P, CGRP, and neuropeptide Y. Nerve fibers have also been found in subchondral bone and intraarticular inclusions of l-z joints, signifying that facet-mediated pain may originate in structures besides the joint capsule.

PAIN REFERRAL PATTERNS

Pain emanating from upper facet joints tends to extend into the flank, hip, and upper lateral thigh, whereas pain from the lower facet joints is likely to penetrate deeper into the thigh, usually laterally and/or posteriorly.

Clinical Findings. The clinical presentation of l-z joint–mediated back pain overlaps considerably with the presentation of LBP due to other etiologies. Although l-z joint pain is not associated with neurologic deficits, patients experiencing this type of referred somatic pain may demonstrate pain-inhibited weakness, nondermatomal extremity sensory loss, and other referred sensory complaints as far distal as the foot.

A review of the relevant literature suggests a lack of specificity of radiographic facet joint abnormalities for facet-mediated pain. Although computed tomography (CT) is a sensitive tool for demonstrating anatomic abnormalities of the l-z joint, a review of the relevant literature indicates a lack of specificity of these findings for the experience of facet-mediated pain.

Because no noninvasive pathognomonic finding or constellation of findings can definitively distinguish l-z joint–mediated pain from other sources of CLBP, it is a diagnosis ventured by exclusion of other causes and confirmed with controlled analgesic injections. These blocks can be accomplished in one of two ways. First, intraarticular injections of an anesthetic agent can be

performed after obtaining an appropriate arthrogram of a specified joint. However, these injections have never been tested for validity. The second, more reliable method, targets the small nerve fibers branching from the dorsal spinal root known to innervate the facet joints, with the so-named medial branch block. It has been suggested that performing controlled comparative blocks at more than one level to prove zygapophyseal joint pain is more reliable because single diagnostic blocks carry a high false-positive rate.

Management. Although these joints are increasingly the target of surgical and interventional approaches, controlled, prospective studies comparing treatment of l-z joint pain are limited. No form of conservative treatment including medications, physical therapy, or manual therapy has been specifically evaluated for analgesic efficacy in l-z joint pain, although these

modalities are routinely used as a first-line treatment in acute-onset LBP.

Based on the existing evidence, including basic science studies demonstrating inflammatory mediators to be present in and around degenerated facet joints, it can be concluded that intraarticular steroid injections may provide intermediate-term relief to a small subset of patients with l-z joint pain associated with an active inflammatory process.

The most studied intervention to date with the most evidence-based support is lumbar medial branch neurotomy (LMBN). The thermal coagulation employed by way of a medial branch neurotomy denatures nerve proteins, offering a far longer lasting clinical effect than a simple medial branch anesthetic block. Several RCTs have been published to date demonstrating LMBN efficiency in the treatment of l-z joint pain.

Facet joint
Joint capsule
Bilevel innervation of synovial membrane and capsule of facet joint

Superior articular process
Facet joint
Inferior articular process

Facet joint and capsule innervated by dorsal rami from two spinal levels

Facet joint, composed of articular processes of adjacent vertebrae, limits torsion and translation

Lumbar spine region

Joint space
Articular cartilage
Superior articular process
Inferior articular process

Trochanteric region

Gluteal region

Synovial membrane
Joint capsule
Innervation of synovial membrane and capsule

Posterior thigh region

Lateral thigh region

Degeneration of articular cartilage with synovial inflammation or capsular swelling may result in referred pain.

Cartilage degeneration
Synovial inflammation
Capsular swelling

Osteophytes
Osteophytic overgrowth of articular processes of facet joint may impinge on nerve root.

LOW BACK PAIN AND EFFECTS OF LUMBAR HYPERLORDOSIS AND FLEXION ON SPINAL NERVES

Hyperlordosis, also known as saddleback or swayback, is an excessive vertebral curvature (lordosis). The lumbosacral region plays a pivotal role in terms of mobility and weight-bearing potential; any postural aberrations affecting the lumbosacral angle may lead to LBP. Hyperlordotic posture is a possible contributor to chronic nonspecific LBP syndromes. Common causes include pregnancy, tight low back muscles, obesity, and congenital disorder.

Lumbar hyperlordosis is 50% more accentuated when standing rather than sitting. This may cause nonspecific LBP localizing to somatic tissues (e.g., paraspinal muscles, facet joints) mediated by inflammatory mechanisms. In extreme hyperlordosis, exiting nerve root entrapment secondary to intervertebral foramen narrowing with this posture may cause radicular irritation or a frank radiculopathy with sensorimotor deficits. Patients with lumbar spinal stenosis (LSS) have reduced anteroposterior central canal and lateral recess dimensions with hyperlordosis. Associated compromise of microvascular perfusion of the cauda equina possibly accounts for posture-precipitated pain while standing and walking, known as neurogenic claudication (NC). LSS nerve root injury may cause radicular pain characterized by sharp, lateralized pain conforming to dermatomal distributions, a radiculopathy, or NC. Straight-leg raising stretches the sciatic nerve, simulating radicular traction that provokes pain in an inflamed or otherwise sensitized nerve root.

In the lumbar spine, the primary motion is flexion/extension with very little segmental rotation. Lumbar flexion opens the foramen more widely, reducing nerve root compression. The amount of compressive force and tension on the nerve root decreases with spinal flexion and increases with spine extension.

Lordosis typically occurs maximally at L4–S1. A simple radiographic image to determine the extent of lordosis may capture the postural status. The normal range of lumbar lordosis is 20 degrees to 50 degrees, whereas hyperlordosis is defined as greater than 60 degrees. Patients with LSS have physical examination findings denoting loss of lumbar lordosis. Another test for NC is the stoop test; here the patient walks with an exaggerated lumbar lordosis until NC symptoms appear or are worsened. The patient is then instructed to lean forward at the waist; reduction in symptom intensity is considered suggestive of NC.

A radiographic study of sagittal lumbar spine measurements of 552 asymptomatic subjects with lordosis found that, in pain-free subjects, 65% of lordosis occurs between L4 and L5, and 35% occurs above L4. This study also demonstrated that hyperlordotic patients tended to have acute LBP, whereas patients with CLBP were hypolordotic.

A systematic review of randomized clinical trials of conservative treatment for acute LBP and CLBP supports the use of muscle relaxants, NSAIDs, acetaminophen, manipulation, and active exercise therapy in the treatment of acute LBP. Hyperlordosis is not always associated with painful symptoms, and this, per se, is not an indication for treatment. Analysis of CLBP therapies has shown stronger evidence of the effectiveness of exercise and manipulation therapy compared with behavior therapy. NSAIDs may accelerate the process of returning to usual activities or work. Of interest, other popular treatment options, including

Effects of lumbar hyperlordosis on spinal nerve roots

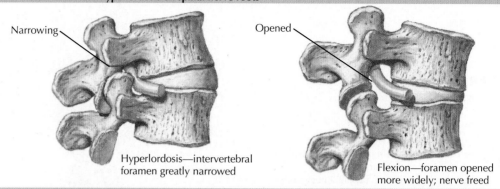

Narrowing

Opened

Hyperlordosis—intervertebral foramen greatly narrowed

Flexion—foramen opened more widely; nerve freed

Treatment of lumbar strain

Acute	Chronic and prophylactic
Absolute bed rest	Reduction of weight
Warm tub baths, heat pad, hydrocollator	Correction of posture
Sedation	Firm mattress, bed board
Firm mattress, bed board	Daily low back exercises
Diathermy, massage	Regular sports activity compatible
Local anesthetic infiltration to trigger zones	with age and physique
Occasionally corset, brace, or strapping	

Exercises for chronic lumbar strain (starting positions in outline)

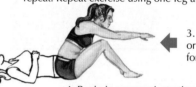

1. Lie on back, arms on chest, knees bent. Press small of back firmly down to floor, tightening muscles of abdomen and buttocks, thus tilting pubis forward; exhale simultaneously. Hold for count of 10, relax, and repeat.

2. Lie on back, arms at sides, knees bent. Draw knees up and pull them firmly to chest with clasped hands several times. Relax and repeat. Repeat exercise using one leg at a time.

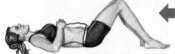

3. Lie on back, knees bent, arms folded on chest or at sides. Sit up using abdominal muscles and reach forward. Return slowly to starting position.

4. Begin in a runner's starting position (one leg extended, the other forward as shown, hands on floor). Press downward and forward several times, flexing front knee and bringing abdomen to thigh. Repeat with legs reversed.

5. Stand with hands on back of chair. Squat, straightening hollow of back. Return to starting position and repeat.

6. Sit on chair, hands folded in lap. Bend forward, bringing chin between knees. Return slowly to starting position while tensing abdominal muscles. Relax and repeat.

Exercises are best done on hard, padded surface like carpeted floor. Start slowly. Do each only once or twice a day, then progressively to 10 or more times within limits of comfort. Pain, but not mild discomfort, is indication to stop.

transcutaneous electrical nerve stimulation, electromyographic biofeedback, acupuncture, and orthoses, have not proved to be useful.

Conservative treatment, such as physical therapy, is recommended for patients with LSS or hyperlordosis. Lumbar extension exercises should be avoided in these patients because spinal extension and increased lumbar lordosis are known to worsen LSS. Flexion exercises for the lumbar spine are emphasized because these methods increase the spinal canal dimension and decrease stress on the spine, thereby reducing lumbar lordosis. Strengthening exercises include back hyperextensions, hip flexor, and gluteus and hamstring stretches, along with abdominal exercises. Avoiding a sedentary lifestyle, such as sitting for long

periods of time, and wearing a lumbar brace may also be helpful. Short-term pain relief can be achieved with the use of NSAIDs. A study published in 2005 demonstrated the greater benefit of Iyengar yoga (significant reduction in self-reported disability and pain and reduced use of pain medication) than educational programs in the management of patients with CLBP. For CLBP, positions that include twists and inversions may alleviate hyperlordotic pain. Twisting motions involve the deeper layer of back muscles and reduce the pain symptoms by realigning the vertebra, increasing intervertebral disk space, and decreasing possible impingement of nerve roots, whereas inversions reverse the compressive effects of gravity on the intervertebral disk space.

Plate 8.16

Pain

EXAMINATION OF THE PATIENT WITH LOW BACK PAIN

Musculoskeletal LBP is defined as pain localized predominantly between the twelfth rib and the inferior gluteal folds. LBP syndromes are highly prevalent, constituting the fifth leading reason for doctor visits. The majority of cases remit in days to weeks and are often regarded as "nonspecific" because of the absence of image-based anatomic abnormality or laboratory evidence of inflammation. Imaging has been shown not to be sensitive or specific for the experience of LBP at many time points in the absence of traumatic onset or infectious prodrome. For this reason, such studies are often not obtained in the acute setting. Emerging lines of evidence suggest that nociplastic mechanisms characteristic of central sensitization such as neuronal hyperactivity, changes in membrane excitability, and altered gene expression may perpetuate pain in the absence of nociceptive stimuli in chronic musculoskeletal LBP syndromes. However, specific LBP causes may be a result of a multitude of pathologic processes, including degenerative diseases, inflammatory conditions, systemic or local infection, neoplasms, metabolic bone disease, referred pain, occult trauma, and congenital disorders. Because of this wide array of etiologies, clinical assessment of the patient's condition is essential to establishing the correct diagnosis.

CLINICAL EVALUATION

A focused history and physical examination are fundamental elements in the assessment of LBP. They are especially helpful in the preliminary classification of acute LBP into one of three groups: (1) acute or chronic musculoskeletal LBP; (2) LBP potentially associated with radiculopathy, radiculitis, or spinal stenosis; or (3) LBP potentially associated with systemic disease. The latter category includes the small proportion of patients with serious or progressive neurologic deficits or underlying conditions requiring prompt evaluation (such as tumor, infection, or the cauda equina syndrome) as well as patients with other conditions that may respond to specific treatments (such as ankylosing spondylitis or vertebral compression fracture). The vast majority of patients experience nociceptive pain referred from somatic structures (i.e., paraspinal muscle, ligament, tendon, facet joint, intervertebral disk). The most common clinical picture is one of axial predominance, whereas radicular impingement or irritation typically involves leg symptoms in a unilateral or, less commonly, bilateral distribution.

The physical exam of a patient with LBP involves assessment of motor, sensory, and reflex function as well as strength, range of motion, and neurologic deficits. It should begin with the collection of vital signs and a systemic survey aimed at identifying evidence of nonmechanical and visceral causes of LBP, such as nephrolithiasis, pancreatitis, or aortic aneurysm, or systemic diseases, such as endocarditis or metabolic bone disease. A thorough inspection and palpation of the affected area should follow, with careful attention to the presence of deformities or radiation of pain. All patients should be evaluated for the presence of red flags, which may indicate a serious condition. Neurologic findings, such as saddle anesthesia, bilateral radiculopathy, bilateral leg weakness, urinary retention, and fecal incontinence, are consistent with the diagnosis of cauda equina syndrome and require immediate attention. Malignancy may be suspected in patients with LBP after a minor trauma, unrelenting night or rest pain, unexplained weight loss,

and progressive neurologic deficit. Chronic steroid use, immunosuppression, intravenous drug abuse, recent urinary infection, or skin infection near the spine should direct the differential diagnosis toward infectious etiology. Finally, fracture is a possible diagnosis in the setting of trauma, osteoporosis, or chronic steroid use.

If no neurologic deficit is present and pain is localized to the lumbar spine and buttocks, lumbar strain localizing to soft tissues or inflammatory processes at the level of disk, facet joints, or bony endplates is more likely.

RANGE OF MOTION

Range of motion in the lumbar spine is dependent on the resistance to movement of the intervertebral disks and the size of the articular surfaces. The most significant degree of motion is in the thickest disks and largest joint surfaces, mostly between L5 and S1. Tests for range of

motion include flexion, extension, lateral bending, and rotation. One has to bear in mind, though, that limitation of spinal range of motion is a nonspecific finding that is not strongly associated with any particular diagnosis.

Flexion

With the patient standing, have the patient fold forward with the knees straight and touch their toes. Measure the distance from the fingertips to the floor. Lumbar pain may prevent full range of motion.

Extension

With the patient standing, place your palm on the patient's posterior superior iliac spine and have the patient bend backward as far as possible. Assess the degree of extension. This motion aggravates the pain experienced by patients with spondylolisthesis, whereas flexion results in pain relief.

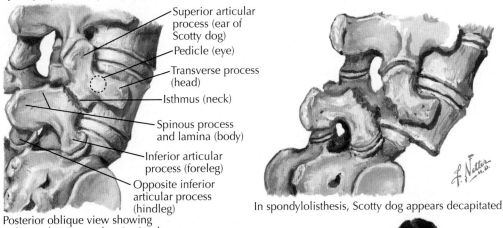

Spondylolysis and Spondylolisthesis

Superior articular process (ear of Scotty dog)

Pedicle (eye)

Transverse process (head)

Isthmus (neck)

Spinous process and lamina (body)

Inferior articular process (foreleg)

Opposite inferior articular process (hindleg)

Posterior oblique view showing radiographic Scotty dog. In simple spondylolysis, dog appears to be wearing a collar

In spondylolisthesis, Scotty dog appears decapitated

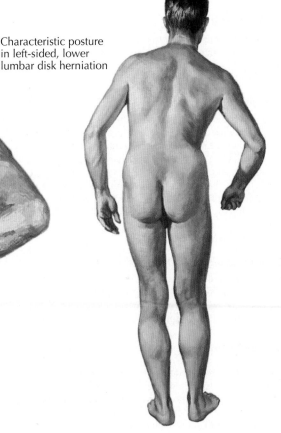

Characteristic posture in left-sided, lower lumbar disk herniation

Lower back pain

EXAMINATION OF THE PATIENT WITH LOW BACK PAIN (Continued)

Rotation

Place one hand on the pelvis and the other on the opposite shoulder. Rotate the pelvis and shoulder posteriorly and repeat on the other side; note any asymmetry in motion.

SPECIFIC TESTS

Two specific tests include the straight-leg raise test and the crossed straight-leg raise test. These are valuable diagnostic tools for disk herniation and lumbosacral radiculopathy.

Straight-Leg Raise Test

Have the patient lie supine with their legs relaxed. Lift the patient's leg upward by supporting the heel with one hand and ensuring that the knee remains straight with the other. When the patient experiences pain, lower the leg slightly and dorsiflex the foot to stretch the sciatic nerve. Note the degree of elevation, description and location of pain, and effect of dorsiflexion. The test is positive if pain is felt in the low back or along the sciatic nerve. A positive test is indicative of lumbosacral radicular inflammation.

Crossed Straight-Leg Raise Test

Have the patient lie supine with their legs relaxed, then raise the unaffected leg. If back or sciatic pain is felt in the opposite leg, this is suggestive of a lesion, such as a herniated disk, in the lumbar region.

REFLEX TESTING

The *patellar deep tendon reflex* arises predominantly from L4 nerve roots, although innervation is also supplied by L2 and L3 segments of the spinal cord. Damage to the L4 nerve will elicit a significantly decreased patellar reflex due to L2 and L3 involvement.

The *Achilles deep tendon reflex* typically involves the S1 nerve root. Dorsiflex the foot and strike the tendon to elicit plantar flexion of the foot.

IMPORTANT FINDINGS

Mechanical LBP characterized by aching pain in the lumbosacral region presents with paraspinal muscle or facet tenderness but no evidence of motor, sensory, or reflex deficits.

Radicular LBP is described as low back pain that extends below the knee into the lateral leg or back of the calf. Clinical findings in sciatica due to disk herniation include calf wasting, decreased ankle dorsiflexion, no ankle jerk, and positive crossed straight-leg raise test.

Positive signs of *lumbar spinal stenosis* are weakness in lower extremities and decreased reflex with a negative straight-leg raise test. Patients report pain with standing or walking that is relieved with rest or flexion and may have paresthesia of the legs.

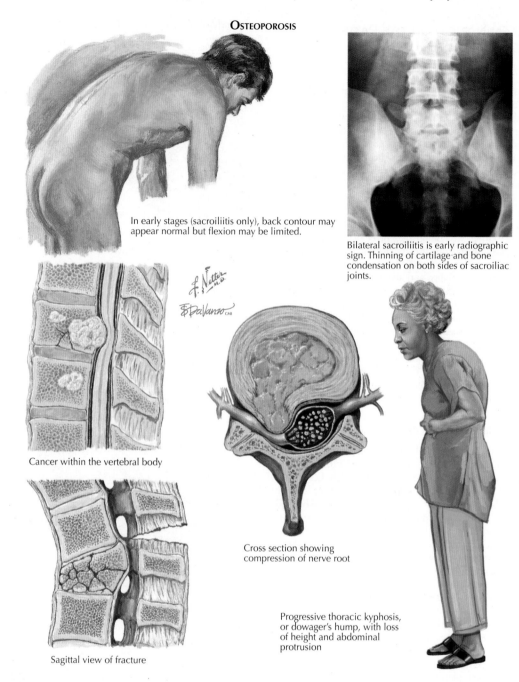

OSTEOPOROSIS

In early stages (sacroiliitis only), back contour may appear normal but flexion may be limited.

Bilateral sacroiliitis is early radiographic sign. Thinning of cartilage and bone condensation on both sides of sacroiliac joints.

Cancer within the vertebral body

Cross section showing compression of nerve root

Sagittal view of fracture

Progressive thoracic kyphosis, or dowager's hump, with loss of height and abdominal protrusion

DIAGNOSTIC IMAGING

Although imaging or other diagnostic tests should not be obtained routinely in patients early in the course of acute or subacute nonspecific LBP, they are irreplaceable in the management of patients with severe or progressive neurologic deficits or with other serious underlying conditions.

Plain radiography is of limited use because it fails to depict a detailed picture of the disease; however, it has been recommended for initial evaluation of possible vertebral compression fracture in patients with a history of osteoporosis or steroid use.

CT scans are particularly valuable in regard to detecting traumatic and degenerative changes in cortical bone and have been shown to have similar sensitivity and specificity as MRI in detecting herniated disks. This modality also demonstrates pars defects that may be associated with spondylolisthesis and foraminal and extraforaminal nerve root impingement and is superior to radiography in detecting infection and neoplasm.

Finally, *MRI* provides superior soft tissue detail compared with CT and plain radiography. It is the method of choice for detecting malignancy and infection in the spine and provides better visualization of intrathecal nerve roots and bone marrow; however, it may be less useful in detecting acute fracture.

LABORATORY EVALUATION

Laboratory testing for LBP is only useful in the setting of red flags that suggest visceral or other nonmechanical causes for the pain. Initial studies should include a complete blood count, erythrocyte sedimentation rate, and C-reactive protein, whereas urinalysis, prostate-specific antigen, or alkaline phosphatase should be reserved for the presence of specific red flags, such as urinary infection, or clinical clues for malignant or metabolic disease.

Plate 8.18

Pain

DIAGNOSIS OF LOW BACK, BUTTOCK, AND HIP PAIN

Discriminating among patterns of referred and neurogenic pain from the lumbar region is a common clinical challenge. In the context of concomitant hip and spine pathology, identifying the cause of pain is especially difficult. These patients may present with radiating pain below the knee, back pain, or symptoms evoked by internal rotation of the hip. Certain combinations of signs and symptoms favor one localization over another. Reported odds ratios in one study suggest that signs and symptoms of a limp, groin pain, and limited internal rotation of the hip are all much more likely to be present in a patient with a hip disorder. Similarly, in a comparison of patients diagnosed with a hip disorder versus those with a spine disorder or both, patients with a positive femoral stretch test are 4.76 times more likely to have a spine disorder or a hip and spine disorder.

In general, true hip pain manifests as groin pain that sometimes radiates to the knee. Thigh pain, buttock pain, and pain radiating below the knee are more often attributable to disorders of the lumbar spine or buttock and proximal thigh musculature.

LOW BACK PAIN

Chronic nonspecific LBP may result from peripheral injury to various neural and nonneural anatomic structures in the lumbar region. Pain generators may include the vertebral column, surrounding muscles, tendons, ligaments, and fascia or the neural structures such as the lumbosacral roots. Hip osteoarthritis, trochanteric bursitis, ischial bursitis, sacroiliac dysfunction, piriformis syndrome, and osteitis condensans ilii are examples of somatic conditions that will refer pain to and from the low back. Hip joint pathology and bursitis of the greater trochanter can mimic mechanical or radicular LBP in both its onset and symptoms.

It is crucial to distinguish radicular pain from somatic referred pain because their management is significantly different. Somatic referred pain is the result of noxious stimulation of structures in the lumbar spine, such as intervertebral disks, facet joints, or sacroiliac joints, and never of the nerve roots. It has a dull, gnawing quality and is difficult to localize. Conversely, radicular pain is elicited by ectopic discharges from a dorsal root. The most common cause of such pain is disk herniation complicated by the inflammation of the affected nerve. It is described as lancinating or shocking, and it can involve allodynia in case of nerve damage and neuropathy. Finally, radiculopathy is a condition characterized by motor and sensory loss in dermatomal distribution due to conduction block along the nerve, and it often accompanies radicular pain.

LBP associated with lumbosacral radiculitis is classically characterized by unilateral lower extremity pain and paresthesias. The onset of pain or paresthesias is typically abrupt and often reported as more severe in the leg versus the low back region. The patient may exhibit decreased truncal range of motion.

Lumbar spinal stenosis is a distinctive syndrome in which the cauda equina and exiting nerve roots are compromised because of degenerative changes. The distinctive experience of pain evoked with standing and walking is known as neurogenic claudication. In contrast to radiculitis, this pain typically remits in the seated (and recumbent) posture or with forward flexion at the waist. This symptom pattern is the leading indication for spine surgery in older adults.

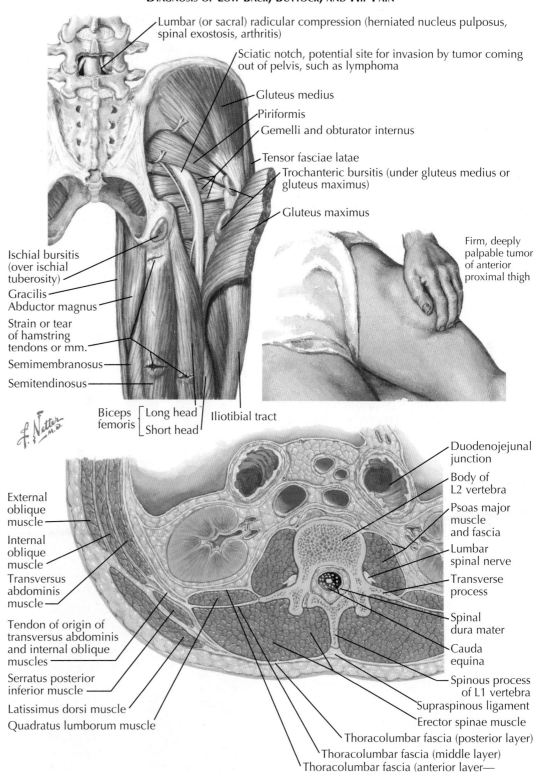

DIAGNOSIS OF LOW BACK, BUTTOCK, AND HIP PAIN

Lumbar (or sacral) radicular compression (herniated nucleus pulposus, spinal exostosis, arthritis)

Sciatic notch, potential site for invasion by tumor coming out of pelvis, such as lymphoma

Gluteus medius

Piriformis

Gemelli and obturator internus

Tensor fasciae latae

Trochanteric bursitis (under gluteus medius or gluteus maximus)

Gluteus maximus

Firm, deeply palpable tumor of anterior proximal thigh

Ischial bursitis (over ischial tuberosity)

Gracilis

Abductor magnus

Strain or tear of hamstring tendons or mm.

Semimembranosus

Semitendinosus

Biceps femoris [Long head / Short head]

Iliotibial tract

External oblique muscle

Internal oblique muscle

Transversus abdominis muscle

Tendon of origin of transversus abdominis and internal oblique muscles

Serratus posterior inferior muscle

Latissimus dorsi muscle

Quadratus lumborum muscle

Duodenojejunal junction

Body of L2 vertebra

Psoas major muscle and fascia

Lumbar spinal nerve

Transverse process

Spinal dura mater

Cauda equina

Spinous process of L1 vertebra

Supraspinous ligament

Erector spinae muscle

Thoracolumbar fascia (posterior layer)

Thoracolumbar fascia (middle layer)

Thoracolumbar fascia (anterior layer—quadratus lumborum fascia)

Spondylolisthesis is a common, painful condition that exists when there is disruption of the normal segmental alignment of a vertebral body in relation to the adjacent level, usually from failure (e.g., fracture of the pars interarticularis) of the posterior vertebral elements. Patients may present with dull, achy back pain that radiates posteriorly to or below the knees. Lumbosacral tenderness, reduced lateral bending, and hamstring tightness are also common findings.

Vertebral compression fractures are also a common cause of LBP, especially in the elderly. Point tenderness is common in early fractures and often is associated with muscle spasm.

BUTTOCK PAIN

In the low back, referral pain patterns commonly manifest with hip or leg symptoms. A classic example of a

Diagnosis of Low Back, Buttock, and Hip Pain (Continued)

referral pain pattern in the lumbosacral spine is LBP associated with aching buttock pain. The lumbosacral region and buttocks are both innervated by L4–S1. However, the buttock is innervated by the ventral rami of these nerve roots (the superior and inferior gluteal nerves), and the lumbosacral region is innervated by the dorsal rami.

Spinal causes for buttock symptoms include facet joint injury and lateral fissure in the lumbar disk. In older patients, lateral recess stenosis and degenerative spondylolisthesis may cause buttock pain.

Muscular or myofascial syndromes can arise in gluteus maximus and medius, quadratus lumborum, and the soleus muscle, all producing strong referral patterns of pain in the region of the sacroiliac joint. This diagnosis may be supported by injecting local anesthetic into a trigger point at which myofascial palpation reproduces the primary symptom pattern.

HIP PAIN

Limited internal rotation of the hip, antalgic gait, and groin pain have been identified as the best predictors of identifying hip disorders. Pain in the groin or hip with single-leg stance, the Patrick test (also known as the FABER test [hip *flexion*, *ab*duction, and *external rotation*]), along with the presence of a leg length discrepancy, are useful for detecting an underlying hip disorder, sacroiliac dysfunction, or greater trochanteric bursitis. Hip internal rotation also can cause increased LBP in patients with piriformis syndrome when this muscle is stretched. The pain is often ameliorated by external rotation of the hip in this condition, along with abductor weakness. The groin should be examined for femoral or inguinal hernias. Osteitis pubis, athletic pubalgia, and adductor tendonitis can produce groin pain that mimics pain associated with disorders of the hip. Persistent hip pain can originate from intraarticular disorders, such as avascular necrosis, osteoarthritis, loose bodies, labral tears, or pyarthrosis. It can also be secondary to lumbar spine disorder. Nerve entrapment syndromes involving the ilioinguinal, genitofemoral, and lateral femoral cutaneous nerve of the thigh may manifest as hip pain or paresthesias.

Osteoarthritis is a common condition affecting the hip in adults. Motion in the hip becomes progressively restricted because of synovitis, soft tissue contractures, and loss of joint congruency. Patients complain of pain in the groin, buttock, anterior thigh, or knee and often have an antalgic gait. Examination of the hip shows limited range of motion and a flexion contracture.

The so-called piriformis syndrome has been attributed to compression of the sciatic nerve as it exits the pelvis under the piriformis muscle. Patients are said to report a dull ache in the low back and midbuttock region and pain with walking upstairs, prolonged sitting, or walking. There are no sensitive or specific imaging correlates of this putative site of entrapment. As such, this syndrome remains a controversial clinical diagnosis.

Hamstring syndrome is a pain radiating from the ischial tuberosity down the posterior aspect of the thigh into the popliteal fossa. Physical examination reveals tenderness over the ischial tuberosity and pain with resisted leg extension.

HIP JOINT INVOLVEMENT IN OSTEOARTHRITIS

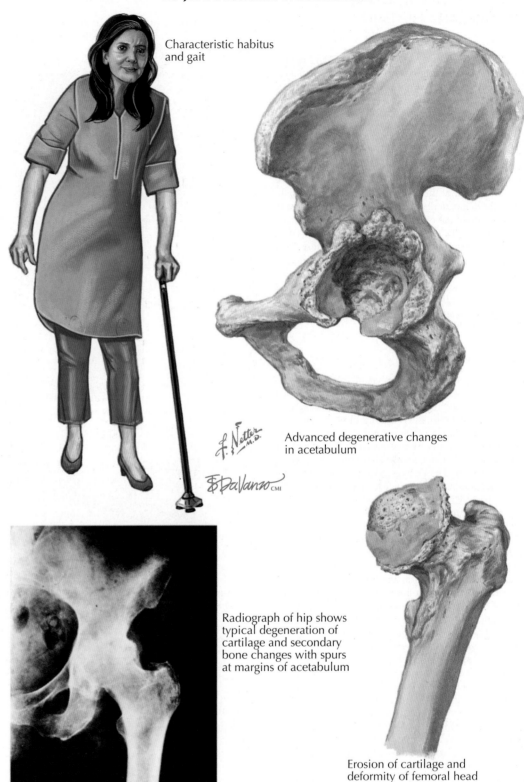

Characteristic habitus and gait

Advanced degenerative changes in acetabulum

Radiograph of hip shows typical degeneration of cartilage and secondary bone changes with spurs at margins of acetabulum

Erosion of cartilage and deformity of femoral head

Bursitis is a common cause of hip pain related to inflammation of one of the three main bursae of the hip. It may be caused by overuse or degenerative changes in the bursae. Patients with trochanteric bursitis present with pain over the greater trochanter that is exacerbated by hip adduction. Ischiogluteal bursitis is often associated with sitting for long periods.

Osteitis condensans ilii is a benign cause of LBP usually found in postpartum women and is thought to develop as a result of mechanical strain placed on the sacroiliac joint during pregnancy. The physical examination is unrevealing, except for localized pain in the low back.

Plate 8.20

Pain

PAINFUL PERIPHERAL NEUROPATHY

The most common causes of painful peripheral neuropathy include diabetes, toxin exposure, alcohol abuse, immune-mediated conditions, human immunodeficiency virus (HIV) infection, and certain medications; however, in up to half of patients the cause remains unknown. Painful neuropathies (PNs) are often characterized by a progressive loss of nerve fibers, which results in pain and paresthesia of the affected areas. The prevalence of PN in persons over the age of 40 is nearly 15%, with the incidence being significantly higher in patients with diabetes.

The underlying mechanisms of nerve injury in PN are highly variable, as are the clinical phenotypes that may present in a distal symmetric pattern, widespread pattern as in the case of small-fiber neuropathies, or in multifocal distributions as is common in inflammatory neuropathies. Axons require their cell bodies to maintain homeostasis of the nerve along its span. One classic pattern of neuronal damage is associated with distal axonal degeneration. The cell body remains intact and begins a process to redirect growth of the remaining axon to reestablish connection or form new ones. Additionally, loss of blood supply from the vasa nervorum results in ischemia of the peripheral nerve, leading to similar injury.

PATHOPHYSIOLOGY OF DIABETIC PERIPHERAL NEUROPATHY

The pathogenesis of diabetic peripheral neuropathy (DPN) is attributed to increased oxidative stress, accumulation of sorbitol, and decreased NO leading to microvascular damage. Oxidative stress results from hyperactivity of the polyol pathway, causing the accumulation of polyol in cells. Nerve cells are permeable to glucose independent of insulin, and aldose reductase converts the glucose into sorbitol and polyol within the cell. Because polyol cannot diffuse out of the cell, it accumulates in the neuron, making the cell osmotically active to excess salt and water influx. In turn, sorbitol is converted to fructose, and its increased levels lead to advanced glycosylation end product (AGEs) precursors. AGEs, in turn, accumulate on neurovascular proteins and damage tissues. These two pathways lead to a reduction in the cell's Na⁺/K⁺ adenosine triphosphatase (ATPase) activity further impairing endothelial function. Additionally, NO is a key modulator of Na⁺/K⁺-ATPase, and endothelial superoxide radicals from the excess glucose reduce NO stimulation on the ion pump via decreased NO synthase activity.

Other cellular changes include protein kinase C activation and alterations in fatty acid metabolism, which also contribute to vascular damage.

Decreased perfusion of the nerve itself is another cause of PN in that hyalinization and hyperplasia of the vasa nervorum impair nerve fibers, particularly unmyelinated fibers that innervate arterioles needed to shunt arteriovenous supply within the nerve. This leads to damage by hypoxia and ischemic insult. These metabolic changes, oxidative stressors, and hypoperfusion are responsible for the endothelial and nerve damage observed in DPN.

The degree of hyperglycemia only affects the overall severity of neuropathy, and it is not related to its development. Furthermore, in studies comparing morphometric parameters between patients with diabetes with and without peripheral neuropathy, there was no

significant difference in the degree of myelinated nerve fiber loss, although there was a trend toward more active degeneration of unmyelinated fibers in patients with peripheral diabetic neuropathy. Studies involving skin biopsy to determine intraepidermal nerve fiber (IENF) density have demonstrated more severe loss of IENF in patients with neuropathic pain, suggesting that IENF damage may partially explain pain in this condition. IENF density measurement from skin biopsy can be used to evaluate small-fiber involvement and has been shown to detect early changes in patients with diabetes.

CLINICAL MANIFESTATIONS

The characteristic features of chronic PN include burning, shooting, or stabbing sensations (with or without

"pins and needles") that are particularly prominent in the evening and while trying to get to sleep, sometimes frequently awakening patients from their sleep. The pain can be severe, compromising the patient's ability to walk and producing an *antalgic gait*. These individuals walk gingerly, trying to avoid pressure-induced painful feet. The rate of disease onset and evolution provides key differential diagnostic features. A thorough history and physical exam are critical in the diagnostic process, and key findings include decreased sense of vibration and temperature and distinction of sharp pressure. Distal symmetrical polyneuropathy, the prevalent form of DPN, is characterized by numbness and paresthesia beginning in the toes and spreading upward to the legs and hands in a "stocking and glove" pattern. Ataxia and motor and autonomic deficits may also present in later stages of the disease.

PERIPHERAL NERVES OF FEET, MOST COMMON SITE OF PAINFUL PERIPHERAL NEUROPATHIES

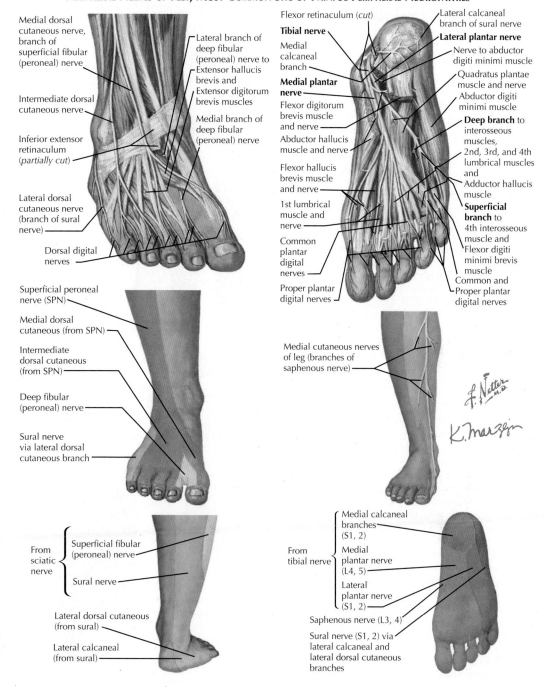

PAINFUL PERIPHERAL NEUROPATHY (Continued)

Acute PN, which may follow initiation of insulin treatment in poorly controlled diabetes, features severe pain symptoms, accompanied by hyperesthesia; however, no alterations to the motor or sensory modalities are present. In contrast, slowly progressive, long-standing neuropathy associated with muscle wasting and foot abnormalities often requires genetic testing to characterize the underlying mechanism of nerve injury. Neuropathy with multifocal symptoms, whether acute or rapidly progressive, that manifests with neuropathic pain and autonomic symptoms will require detailed diagnostic evaluation to exclude vasculitis, amyloidosis, or paraneoplastic syndrome. Genetic testing is increasingly important in patients whose history points to a hereditary origin such as axonal Charcot-Marie-Tooth (CMT) disease or transthyretin amyloidosis. Nerve ultrasound is an emerging diagnostic tool that may identify increase in cross-sectional area in immune-mediated neuropathy or CMT type 1A.

PN related to HIV infection will usually present with pain mostly on the soles and dorsum of the feet, decreased primary sensory modalities in the feet, decreased ankle reflexes, and minimal intrinsic foot weakness.

TREATMENT

The treatment for PN pain largely depends on the primary condition. Novel therapeutic strategies aim to address the underlying neurophysiologic alterations because many recent studies have demonstrated the differences in drug efficacy depend on the cause of neuropathy. The development of specific treatment approaches for inherited neuropathies by RNA interference and antisense oligonucleotides underscores the importance of establishing a diagnostic etiology where possible.

Diabetic PN requires a multimodal approach. Several open-label, uncontrolled studies have suggested that achieving stable normoglycemic state is helpful in the management of the symptoms, and according to general recommendations, intensive diabetes therapy should be the first step in the treatment of any form of diabetic neuropathy.

Anticonvulsants, such as gabapentin and pregabalin, are widely used for neuropathic symptoms. Large RCTs have confirmed their utility in the treatment of DPN because they influence pain as well as sleep patterns, mood disturbances, and overall quality of life.

Topical capsaicin has been proven effective in pain relief in randomized controlled studies. Long-term application of capsaicin leads to depletion of axonal substance P (C-fiber neurotransmitter), thus reducing the transmission of painful stimuli.

Lidocaine, targeting the hyperexcitable superficial free nerve endings, has also been proven successful in self-limited forms of neuropathy.

The latest research focuses on selective serotonin and norepinephrine reuptake inhibitors (SSNRIs) as the first line of DPN treatment. Duloxetine, approved by the US Food and Drug Administration in the treatment of PNs, has been shown to be efficacious in the treatment of DPN. Venlafaxine, another SSNRI, has also been found to improve pain, mood, and quality of life when added to gabapentin treatment.

Tricyclics, such as amitriptyline and imipramine, possibly alleviate pain through inhibition of norepinephrine and/or serotonin reuptake and the antagonism of NMDARs (responsible for hyperalgesia and allodynia). An alternative treatment commonly used in Europe with mixed evidence is alpha-lipoic acid, which is thought to stabilize NO metabolites to increase neuronal perfusion. Recent studies of moderate rigor demonstrate evidence of the effectiveness of SCS for the pain associated with diabetic neuropathy.

Treatment of HIV-related PN poses more problems for the clinicians. So far, there have been no positive studies in patients with HIV-related neuropathy. The most recent randomized, double-blind clinical trial on the effectiveness of amitriptyline and mexiletine, successfully used in other types of neuropathic pain, has demonstrated no significant benefit in pain relief in these patients. Similarly, a trial of pregabalin found that this therapy did not significantly reduce pain intensity in this population compared with placebo.

For etiologies such as alcoholism and chemotoxic side effects, the mainstay of treatment would be replenishment of vitamin B and folate, which are deficient in alcoholic-induced PN, and dosage reduction or change in the medications causing PN.

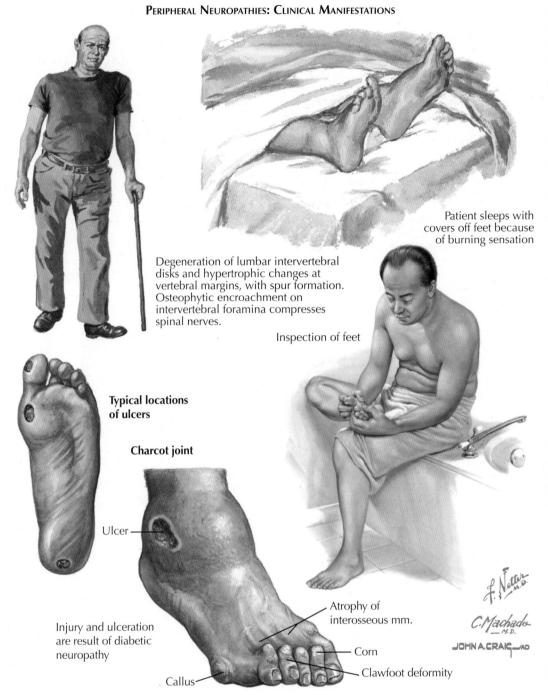

PERIPHERAL NEUROPATHIES: CLINICAL MANIFESTATIONS

Patient sleeps with covers off feet because of burning sensation

Degeneration of lumbar intervertebral disks and hypertrophic changes at vertebral margins, with spur formation. Osteophytic encroachment on intervertebral foramina compresses spinal nerves.

Inspection of feet

Typical locations of ulcers

Charcot joint

Ulcer

Injury and ulceration are result of diabetic neuropathy

Atrophy of interosseous mm.

Corn

Clawfoot deformity

Callus

Plate 8.22

Pain

FUNCTIONAL NEUROLOGIC DISORDERS

As in other diseases of the nervous system, neurologic symptoms that are not explained by identifiable pathology may be severe, adversely affect function, and reduce quality of life. The symptoms of functional neurologic disorders (FNDs) differ from those that are intentionally produced in conditions such as malingering and factitious disorder. The symptoms may affect voluntary motor or sensory function and resemble neurologic or medical disease. In contrast to most acute pain syndromes, chronic pain states often lack a clear pathoanatomic or pathophysiologic correlate. Our limited understanding of pain mechanisms informs a tendency to attribute poorly understood variation in pain intensity and activity limitation to psychogenic origins or motives. A dualistic model of chronic pain, perceived as either wholly organic or psychogenic, is not supported by prevailing basic science or clinical models of pain pathophysiology. Diagnostic constructs such as conversion disorder are rapidly falling out of use in clinical practice because of the implicit inference of causative psychosocial stressors that may be absent or not readily identifiable.

The biopsychosocial model of pain, as conceived nearly a half century ago, is the most widely called upon heuristic to characterize the experience of chronic pain. Viewed as complex interplay of biologic, psychological, and social factors, this model embraces concepts of both disease and illness. Disease is defined as an objective biologic event involving the disruption of specific body structures or organ systems, whereas illness refers to the subjective experience or self-attribution that a disease is present.

Accordingly, the biopsychosocial model distinguishes between nociception and pain. Nociception is defined as the stimulation of nerves that relay information about potential tissue damage to the brain. Conversely, pain is the subjective perception resulting from transduction, transmission, and modulation of sensory information.

Finally, this model incorporates concepts of suffering (such as the fear and apprehension about the future triggered by nociception) and pain behaviors, which are forms of overt communication of pain and distress.

PSYCHOLOGIC FORMULATIONS OF PAIN BEHAVIOR AND "CONVERSION" DISORDERS

Pain behaviors serve not only to gain attention or avoid undesirable consequences but may also be considered as pain-reducing strategies or as protective strategies to diminish exacerbation of pain. So-called *abnormal illness behavior* describes patients who present with symptoms in the absence of physical pathology or who present with exaggerated illness behavior. It is considered a social mechanism that exempts a patient from

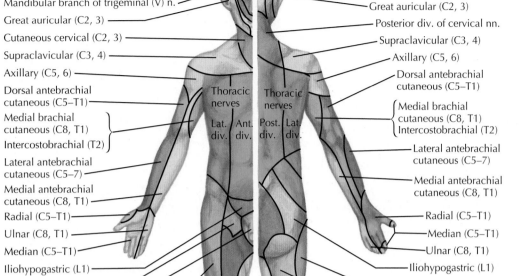

CUTANEOUS DISTRIBUTION OF PERIPHERAL NERVES (AFTER DEJONE)

Ophthalmic branch of trigeminal (V) n.
Maxillary branch of trigeminal (V) n.
Mandibular branch of trigeminal (V) n.
Great auricular (C2, 3)
Cutaneous cervical (C2, 3)
Supraclavicular (C3, 4)
Axillary (C5, 6)
Dorsal antebrachial cutaneous (C5–T1)
Medial brachial cutaneous (C8, T1)
Intercostobrachial (T2)
Lateral antebrachial cutaneous (C5–7)
Medial antebrachial cutaneous (C8, T1)
Radial (C5–T1)
Ulnar (C8, T1)
Median (C5–T1)
Iliohypogastric (L1)
Genitofemoral (L1, 2)
Ilioinguinal (L1)
Lateral femoral cutaneous (L2, 3)
Femoral (L2–4)
Obturator (L2–4)
Common peroneal (L4–S2)
Saphenous (L3, 4)
Superficial peroneal (L4–S1)
Sural (S1, 2)
Deep peroneal (L4, 5)
Lateral plantar (S1, 2)

Ophthalmic branch of trigeminal (V) n.
Greater occipital (C2)
Lesser occipital (C2, 3)
Great auricular (C2, 3)
Posterior div. of cervical nn.
Supraclavicular (C3, 4)
Axillary (C5, 6)
Dorsal antebrachial cutaneous (C5–T1)
Medial brachial cutaneous (C8, T1)
Intercostobrachial (T2)
Lateral antebrachial cutaneous (C5–7)
Medial antebrachial cutaneous (C8, T1)
Radial (C5–T1)
Median (C5–T1)
Ulnar (C8, T1)
Iliohypogastric (L1)
Lateral femoral cutaneous (L2, 3)
Posterior femoral cutaneous (S1–3)
Obturator (L2–4)
Femoral (L2–4)
Common peroneal (L4–S2)
Saphenous (L3, 4)
Superficial peroneal (L4–S1)
Sural (S1, 2)
Calcaneal (S1, 2)
Medial plantar (L4, 5)
Lateral plantar (S1, 2)

Thoracic nerves
Thoracic nerves
Lat. div. Ant. div. Post. div. Lat. div.

Anterior aspect   Posterior aspect

JOHN A. CRAIG—AD

Loss of sensory modalities is based on the anatomic location of the inciting lesion. The pattern of loss may follow either a spinal dermatome pattern or one based on peripheral nerve damage. Because exact peripheral nerve distribution varies among individuals, patterns may differ.

Note that isolated islands of anesthesia (e.g., axillary and deep peroneal) can exist on an anatomic basis.

certain responsibilities, concurrently establishing an obligation to seek treatment and cooperate in the healing process. In other words, pain behavior may offer a more socially legitimate way to express distress or anxiety. In contrast, psychoanalytic explanations of *conversion* emphasize unconscious drives, including sexuality, aggression, or dependency, and the internalized prohibition against their expression. Other psychoanalytic explanations focus on the need to suffer or identification with a lost object.

Other theories emphasize the role of fear-avoidance beliefs and catastrophizing (tendency to engage in negative thinking and worry about pain) as the catalysts of persistent pain and disability. Studies have demonstrated that catastrophizing is a strong risk factor for increased pain, increased illness behavior, and the development of both physical and psychological disability. Fear-avoidance beliefs stem from a conviction that pain is synonymous with harm and that any activity should thus be avoided; such beliefs have been shown to be predictive of pain chronicity and disability.

The neuromatrix model of pain proposes that pain experience results from the integration of outputs from perceptual, behavioral, and homeostatic systems in response to injury and chronic stress. It is the output of the diffuse brain neural networks rather than a direct response to sensory information. Neuroimaging studies have begun to delineate the neural processes implicated in the somatoform disorders. The cortical correlates of the touch and pain pathways include the SI and SII cortexes, insula, and ACC. However, additional cortical regions associated with attention, such as the posterior parietal cortex (PPC), prefrontal cortex, and temporoparietal junction, can also affect or be influenced by somatosensory processing. Furthermore, attentional state can modulate sensory-evoked responses. Somatosensory inputs to circuits are also involved in the processing of emotional or other aspects of psychosocial behavior that may then feed back to somatosensory or motor circuits. In one study, functional MRI during stimulation of the symptomatic limb revealed prominent abnormalities in somatosensory areas; namely,

FUNCTIONAL NEUROLOGIC DISORDERS (Continued)

lack of activations, novel activations, and stimulus-related deactivations in the SI, SII, and PPC. One notable activation during unperceived noxious stimulation was found in the rostral and perigenual ACC, which are thought to be involved more generally in cognitive processes and emotion.

DIAGNOSIS

Pain behavior in the context of chronic pain has a wide differential diagnosis that requires the clinician to incorporate historical elements as well as examination findings into the global assessment. Sensory findings such as midline splitting, vibration sense splitting, and laterality of symptoms may have proved useful contexts to weigh the role of psychosocial factors in modulating pain intensity. However, the value of these localizing assumptions must take into account that certain painful symptom patterns, such as those related to a thalamic stroke or postherpetic neuralgia, may in fact respect the midline.

The concept of "belle indifference," as it was first described, also applied to patients who were unaware of sensory loss found on examination. The term has also been used to describe a certain indifference of the patient to their symptoms; however, studies have demonstrated that this finding performs poorly as a discriminator of organic disease.

TREATMENT

Treatment of FND begins with explanation of the diagnosis in a way that facilitates patient understanding by disclosing how this determination was made. Therapeutic success hinges on validation of neurologic symptoms, a high level of confidence in the diagnosis, cultivation of a therapeutic alliance, and shared understanding of the rationale for a multimodal approach including psychological interventions. The biopsychosocial model of pain stresses the multitude of factors that influence a person's perception of pain and response to it. In accord with this conception, it is theorized that a multidimensional approach to chronic pain syndromes and abnormal pain behaviors is most effective at reducing symptoms and associated loss of function. Medical and surgical treatments may address the biologic underpinnings of pain experience, though their utility in the treatment of abnormal pain behaviors is controversial. As yet, there is no firm evidence that antidepressants or any other pharmaceutical agent can be regarded as the best approach for treating FNDs. There is also no information on the optimal dose, duration of treatment, or long-term outcome in patients treated with such medication for this indication.

Comorbid conditions such as depression, anxiety, and sleeping disorders reinforce the undesirable effects of pain, and these psychological factors may interfere with successful rehabilitation. There has been growing evidence that cognitive-behavioral therapy (CBT) improves long-term rehabilitation success in patients with chronic pain symptoms. The primary aim of such interventions is to improve daily functioning, self-efficacy, and quality of life. In case of abnormal pain behaviors, CBT also helps to diminish fear-avoidance beliefs, catastrophizing, and other behavioral responses to pain, thus modifying the pain experience.

Family therapy or psychodynamic psychotherapy may prove effective as well because it addresses the social aspect of pain behaviors. However, no systematic reviews have assessed the efficacy of these methods.

Conversion symptoms, especially when acute, may undergo spontaneous resolution after explanation and suggestion. Some patients may benefit from education about the patterns of sensorimotor disturbance associated with alteration in neurotransmission, as in the case of major depression, thereby providing a cognitive framework for treatment. Hypnosis is also a potential intervention in the management of the disorder. The goals of such hypnosis include symptom reduction and exploration. It can also be used to evoke memories of a traumatic event that has a positive link with the symptoms. Although there are many anecdotal accounts of the efficacy of hypnosis in conversion disorder, one RCT found that hypnosis had no additional effect on treatment outcome.

SOMATOFORM CONVERSION REACTIONS

Hemianesthesia

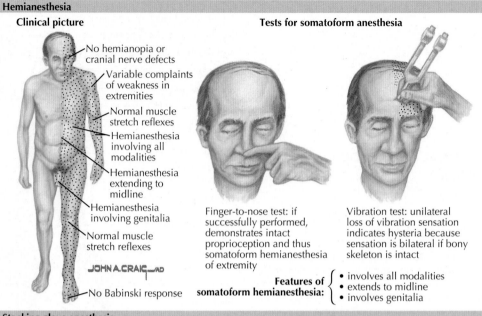

Clinical picture

- No hemianopia or cranial nerve defects
- Variable complaints of weakness in extremities
- Normal muscle stretch reflexes
- Hemianesthesia involving all modalities
- Hemianesthesia extending to midline
- Hemianesthesia involving genitalia
- Normal muscle stretch reflexes

JOHN A. CRAIG—AD

- No Babinski response

Tests for somatoform anesthesia

Finger-to-nose test: if successfully performed, demonstrates intact proprioception and thus somatoform hemianesthesia of extremity

Vibration test: unilateral loss of vibration sensation indicates hysteria because sensation is bilateral if bony skeleton is intact

Features of somatoform hemianesthesia:
- involves all modalities
- extends to midline
- involves genitalia

Stocking-glove anesthesia

Demarcation

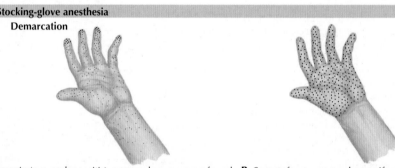

A. Organic (e.g., polyneuritis): sensory loss more profound distally; gradual transition to area of normal sensation

B. Somatoform: sensory loss uniform; sharp demarcation from area of normal sensation, usually at external anatomic landmark (e.g., joint, skinfold) rather than along a nerve distribution

Dissociation

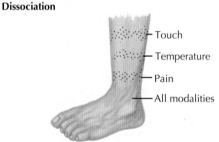

- Touch
- Temperature
- Pain
- All modalities

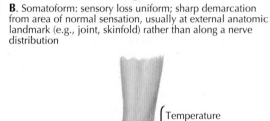

- Temperature
- Touch
- Pain

A. Organic: different level of loss for each sensory modality **B.** Somatoform: single level of loss for all sensory modalities

FLOPPY INFANT

NEONATAL HYPOTONIA

Neonatal hypotonia, often referred to as the "floppy infant," is the main presenting clinical feature of most neuromuscular diseases of early life. However, disorders of the central nervous system (CNS) may also manifest with hypotonia.

Two types of muscle tone can be assessed clinically: postural and phasic. *Postural* (antigravity) tone is a sustained, low-intensity muscle contraction in response to gravity. It is mediated by both gamma and alpha motor neuron systems in the spinal cord, and it is assessed clinically by passive manipulation of the limbs. *Phasic* tone is a brief contraction in response to a high-intensity stretch. It is mediated by the alpha motor neuron system alone and is examined clinically by eliciting the muscle stretch reflexes. Hypotonia is defined as reduction in postural tone, with or without a change in phasic tone. When postural tone is depressed, the trunk and limbs cannot overcome gravity, and the child appears hypotonic or floppy.

PHYSICAL EXAMINATION AND ASSESSMENT

After a careful general physical examination, the neurologic assessment should include an evaluation of primary neonatal reflexes, a sensory examination, and, most importantly, a motor examination. Muscle tone is assessed by passive manipulation of the infant's limbs.

Muscle tone can be evaluated further by performing the traction response, vertical suspension, and horizontal suspension maneuvers. A floppy infant exhibits "head lag," "slips through" the examiner's hands on vertical suspension, and "drapes over" the examiner's hand, like a rag doll, on horizontal suspension.

DIFFERENTIAL ANATOMIC DIAGNOSIS

Neonatal hypotonia may be the manifestation of pathology involving the CNS, the peripheral nervous system (i.e., lower motor unit), or both. In infants with *cerebral* or *central hypotonia* (nearly two-thirds of cases), the perinatal or prenatal history may suggest a CNS insult. There may also be associated global (rather than isolated gross motor) developmental delay, occasionally seizures, microcephaly, dysmorphic features, and/or malformation of the brain and/or other organs. Central hypotonia may be associated with brisk and/or persistent primitive reflexes, normal or brisk muscle stretch reflexes, clonus, and, in older children, Babinski signs. The degree of weakness noted in these infants is usually less than expected for the degree of hypotonia ("nonparalytic" hypotonia).

In *lower motor unit hypotonia* or *peripheral hypotonia*, developmental delay is primarily gross motor and is associated with absent or depressed muscle stretch reflexes and/or muscle atrophy and fasciculations of the tongue. In general, antigravity limb movements are decreased and cannot be elicited via postural reflexes. In these infants, the degree of weakness is proportional to or more than the degree of hypotonia ("paralytic" hypotonia). Trauma to the high cervical cord due to traction in breech or cervical presentation may also initially manifest itself as flaccid paralysis, which may be asymmetric, and initially absent muscle stretch reflexes; however, upper motor neuron signs develop later.

Because muscle tone is also determined by the viscoelastic properties of muscle and joints, connective tissue disorders, such as *Marfan* and *Ehlers-Danlos* syndromes, osteogenesis imperfecta, and benign ligamentous laxity, can present with hypotonia. In addition, *combined cerebral and lower motor unit hypotonia* occurs in infants and older

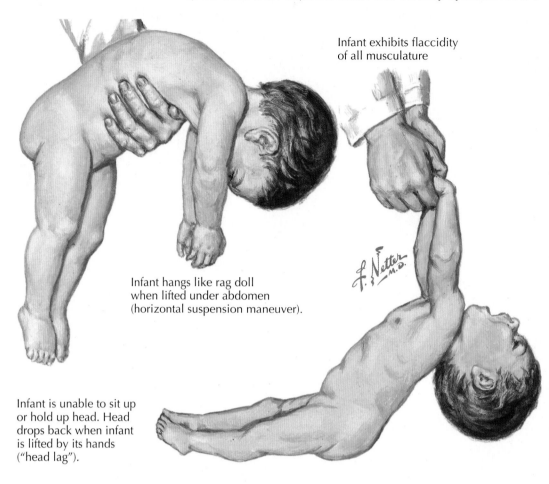

Infant exhibits flaccidity of all musculature

Infant hangs like rag doll when lifted under abdomen (horizontal suspension maneuver).

Infant is unable to sit up or hold up head. Head drops back when infant is lifted by its hands ("head lag").

Muscle biopsy specimens in different cases

Nemaline rod	Central core	Centronuclear/myotubular

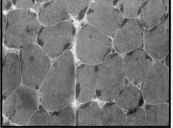

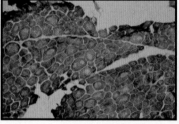

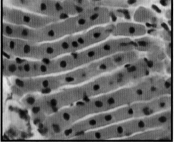

Histochemical staining of muscle biopsy frozen section reveals nemaline rods in almost all fibers (trichrome stain).

Muscle fibers show well-defined "cores" that are not enzymatically active, mostly in a central location (NADH stain).

Large central nuclei in small-diameter muscle fibers resemble fetal myotubes (longitudinal section; H&E stain).

children as a presenting manifestation of congenital myotonic dystrophy, some congenital muscular dystrophies, peroxisomal disorders, mitochondrial encephalomyopathies, neuroaxonal dystrophy, leukodystrophies (e.g., globoid cell leukodystrophy), familial dysautonomia, and asphyxia secondary to motor unit disease. Further, hypotonia without significant weakness may be a feature of systemic disease, such as sepsis, congenital heart disease, hypothyroidism, rickets, or renal tubular acidosis.

Neuromuscular diseases in infancy manifest primarily with hypotonia and weakness; however, infants with severe hypotonia but only marginal weakness usually do not have a disorder of the lower motor unit (anterior horn cell, peripheral and cranial nerves, neuromuscular junction [NMJ], and muscle). These infants may have genetic conditions, metabolic disturbances, or as discussed above, systemic disorders (e.g., congenital heart disease, renal failure).

Plate 9.2

Floppy Infant

CONGENITAL MYOPATHIES

Shy and Magee introduced the term *congenital myopathy* to describe central core disease (CCD) and myopathy present at birth, excluding muscular dystrophy. Clinical distinction from the muscular dystrophies is blurred by conditions such as nemaline and centronuclear myopathies, but these are distinct at a pathologic level. The muscle biopsy findings in congenital myopathies show distinct myopathologic features without dystrophic changes such as significant fibrosis, muscle fiber degeneration, or replacement with adipose tissue. Over time, the specificity of distinguishing pathologic features in congenital myopathies has declined with the inclusion of conditions with similar, but not identical, histologic features, such as multicore or minicore disease, and the discovery of gene mutations causing congenital myopathies with mixed myopathologic features.

Hypotonia and weakness are the major clinical features. Other characteristic features such as scoliosis, ptosis, and ophthalmoplegia may not be apparent at birth, and diagnosis may be delayed until gross-motor developmental delay and associated weakness develop in late infancy or early childhood. The serum creatine kinase (CK) level is usually normal or slightly elevated, and diagnosis is heavily dependent on muscle biopsy.

NEMALINE MYOPATHY

The term nemaline (Greek *nema*, thread) characterizes the presence of rods or thread-like structures seen in the muscle biopsies of patients with this type of congenital myopathy. The neonatal type is the most severe, presenting with hypotonia, diminished spontaneous activity, history of poor fetal movements, and early respiratory distress. More commonly, presentation is delayed until after the newborn period when gross-motor delay with proximal weakness develops.

The nemaline bodies on muscle biopsy originate from the Z disks and tend to cluster under the sarcolemma. To date, more than 10 genes have been involved in the pathogenesis of nemaline myopathy (gene products α-tropomyosin-3, nebulin, α-actin, β-tropomyosin, troponin T type I, cofilin-2, and others). It is transmitted by autosomal dominant or recessive inheritance.

CENTRAL CORE DISEASE

Most patients with CCD present with hypotonia in early infancy and childhood and a subsequent delay in motor milestones. Rarely, severe hypotonia and marked contractures are present at birth. Skeletal abnormalities are also present. The clinical course varies from nonprogressive to slowly progressive. An association between CCD and malignant hyperthermia has been observed. On muscle biopsy, central cores appear to be packed with myofiber material and depleted of organelles.

CCD is an autosomal dominant or recessive condition. Mutations of the ryanodine receptor-1 have been detected in families with susceptibility to malignant hyperthermia and patients with CCD.

CENTRONUCLEAR/MYOTUBULAR MYOPATHY

The mode of inheritance of centronuclear/myotubular myopathy can be X-linked recessive, autosomal dominant, or recessive. Early-onset cases are the most common form

Hypotonic infant can sit with support but cannot stand and has respiratory problems and difficulty holding up head. Some toes may be foreshortened.

High-arched palate may be associated finding

Teenage girl with characteristic elongated facies, mild muscular weakness, and early-onset progressive scoliosis

Electron micrographs show sections of muscle biopsy specimens (osmium fixed). *Above*, longitudinal section showing nemaline body that is somewhat longer than a sarcomere (30,000). *Right*, cross section of rods (145,000).

and present with severe hypotonia, weakness, and respiratory distress. Affected infants are very weak and have major feeding difficulties, facial diplegia, bilateral ptosis, and limitation of eye movements (external ophthalmoplegia). Despite intensive respiratory support, infants rarely survive or have improved motor function. The muscle biopsy shows central nuclei present in many muscle fibers and type I fiber predominance. The gene product in the X-linked recessive variety (MTM1) was designated myotubularin. Dynamin-2, amphiphysin (B1N1), titin, and RYR1 mutations have also been described in patients with centronuclear myopathy.

CONGENITAL FIBER-TYPE DISPROPORTION

Congenital fiber-type disproportion (CFTD) typically presents with hypotonia and weakness at birth or in the neonatal period. There is delay in acquisition of motor milestones. Serum CK is normal, and electromyography (EMG) may be normal or myopathic. Muscle biopsy shows type I fiber predominance but also nonspecific type I fiber atrophy seen in other clinically diverse conditions. Therefore the existence of CFTD as an entity has been debated. α-Actin (ACTA1), RYR1, α-tropomyosin, selenoprotein N (SEPN1), and other gene mutations have been described in patients with CFTD.

OTHER CONGENITAL MYOPATHIES

In addition to these common congenital myopathies, there are uncommon types with similar clinical characteristics but less well-defined patterns of inheritance. Their names reflect their myopathologic features and include (1) actin myopathy (non-nemaline), (2) fingerprint body myopathy, (3) sarcotubular myopathy, (4) hyaline body myopathy, (5) reducing body myopathy, (6) cytoplasmic body myopathy, (7) myopathy with myotubular aggregates, (8) zebra body myopathy, (9) core-rod myopathy, (10) cap myopathy, and (11) trilaminar myopathy. The mutated genes are known in some of them, but diagnosis is made by muscle biopsy.

SPINAL MUSCULAR ATROPHY

Spinal muscular atrophy (SMA) is an autosomal recessive hereditary illness. Rare variant forms exist, including X-linked and dominant forms. It is one of the two most common causes of a floppy infant secondary to lesions of the peripheral motor unit. The most common form of SMA is the proximal recessive type, which includes a broad range of subtypes ranging from the severe infantile variant to ambulatory forms with adult onset.

At birth, many infants with SMA type I appear normal; if left untreated, within a few weeks to months generalized hypotonia and neuromuscular weakness develop. A classic hypotonic posture characterized by abducted hips, internal rotation of the forearms, and frog-legged and jug-handle habitus is typical. Respiratory pattern is characterized by paradoxic chest and abdomen movement as a result of selective intercostal muscle weakness with preserved diaphragm function. Without supportive treatment, such infants subsequently develop characteristic bell-shaped deformities of the thorax. Progressive bulbar and respiratory insufficiency results in a vulnerability to both aspiration and infectious pneumonias.

Extraocular and facial movements are preserved; these infants typically have a bright, attentive countenance. Careful evaluation of the tongue reveals tongue fasciculations. In contrast to adult motor neuron disorders, fasciculations in limbs are difficult to appreciate due to excessive subcutaneous infantile fat. Before newborn screening for this condition, which takes place in almost all of the United States and in many other countries, abnormal motor milestones with poor head control and the inability to roll and to achieve independent sitting, as expected during the first few months, led to investigation and eventual diagnosis of SMA type I. In a most severe subset, reduced fetal movements are detected prenatally; these infants are born with generalized hypotonia, weakness, respiratory insufficiency, bulbar dysfunction, and proximal joint contractures.

SMA with respiratory distress (SMARD) is distinguished by early respiratory failure due to diaphragm involvement, especially in association with more distal presentation of limb weakness. X-linked SMA manifests as a severe infantile SMA variant predominantly affecting males.

Infants with SMA type II initially can sit but without treatment never become able to walk; before newborn screening, they were usually diagnosed at ages 6 to 24 months. Kugelberg-Welander disease, or SMA type III, typically shows signs of proximal weakness between ages 2 and 14 years if untreated. These children may have mild elevations of serum CK (<1000 IU/L).

More than 95% of individuals with SMA have a homozygous deletion/mutation of exon 7 of the *SMN1* gene. *SMN2* is a highly homologous copy of *SMN1* apart from a single base pair mutation that prevents incorporation of exon 7. *SMN1* and *SMN2* lie within the telomeric and centromeric halves, respectively, of a large, inverted duplication on chromosome 5q13. Both SMA II and SMA III have the same genetic defects as type I. Roughly 90% of patients with SMA I will have two copies of *SMN2*, whereas the rest will have three or

Infant with typical bell-shaped thorax, frog-leg posture, and "jug-handle" position of upper limbs

Boy with much milder, late-onset form of Kugelberg-Welander disease, with marked lordosis and eversion of feet

Muscle biopsy specimen showing groups of small atrophic muscle fibers and areas of normal or enlarged fibers (group atrophy) (trichrome stain)

Baseline tremor in otherwise normal electrocardiogram

Electromyography (motor units during active contraction)

Normal

Werdnig-Hoffman disease

even four copies. Almost 90% of those with SMA II will have three copies, whereas the rest will have two copies. Of those with SMA III, two-thirds will have four copies of *SMN2*, 30% will have three copies, and the rest will have two copies or, rarely, more than four. Infants who do not have this deletion identified may have a non–chromosome 5 SMA or a mutation in the *SMN* gene not detectable with the currently used polymerase chain reaction–based methods.

EMG is a very sensitive primary diagnostic tool, but it has been largely supplanted by DNA analysis. However, when DNA testing is normal and significant weakness is manifest, the EMG findings are distinct in SMA I, demonstrating diffuse fibrillations in virtually all muscles in association with markedly reduced recruitment of small motor units in the absence of the typical large complex motor units characteristic of reinnervation in milder, more chronic forms of the

disorder. Muscle biopsy demonstrates findings typical of neurogenic atrophy, although the reduced reinnervation capacity in SMA I often results in a predominance of small, rounded fibers within entirely denervated fascicles.

Other lesions in the motor unit can mimic Werdnig-Hoffmann disease (WHD), but, as a rule, they can be differentiated by clinical and EMG findings and examination of muscle biopsy specimens if genetic and/or neurophysiologic testing are not definitive. Differential diagnosis includes the very rare recessive inherited peripheral neuropathy variants, such as congenital hypomyelinating neuropathy, that may clinically mimic WHD, even to the point of tongue fasciculations. More distally within the motor unit, NMJ disorders, including transient neonatal myasthenia gravis and infantile botulism, as well as the various congenital myopathies and dystrophies, may present as a floppy infant.

Plate 9.4

Floppy Infant

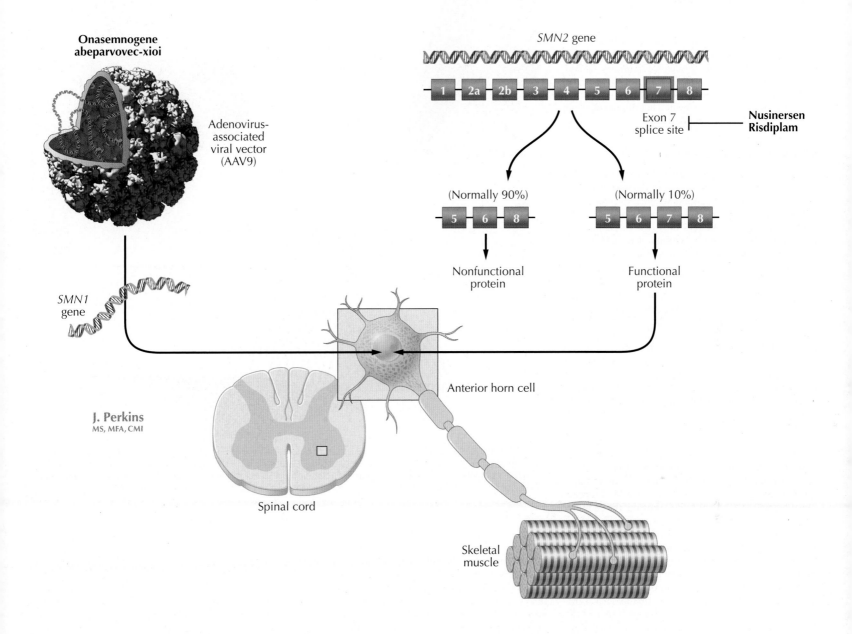

Onasemnogene
abeparvovec-xioi

Adenovirus-
associated
viral vector
(AAV9)

SMN2 gene

| 1 | 2a | 2b | 3 | 4 | 5 | 6 | 7 | 8 |

Exon 7
splice site

**Nusinersen
Risdiplam**

(Normally 90%)

| 5 | 6 | 8 |

Nonfunctional
protein

(Normally 10%)

| 5 | 6 | 7 | 8 |

Functional
protein

SMN1
gene

Anterior horn cell

J. Perkins
MS, MFA, CMI

Spinal cord

Skeletal
muscle

TREATMENT FOR SPINAL MUSCULAR ATROPHY

Treatment of SMA marks one of the most successful implementations of genetically targeted therapeutics, with three medications approved by the US Food and Drug Administration (FDA) between 2016 and 2020. Currently three medications are approved to either provide a working copy of SMN1 or improve the production of full-length protein from SMN2.

The first is the antisense oligonucleotide nusinersen, which is delivered intrathecally every 4 months after an initial loading phase. Its mechanism of action is blocking a splice site that leads to exclusion of exon 7 from the SMN2 gene, thus increasing inclusion of exon 7 and formation of more stable SMN protein product. Nusinersen was approved for use in all types of SMA and all ages of onset. The most dramatic treatment responses have been observed in children with presymptomatic

SMA, which was a major factor in launching newborn screening for SMA in most states. Nusinersen is generally well tolerated, with most adverse events being related to lumbar punctures, which may need to be done under fluoroscopy in those patients with severe spinal deformities and/or spinal hardware from surgical fusion.

The second approved therapy for SMA is an intravenous gene therapy, onasemnogene abeparvovec-xioi, which uses an adenovirus-associated viral vector to deliver SMN1 to motor neurons. This medication was approved by the FDA in 2019 as a single-dose intravenous infusion for children under 24 months, although clinical trials showed the most robust responses in children treated presymptomatically or in the first months of life. After infusion, patients may experience elevated serum transaminases and/or troponins. For this reason, treatment with corticosteroids is started the day before infusion and continued for at least 1 month. Clinical trials are ongoing for intrathecal infusion in older children and adults with SMA.

The third treatment for SMA, approved by the FDA in 2020 for patients older than 2 months, is risdiplam, an oral splicing modifier that, like nusinersen, increases incorporation of exon 7 into SMN2 mRNA, leading to increased expression of the more stable, full-length SMN protein product. This daily medication was approved after trials of multiple SMA subtypes in children and young adults showed improvements in motor outcomes. Adverse effects can include diarrhea, constipation, abdominal discomfort, body aches, and headache.

The development of these therapies, in combination with newborn screening, has dramatically changed the outcome of patients with this disease. Although it is too soon to know the full impact of these therapies, many treated patients do not develop the need for respiratory support and are able to make developmental milestones throughout the years. Studies looking at combination therapies are ongoing as well to determine whether these outcomes can be improved even further.

INFANTILE NEUROMUSCULAR JUNCTION DISORDERS

In rare cases, infants may develop acute NMJ disorders, including neonatal myasthenia gravis (MG), infantile botulism, and congenital myasthenic syndromes (CMSs). Historically, magnesium sulfate treatment for maternal eclampsia was reported to be a cause of impaired neuromuscular transmission in neonates, but this has not been studied extensively in recent decades.

NEONATAL MYASTHENIA GRAVIS

Mothers with acetylcholine receptor (AChR) antibody–related MG have a 15% incidence of having babies with neonatal MG, although all infants born to seropositive mothers have been reported to have circulating AChR antibodies. These antibodies cross the placenta, enter the fetal circulation, and then bind to fetal NMJs. Once an affected mother has an infant with neonatal MG, her subsequent children have a higher risk of also developing this disorder.

Infants with neonatal MG sometimes have a preceding history of weak fetal movements or fetal distress during delivery. Severe hypotonia may develop shortly after birth. Other manifestations include facial diplegia, poor suck/feeding, a weak cry, intermittent cyanosis (especially during feeding), and respiratory weakness and/or failure. Muscle stretch reflexes, sphincter function, and sensation are generally preserved. Ptosis and external ophthalmoplegia are seen less frequently than in juvenile MG. Typically, symptoms are transient, lasting 3 to 12 weeks.

Traditionally, improvement in response to edrophonium or neostigmine injection would support this diagnosis, but edrophonium is no longer available in several countries, including the United States, and this test does not distinguish among different types of NMJ disorders. The presence of AChR antibodies provides the definitive diagnosis of neonatal MG in the appropriate clinical setting. Postnatally, there is no clinically meaningful transmission of maternal AChR antibodies, including in breast milk. Supportive treatment is the primary therapeutic modality and is necessary until symptoms clear. Some infants require transient intubation (mechanical ventilation). Acetylcholinesterase inhibitors such as pyridostigmine or neostigmine methylsulfate may be helpful in some cases. Both intravenous immunoglobulin and plasma exchange provide therapeutic alternatives for severe cases.

INFANT BOTULISM

This rare disorder typically occurs in previously healthy infants, particularly in the mid-Atlantic states, Utah, and California, although it is occasionally seen in other regions. It is not a contagious disease. *Clostridium botulinum* is an obligatory anaerobic, gram-positive, spore-forming, rod-shaped bacterium that thrives within the immature gut of infants. The bacteria release a toxin affecting presynaptic ACh release from the NMJ. In economically developed settings, this is the most common form of human botulism. The *C. botulinum* spores are often ingested from contaminated soil or honey. Because parents are advised not to feed honey to infants, this is currently a rare source of infant botulism.

Infant botulism usually has a fairly stereotyped clinical presentation. Typically, a previously healthy infant between 10 days and 6 months old develops

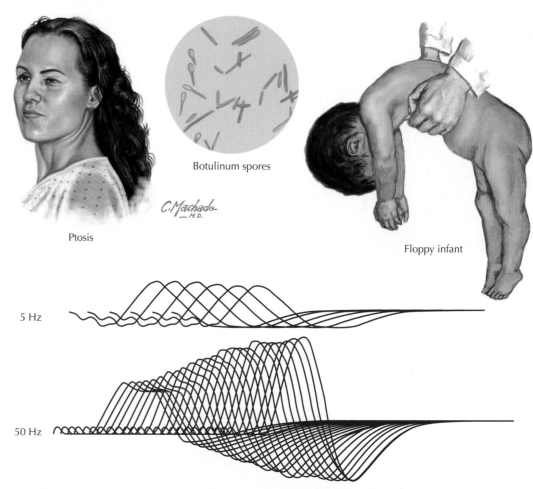

Botulinum spores

C. Machado
—M.D.

Ptosis

Floppy infant

5 Hz

50 Hz

Repetitive stimulation at 5 Hz of a hypotonic baby's ulnar nerve; recording at the hypothenar eminence demonstrates no facilitation or decrement in the response, whereas 50-Hz stimulus promotes an almost 100% facilitation in the eventual amplitude of the recorded response. Facilitation on 50-Hz stimulation is the characteristic and diagnostic finding of a presynaptic defect in neuromuscular transmission as occurs with infant botulism.

acute hypotonia, generalized weakness, poor feeding secondary to bulbar dysphagia, and poor suck that impairs feeding; there is also potential for a life-threatening respiratory crisis. The parents may note in retrospect that their infant was constipated before the development of other symptoms. An affected infant admitted to the hospital will typically be alert, afebrile, and nonirritable but have poorly reactive pupillary light reflexes, ophthalmoparesis, symmetric facial bulbar weakness, and generalized hypotonia. The face is typically expressionless with sialorrhea, and there may be a high-pitched cry. Infant botulism should be considered in the differential diagnosis of unexplained respiratory distress in any infant up to 6 months old, and in some cases in slightly older infants.

Electrodiagnostic studies and stool testing for botulinum toxin are the key diagnostic studies for diagnosing infant botulism; high-frequency repetitive motor nerve stimulation (20 or 50 Hz) demonstrates significant incremental responses (23%–313%). This is in keeping with a presynaptic defect in ACh release, resulting in impaired neuromuscular transmission. Electrodiagnostic changes may not be present early in the disease course.

The mainstays of treatment are ventilatory support, if needed, and human-derived botulinum immunoglobulin administered as early as possible. With good management, most children recover without long-term sequelae.

CONGENITAL MYASTHENIC SYNDROMES

CMSs are a group of widely differing, rare familial infantile NMJ disorders, each characterized by compromised neuromuscular transmission safety margins leading to fatigable weakness.

These genetically determined "myasthenic" disorders usually manifest during the first years of life. Clinically, ptosis and extraocular weakness are often more subtle than in juvenile MG. In addition, bulbar, neck, and extremity weakness occur, sometimes within a restricted distribution.

Respiratory distress, either constant or episodic, occurs in some subtypes of CMS. When episodic apnea occurs in infants with CMS, these events may be life-threatening. Some babies have fluctuating ptosis, poor suck and cry, feeding difficulty, and secondary respiratory infections.

Electrodiagnostic studies typically demonstrate abnormalities suggestive of disorders of neuromuscular transmission. The exact pattern of abnormalities depends on whether the physiologic defect is presynaptic, synaptic, or postsynaptic.

Certain medications are beneficial in specific subtypes of CMS. Some of these medications will worsen symptoms in other subtypes, so it is important to arrive at a specific subtype diagnosis, ideally confirmed by genetic testing, for optimal medical management.

Plate 9.6

Floppy Infant

Arthrogryposis Multiplex Congenita

Arthrogryposis is defined as the presence of a congenital joint contracture. Arthrogryposis multiplex congenita (AMC) is, by extension, a syndrome in which an infant is born with congenital contractures at two or more major joints. The incidence is estimated to range from 1 in 3000 to 1 in 12,000 live births. Approximately 150 causes of AMC are defined, including maternal factors, genetic disorders, and cryptic etiologies. A prolonged period of fetal immobility provides the final common pathway shared by all the pathologic processes that lead to the clinical phenotype of AMC. Vigorous and frequent fetal movements are needed to maintain a normal range of motion across joints.

The maternal conditions that put an infant at risk for AMC are those that restrict fetal movements. They include oligohydramnios, placental insufficiency, and structural abnormalities such as bicornuate uterus. Medical conditions, such as maternal MG, may also cause prolonged prenatal weakness. A wide variety of genetic disorders can lead to AMC; some of these affect the CNS and lead to decreased fetal motor abilities. Chromosomal aneuploidies are occasionally associated with AMC but account for a small fraction of cases. Inherited peripheral nervous system disorders cause AMC if they prevent a fetus from moving normally, and they account for a significant proportion of cases. These include motor neuron disease (including variants of SMA), CMS, congenital myopathy, congenital muscular dystrophy, and congenital myotonic dystrophy. Among the neuromuscular etiologies, a form of motor neuron disease is the most common; these cases tend to be non-5q forms of SMA (i.e., not associated with deletions or other pathogenic variants in *SMN1*).

The diagnostic evaluation of AMC starts with a thorough history, including details of gestation. If a maternal issue, such as oligohydramnios or uterine structural abnormalities, is identified and no findings in the infant suggest an endogenous disease process, the infant may not require an extensive evaluation. If no clear maternal factor is defined, then a diagnostic evaluation for an endogenous disease should be initiated. Certain findings on history and examination, such as cognitive delays, dysmorphic features, and microcephaly, may suggest a CNS localization or generalized genetic syndrome. In such cases, basic screening tests that may be useful include karyotype, chromosomal microarray, and brain magnetic resonance imaging. Additional studies may be indicated depending on the individual presentation.

The presence of muscle weakness, considering the limitations in range of motion, is strongly suggestive of a peripheral nervous system etiology. The presence or absence of muscle stretch reflexes may in some cases help differentiate between central and peripheral motor unit disorders; however, reflexes are not as accurate as the presence or absence of weakness in making this distinction. In cases where a peripheral motor unit process is suspected, a serum CK level should be obtained, although it should be noted that these levels are sometimes artifactually elevated in the first several days of life.

Whenever possible, both an electrodiagnostic study and muscle biopsy should be obtained because these

Typical rigid deformities of all four limbs seen in an infant with arthrogryposis

Radiograph of pelvis and hips of 2-week-old infant shows advanced changes typical of teratologic dislocation of hips.

Intractable foot deformities and hip dislocations; hyperextension of knees

Deformities of upper limbs in older child

Hand deformities

tests are most accurate when they are concordant with each other. There are some conditions, such as certain subtypes of congenital muscular dystrophy, in which both the central and peripheral nervous systems are affected, and thus the infant may have clinical features suggestive of both. Some endogenous causes are not neurologic in origin; these may include connective tissue disorders such as multiple pterygium syndrome, developmental disorders such as amyoplasia, and genetic arthrogryposis syndromes such as Pena-Shokeir syndrome. In some cases, a specific etiology cannot be identified after a thorough evaluation. Genetic diagnoses may be identified in an increasing proportion of affected infants with central or peripheral nervous system localizations. This is due to the widespread adoption of large next-generation genetic

test panels and exome sequencing, and the emerging adoption of genome sequencing, including long-read sequencing.

The treatment of AMC is largely supportive because the injuries to the affected joints occur prenatally and are difficult to reverse. Physical therapy is needed on a long-term basis. A skilled orthopedic surgeon familiar with arthrogryposis, or at least with contractures in children, will need to be involved because these patients often need multiple surgeries to help alleviate some of the joint limitations. Molecular therapies are being developed for more and more orphan diseases, including some of the ones associated with arthrogryposis. A notable success story is the approval of three different therapies for SMA by the FDA since 2016.

MOTOR NEURON AND ITS DISORDERS

PERIPHERAL NERVOUS SYSTEM: OVERVIEW

The major functions of the nervous system are processing information and communicating signals in response to external and internal stimuli. These functions rely on propagation of electrical signals between the peripheral nervous system and the central nervous system. The somatic peripheral nervous system is composed of afferent (sensory) neurons (green in the figure) and efferent (motor) neurons (red in the figure). The first-order somatic sensory neurons transmit the initial electrical signals generated by a sensory stimulus. For example, a sensory stimulus to the skin initiates sensory processing by activating the local specialized sensory receptors within the skin. A sensory nerve action potential (electrical signal) is generated and propagates along the afferent sensory axons within a peripheral nerve, toward the spinal cord. The final-order somatic (lower) motor neurons are depolarized by central or peripheral signals to the anterior horn of the spinal cord. The action potentials then propagate away from the anterior horn of the spinal cord via the motor axons, through the neuromuscular junction (NMJ), and into the muscle, ultimately leading to muscle contraction.

The somatic sensory and motor neurons have several morphologic differences. The *peripheral somatic sensory neurons* are pseudounipolar neurons. The sensory neuron cell bodies reside in the dorsal root ganglion situated posterolateral to the spinal cord near the intervertebral foramen. Extending out from the cell body are axons that split into two branches. One branch extends distally toward the hands, feet, and periphery, and the other extends proximally through the dorsal root into the posterior horn of the spinal cord. Axons from either branch undergo wallerian degeneration if they are separated from their neuron cell bodies. As a result, an injury to the dorsal nerve root affecting the proximal branch will lead to sensory deficits even though the distal branch axons remain intact. The clinical implications of this occur during electrophysiologic testing with sensory nerve conduction studies. In the presence of sensory loss in a limb, a preserved or normal distal sensory nerve conduction study response suggests that the sensory loss is caused by a disorder involving the sensory pathway sparing the distal branch axons, which implies the lesion lies either in the dorsal root (proximal to the ganglion) or the central somatosensory conduction pathways.

The functions of somatic nerve fibers differ depending on their structure. The largest caliber sensory neurons are type Ia and Ib (Aα) fibers, which are large, myelinated fibers whose function is to rapidly transmit proprioceptive signals from muscle spindle endings and Golgi tendon organs in response to stretches in muscle fibers. Type II (Aβ) fibers are large, myelinated fibers that transmit signals from muscles and joints at rest, and skin mechanoreceptors perceiving fine touch and pressure. Type III (Aδ) fibers are smaller, thinly myelinated fibers that play a role in pain, cold temperature, touch, pressure, and visceral sensations. The smallest and slowest conducting, type IV (C), fibers are unmyelinated and transmit sensations of heat and pain.

Somatic motor neurons are unipolar neurons. The motor neuron cell bodies reside in the anterior gray matter (anterior horns) of the spinal cord. A single axon extends distally from each anterior horn cell, through the ventral root, and joins the peripheral nerve that innervates individual muscles. The motor conduction pathway continues along the nerve to the nerve terminal. At this site, an action potential traveling through the motor axon to the nerve terminal leads to a cascade of reactions at the NMJ, where the nerve terminal is adjacent to the muscle fiber. Through these reactions, an action potential is generated along the muscle fibers, resulting in muscle fiber contraction. The integrity of the motor unit (an anterior horn cell and its axon, nerve terminal, NMJ, and innervated muscle fibers) can be tested during electrophysiologic testing with motor nerve conduction studies and electromyography (EMG).

Motor neurons are typically large in diameter and myelinated. The major type of motor neuron, the alpha motor neuron, innervates the *extrafusal striated muscle fibers* and, primarily, is responsible for muscle fiber contraction. Smaller, myelinated gamma motor neurons innervate the *intrafusal fibers of muscle spindles*.

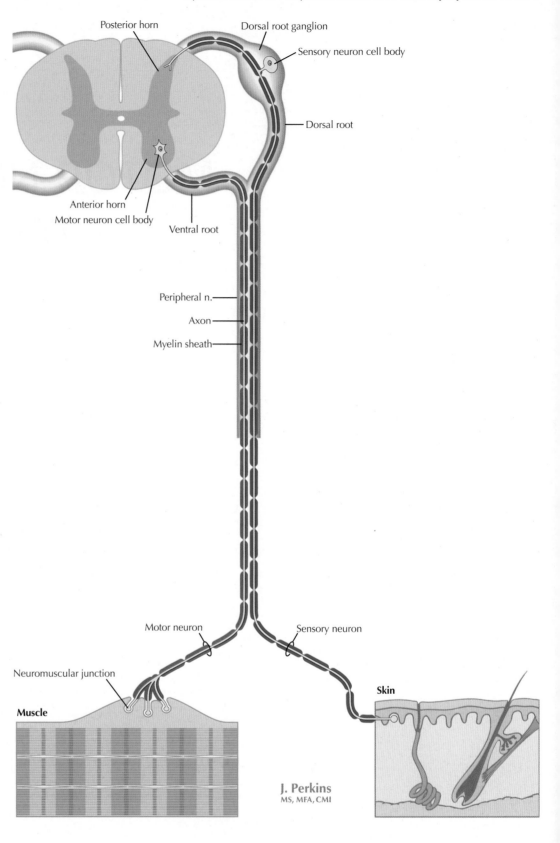

Posterior horn • Dorsal root ganglion • Sensory neuron cell body • Dorsal root • Anterior horn • Motor neuron cell body • Ventral root • Peripheral n. • Axon • Myelin sheath • Motor neuron • Sensory neuron • Neuromuscular junction • **Muscle** • **Skin**

J. Perkins
MS, MFA, CMI

Plate 10.2

Motor Neuron and Its Disorders

SPINAL CORD AND NEURONAL CELL BODY WITH MOTOR, SENSORY, AND AUTONOMIC COMPONENTS OF THE PERIPHERAL NERVE

The cell body (soma) is the metabolic center of the neuron and performs numerous functions necessary to maintain the health and function of the neuron. The motor neuron cell body resides in the ventral (anterior) horn of the spinal cord or in the cranial nerve nuclei within the brainstem. Within the cell body are numerous organelles, each of which serves a particular role for the neuron. The nucleus and nucleolus contain the cell's deoxyribonucleic acid (DNA). The mitochondria play the important role of energy metabolism within the neuron and produce adenosine triphosphate, which is necessary for other metabolic processes within the cell to occur. The rough endoplasmic reticulum, along with the Nissl substance and its associated ribosomes, synthesize proteins that are then secreted through and modified by the smooth endoplasmic reticulum and Golgi apparatus. The proteins are subsequently packaged into vesicles that store and transport proteins throughout the cell. Lysosomes are organelles that are responsible for degradation of molecules within the cell.

Each neuronal cell body contains many dendrites, which are peripheral extensions from the cell body that, along with the smaller dendritic spines (gemmules), receive input from other neurons. Each dendrite receives *excitatory or inhibitory potentials* from the nerve terminals of neighboring neurons at the *axodendritic synapses*. The dendrites and the cell body of a single neuron may have hundreds of synapses from many different neurons. Each of the postsynaptic excitatory or inhibitory potentials are summated to determine whether an action potential will or will not be initiated within the neuron. When initiated, an action potential usually originates at the axon hillock, the region of the cell body at which the axon originates. The axon is a neuronal process extending beyond the cell body and conducts electrical activity and trophic factors away from the cell body and toward other neurons or organs. The course of the axons and route of conduction of the electrical signals vary according to the type of neuron and its function.

The somas of the somatic sensory neurons are located in the dorsal root ganglion, just lateral to the spinal cord and typically within the intervertebral foramen. The somatic sensory neurons are pseudounipolar neurons with axons that branch in two directions, one branch conducting impulses from the sensory receptors of the limbs and organs toward the dorsal root ganglion through the somatic nerves, and the other branch traversing proximally from the dorsal root ganglion through the dorsal root into the dorsal column of the spinal cord.

The cell bodies (anterior horn cells) of the somatic motor neurons are located in the anterior gray matter of

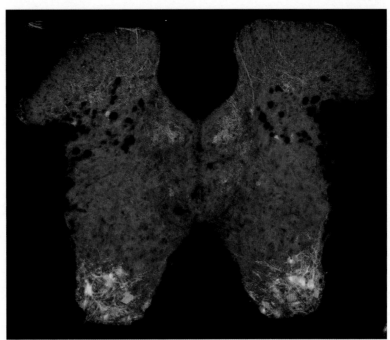

Image of the upper thoracic spinal cord of a Brainbow transgenic mouse. Individual motor neurons in the ventral spinal cord express randomized amounts of a red, green, and blue fluorescent protein. The colors are generated by genetic recombination using a recombinase enzyme that is specifically activated in motor neurons but in few other spinal neurons. This method allows researchers to track the connections of individual neurons by tracing the nerve cell's processes through multiple serial sections of brain and spinal cord tissue. *(Courtesy Dawen Cai, Joshua Sanes, and Jeff Lichtman, Harvard University.)*

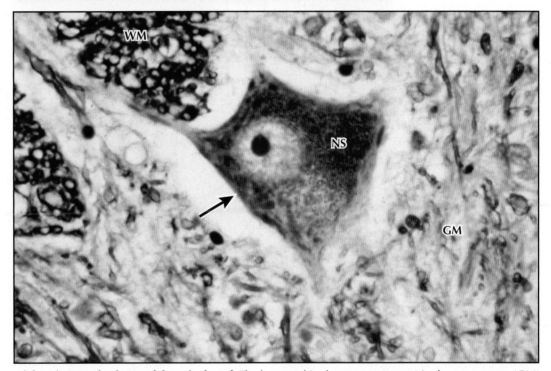

Light micrograph of part of the spinal cord. The large multipolar neuron *(arrow)* in the gray matter *(GM)* has an irregularly shaped soma with dispersed Nissl substance *(NS)*, which makes the cytoplasm basophilic. A lightly stained, spheric nucleus is eccentrically placed and contains a prominent, dark nucleolus. The neuron is close to the white matter *(WM)*, consisting of bundles of myelinated nerve fibers. Small round nuclei in the gray matter are those of glial cells. 750×. Luxol fast blue and cresyl violet. *(From Ovalle W, Nahirney P. Netter's Essential Histology. Elsevier; 2008).*

the spinal cord. The motor neurons are unipolar neurons, and each neuron has an axon that extends through the ventral root and then through either the dorsal ramus (innervating paraspinal skeletal muscles) or the ventral ramus (innervating limb and peripheral skeletal muscles) and into individual nerves.

The cell bodies of the sympathetic autonomic peripheral neurons are located in the spinal cord. The preganglionic sympathetic neurons extend through the ventral roots and the white rami communicantes, and they synapse in peripherally located ganglia—either the sympathetic chain adjacent to the spinal cord or the collateral sympathetic ganglia near the organs that the neurons supply. After synapsing at either site, the postganglionic sympathetic neurons course to the end organs, including vascular smooth muscle, sweat glands, and arrector pili muscles in the skin or the smooth muscles and glands of other organs.

MOTOR UNIT

The outward expression of all human behavior requires the communication of thoughts, reactions, and ideas through the neuromuscular system, where nerves emanating from the spinal cord and brainstem connect to skeletal muscles and translate these thoughts, ideas, and expressions into locomotion. There are more than 650 named skeletal muscles in the human body. The face and hands have the greatest density of individual muscles, allowing us to express emotions, communicate, and eat. These skeletal muscles provide humans with the civilization-forming capabilities of writing and speech, the strength to climb mountains and run a marathon, the finesse to perform the most intricate surgical movements or grandest artistic dance, and the expression of music through vocal cords and handcrafted musical instruments.

The motor unit is the "final efferent pathway" of the peripheral somatic motor pathway. A *motor unit* is defined as a single anterior horn cell or brainstem motor neuron, its axon, and all the muscle fibers innervated by that axon. All the muscle fibers within a single motor unit are of the same fiber type. The *motor units* are very small for some muscles that require very fine control or miniscule movements, such as the muscles of the eyes, eardrum, larynx, and finger muscles, where motor units may be composed of only 10 to 100 muscle fibers. By contrast, other motor units are much larger and innervate hundreds to thousands of muscle fibers for massive postural, girdle, and limb muscles (e.g., erector spinae, gluteus maximus, and gastrocnemius muscles).

When muscles are activated, motor units are sequentially recruited in a fixed order. Typically, the weakest motor units causing the smallest muscle twitches are recruited first. If more force is required, additional motor units are activated, each progressively producing larger amounts of muscle tension. In this way, there is fine control of small muscle contractions and less control as muscle contraction force is increased. All muscle fibers within a single motor unit have similar contraction properties because they have similar subtypes of the contraction protein, *myosin.*

Within a small section of muscle, the fibers of several (up to 10 or more) different motor units are interspersed with each other (Plate 10.3, bottom). This figure illustrates the anatomy of three different motor units forming the final peripheral components of the descending motor pathway that emanates from a single anterior horn motor neuron cell body and all axons and

muscle fibers innervated by that single neuron. The cell bodies of the motor units lie within the brainstem for motor cranial nuclei, serving the somatic cranial muscles, such as the extraocular, facial, and pharyngeal muscles, and within the anterior horn cells of the spinal cord for the motor neurons serving somatic motor function to the noncranial muscles.

Cells bodies of each of three motor units originate within spinal cord anterior horn gray matter. The peripheral axon arising from each *anterior horn cell* leaves the spinal cord through the ventral nerve root, forming a peripheral nerve that adjoins the muscle distally. At these junctions, the nerve terminals of different motor units are positioned in a relatively confined intramuscular area named the *endplate zone* or *motor point.* At

this site, there are high concentrations of acetylcholine receptors attached within the muscle fibers. It is here, usually toward the middle of a muscle, that muscle fiber action potentials are generated after acetylcholine is released and bound to the receptors.

The *first motor units* recruited generally activate muscle fibers having "slow twitch" fatigue-resistant myosin that cause slow contractions. The *last motor units* to be recruited tend to activate "fast twitch" muscle fibers with fast myosin but are highly fatigable. It is possible to see positions of all muscle fibers within each of the motor units in one muscle. Such descriptions reveal "connectomes" that are complete maps of all the positions of all the motor axons and their connections within a muscle.

Plate 10.4

Motor Neuron and Its Disorders

MOTOR UNIT POTENTIALS

Needle EMG assesses the electrical signals from muscle fibers within a muscle. This is one of the two major components of the clinical EMG evaluation; nerve conduction studies are complementary. During voluntary activation, when a cranial nerve motor nucleus or an anterior horn cell is activated from within the brainstem or spinal cord, an action potential is generated and propagates along the main axon through its terminal branches to the NMJ, releasing acetylcholine and leading to depolarization of all the muscle fibers innervated by that specific anterior horn cell. When a recording needle electrode is placed within the muscle in the region of an activated motor unit, the action potentials of each of the muscle fibers in the recording range of the electrode (usually 1–2 mm) are recorded and summated to record the *motor unit potential* (MUP). In a typical individual, the axon branches of each motor unit conduct the action potential at a similar rate; therefore the firing of the individual muscle fiber action potentials is relatively synchronous. Because the muscle fiber action potentials fire at a similar time, the MUP has a relatively short duration (usually 8–12 msec) and summated amplitude that typically varies between 400 to 1000 microvolts (Plate 10.4, *A*).

Pathologies of nerves or muscles lead to changes within the motor unit structure and function. These changes, which are recorded with a needle electrode, are reflected in the MUP. *Neuropathic disorders* are associated with specific changes in the MUP character that develop temporally in several stages. Initially, as loss of anterior horn cells or axons occurs, there is a reduction in the number of functioning motor units innervating an individual muscle. In this *acute stage*, characterized by the loss of motor units, the MUP recorded during needle EMG appear morphologically normal, although fewer MUPs are activated despite increasing effort. This reduction in recruitment of MUPs with effort can be recognized by an increased firing rate of seemingly healthy MUPs relative to the number of MUPs activated within the region of the recording electrode.

As *recovery* begins, newly formed collateral axons derived from the remaining healthy anterior horn cells reinnervate those affected muscle fibers that have lost their normal innervation. The reinnervated motor unit consists of an increased number and density of muscle fibers within a region of the muscle compared with the original motor unit. Because the collateral nerve sprouts may not be adequately or completely myelinated and as a result of the wider distribution of innervated fibers within the muscle, the synchrony of firing of the individual muscle fibers is reduced. The resultant effect of these changes is a recorded MUP that is of higher amplitude, is of longer duration, and may have multiple phases leading to a polyphasic appearance. In an attempt to compensate, these fire more rapidly (Plate 10.4, *B*).

A classic example of neuropathic MUPs is seen in patients who survived poliomyelitis that caused paralysis as young persons. The surviving anterior horn cells provided a means to develop collateral reinnervation and thus partial recovery. In this instance, needle EMG demonstrates just a few remaining MUPs. However, these high-amplitude MUPs fire at much greater rates to provide compensation and ability to move the limb once again. Amyotrophic lateral sclerosis (ALS; also called motor neuron disease [MND] or Lou Gehrig disease) provides a different example of this process. Here, although there is an

B. Neuropathic motor unit potential

A. Normal motor unit potential

C. Myopathic motor unit potential

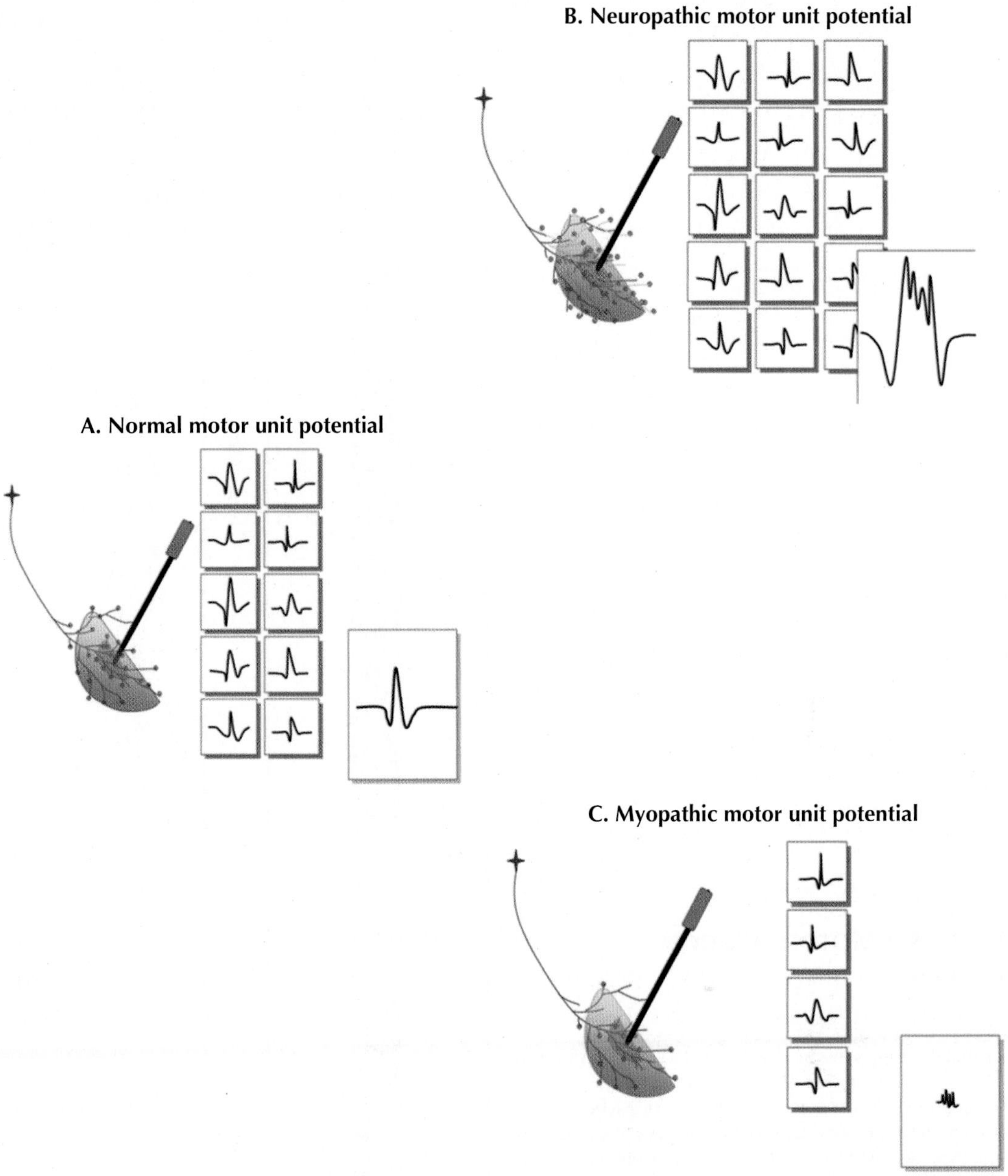

Three different motor unit potentials recorded from needle EMG (normal, neurogenic, myopathic). Each image illustrates the schematic of a single motor unit: the anterior horn cell, an axon, and a group or muscle fibers (in red) innervated by the axon. The gray area is the recording area from the needle electrode. Each small box contains the representation of a single muscle fiber action potential. The larger box illustrates the summation of all of the single muscle fiber action potentials in the needle recording area. In a chronic, neurogenic process, where collateral sprouting and reinnervation has occurred, there are more muscle fibers in the needle recording area, resulting in a large, motor unit potential (MUP). In a myopathic process, with loss of muscle fibers, there are fewer fibers in the needle recording area, resulting in a smaller MUP. Both the neurogenic and myopathic processes also result in asynchronous firing of the muscle fiber action potentials, which manifests on the needle examination as increased phases of the MUPs (i.e., polyphasic MUPs).

initial consistent attempt to provide collateral reinnervation, the continued decline in the number of healthy anterior horn cells can no longer provide compensatory reinnervation, and the patient becomes progressively weaker and paralyzed.

In contrast to neuropathic disorders, myopathies are disorders characterized by a reduction in functioning muscle fibers within a motor unit with normal nerves (e.g., muscular dystrophy or inflammatory myopathy). In myopathic disorders, there are diminished numbers of healthy muscle fibers within a motor unit. Therefore fewer muscle fibers remain within in the region of the

recording needle electrode, leading to a summation of fewer muscle fiber action potentials. In addition, those small remaining MUPs need to have their anterior horn cells fire in increased numbers to generate sufficient contractile force. The resultant myopathic MUP has shorter duration and lower amplitude, and it is polyphasic secondary to asynchronous activation (Plate 10.4, *C*). To compensate, an increased firing of anterior horn cells occurs to generate required forces. This causes patients with myopathies to characteristically demonstrate rapid recruitment of many low-amplitude, short-duration, polyphasic MUPs.

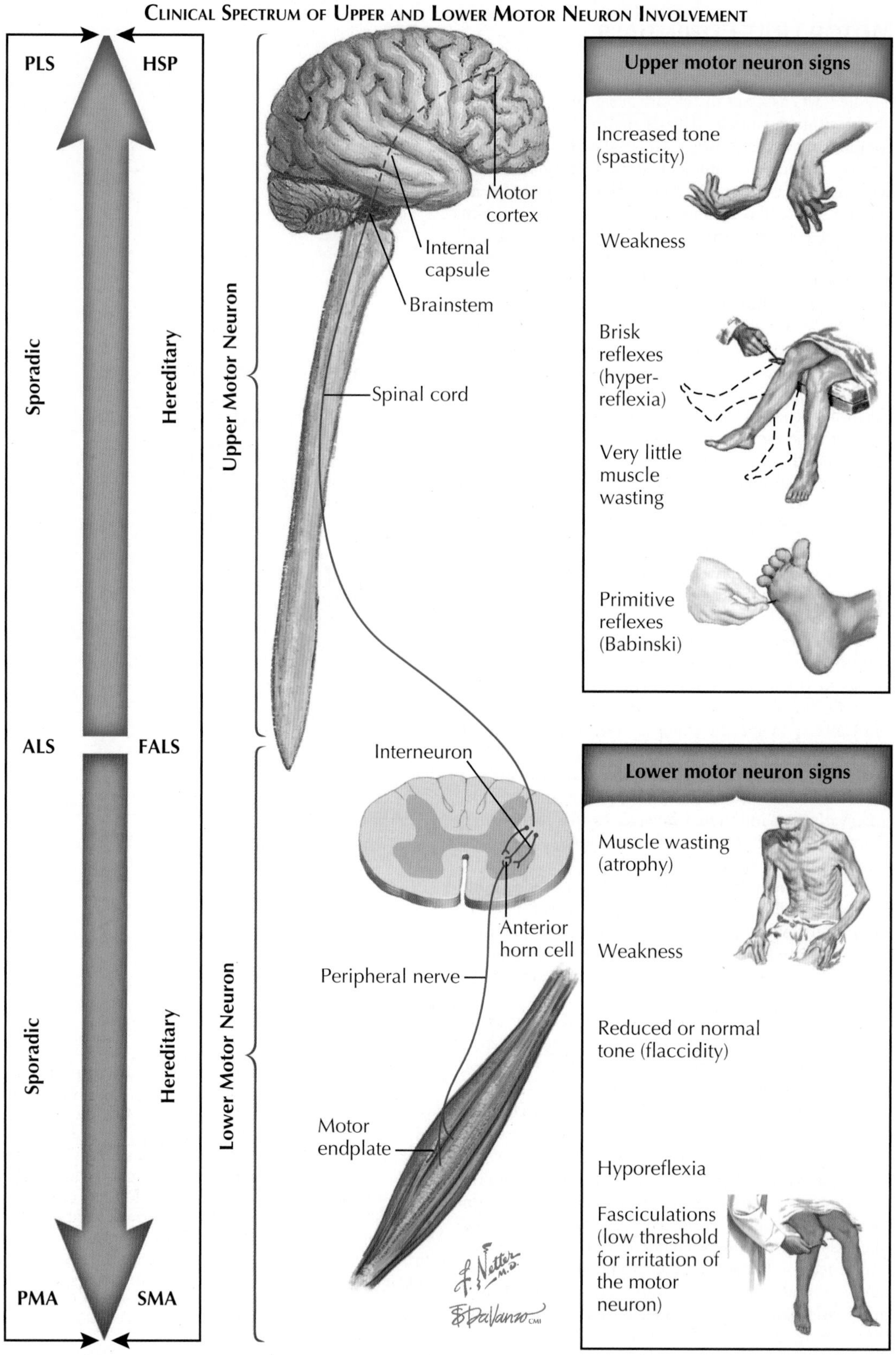

CLINICAL SPECTRUM OF UPPER AND LOWER MOTOR NEURON INVOLVEMENT

PLS   HSP

Sporadic   Hereditary

ALS   FALS

Sporadic   Hereditary

PMA   SMA

Upper Motor Neuron

Lower Motor Neuron

Motor cortex
Internal capsule
Brainstem
Spinal cord

Interneuron
Anterior horn cell
Peripheral nerve
Motor endplate

Upper motor neuron signs

Increased tone (spasticity)

Weakness

Brisk reflexes (hyper-reflexia)

Very little muscle wasting

Primitive reflexes (Babinski)

Lower motor neuron signs

Muscle wasting (atrophy)

Weakness

Reduced or normal tone (flaccidity)

Hyporeflexia

Fasciculations (low threshold for irritation of the motor neuron)

PRIMARY MOTOR NEURON DISEASE

Primary motor neuron diseases (MND) have protean clinical manifestations. The pathology involves the motor neurons of the spinal cord, cerebral cortex, brainstem (except for brainstem nuclei subserving eye movements), and the associated corticospinal and corticobulbar tracts. Classically, these diseases are grouped into several categories according to the predominant clinical manifestations at onset and whether the disorder is inherited or sporadic: (1) sporadic lower motor neuron (LMN) disorders, such as progressive muscular atrophy (PMA); (2) sporadic upper motor neuron (UMN) disorders, such as primary lateral sclerosis (PLS); (3) hereditary LMN disorders, such as spinal muscular atrophy (SMA) or spinal bulbar muscular atrophy (SBMA); (4) hereditary UMN processes, such as hereditary spastic paraparesis (HSP); and (5) ALS, the most common MND, which manifests with various degrees of degeneration of the UMNs in the cortex associated with corticospinal tract involvement superimposed on degeneration of the LMNs within the spinal cord. Familial ALS (FALS), defined as ALS with a clear inheritance pattern, represents 10% of cases of ALS. Of these FALS cases, two-thirds can be explained by one or more than 20 known ALS genes. The remaining 90% of cases are considered sporadic with no clear family history, of which 11% are associated with a known causative ALS gene.

The signs and symptoms characteristic of many of these diseases (e.g., PMA, PLS) eventually evolve in most patients to demonstrate mixed UMN and LMN involvement and thus a diagnosis of ALS. Notable exceptions include HSP, SMA, and SBMA.

ALS characteristically involves a mixture of LMN findings (weakness, atrophy, fasciculations) and UMN features (spasticity, brisk reflexes, upgoing toes). Estimates suggest that one to two new cases per year are diagnosed per 100,000 people in the United States and Europe, with a prevalence of 3 to 5 per 100,000. The cumulative risk of ALS is 1 in 400 in these areas, with an increased incidence and prevalence of ALS with each decade of life. The affected male to female ratio in sporadic ALS approaches 2:1, whereas the ratio in FALS is closer to 1:1. Onset is insidious and usually in middle to late life, although symptoms can rarely begin in the second or third decade.

CLINICAL MANIFESTATIONS OF AMYOTROPHIC LATERAL SCLEROSIS

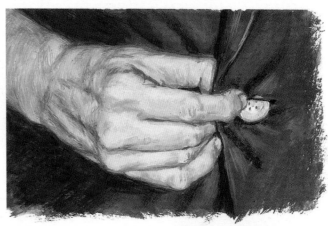

Fine movements of hand are impaired; prominent metacarpal bones indicate atrophy of interossei muscles.

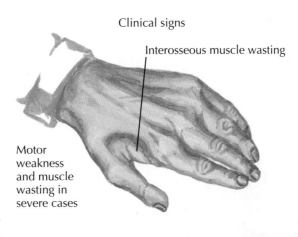

Clinical signs

Interosseous muscle wasting

Motor weakness and muscle wasting in severe cases

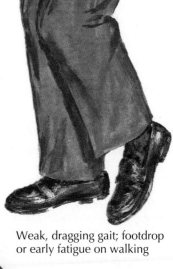

Weak, dragging gait; footdrop or early fatigue on walking

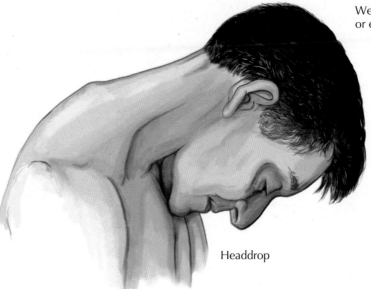

Headdrop

AMYOTROPHIC LATERAL SCLEROSIS

The most common presentation of ALS is painless progressive weakness of a limb in the absence of sensory disturbance. In approximately 25% of patients, symptoms may be initially confined to the motor nuclei of the brainstem, except for the nuclei that supply the extraocular muscles. Progressive difficulty with articulation, inability to move the tongue, and failure of the palate to rise on phonation results in stiff, breathy speech that is characteristic of ALS (a mixed spastic/flaccid dysarthria). Early pharyngeal involvement makes swallowing difficult. The term *progressive bulbar palsy* has been used to describe these patients. Some patients initially develop regional variants, such as the bibrachial amyotrophic diplegia phenotype characterized by a predominantly LMN syndrome affecting both arms, often remaining confined to the arms for several years before advancing to more typical ALS. A lower extremity diplegia phenotype has also been described.

Cognitive dysfunction is present in up to 50% of patients with ALS and can range from mild impairment of word fluency to frontotemporal lobe dementia (FTD). From 10% to 15% of patients with ALS also meet diagnostic criteria for FTD. This discovery has led to the recognition of ALS as a multisystem disorder extending beyond the motor neurons.

The pathophysiologic basis underlying the progressive degeneration of motor neurons in these disorders is incompletely understood. A complex interplay of RNA and protein homeostasis, changes in cytoskeletal dynamics, and trafficking of RNA have been detected in both familial and sporadic ALS. Each of these factors can initiate a cascade of additional cellular abnormalities (e.g., mitochondrial dysfunction, endoplasmic reticulum stress) that can in turn activate nonneuronal cells (e.g., microglia, astrocytes, oligodendrocytes) to adversely affect subcellular compartments (e.g., axons, NMJ).

PMA is an MND variant that accounts for approximately 5% of adult-onset acquired MND. Patients with PMA initially report symptoms of weakness and muscle atrophy, sometimes associated with cramping. Most commonly, onset is asymmetric and in the distal musculature, beginning in either the upper or the lower extremity. Fine movements of the hands may be impaired, or a foot may become weak. Sensory symptoms and pain are absent. Patients may also note spontaneous twitching (fasciculations) of muscles at rest. Some patients with apparent PMA develop UMN symptoms over time, requiring reclassification as ALS. Even in the absence of clinical UMN signs, approximately half of the patients diagnosed with PMA have autopsy evidence of corticospinal tract involvement, again implying ALS. Whether these disorders represent distinct entities or points on a continuum is unclear.

CLINICAL MANIFESTATIONS OF AMYOTROPHIC LATERAL SCLEROSIS (CONTINUED)

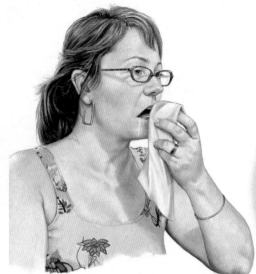

Salivary drooling due to impaired swallowing and poor facial muscle tone

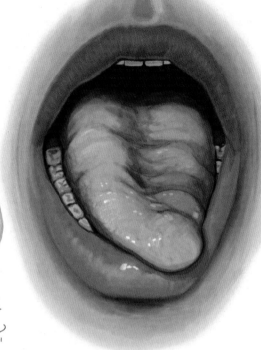

Asymmetric (left greater than right) atrophy, weakness, and fasciculations of the tongue, with deviation to the left on protrusion

Difficulty in chewing and/or swallowing

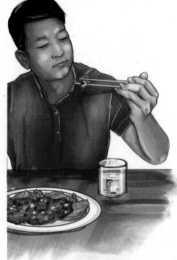

Variable speech impairment due to weakness of tongue, soft palate, and/or larynx or respiratory muscles. Patient may resort to writing (often also impaired) to communicate.

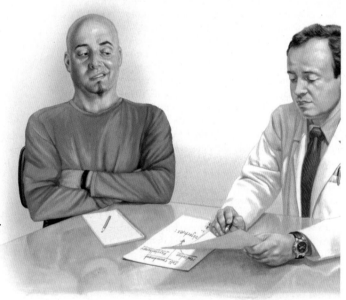

AMYOTROPHIC LATERAL SCLEROSIS (Continued)

PLS is a syndrome of progressive UMN dysfunction. It is an uncommon diagnosis and accounts for less than 5% of patients with MND. PLS is pathologically characterized by corticospinal degeneration, with sparing of the anterior horns that distinguishes it from ALS. The typical clinical presentation is characterized by leg weakness and spasticity or predominant bulbar involvement, with an upper extremity presentation less common. Symptoms usually start unilaterally and tend to spread to the contralateral side first, before involving a new region. Stiffness, clumsiness, and poor coordination are prominent symptoms. A patient with a MND who presents with idiopathic spasticity and does not develop wasting and other clinical or electrophysiologic evidence of LMN involvement within 4 years likely has PLS; before 4 years has elapsed, it is more uncertain whether such a patient will eventually evolve to a diagnosis of ALS (i.e., a diagnosis of UMN-predominant ALS). The course of PLS is slowly progressive, with average disease duration of 8 years or more, in contrast to a shorter average life span for patients with ALS.

MIMICS OF AMYOTROPHIC LATERAL SCLEROSIS

The differential diagnosis for a patient with possible ALS varies depending on the clinical characteristics of the patient. Common considerations include inclusion body myositis (IBM), cervical myelopathy plus radiculopathy, multifocal motor neuropathy (MMN), HSP, and juvenile monomelic amyotrophy (JMA). Recognition of the specific clinical features and appropriate diagnostic testing almost always allow for a focused differential diagnosis and efficient diagnosis. HSP and JMA are discussed below. Other mimics, IBM and MMN, are discussed in Sections 12 and 6, respectively.

JMA is characterized by insidious onset of unilateral or asymmetric muscular atrophy and weakness of the hand and forearm in the absence of sensory or pyramidal signs. JMA predominantly affects young men between 15 and 25 years of age. The manifestations are often unilateral, although bilateral, asymmetric involvement may occur. The clinical course is initially progressive for a few years, followed by spontaneous stabilization. Although disputed, some specialists

believe that the pathophysiology of JMA may be related to abnormal movement of the lower cervical spinal cord during neck flexion, which either directly or via microcirculatory insufficiency damages the anterior horn cells of the lower cervical spinal cord, leading to a focal motor neuronopathy manifesting as weakness and atrophy of lower cervical segment–innervated muscles. Treatment options for JMA may include patient education to avoid neck flexion, wearing a soft cervical collar,

MIMICS OF AMYOTROPHIC LATERAL SCLEROSIS

Hirayama disease	Hereditary spastic paraparesis

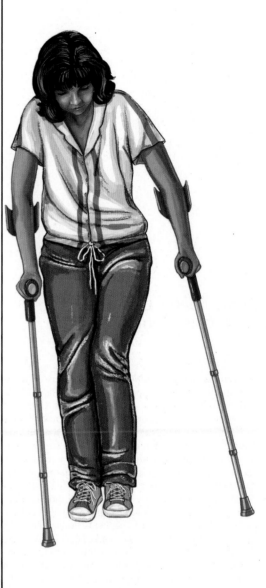

Asymmetric atrophy of
intrinsic hand muscles

Asymmetric atrophy
of forearm muscles
with sparing
of brachioradialis

AMYOTROPHIC LATERAL SCLEROSIS (Continued)

and surgical decompression. Most patients show spontaneous arrest of progression within 3 to 5 years. However, hand weakness and atrophy are permanent.

HSP, also known as familial spastic paraparesis, is a genetic disorder that may mimic PLS. HSP symptom onset can occur from infancy to late adulthood. Clinical features include relatively symmetric, progressive limb spasticity, progressive gait disturbance, and variable bladder disturbances. Clinical examination demonstrates spasticity and pathologically brisk reflexes. Lower extremity spasticity progresses very gradually over time and sometimes spreads to the arms and, rarely, the bulbar region (e.g., spastic dysarthria). Other features may include mild impairment of vibratory and joint position sense and pes cavus malformation. Less common accompaniments for some forms of complicated HSP include optic atrophy, intellectual disability, peripheral neuropathy, dementia, and deafness. It is sometimes difficult to confidently differentiate apparently sporadic HSP from PLS based on clinical characteristics alone. HSP usually does not cause early bulbar manifestations, whereas this is common in PLS. HSP is also relatively symmetric, with manifestations beginning first in the lower extremities; PLS, on the other hand, may manifest first in any limb and is usually asymmetric. HSP tends to progress more slowly than PLS. A detailed family history is necessary, and genetic testing can be helpful. The pattern of inheritance can be autosomal dominant, autosomal recessive, X-linked, or apparently sporadic. There are currently more than 70 different genetic mutations or loci identified for various families with HSP. Cerebral and spinal magnetic resonance imaging help exclude nongenetic causes of spasticity.

DIAGNOSIS

In a patient with symptoms of footdrop or an atrophied hand, the diagnosis usually considered is an isolated lesion of a peripheral nerve or nerve root. If such a lesion is the initial sign of early MND, careful testing of other muscles often reveals more diffuse motor weakness, typically in a myotomal pattern. Fasciculations and widespread evidence of atrophy on examination are useful additional diagnostic signs. Atrophy and fasciculations of the tongue may be the first sign of cranial nerve involvement. Reflexes may vary from depressed to brisk. The Babinski sign may be extensor or plantar, depending on whether LMN or UMN involvement predominates. Sensory examination must be thorough and detailed, and results should be normal if MND is present. The coexistence of both UMN (increased tone, brisk reflexes) and LMN (atrophy, fasciculations) signs in the same limb is strongly suggestive of ALS.

DIAGNOSIS OF AMYOTROPHIC LATERAL SCLEROSIS

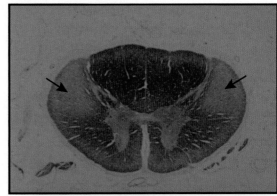

Cross-section of spinal cord. From patient with amyotrophic lateral sclerosis showing bilateral degeneration of corticospinal tracts *(arrows)*.

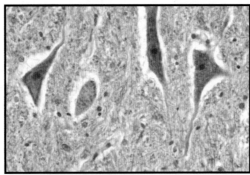

Anterior horn of spinal cord. With normal motor neurons (Luxol fast blue with H&E stain).

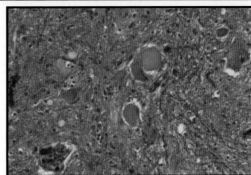

Degeneration of anterior horn cells. In amyotrophic lateral sclerosis (same stain).

AMYOTROPHIC LATERAL SCLEROSIS (Continued)

Electromyography and nerve conduction studies (collectively known as *EMG*) are the most useful diagnostic techniques for supporting the diagnosis of MND and excluding potential mimics, such as IBM and MMN. In ALS, motor conduction studies may demonstrate no more than minimal slowing of conduction velocity and a mild to moderate decrease in the compound action potential amplitude. Sensory conduction studies are normal. Signs of active (fibrillation potentials [FPs] and positive sharp waves [PSWs]) and chronic (high-amplitude, long-duration motor units) neurogenic changes should be demonstrated in at least two of four neuroanatomic segments (bulbar, cervical, thoracic, lumbosacral) on the needle EMG study. Some diagnostic criteria permit the substitution of fasciculation potentials for FPs/PSWs in the presence of chronic changes. When bulbar symptoms predominate, checking for the presence of acetylcholine receptor binding antibodies and muscle-specific kinase antibodies, and performing repetitive nerve stimulation studies or single-fiber EMG, could be done to exclude the possibility of myasthenia gravis. Occasionally, cervical spine imaging may be indicated to exclude a structural cervical myeloradiculopathy. Rarely, a muscle biopsy specimen is taken to exclude an inflammatory myopathy in the patient who has weakness of the proximal musculature, although EMG is also helpful in differentiating this disorder.

Electromyography

Normal — At rest — Voluntary contraction

Silent | Motor units closely spaced, 0.5–1.0 mV | 0.01 sec | 1 mV

Amyotrophic lateral sclerosis

Fibrillations and fasciculations | Motor units decreased in number, high amplitude, long duration, polyphasic | 0.01 sec | 8 mV

TREATMENT

To date, there are two drugs approved by the US Food and Drug Administration for the treatment of ALS. Several randomized trials have demonstrated that oral riluzole prolongs the life of patients with ALS by 2 to 3 months. Edaravone, an intravenous free radical scavenger, showed a slowing of disease progression by 33% (as measured by a particular functional rating scale) over a 6-month period in a select population of patients with ALS. Until more effective drug therapies are discovered, symptomatic control and emotional support are the primary therapeutic goals because these diseases usually progress relentlessly to death in 2 to 10 years. Fortunately, there have been significant advances in the realm of supportive therapy for ALS.

Feeding difficulties are frequently related to an inability to move food about in the mouth and to swallow effectively. Some patients may manage food prepared in a blender or use thickening agents for liquids. Instructing the patient in chin tuck and other mechanical maneuvers can facilitate safe swallowing. When oral intake becomes unsafe or ineffective at maintaining weight, a feeding gastrostomy tube can be placed.

TREATMENT OF AMYOTROPHIC LATERAL SCLEROSIS

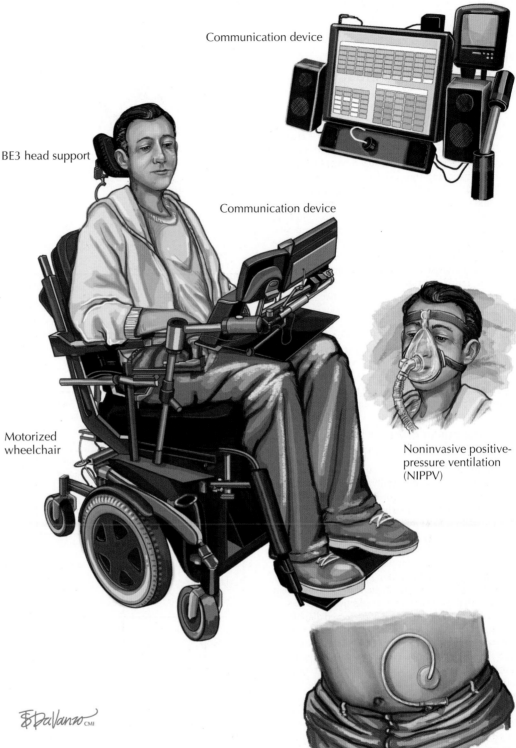

Communication device

BE3 head support

Communication device

Motorized wheelchair

Noninvasive positive-pressure ventilation (NIPPV)

Percutaneous endoscopic gastrostomy (PEG)

AMYOTROPHIC LATERAL SCLEROSIS (Continued)

Numerous adaptive devices and machines can facilitate functional independence. Mobility can be maintained with scooters and motorized wheelchairs. Transfers can be facilitated with ramps, lifts, and boards. Grab bars, commodes, and structural adjustments to the home environment can improve access. Several adaptive devices, including strategic foot bracing, arm boards, and foam grips, can enhance function. Physical therapy regimens can maintain flexibility and avoid frozen joints.

One of the many consequences of MND is the patient's loss of ability to speak understandably. Numerous augmentative devices using digital technology can maintain effective communication no matter how impaired the patient. Such devices can be controlled with slight finger movements, eye movements, or minimal head movements.

Respiratory failure is the cause of death in most patients. Early in the course of the illness, the patient should be warned against the use of respiratory depressants such as sedatives, particularly in combination with alcohol. The patient should be prophylactically immunized against influenza and pneumococcal infections. Pulmonary function testing should be regularly assessed at each clinic visit. When the patient develops symptoms of early respiratory failure (excessive daytime fatigue, orthopnea, early-morning headaches, dyspnea on exertion or at rest) or the vital capacity falls below 50% of predicted, noninvasive positive-pressure ventilation (NIPPV) should be considered. NIPPV has been shown to prolong life and improve quality of life in patients with ALS. Initially, NIPPV can be confined to nighttime use during sleep but can eventually be extended to daytime use as needed. Ultimately, some patients opt for tracheostomy and mechanical ventilation.

Pseudobulbar affect, characterized by unexpected outbursts of laughing and crying, can be managed with a combination of dextromethorphan and quinidine, tricyclics, or selective serotonin reuptake inhibitors. Troubling sialorrhea can be treated with numerous oral agents (e.g., atropine, nortriptyline, guaifenesin), scopolamine patches, or botulinum toxin injections. Portable suction devices and cough-assist machines can also assist in secretion management. Depression and anxiety can be managed pharmacologically.

Most important is the providers' honest and compassionate approach to the whole patient and the caregivers. Care is best delivered by a multidisciplinary team. The care team should never destroy the patient's hope but should provide optimal symptomatic treatment and family- and patient-centered counseling throughout the disease process.

SPINAL MUSCULAR ATROPHY AND SPINAL BULBAR MUSCULAR ATROPHY

Spinal bulbar muscular atrophy (SBMA, or Kennedy disease), is produced by a trinucleotide repeat mutation disrupting the gene for the androgen receptor. Inheritance is X-linked and thus affects males only. Onset is typically in the 40s, with a nasal LMN dysarthria, dysphagia, and proximally predominant weakness. Reflexes are depressed or absent and fasciculations common; perioral fasciculations are characteristic. Gynecomastia, diabetes, and testicular atrophy may be seen. Creatine kinase is elevated. Electrodiagnostic studies demonstrate findings consistent with MND, including reduced compound muscle action potentials with preserved latencies and velocities, and signs of active (FPs and PSWs at rest) and chronic (high-amplitude, long-duration MUPs) denervation on needle EMG. However, unlike other MNDs, the EMG in SBMA reveals an associated sensory neuronopathy manifested as a global reduction or absence of sensory nerve conduction responses. Differentiating SBMA from ALS is important for reasons of family counseling and prognosis (SBMA has a much slower progression). Gene testing is diagnostic.

SPINAL MUSCULAR ATROPHY TYPE I (WERDNIG-HOFFMANN DISEASE)

In the healthy newborn, the purposeless movements of the extremities are associated with a well-defined muscular tone despite the lack of coordinated motor function. In addition, the full-term newborn has a well-developed suck and swallow. Most infants with SMA type I demonstrate normal muscular tone, motor function, and bulbar function at birth. However, within the first few weeks to months after birth, they develop generalized hypotonia and weakness. In addition, they manifest a respiratory pattern characterized by paradoxic chest and abdomen movement that results from the selective weakness of intercostal muscles in the setting of preserved diaphragm function. Without supportive treatment, infants subsequently develop the characteristic bell-shaped deformity of the thorax. In addition, they manifest a hypotonic posture characterized by abducted hips and internal rotation of the forearms (frog-legged and jug-handle habitus). Progressive bulbar and respiratory insufficiency results in a vulnerability to both aspiration and infectious pneumonias. Extraocular movements and facial movements are preserved until late. Careful evaluation of the tongue reveals evident tongue fasciculations. In contrast to adults, fasciculations in limbs are difficult to appreciate due to excessive subcutaneous fat in infants. In milder cases, normal motor milestones, such as head control and ability to roll and sit, are not acquired as expected during the first few months. Ultimately, however, SMA I is defined clinically by the inability of all such infants to achieve independent sitting. In a subset of the most severe cases, reduced fetal movement occurs before birth, and the infant is born with generalized hypotonia, neuromuscular weakness, respiratory insufficiency, bulbar dysfunction, and proximal joint contractures.

SMA is a hereditary illness, most often of autosomal recessive inheritance, although other variant forms exist, including X-linked and dominant forms. The most

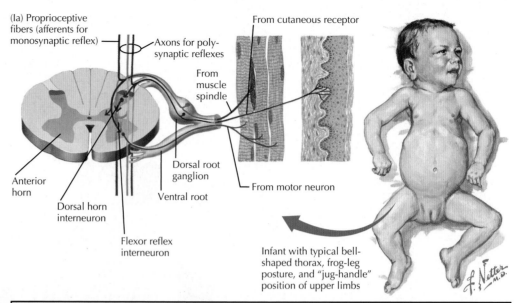

Infant with typical bell-shaped thorax, frog-leg posture, and "jug-handle" position of upper limbs

Spectrum of phenotypic manifestations in proximal spinal muscular atrophy				
SMA Type	Typical age of onset	Typical life span	Also called	Clinical characteristics Maximum milestones achieved
0	Prenatal	<6 months	SMA-arthrogryposis multiplex congenita type	Congenital hypotonia, weakness, respiratory failure, proximal joint contractures Unable to breathe unsupported
I	Birth–6 months	~32% survival probability >2 years	Werdnig-Hoffmann disease	Infantile onset of generalized hypotonia weakness, impaired bulbar function, respiratory insufficiency Unable to sit unsupported
II	6–12 months	~70% survival to adulthood	SMA, Dubowitz type	Able to sit independently Onset of limb weakness as infants or toddlers Progressive weakness, respiratory insufficiency, scoliosis, joint contractures in childhood
IIIa	After 12 months	Normal	Kugelberg-Welander disease	Onset of proximal muscle weakness in childhood Able to walk independently, although 50% with type IIIa lose independent ambulation by 12 years of age
IIIb	After 3 years			
IV	Adulthood	Normal		Onset of proximal leg weakness in adulthood, able to walk independently

common form of SMA is the proximal recessive type, which includes a broad range of subtypes ranging from the severe infantile variant to ambulatory forms with adult onset.

EMG as a primary diagnostic tool has been largely replaced by genetic testing in most cases because more than 95% of such infants have a homozygous deletion/mutation of exon 7 of the *SMN1* gene. Once significant weakness is manifest, the EMG findings are distinct in type I, demonstrating diffuse fibrillations in virtually all muscles in association with markedly reduced recruitment of small motor units in the absence of the typical large complex motor units characteristic of reinnervation in milder, more chronic forms of the disorder. Muscle biopsy shows findings typical of neurogenic atrophy. Other lesions in the motor unit can mimic Werdnig-Hoffmann disease but, as a rule, can be differentiated by

clinical and EMG findings and examination of muscle biopsy specimens if genetic and/or neurophysiologic testing is not definitive. Differential diagnosis for presentation in infancy includes SMA with respiratory distress (SMARD), which is distinguished by early respiratory failure due to diaphragm involvement, especially in association with more distal presentation of limb weakness. X-linked SMA manifests as a severe infantile SMA variant predominantly affecting males. Diseases of the NMJ, such as transient neonatal myasthenia gravis and infantile botulism, and rare recessive inherited peripheral neuropathy variants, such as congenital hypomyelinating neuropathy, should be considered in the differential diagnosis.

Highly effective medications are now available to arrest or slow the course of this otherwise fatal condition (see Plate 9.3).

NEUROMUSCULAR JUNCTION AND ITS DISORDERS

STRUCTURE OF NEUROMUSCULAR JUNCTION

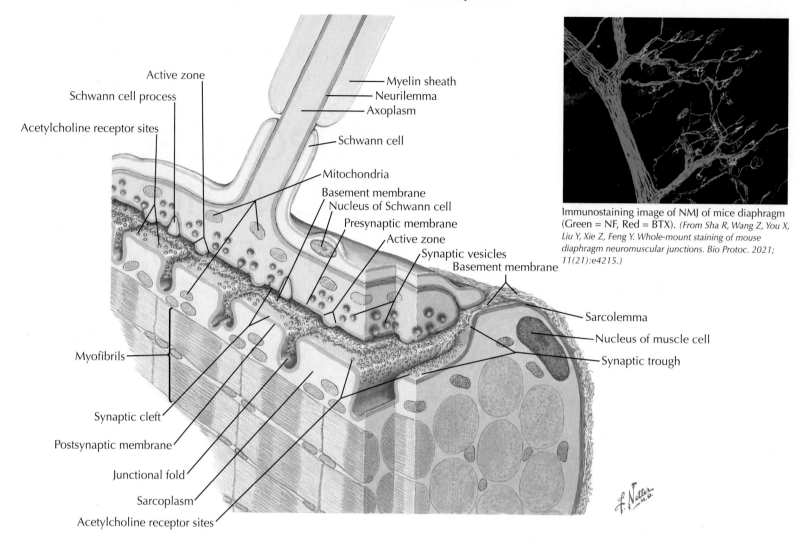

Active zone
Schwann cell process
Acetylcholine receptor sites

Myelin sheath
Neurilemma
Axoplasm

Schwann cell

Mitochondria
Basement membrane
Nucleus of Schwann cell
Presynaptic membrane
Active zone
Synaptic vesicles
Basement membrane

Myofibrils

Sarcolemma
Nucleus of muscle cell
Synaptic trough

Synaptic cleft
Postsynaptic membrane
Junctional fold
Sarcoplasm
Acetylcholine receptor sites

Immunostaining image of NMJ of mice diaphragm (Green = NF, Red = BTX). *(From Sha R, Wang Z, You X, Liu Y, Xie Z, Feng Y. Whole-mount staining of mouse diaphragm neuromuscular junctions. Bio Protoc. 2021; 11(21):e4215.)*

NEUROMUSCULAR JUNCTION

The outflow of nearly all behavior depends on the neuromuscular system, where nerves emanating from the spinal cord and brainstem make connections with skeletal muscles that allow us to move, stand, and express ourselves. The number of skeletal muscles in the human body is daunting, at somewhere between 500 and 1000. The face alone has enormous numbers of muscles that allow us to express our emotions, articulate our words, and eat our food. Our hands are the second most "muscular" parts, giving us the finesse to play musical instruments, communicate with sign language, and write. Some muscles are huge. The gluteus maximus, for example, has many thousands of muscle fibers and is essential for walking. Other muscles are miniscule, designed to produce the slightest movements of the eardrum or the larynx and have a few hundred muscle fibers or less. The set of muscle fibers innervated by a motor neuron through an axon (a motor unit) is very small in muscles that require very fine control, such as the extraocular and finger muscles, where the number of motor units can be fewer than 10, or very large (hundreds or thousands) in postural (back musculature) and girdle muscles (gluteus maximus). Despite the functional and structural diversity of muscles, however,

the communication between the nervous system and muscles is much the same throughout the body. In humans and other mammals, muscles are composed of many muscle fibers, and each muscle fiber is typically innervated by only one motor neuron, with innervation focused on a small region of the muscle fiber known as the *neuromuscular junction* (NMJ). An NMJ may occupy less than 0.1% of the muscle fiber's surface area and yet is sufficient, without fail, to cause the muscle fiber to twitch each time an electrical impulse travels from the motor neuron cell body in the central nervous system to the muscle via the peripheral nerve. Thus the NMJ is among the most reliable and powerful synapses within the body.

The structure of the NMJ explains why it is so powerful. An axon terminates in a branched structure that is laden with mitochondria, synaptic vesicles, and several special features. The main constituent of these synaptic vesicles is acetylcholine (ACh), the neurotransmitter for all skeletal muscle NMJs. When an action potential invades the axon terminal, a sequence of events is set in motion leading to the fusion of synaptic vesicles with the presynaptic membrane and release of ACh into the synaptic cleft. The released ACh molecules diffuse across the synaptic cleft, which is 10 to 20 nm wide. It takes roughly 1 microsecond for an ACh molecule to traverse the cleft and reach the synaptically specialized

membrane of the muscle fiber, known as the postsynaptic membrane.

However, at least half of the released ACh molecules never reach the postsynaptic membrane because there is a high concentration of an enzyme on the cleft that inactivates ACh, cleaving it into acetate and choline. The large amount of ACh released from hundreds of synaptic vesicles means that there are far more ACh molecules available than are normally required to cause the muscle fiber to contract when an electrical impulse arrives at the axon terminal. This "safety factor" means that in normal use it is very unlikely that the available neurotransmitter will fail to cause the muscle to contract. The muscle contraction is initiated by the binding of ACh molecules to the acetylcholine receptors (AChRs) on the postsynaptic membrane. The AChRs are packed into the postsynaptic membrane at as high a concentration as their size permits, about 10,000 receptors per square micron of membrane.

The AChR is a typical *ligand-gated ion channel*. Thus, when ACh (the ligand) binds to the AChR, the receptor becomes an ion channel that allows cations to pass through a central pore. The main cations are *sodium* (Na^+) and *potassium* (K^+). The high concentration of Na^+ outside and the inside negative resting membrane potential drive Na^+ into the cytoplasm of the muscle fiber. The *positive charges* that enter the muscle fiber depolarize the muscle's

Plate 11.2   Neuromuscular Junction and Its Disorders

PHYSIOLOGY OF NEUROMUSCULAR JUNCTION

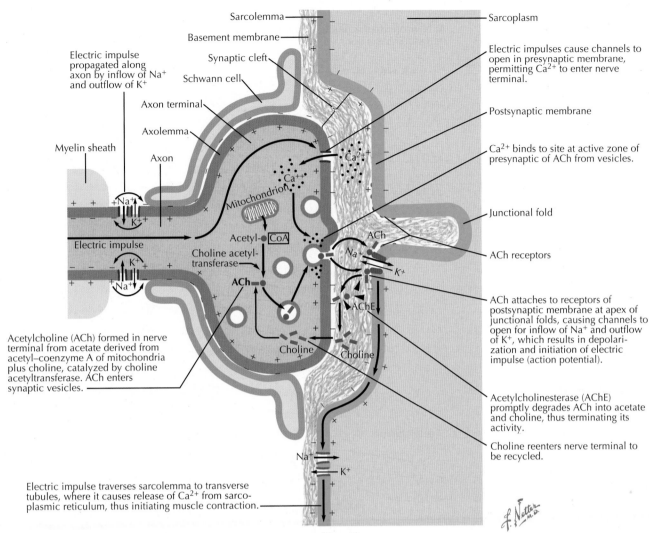

NEUROMUSCULAR JUNCTION
(Continued)

membrane potential from a negative value to a much less negative value. This depolarization initiates a muscle fiber action potential that propagates away from the NMJ in both directions to transverse tubules, where it causes a release of calcium from sarcoplasmic reticulum, rapidly causing the muscle fiber to contract.

The esterase in the synaptic cleft prevents the same ACh from rebinding multiple times to AChRs so that each single nerve impulse in the axon leads to exactly one action potential in the muscle fiber. The esterase plays a second essential role: the choline created from ACh breakdown is taken back (reuptake) by the nerve terminal to make additional ACh via an intracellular enzyme (choline acetyltransferase [ChAT]).

The NMJ is thus a highly regulated site where a nerve terminal, muscle fiber, and several supporting glial cells are juxtaposed. A wide range of pharmacologic agents, natural toxins, and electrolyte imbalances associated with disease have profound effects on the function of this synapse. For example, *NMJ function can be blocked* by agents that affect the muscle's AChRs, the nerve terminal vesicle release machinery, or the synaptic cleft. Venom from certain poisonous snakes has a component (alpha bungarotoxin) that blocks the ability of ACh to bind to the AChR and is thus paralytic. Anaerobic

Clostridia bacteria make a factor (botulinum toxin) that paralyzes by blocking the ability of synaptic vesicles to fuse with the presynaptic nerve membrane, thus preventing ACh release. Insecticides can block the function of the acetylcholinesterase (AChE), causing abnormally large amounts of ACh molecules to reach the muscle fiber. Muscles protect themselves from excessive depolarization by inactivating AChRs, which also has the effect of paralysis.

Alpha bungarotoxin has another use. Because it binds tightly to the AChR, it provides a means of visualizing each muscle fiber's postsynaptic site. This is accomplished by tagging bungarotoxin with a small organic fluorescent dye so that the alpha bungarotoxin (red in Plate 11.2) clearly delineates the postsynaptic site. A protein that gives certain jellyfish their green bioluminescent glow, known as green fluorescent protein (GFP), has been modified to allow its insertion into the genome of mammals such as mice. The transgenic mice are engineered by molecular biologists to express the GFP in neurons selectively. In this way, a transgenic mouse can express GFP in its motor nerves, whereas the AChRs are labeled with red alpha bungarotoxin. The two distinct colors in the nerve (green) and the muscle membrane (red) show the remarkably precise

alignment of the nerve's release sites and the muscle's AChRs (see inset, Plate 11.1). The fluorescent protein expression also allows visualization and identification of all the muscle fibers innervated by a single axon.

Motor units are recruited in a fixed order when muscles are used. Typically, the weakest motor units that cause the smallest muscle twitches are recruited first. If these are insufficient for the task, additional motor units are recruited so that each gives rise to progressively larger amounts of muscle tension. In this way, there is fine control of small muscle contractions and less control as the force of muscle contraction is increased. All the muscle fibers within a single motor unit have very similar contraction properties because they have the same subtype of the contraction protein myosin. The first motor units recruited comprise muscle fibers having "slow" fatigue-resistant myosin that causes slow contractions. The last motor units to be recruited activate muscle fibers that have fast contractions, thanks to fast myosin, but are highly fatigable. It is possible to see positions of all muscle fibers in each of the motor units in one muscle. Such descriptions reveal connectomes, which are complete maps of all the positions of all the motor axons and their connections within a muscle.

SOMATIC NEUROMUSCULAR TRANSMISSION

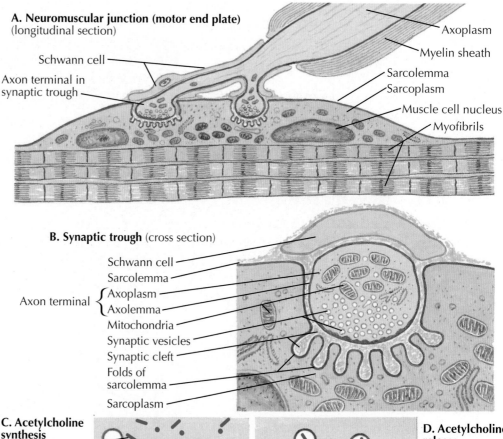

A. Neuromuscular junction (motor end plate)
(longitudinal section)

Schwann cell

Axon terminal in synaptic trough

Axoplasm

Myelin sheath

Sarcolemma

Sarcoplasm

Muscle cell nucleus

Myofibrils

B. Synaptic trough (cross section)

Schwann cell

Sarcolemma

Axon terminal { Axoplasm

Axolemma

Mitochondria

Synaptic vesicles

Synaptic cleft

Folds of sarcolemma

Sarcoplasm

SYNAPTIC TRANSMISSION

Normal somatic motor nervous system function requires rapid and efficient electrical impulse transmission. These electrical signals initially propagate along peripheral nerves to the nerve terminals where they release ACh through a complex series of electrochemical processes. The released ACh binds to the receptors at the postsynaptic NMJ, generating electrical impulses that propagate along the muscle fiber. The subsequent muscle fiber action potentials couple with the muscle cell's inherent contractile mechanism, producing muscle contraction. The physiologic steps of synaptic transmission are divided into those that occur in the (1) presynaptic nerve terminal, (2) the synaptic cleft, and (3) the postsynaptic muscle membrane.

The presynaptic nerve terminal is the site of synthesis, release, and reuptake of the neurotransmitter ACh, the chemical responsible for neuromuscular transmission. ACh is synthesized in the peripheral nerve axon terminals when acetate derived from acetyl–coenzyme A within the mitochondria and choline that has been recycled and taken up from the synaptic cleft is catalyzed by the enzyme ChAT. The newly formed ACh is then packaged into synaptic vesicles within the nerve terminal. Some ACh vesicles are located immediately adjacent to the nerve terminal membrane and are available for immediate release, whereas others are localized a short distance from the terminal nerve membrane and mobilized for rapid release.

ACh mobilization and release are triggered by calcium influx into the nerve terminal. As a propagating nerve action potential reaches the nerve terminal, the depolarization activates voltage-gated calcium channels (VGCCs) in the active zones of the terminal membrane, resulting in an influx of calcium (Ca^{2+}) ions into the axon terminal. The Ca^{2+} binds to active zones within the nerve terminal lying in juxtaposition to the muscle postsynaptic ACh receptors. This allows for synaptic vesicle membrane fusion to the nerve terminal membrane, with ACh release into the synaptic cleft.

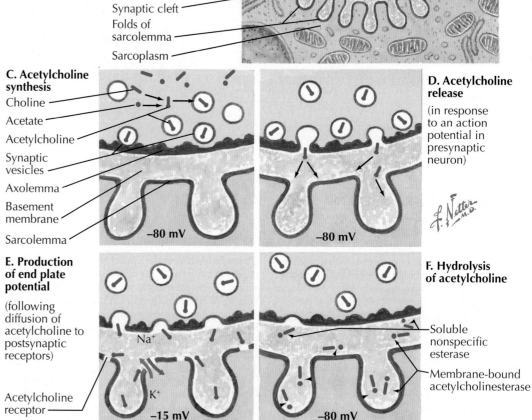

C. Acetylcholine synthesis

Choline

Acetate

Acetylcholine

Synaptic vesicles

Axolemma

Basement membrane

Sarcolemma

−80 mV

D. Acetylcholine release

(in response to an action potential in presynaptic neuron)

E. Production of end plate potential

(following diffusion of acetylcholine to postsynaptic receptors)

Acetylcholine receptor

Na^+

K^+

−15 mV

F. Hydrolysis of acetylcholine

Soluble nonspecific esterase

Membrane-bound acetylcholinesterase

−80 mV

The synaptic cleft is the site where ACh released from the nerve terminal crosses and eventually binds to postsynaptic muscle membrane ACh receptors. The time required for ACh to move across the synaptic cleft is slower than electrical impulse transmission along the axon or muscle fiber membrane. Unlike action potential transmission, movement of ACh across the cleft is unidirectional. ACh remaining within the cleft, either before or after attachment to the ACh receptors, is rapidly degraded within the synaptic cleft into acetate and choline by AChE, thus terminating its activity. Subsequently, choline is redirected into the nerve terminal and recycled to form new ACh transmitters.

Plate 11.4

Neuromuscular Junction and Its Disorders

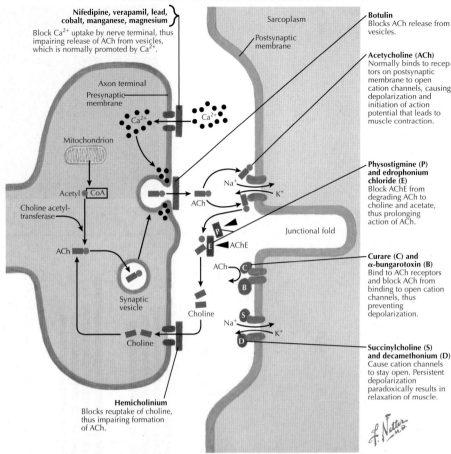

PHARMACOLOGY OF NEUROMUSCULAR TRANSMISSION

Nifedipine, verapamil, lead, cobalt, manganese, magnesium
Block Ca²⁺ uptake by nerve terminal, thus impairing release of ACh from vesicles, which is normally promoted by Ca²⁺.

Sarcoplasm

Postsynaptic membrane

Botulin
Blocks ACh release from vesicles.

Acetycholine (ACh)
Normally binds to receptors on postsynaptic membrane to open cation channels, causing depolarization and initiation of action potential that leads to muscle contraction.

Axon terminal
Presynaptic membrane

Mitochondrion

Acetyl CoA

Choline acetyl-transferase

ACh

Synaptic vesicle

Choline

Physostigmine (P) and edrophonium chloride (E)
Block AChE from degrading ACh to choline and acetate, thus prolonging action of ACh.

Junctional fold

Curare (C) and α-bungarotoxin (B)
Bind to ACh receptors and block ACh from binding to open cation channels, thus preventing depolarization.

Succinylcholine (S) and decamethonium (D)
Cause cation channels to stay open. Persistent depolarization paradoxically results in relaxation of muscle.

Hemicholinium
Blocks reuptake of choline, thus impairing formation of ACh.

SYNAPTIC TRANSMISSION
(Continued)

The postsynaptic muscle fiber membrane is composed of junctional folds within the membrane, and the receptors that bind the ACh (AChRs) are concentrated at the apex of the folds. The nicotinic AChR contains five subunits arranged radially around a transmembrane ion channel. When ACh released from the nerve terminal binds to ACh receptors, muscle fiber membrane sodium channels open, resulting in Na⁺ influx into the muscle fiber with depolarization of the muscle membrane and generation of muscle fiber action potentials.

In certain diseases, such as myasthenia gravis (MG), antibodies are primarily directed against the AChR alpha subunit. These antibodies may bind at or near the ACh binding site, directly preventing ACh binding, or may alter receptor function through other mechanisms, such as increased receptor degradation or complement-mediated receptor lysis. Other receptors (muscle-specific kinase [MuSK], agrin, and rapsyn) are required for NMJ formation and appropriate function. MuSK receptor is important for clustering of AChRs during NMJ development by allowing binding to the receptor's skeletal muscle cytoplasmic domain. Agrin binds several other proteins on the surface of muscle, including dystroglycan and laminin. Rapsyn anchors or stabilizes the AChR at synaptic sites linking the receptor to the underlying postsynaptic cytoskeleton. Dysfunction of any of these receptor stabilizing proteins may lead to impaired neuromuscular transmission.

Acquired MG develops because of antibodies primarily to the alpha-1 postsynaptic NMJ immunogenic regions (epitopes). AChR antibodies trigger immune-mediated AChR degradation. The loss of large numbers of functional AChRs decreases the number of muscle fibers available for depolarization during motor nerve terminal activation, resulting in decreased generation of muscle fiber action potentials and subsequent muscle contraction, leading to clinical weakness.

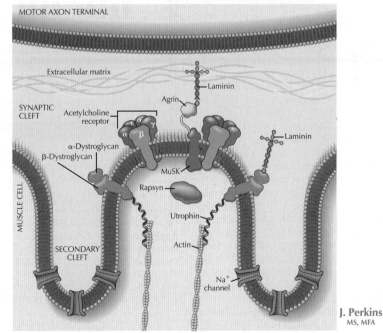

MOTOR AXON TERMINAL

Extracellular matrix

Laminin

Agrin

SYNAPTIC CLEFT

Acetylcholine receptor

α-Dystroglycan

β-Dystroglycan

Laminin

MuSK

Rapsyn

MUSCLE CELL

Utrophin

Actin

SECONDARY CLEFT

Na⁺ channel

J. Perkins
MS, MFA

Representation of the normal neuromuscular junction, adult acetylcholine receptor in the postsynaptic muscle membrane, and other important associated proteins

Some medications have their pharmacologic site of action at the NMJ, subsequently affecting neuromuscular transmission. Several block Ca²⁺ uptake by the nerve terminal, resulting in impaired mobilization of the ACh vesicles and subsequent ACh release. These include calcium channel blockers and heavy metals. Although these agents do not often produce clinically evident NMJ failure in healthy persons, exposure to these medications in patients with a NMJ disease (i.e., MG or Lambert-Eaton myasthenic syndrome [LEMS]) may cause clinical exacerbations. Additionally, toxins such as botulinum toxin impair the presynaptic mobilization and release of ACh, also resulting in muscle weakness.

REPETITIVE MOTOR NERVE STIMULATION

The integrity of neuromuscular transmission can be assessed through electrophysiologic testing using the repetitive motor nerve stimulation (RMNS) technique. When an action potential propagates along a nerve and reaches the nerve terminal, many quanta of ACh are released from the presynaptic nerve ending and bind to the AChR, generating an *endplate potential* (EPP). When the actual EPP amplitude is much larger than the threshold required for muscle fiber action potential generation (the *safety factor* of NMJ transmission), small reductions in the EPP will still result in a muscle fiber action potential generation. However, with a presynaptic or postsynaptic NMJ disorder, this safety factor is much lower and reductions in the EPP result in lack of generation of some muscle fiber action potentials and clinical weakness. RMNS provides a neurophysiologic means to assess neuromuscular transmission.

This motor nerve conduction technique involves supramaximal stimulation of a nerve trunk with surface or needle electrodes while recording the summated compound muscle action potential (CMAP) from the surface of an innervated muscle. Repeated stimuli at certain rates may stress the safety factor by rapidly mobilizing and releasing multiple stores of ACh. With stimulation at 2 to 5 Hz, fewer stores of ACh are released and less ACh is available to bind to the AChR with each stimulus, up to approximately five to six stimuli. By assessing the change in the recorded CMAP after depolarization of all the axons, and therefore all the muscle fibers within a muscle, defects of neuromuscular transmission can be identified.

PATIENT WITH MYASTHENIA GRAVIS

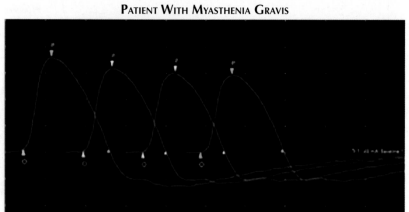

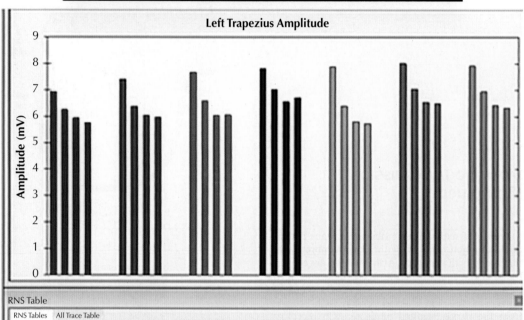

RNS Table

RNS Tables   All Trace Table

Trial #	Label	Amp 1 (mV) O-P	Amp 4 (mV) O-P	Amp % Dif	Area 1 (mV·ms)	Area 4 (mV·ms)	Area % Dif	Rep Rate	Train Length	Pause Time (min:sec)
Tr 1	Baseline 1	6.93	5.75	-17.0	44.89	35.81	-20.2	2.00	4	00:00
Tr 2	Baseline 2	7.40	5.98	-19.2	52.36	40.11	-23.4	2.00	4	00:00
Tr 3	Baseline 3	7.67	6.06	-21.0	61.88	45.38	-26.7	2.00	4	00:00
Tr 5	Immed Post 1min ex	7.81	6.72	-14.0	63.84	49.78	-22.0	2.00	4	00:00
Tr 6	Post ex :30	7.83	5.74	-27.2	69.24	47.50	-31.4	2.00	4	00:00
Tr 7	Post ex 1:00	8.02	6.50	-18.9	66.47	53.18	-20.0	2.00	4	00:00
Tr 8	Post ex 2:00	7.92	6.32	-20.2	65.04	49.52	-23.9	2.00	4	00:00

Repetitive nerve stimulation in a patient with myasthenia gravis. *Top,* a train of 4 stimuli at 2 Hz showing the decrease in the amplitude of the waveform. *Middle,* bar histograms of the compound muscle action potential amplitudes for each train of 4 stimuli at 2 Hz. The first 3 sets at rest show a maximum amplitude decrease of approximately 20%. Set 4 is immediately after 1 minute of exercise, showing slight improvement in the decrement. The final 3 sets are at 30 seconds, 1 minute, and 2 minutes after exercise and demonstrate slight worsening of decrement.

In normal NMJs, the EPP is much larger than the threshold required to initiate an action potential along the muscle fiber. As a result, the reduction in ACh release after repetitive stimulation at slow rates does not reduce the EPP below the threshold for depolarization, and action potentials are initiated in all muscle fibers innervated by the nerve. The resulting CMAP amplitude and area after each stimulus are therefore identical, and no reduction (decrement) of the responses occurs.

When patients have a *presynaptic dysfunction,* such as in LEMS or infantile botulism, the resting EPP is markedly reduced due to a reduction in release of ACh from the presynaptic nerve. The ACh release is

Plate 11.6

Neuromuscular Junction and Its Disorders

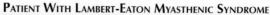

PATIENT WITH LAMBERT-EATON MYASTHENIC SYNDROME

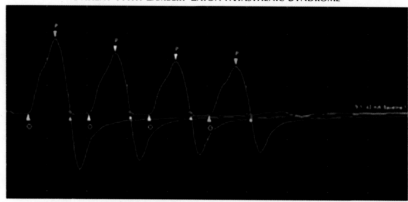

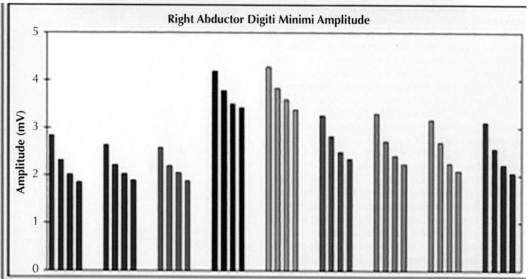

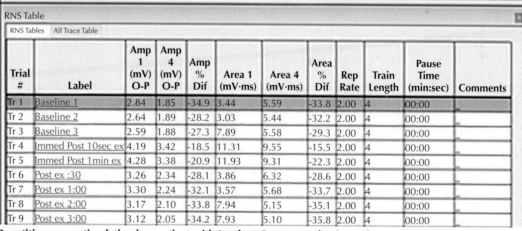

REPETITIVE MOTOR NERVE STIMULATION (Continued)

diminished at the peripheral nerve terminal at the NMJ because of either an autoimmune disorder blocking presynaptic uptake of Ca^{2+} or a specific effect of the botulinum toxin having a similar effect. This EPP is often lower than the threshold for depolarization of the muscle fiber, and therefore a single stimulus will not produce a muscle fiber action potential in many fibers. With standard motor nerve conduction studies, the CMAP amplitude is often low as a result. With slow rates of stimulation during RMNS, there is an additional reduction in the release of ACh stores with each stimulus, and a decrement in the CMAP amplitude and area (similar to that occurring in a postsynaptic NMJ disorder) is seen. However, after brief isometric exercise for 10 seconds or with stimulation at rates of 20 to 50 Hz, the influx of Ca^{2+} and mobilization and release of additional ACh stores result in a significant increase (increment or facilitation) of the CMAP amplitude (Plate 11.6). This facilitation is a characteristic and diagnostic finding in LEMS.

In patients with a much more common *postsynaptic dysfunction,* such as MG, there is an autoimmune disorder leading to accelerated breakdown of the ACh receptors at the postsynaptic (muscle) side of the NMJ as well as a blockade of the ACh at the postsynaptic endplate. This affects the ability of ACh to produce a normal EPP. Therefore the resting EPP may be lower than normal as the safety factor for neuromuscular transmission is reduced. With repeated stimulation during RMNS, there is a further reduction of both the recorded CMAP amplitude and area with each stimulus for the first five to six stimuli (see Plate 11.5). This decrement results from a loss of summated muscle fiber action potentials from those fibers in which the EPP does not reach the threshold for depolarization. Brief isometric exercise for 10 seconds leads to increased Ca^{2+} permeability in the presynaptic nerve terminal, causing mobilization and a release of additional stores of ACh. As a result, the degree of decrement immediately after brief exercise is less than at rest. However, with repeat testing between 1 to 4 minutes later, there is progressive NMJ fatigue, and the degree of deficit defined with RMNS increases up to a maximum at this time and then begins to improve with sequential testing.

Right Abductor Digiti Minimi Amplitude

RNS Table

RNS Tables   All Trace Table

Trial #	Label	Amp 1 (mV) O-P	Amp 4 (mV) O-P	Amp % Dif	Area 1 (mV·ms)	Area 4 (mV·ms)	Area % Dif	Rep Rate	Train Length	Pause Time (min:sec)	Comments
Tr 1	Baseline 1	2.84	1.85	-34.9	3.44	5.59	-33.8	2.00	4	00:00	
Tr 2	Baseline 2	2.64	1.89	-28.2	3.03	5.44	-32.2	2.00	4	00:00	
Tr 3	Baseline 3	2.59	1.88	-27.3	7.89	5.58	-29.3	2.00	4	00:00	
Tr 4	Immed Post 10sec ex	4.19	3.42	-18.5	11.31	9.55	-15.5	2.00	4	00:00	
Tr 5	Immed Post 1min ex	4.28	3.38	-20.9	11.93	9.31	-22.3	2.00	4	00:00	
Tr 6	Post ex :30	3.26	2.34	-28.1	3.86	6.32	-28.6	2.00	4	00:00	
Tr 7	Post ex 1:00	3.30	2.24	-32.1	3.57	5.68	-33.7	2.00	4	00:00	
Tr 8	Post ex 2:00	3.17	2.10	-33.8	7.94	5.15	-35.1	2.00	4	00:00	
Tr 9	Post ex 3:00	3.12	2.05	-34.2	7.93	5.10	-35.8	2.00	4	00:00	

Repetitive nerve stimulation in a patient with Lambert-Eaton myasthenic syndrome. *Top,* the amplitudes of the waveforms on the left are lower than in the patient with myasthenia gravis. *Middle,* bar histograms of the compound muscle action potential amplitudes for each train of 4 stimuli at 2 Hz. The first 3 sets at rest show a maximum amplitude decrease of approximately 27%. Sets 4 and 5 are immediately after 10 seconds and 1 minute of exercise, showing a near doubling of the amplitude (from 2.8 to 4.2 mV). The final 3 sets are at 1, 2, and 3 minutes after exercise and demonstrate slight worsening of decrement.

MYASTHENIA GRAVIS: CLINICAL MANIFESTATIONS

MYASTHENIA GRAVIS

DEMOGRAPHICS

Myasthenia gravis (MG) is a well-characterized and understood autoimmune disorder. It is the most common disorder of neuromuscular transmission resulting from an antibody-mediated immunologic attack on the AChR in the postsynaptic membrane of the NMJ. The hallmark of the disease is fluctuating weakness of ocular, bulbar, neck, limb, and respiratory muscles.

MG is seen in all age groups, with a bimodal distribution, affecting younger adults in their 20s and 30s (with a female predominance) and older adults in their 60s and 70s (slight male predominance). The annual incidence is 10 to 20 new cases per million, and the prevalence is 150 to 200 per million.

The two major clinical forms of autoimmune MG are ocular and generalized. Transitory MG may also occur in infants born to myasthenic mothers—so-called neonatal MG (a cause of floppy infant syndrome) brought about by transplacental maternal antibodies. Myasthenic syndromes may also be congenital and nonimmune in character, presenting in infancy and childhood with ocular weakness and resulting from a genetically determined defect at the NMJ (see Plate 11.11).

CLINICAL PICTURE

The cardinal feature of MG—the one that helps distinguish it from other neuromuscular disorders—is fluctuating weakness. The degree of weakness often varies throughout the day, is typically most pronounced with activity later in the day or evening, and is often mild in the morning after a period of rest (i.e., diurnal).

More than 50% of patients initially present with ocular weakness, with reports of double vision and eyelid droop. If there is bulbar and facial muscle involvement, patients have trouble chewing, speaking, swallowing, and making facial expressions. Neck extensors and flexors often become involved, causing headdrop. Limb weakness has a predilection for the shoulder and hip girdle muscles and the proximal muscles of the arms and legs so that difficulties washing and drying hair or climbing stairs are commonly reported complaints. Shortness of breath is a sign of diaphragmatic weakness and may herald respiratory insufficiency, leading to respiratory failure and ultimately the life-threatening situation of "myasthenic crisis" that requires mechanical ventilation.

On physical examination, ocular involvement is revealed by (1) eyelid ptosis, which may be unilateral or bilateral and may worsen (or be unmasked) during sustained (>60 seconds) upgaze, and (2) extraocular muscle weakness (sparing the pupil), with the patient noting binocular diplopia or blurry vision. Facial weakness is typically characterized by both an inability to bury the eyelashes with forced eye closure and the "myasthenic snarl." In the latter, there is weakness of the orbicularis oris and inability to turn the corners of the mouth upward when the patient is asked to smile. This manifestation

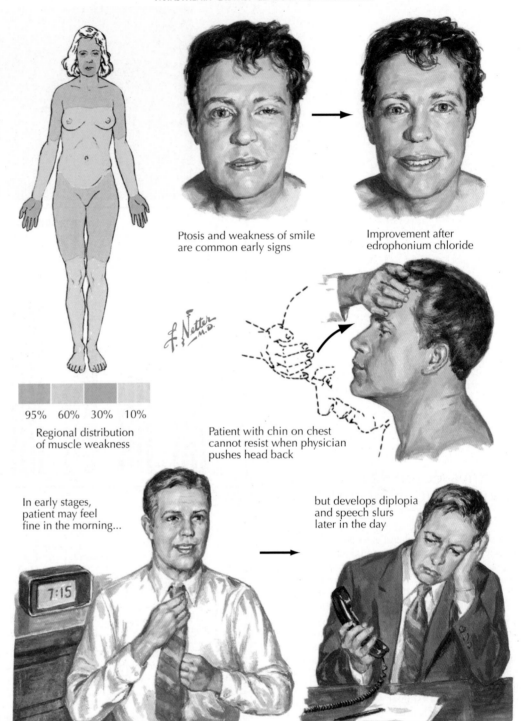

95% 60% 30% 10%

Regional distribution of muscle weakness

Ptosis and weakness of smile are common early signs

Improvement after edrophonium chloride

Patient with chin on chest cannot resist when physician pushes head back

In early stages, patient may feel fine in the morning...

but develops diplopia and speech slurs later in the day

leads to a "smile" that is transverse and appears almost angry. Patients may also develop jaw weakness (with difficulty in keeping the jaw closed); changes in speech (nasal quality from palatal weakness or low quality/hypophonic); neck extensor weakness, causing the head to be propped up using the hand under the chin; and proximally predominant arm and leg weakness.

DIFFERENTIAL DIAGNOSIS

Disorders that may be confused with ocular MG and cause ptosis and/or diplopia include thyroid ophthalmopathy, myotonic dystrophy, oculopharyngeal muscular dystrophy, chronic progressive external ophthalmoplegia

from mitochondrial disorders, and brainstem pathology. Conditions that mimic generalized MG include motor neuron disease, myopathy, and LEMS. In most instances, however, these disorders are recognized by their distinctive clinical and laboratory features, and unlike MG, they do not demonstrate true fatigability with diurnal fluctuating weakness.

DIAGNOSIS

Testing for autoantibodies specifically directed against AChR and MuSK are the MG diagnostic studies of choice; rarely, low-density lipoprotein receptor-related protein 4 (LRP4) antibodies are detected. When any of

Plate 11.8

Neuromuscular Junction and Its Disorders

MYASTHENIA GRAVIS: ETIOLOGIC AND PATHOPHYSIOLOGIC CONCEPTS

MYASTHENIA GRAVIS
(Continued)

these autoantibodies is positive, the other studies subsequently mentioned are not usually required. The one drawback to these studies is that they are not immediately available in the acutely ill patient. AChR antibodies (AChRAbs) are found in 85% of patients with generalized MG and 50% of patients with purely ocular involvement. These complement-fixing antibodies originate in hyperplasic germinal centers of the thymus gland and bind to AChR. The binding of antibody to receptor—each divalent immunoglobulin G (IgG) antibody cross-linking two receptor molecules—triggers a cascade of events resulting in loss of skeletal muscle postsynaptic AChR. The membrane attack complex of the complement cascade leads to loss and simplification (marked reduction of surface area) of the postsynaptic membrane.

Approximately 40% of patients with negative AChR antibodies (or 5% of patients with MG overall) harbor antibodies directed against the protein MuSK; 1% of patients with MG will be seropositive for LRP4 antibodies. MuSK plays a role in the clustering of AChRs during NMJ development. MuSK and LRP4 antibodies have a deleterious effect on neuromuscular transmission and are responsible for myasthenic weakness. Clinical differences are noted in the MuSK subgroup of patients; in particular, these individuals may have tongue atrophy mimicking a lower motor neuron cranial neuropathy as seen with motor neuron disease.

A presumptive diagnosis of MG in the past could be supported during outpatient assessment by a test dose of edrophonium chloride, but the drug is not currently available in the United States. A less specific bedside test involves placing an ice bag over a ptotic eyelid for 1 to 2 minutes (cold pack test) and observing for improvement in ptosis.

Traditionally, electrodiagnostic studies have been used to provide support for the diagnosis. In the era of AChRAb testing, these studies are most useful in the setting of new-onset myasthenic crisis while awaiting test results, or when antibody tests are negative or equivocal. RMNS and single-fiber electromyography (SFEMG) are designed to provide evidence for a postsynaptic defect in neuromuscular transmission and are sensitive (75% and 95%, respectively) in generalized MG. RMNS is performed by stimulating a motor nerve 6 to 10 times at low rates (2–3 Hz) and recording the amplitude of the response from the muscle that the nerve supplies. In the normal NMJ, RMNS elicits responses with identical amplitudes from stimulus to stimulus. In MG, however, a decrement (>10%) in the amplitude may be seen from the first to the subsequent stimuli, especially if the muscle is weak. SFEMG is technically challenging, but highly sensitive, and uses a needle electrode to measure the variability in time of one action potential to reach threshold relative to another action potential from different muscle fibers innervated by the same axon. This variability, or "jitter," is increased when transmission at the NMJ is compromised.

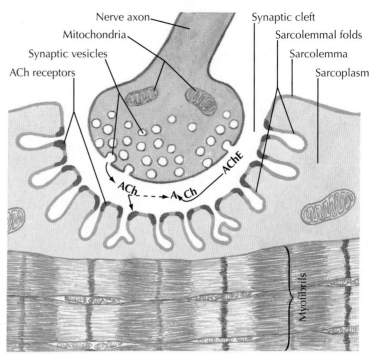

Normal neuromuscular junction. Synaptic vesicles containing acetylcholine (ACh) form in nerve terminal. In response to nerve impulse, vesicles discharge ACh into synaptic cleft. ACh binds to receptor sites on muscle sarcolemma to initiate muscle contraction. Acetylcholinesterase (AChE) hydrolyzes ACh, thus limiting effect and duration of its action.

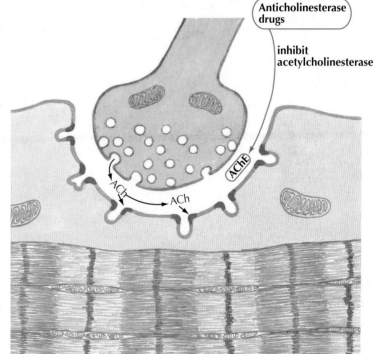

Myasthenia gravis. Marked reduction in number and length of subneural sarcolemmal folds indicates that underlying defect lies in neuromuscular junction. Anticholinesterase drugs increase effectiveness and duration of ACh action by slowing its destruction by AChE.

Patients with MG have an increased incidence of thymoma; although usually benign, a small percentage of these tumors are malignant. Therefore evaluation for the presence of thymoma should be done in all patients with MG by imaging the mediastinum with computed tomography (CT) or magnetic resonance imaging.

Treatment of MG consists of symptomatic control, immunosuppressive and/or immunomodulating therapy, and thymectomy in appropriate patients. For patients with mild symptoms, pyridostigmine may provide an adequate response. For patients with bulbar or limb involvement, corticosteroids and other immunosuppressive agents are necessary. Complement inhibitors have been demonstrated to effectively control symptoms in patients with MG refractory to other treatments.

Patients with rapidly progressive and severe symptoms such as dysphagia and respiratory insufficiency require critical care. Treatments such as intravenous immunoglobulin globulin (IVIG) and plasmapheresis provide the fastest initial response, often within 1 to 2 weeks.

Thymectomy is required in the presence of thymoma. In those without thymoma who are younger than 65 years, thymectomy has been shown to increase the probability of remission.

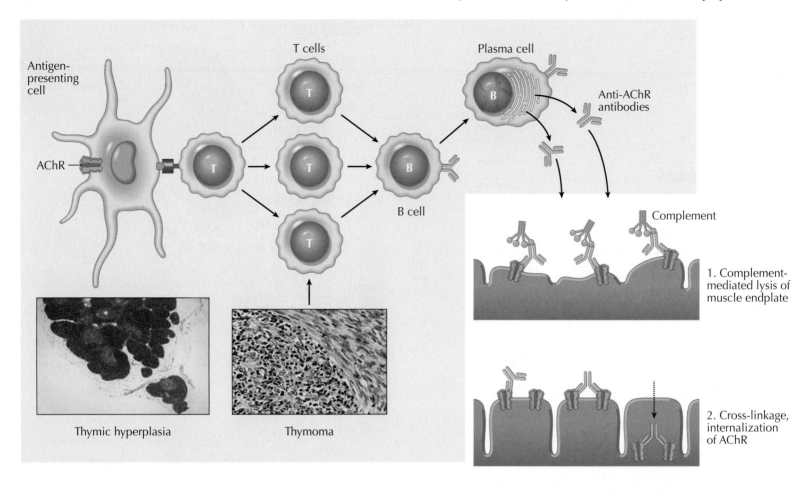

Thymic hyperplasia   Thymoma

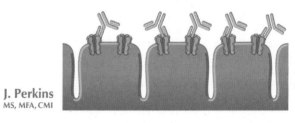

1. Complement-mediated lysis of muscle endplate

2. Cross-linkage, internalization of AChR

3. Blockage of AChR by antibodies

J. Perkins
MS, MFA, CMI

IMMUNOPATHOLOGY OF MYASTHENIA GRAVIS

MG is a chronic autoimmune disorder of the postsynaptic NMJ. Approximately 85% of patients with generalized MG have autoantibodies to the AChR. In those patients, anti-AChR antibodies, usually of the IgG1 or IgG3 isotype, bind to the extracellular domain of the AChR molecule, activating complement and causing destruction of the muscle endplate. Complement-mediated lysis of the muscle endplate causes morphologic damage to the endplate, resulting in simplification of what was previously a highly folded muscle membrane. The morphologic changes to the endplate result in a reduction in the number and function of AChR channels, impairing the EPP amplitudes generated during neuromuscular transmission. This reduces the probability that the EPP generated will be sufficient to activate an all-or-nothing muscle fiber action potential. The morphologic changes at the endplate also result in a reduction of the function of the

voltage-gated sodium channels, which results in a hyperpolarization of the muscle fiber action potential. In addition to the anti-AChR antibodies causing simplification of the muscle endplate, cross-linkage of AChRs by divalent antibodies causes internalization and degradation of AChRs. Furthermore, direct blockage of the AChRs by antibodies directed at the AChR binding sites likely contributes to functional loss of AChR, at least in some patients.

The autoimmune events of MG are also influenced by T cells, with CD4 T cells facilitating B cells in the production of pathogenic antibodies. Approximately 7% of patients with generalized MG have autoantibodies to MuSK and not to AChR. Anti-MuSK antibodies are mainly the IgG4 isotype and do not activate complement. Although less is currently known about the specific role of anti–MuSK antibodies, such antibodies appear to impair the maintenance of clustering of AChR at the muscle endplate.

The thymus gland plays a central role in the development of AChR-antibody MG, particularly for

early-onset cases of MG (e.g., patients younger than 50 years). Hyperplastic thymus glands of patients with MG contain T cells, B cells, plasma cells, and muscle-like ("myoid") cells that express AChR. It is generally believed that the autoimmune response begins in the thymus and is subsequently exported to the periphery, where damage to the postsynaptic muscle endplate occurs, as described previously. In early-onset MG, most patients have hyperplastic thymus glands (i.e., lymphofollicular thymic hyperplasia). In late-onset MG, patients often do not have thymic abnormalities, and the role of the thymus in late-onset MG is less clear. Approximately 10% to 15% of patients with generalized MG are found to have a thymoma that produces abundant autoreactive T cells. These autoreactive T cells are exported to the periphery and facilitate pathogenic B cells and their autoantibodies. Patients with MuSK-antibody MG tend to lack thymus pathology, and the role of the thymus in MuSK-antibody MG, if any, is unknown.

Plate 11.10

Neuromuscular Junction and Its Disorders

Presynaptic Neuromuscular Junction Transmission Disorders: Lambert-Eaton Myasthenic Syndrome and Infantile Botulism

Presynaptic neuromuscular transmission disorders (PNMTDs) are uncommon. LEMS is the most frequent adult PNMTD. It is the pathoanatomic mirror image of postsynaptic MG. Infantile botulism is the pediatric acquired PNMTD.

LEMS is caused by autoantibodies against VGCCs located on the presynaptic nerve terminal. Dysfunction of VGCCs leads to reduced Ca^{2+} influx into the nerve terminal, which ultimately leads to reduced release of ACh into synapse or the NMJ. LEMS can be paraneoplastic or nonparaneoplastic (nontumor LEMS). Approximately 50% of patients with LEMS have small cell lung cancer (SCLC), often not clinically evident at the inception of neuromuscular symptoms. Presumably, the immune response leading to LEMS begins early in tumor evolution. SCLC is more likely in patients with weight loss of 5% or greater, bulbar involvement, or erectile dysfunction; in patients older than 50 years; and in patients who actively smoke. Primary autoimmune, nonparaneoplastic LEMS occurs in younger adults, is very rare in children, and tends to progress faster.

The initial LEMS clinical manifestations often begin months to a few years before SCLC is recognized. Sometimes, however, the cancer precedes LEMS. Classic symptoms include fatigue, proximal muscle weakness, dry mouth sometimes presenting as increased thirst, and, in males, erectile dysfunction. The motor components relate to reduction of the nicotinic AChR function at the NMJ, and muscarinic symptoms result from similar effects on the ACh-dependent autonomic nervous system receptors. The fluctuating symptoms and absence of neurologic deficits on exam early in the disorder at times are misinterpreted as psychogenic. Occasionally, patients observe symptom improvement after brief exercise, as exemplified by experiencing increased strength near the top of stairs. Less frequently, symptoms of LEMS can mimic MG, including mild diplopia, ptosis, difficulty chewing, dysphagia, and dysarthria.

Neurologic examination demonstrates proximal weakness, sometimes initially noted by the examining physician when the patient arises from a chair. On repetitive contraction of a weak muscle there may be transient strengthening followed by return of baseline weakness. Similarly, muscle stretch reflexes (MSRs) are usually diminished or absent, but on brief forceful exercise of the associated muscle the reflex may return transiently. This finding is the clinical correlate of the postexercise facilitation seen in PNMTD during nerve conduction studies for LEMS. Some patients with LEMS develop gait ataxia out of proportion to the degree of weakness. This may be related to LEMS-related hip girdle weakness, but it may be the feature of a superimposed cerebellar disorder from a separate but concurrent paraneoplastic disorder.

Electrodiagnosis provides a means to confirm the presence of a PNMTD. Motor nerve conduction studies demonstrate low-amplitude CMAPs with postexercise facilitation of the amplitude after voluntary

X-ray film showing large tumor in hilum of lung

Acetylcholine (ACh) release at neuromuscular junction decreased; sparse, disorganized active zones for ACh release

Inhibition

Synaptic cleft

Muscle

Nerve axon

Synaptic vesicles

ACh

Difficulty in climbing stairs or arising from chair often early symptoms due to weakness of pelvic girdle muscles

Dryness of mouth due to decreased saliva secretion

Areflexia

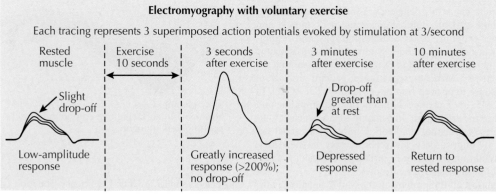

Electromyography with voluntary exercise

Each tracing represents 3 superimposed action potentials evoked by stimulation at 3/second

Rested muscle	Exercise 10 seconds	3 seconds after exercise	3 minutes after exercise	10 minutes after exercise
Slight drop-off			Drop-off greater than at rest	
Low-amplitude response		Greatly increased response (>200%); no drop-off	Depressed response	Return to rested response

exercise for 10 to 30 seconds. With LEMS, the CMAP at least doubles in amplitude immediately postexercise. CMAP amplitude then decreases back to baseline. There is also a significant decrement on RMNS, similar to MG.

Antibodies against VGCC are detected in 90% of patients with either paraneoplastic or primary autoimmune LEMS. In most patients, antibodies are directed against the P/Q subtype of VGCC. Rarely antibodies are detected against N subtype, the clinical significance of which is not clear. Because SCLC is found in 50% of patients with LEMS, chest CT is required to search for

an occult tumor. If negative, positron emission tomography may increase the sensitivity of tumor detection. If negative, repeat studies over time are appropriate, especially with a personal history of tobacco use.

In the presence of malignancy, aggressive treatment of the tumor can result in muscle strength improvement. 3,4-Diaminopyridine may provide symptomatic improvement similar to the way pyridostigmine improves symptoms in MG. For moderate or greater weakness, immunomodulating agents, such as prednisone, azathioprine, and IVIG, are useful to control the disorder.

CONGENITAL MYASTHENIC SYNDROMES

Congenital myasthenic syndromes (CMSs) are rare hereditary disorders of the NMJ. These conditions are usually present at birth, sometimes in early childhood and rarely in adulthood, with varying degrees of fatigable and fluctuating weakness involving ocular, bulbar, and limb and trunk muscles. RMNS and SFEMG are consistent with an NMJ transmission defect. Antibodies are not present because they are not immune mediated. Inheritance is autosomal recessive except the dominantly inherited slow-channel CMS (SCCMS) and some rare subtypes.

Although clinical profile alone does not usually distinguish between different forms of CMS, genetic studies allow for precise diagnosis in many but not all cases. Mutations underlying CMS are in genes coding for proteins localized to the presynaptic, basal lamina–associated synaptic, or postsynaptic (most frequently) region of the NMJ. The most common of these is primary AChR deficiency, followed by deficiencies of DOK-7, rapsyn, and synaptic AChE in varying order of frequency.

Primary AChR deficiency, mostly due to mutations in the epsilon subunit, is usually benign, with prominent bilateral ptosis, ophthalmoparesis, and little or no diplopia. Onset is usually at birth or infancy, with poor cry/suck and fluctuating ptosis. Bulbar symptoms regress with time, but fatigue and ptosis persist. There is partial response to AChE inhibitors (AChEi) and 3,4-diaminopyridine (3,4-DAP). Fast-channel CMS, a rare kinetic defect of AChR, is similar regarding phenotype and treatment, but unlike AChR deficiency, acute respiratory crises occur frequently in childhood.

Two CMS with phenotypic similarities are postsynaptic SSCMS (another kinetic abnormality of AChR) and synaptic basal lamina AChE deficiency due to mutations in its collagenic tail gene (*COLQ*). Onset is in childhood or adulthood for SCCMS and at birth or infancy for AChE deficiency. Similar clinical findings include variable ophthalmoparesis, neck muscle and upper extremity distal weakness/atrophy, and respiratory insufficiency. In both syndromes, the postsynaptic membrane is exposed to excessive ACh, explaining the repetitive CMAPs present in most patients and lack of response to or even respiratory failure from AChEi. In SSCMS, open channel blockers such as quinidine and fluoxetine are helpful. In synaptic AChE deficiency, albuterol/salbutamol markedly improves functional capacity, and surgery for scoliosis may be necessary. Careful monitoring for respiratory insufficiency is paramount in these two syndromes.

Almost all the proteins in the MuSK signaling pathway have been associated with CMSs. Among them, postsynaptic rapsyn and DOK-7 deficiencies are major causes of CMSs. Rapsyn deficiency is characterized by mild arthrogryposis, strabismus, and frequent respiratory crises. Symptoms usually start at birth and rarely in adulthood. Patients improve with age and respond well to AChEi and 3,4-DAP. *DOK7* mutations are responsible for some cases of limb girdle CMS. Proximal weakness, generally accompanied by ptosis and facial weakness, usually begins in early childhood. Severity of weakness may fluctuate over weeks/months. AChEi are harmful, but response to albuterol/salbutamol is generally favorable.

Glycosylation defects represent another subset of CMS with a limb girdle pattern of weakness and normal eye

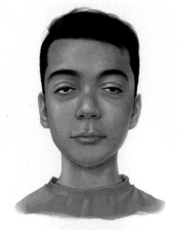

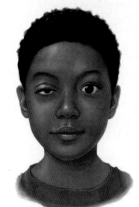

Paul Kim

Marked bilateral ptosis and ophthalmoparesis in a patient with CMS (*top*) vs. unilateral ptosis in a patient with myasthenia gravis (*bottom*)

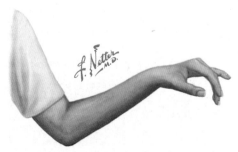

Slow-channel CMS with distal weakness and atrophy (*left*) and repetitive compound muscle action potential (*right*)

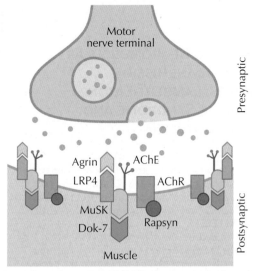

Schematic representation of the neuromuscular junction. Muscle-specific tyrosine kinase (MuSK), activated neurally by the presynaptic protein agrin through low-density lipoprotein (LRP4) and by the postsynaptic downstream of tyrosine kinase 7 protein (DOK-7), associates with rapsyn, leading to the clustering of acetylcholine receptors (AChR) and the formation of the neuromuscular junction.

Main congenital myasthenic syndromes
Presynaptic
• ChAT deficiency
Synaptic
• Endplate AChE deficiency (COLQ deficiency)
Postsynaptic
• AChR deficiency
• AChR kinetic defects
– Slow-channel and fast-channel CMS
• DOK-7 deficiency
• Rapsyn deficiency
Glycosylation defects
• GFPT1 deficiency

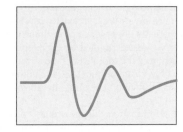

movements similar to DOK-7 deficiency. The most common mutations are in the glutamine-fructose-6-phosphate transaminase 1 gene (*GFPT1*). They respond well to AChEi.

A rare presynaptic CMS, ChAT deficiency, causes episodic apnea, presenting with sudden respiratory insufficiency in infancy or childhood, particularly during infections. Some patients have mild myasthenic symptoms in the interim, whereas others become severely disabled. Prophylactic AChEi are necessary. The risk of sudden respiratory insufficiency requires close observation.

The diagnosis of CMS can be challenging because the clinical and laboratory features overlap with those of congenital myopathies including high-arched palate, joint contractures, kyphoscoliosis, creatine kinase elevation, myopathic electromyography, and myopathic histopathologic changes. CMS should be considered in

prepubertal children diagnosed with seronegative MG, which almost never starts in infancy. Therefore a high index of clinical suspicion is a key step in the diagnosis of CMS.

Once the clinical diagnosis is established, molecular genetic studies help guide therapeutic options, which depend on the specific subtype. Although AChEi are beneficial in most CMSs, it is important to be aware that they can have a detrimental effect in some of them. Addition of ephedrine or albuterol/salbutamol is beneficial in almost all forms of CMS, with the effect increasing over months. Many patients have a good prognosis with appropriate therapy and fare well through adolescence and adulthood.

The spectrum of CMS continues to expand with newly defined rare syndromes.

Plate 11.12

Neuromuscular Junction and Its Disorders

Foodborne Neurotoxins

Diagnosis of a foodborne neurotoxicity requires consideration whenever patients suddenly present with nausea, vomiting, abdominal pain, diarrhea, and fever with concomitant headache, paresthesias, and muscle weakness. Careful history is essential to a foodborne disease diagnosis, that is, which foods and what time interval occurred between ingestion and symptom onset, and whether symptoms and signs are specific. Plate 11.12 highlights three foodborne neurotoxins (botulinum, ciguatera, and saxitoxin) and one infectious disease (trichinosis) that cause distinctive neuromuscular disorders.

Botulism is a rare, life-threatening neuroparalytic syndrome caused by an anaerobic organism, *Clostridium botulinum*, that produces an extremely potent neurotoxin. *C. botulinum* spores are heat resistant; when they germinate, these spores become toxin-producing bacilli. The spores are extremely hardy; in contrast, their toxins are denatured at greater than 80°C. The heat-resistant properties of *C. botulinum* permit home-processed foods to provide a culture medium for spore growth and subsequent neurotoxin production. There are eight distinct *C. botulinum* toxin types (A, B, C1, C2, D, E, F, and G); only types A, B, and E may lead to clinical botulism. There are five acquired forms of botulism: foodborne, infantile, wound, adult enteric infectious, and inhalational. In the United States infantile botulism is the most common form (72% of cases); the foodborne form accounts for 25% of cases. Wound and adult infectious botulism are very uncommon (3% of cases) and can be seen in the setting of IV drug abuse (particularly black tar heroin).

Symptom onset in foodborne botulism begins 12 to 36 hours after toxin ingestion and is characterized by nausea, vomiting, abdominal pain, diarrhea, and dry mouth. Neurologic manifestations develop rapidly, with pronounced cranial nerve paresis and extremity weakness. Pupils are sluggish or fixed. Ptosis, diplopia, dysphagia, dysarthria, and facial weakness develop. A descending muscle paralysis occurs that initially affects arms, then legs, with subsequent diaphragmatic involvement that can lead to respiratory insufficiency.

Diagnosis is primarily clinical but later confirmed by demonstration of toxin in the serum by way of a mouse bioassay performed by specialized laboratories. The toxin can also be found in stool, vomitus, and contaminated food. Electrodiagnostics demonstrate a classic presynaptic NMJ disorder with low-amplitude motor responses and postactivation facilitation.

When there is a high clinical likelihood of the diagnosis, emergent antitoxin therapy is indicated. Equine serum heptavalent antitoxin, available through the Centers for Disease Control and Prevention, contains antibodies to botulism types A through G. Expert respiratory and supportive care keeps mortality very low. Most patients have excellent recoveries within 3 months.

Trichinosis is an acute parasitic infection acquired by ingesting undercooked pork infested with roundworm *Trichinella spiralis* larvae. Typically, acute systemic infectious symptoms develop, including fever, headache, and severe muscle pain and tenderness. Periorbital edema occurs early and is a good clue to diagnosis. Other manifestations include encephalitis, myocarditis,

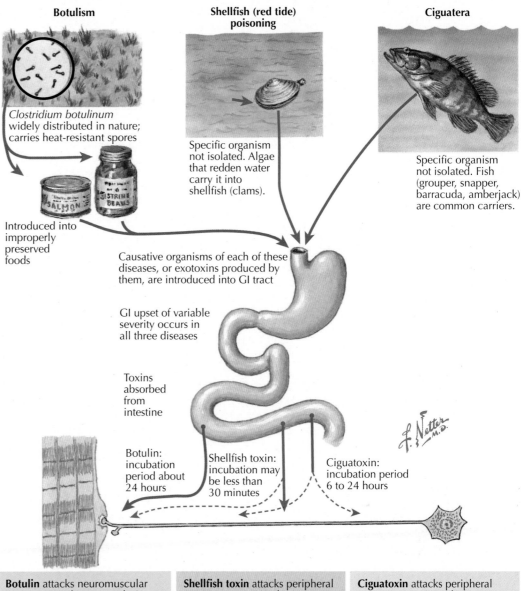

Botulism

Clostridium botulinum widely distributed in nature; carries heat-resistant spores

Introduced into improperly preserved foods

Shellfish (red tide) poisoning

Specific organism not isolated. Algae that redden water carry it into shellfish (clams).

Ciguatera

Specific organism not isolated. Fish (grouper, snapper, barracuda, amberjack) are common carriers.

Causative organisms of each of these diseases, or exotoxins produced by them, are introduced into GI tract

GI upset of variable severity occurs in all three diseases

Toxins absorbed from intestine

Botulin: incubation period about 24 hours

Shellfish toxin: incubation may be less than 30 minutes

Ciguatoxin: incubation period 6 to 24 hours

Botulin attacks neuromuscular junction. Weakness, paralysis, respiratory distress occur. Prognosis variable, may be fatal.

Shellfish toxin attacks peripheral motor neurons. Weakness, paralysis, respiratory distress, paresthesias occur. Prognosis variable, better than in botulism.

Ciguatoxin attacks peripheral nerves, exact site unknown. Weakness, paralysis, radicular pain occur. Prognosis generally good.

and subconjunctival hemorrhages. Leukocytosis with marked eosinophilia is present. Serum creatine kinase is elevated. Cerebrospinal fluid analysis demonstrates a lymphocyte pleocytosis and increased protein. Primary treatment is with mebendazole or albendazole; prednisone will blunt systemic responses to dying *Trichinella*.

Ciguatera is the most common fish food poisoning in tropical coastal regions, accounting for most fish-related foodborne disease outbreaks in the United States. There are several distinct ciguatera toxins; ciguatoxin is the best known. It is a heat-stable neurotoxin that opens voltage-dependent cell membrane sodium channels, triggering depolarization. The toxins are formed in algae-like organisms called dinoflagellates, which are subsequently ingested by large reef fish, including grouper, red snapper, amberjack, and barracuda, which in turn are ingested by humans, causing disease.

Gastrointestinal symptoms develop acutely (3–6 hours) after eating contaminated fish. Neurologic symptoms may begin within 3 to 72 hours. These include paresthesias, nerve palsies, weakness, and hot/cold temperature reversal.

Cardiovascular abnormalities occur within 2 to 5 days, including hypotension, bradycardia, and heart block.

There is no commercially available serum test for ciguatera toxin; diagnosis depends on clinical suspicion. Supportive care is the primary treatment modality when available; mortality is low. After an attack of ciguatoxin, patients are instructed to avoid all fish for at least 6 months because a second attack of ciguatera on the heels of the first may be much worse than the initial episode.

Shellfish poisoning relates to blooms of algae known as *red tides*. There are several toxins, with saxitoxin the best known. Bivalve mollusks, including clams, mussels, scallops, oysters, crabs, and snails, preferentially take up saxitoxin. In humans saxitoxin blocks Na^+ ion channels, leading to rapid evolution of neurologic symptoms, ranging from mild perioral tingling to severe paralysis with respiratory failure that leads to death within hours when ventilatory support is lacking. Treatment is supportive, and patients improve gradually over 12 to 72 hours.

MUSCLE AND ITS DISORDERS

ORGANIZATION OF SKELETAL MUSCLE

MUSCLE FIBER ANATOMY: BASIC SARCOMERE SUBDIVISIONS

The function of skeletal muscle is to move various parts of the body via muscle contraction. Muscle structure is specifically related to function. Muscles are composed of numerous multinucleated muscle cells called *muscle fibers,* or *myofibers.* Myofibers insert into tendons at their ends, at what on the microscopic level is referred to as the *myotendinous junction.* The tendons attach to bones at the origin and insertion points for each muscle. Whole muscles are encased in connective tissue, the *epimysium.* Each muscle is subdivided into smaller bundles of muscle fibers called *fascicles.* The *perimysium* is connective tissue within the muscle that separates one fascicle from another. Within a fascicle, individual muscle fibers are separated by another thin layer of connective tissue, the *endomysium.*

Each muscle fiber is surrounded by a basal lamina, or basement membrane. Lying under the basement membrane are specialized cells called *satellite cells.* Satellite cells are derived from embryonic cells called *myoblasts.* They are likely important in muscle fiber regeneration and are thought to fuse with the muscle fiber during this process. The muscle fiber is surrounded by its cell membrane, called the *sarcolemma.* It forms the membrane under which multiple muscle fiber nuclei reside. Within the boundaries of the sarcolemma, contractile *myofibrils* are contained. They are surrounded by the cytoplasm of the muscle fiber, called the *sarcoplasm.*

Just as muscle contraction depends on numerous muscle fiber contractions, muscle fiber contraction depends on the action of the numerous muscle fiber subunits, the myofibrils that run longitudinally along the length of the muscle fiber. They are collections of thin and thick filaments (myofilaments)—*actin* and *myosin,* respectively. The contractile unit of the muscle is the *sarcomere.* Each sarcomere is bound on either end by the *Z disk,* a proteinaceous structure that is oriented across the myofibril perpendicular to the filaments. When the fibril is viewed longitudinally it is apparent as the *Z band.* Z bands are seen with regular periodicity along the myofibril, defining the several sarcomeres lined up at their ends. The thin filaments, actin, anchor into the Z disk and do not extend along the length of the sarcomere but reside only at the ends.

In contrast, the thick filaments—myosin—are situated at the middle of the sarcomere at the area seen as the A band. A slight enlargement at the middle of the thick filaments, in the midline of the sarcomere, leads to the appearance of the *M band,* or *M line.* The thick filaments overlap the ends of the thin filaments that are not anchored into the Z disk. The thick filaments also do not run the length of sarcomere.

There are two additional areas seen within the sarcomere. On either side of the Z band, there are only thin filaments, and the region straddling the Z disk is the

Two-dimensional graphic of myofilaments. Three-dimensional arrangement shown below.

Cross sections show relationships of myofilaments within myofibril at levels indicated

I band. Likewise, in the middle of the sarcomere at rest there are only thick filaments, which appear as the *H* zone. Therefore traveling from the Z disks to the mid-sarcomere, one sees the Z band, the I band, the A band, the H zone, and the M band.

When seen in cross section, the thick filaments are regularly dispersed throughout the myofibril. Hexagonally arranged around them are the thin filaments. Each thin filament is equally near to three thick filaments. The thick filaments have outwardly oriented

heads that are directed toward the thin filaments and that run along the length of the thick filaments with the exception of the midline. At rest, the heads of the thick filaments are tilted slightly toward their nearest Z disk. During contraction, these thick filaments bind neighboring thin filaments, pulling these toward the sarcomeric midline, developing contractile force. When a sarcomere contracts, the Z disks are drawn toward each other, shortening the sarcomere. When all the sarcomeres in a muscle shorten, the muscle contracts.

Plate 12.2

Muscle and Its Disorders

Actin Troponin Tropomyosin Z band

Myosin head group Thin filament ADP ~ P$_i$

Thick filament (myosin)

At rest, ATP binds to myosin head groups and is partially hydrolyzed to produce a high-affinity binding site for actin on the myosin head group. However, the head group cannot bind because of blocking of the actin binding sites by tropomyosin. Note: Reactions shown occur at only one cross-bridge, but the same process takes place at all or most cross-bridges.

A new molecule of ATP binds to the myosin head, causing it to release from the actin molecule. Partial hydrolysis of this ATP (ADP ~ P$_i$) will "recock" the myosin head and produce a high-affinity binding site for actin. If Ca^{2+} levels are still elevated, the cross-bridge will quickly reform, causing further sliding of the actin and myosin filaments past each other. If Ca^{2+} is no longer elevated, the muscle relaxes.

ATP

Ca^{2+} ADP ~ P$_i$ Ca^{2+}

Ca^{2+} released from sarcoplasmic reticulum in response to action potential binds to troponin, causing tropomyosin to move and expose the myosin binding site on the actin molecule. The cross-bridge is formed.

ADP ~ P$_i$

ADP + P$_i$

ATPase

ADP and P$_i$ are released, the myosin head flexes, and the myosin and actin filaments slide past each other.

MUSCLE FIBER ANATOMY: BIOCHEMICAL MECHANICS OF CONTRACTION

The *sarcomere* is the fundamental contractile unit of skeletal muscle. Multiple sarcomeres align end to end along a muscle fiber, are defined by the *Z disk* at each end of the sarcomere, and give skeletal muscle its striated appearance. *Thin filaments* have a polymeric filamentous *actin* core and anchor to the Z disk. They are not continuous throughout the sarcomere, and only one end of each actin filament is associated with the Z disk. Multiple molecules of *globular actin* self-associate to form *filamentous actin*. Globular actin harbors a *myosin binding site* that is blocked at rest by *tropomyosin* molecules running the length of the thin filament.

Troponin molecules also run the course of the thin filament but occur as complexes bound at regular intervals. Three components comprise troponin: TnI, TnT, and TnC. *TnI* is an inhibitory molecule that *binds actin* itself and the other two troponin elements. *TnT binds tropomyosin*. TnC binds the calcium ion (Ca^{2+}), which then leads to a conformational change, ultimately rotating tropomyosin off and unblocking the myosin binding site on actin. Thick filaments are also a polymer but are composed of numerous myosin molecules. Myosin is a hexamer of two heavy chains and two pairs of light chains. The heavy chain tails also self-associate to form the backbone of the thick filament. The heads of the heavy chains form the myosin heads, which, after self-assembly, protrude in all directions from the thick filament backbone toward the thin filaments that surround the thick filament in a hexagonal arrangement. One segment of the myosin head binds actin and hydrolyzes adenosine triphosphate (ATP), ultimately leading to a conformational change and "power stroke," thus flexing the myosin head and sliding the bound actin filament toward the middle of the sarcomere.

The cross-bridge cycle describes the steps by which myosin, actin, ATP, and Ca^{2+} interact to lead to sarcomere shortening and muscle contraction on an elemental level. At rest, ATP is bound to the myosin head and is partially hydrolyzed to adenosine diphosphate (ADP) and phosphate (P$_i$), the myosin head is "cocked" and available to form a high-affinity bond with actin, but the myosin binding site on actin is obstructed by tropomyosin. After depolarization of the muscle membrane and generation of a muscle fiber action potential, large amounts of Ca^{2+} are released from the sarcoplasmic reticulum. Ca^{2+} binds TnC, causing tropomyosin to "unblock" the myosin binding site on actin. The myosin

head then binds actin, forming the cross-bridge. ADP and P$_i$ are released from the myosin head. The myosin head flexes on its backbone (the "power stroke"), pulling the bound actin toward the middle of the sarcomere. ATP again binds to the myosin head, which dissociates from actin. ATP is hydrolyzed again to ADP and P$_i$, the myosin head "recocks," and the actin binding site on the myosin head is again produced. If Ca^{2+} continues to be available, the sequence of events repeats, and actin is pulled further toward the middle of

the sarcomere. When this happens multiple times over multiple cross-bridges" between multiple myosin-actin molecules in multiple thick and thin filaments, the sarcomere shortens. As this occurs along several sarcomeres in the muscle fiber, the muscle fiber shortens. When multiple muscle fibers shorten within a muscle, the muscle contracts. If Ca^{2+} is no longer available, however, myosin binding sites on actin become blocked by tropomyosin, myosin cannot bind actin, and the muscle relaxes.

MUSCLE MEMBRANE, T TUBULES, AND SARCOPLASMIC RETICULUM

The muscle membrane system includes external (*sarcolemma, transverse [T] tubules*) and internal (*sarcoplasmic reticulum*) components. Although separate, the T tubules and sarcoplasmic reticulum are related in function. The membrane system is specially adapted to propagate the muscle membrane action potential and couple it to Ca^{2+} release into the *sarcoplasm*, leading to excitation-contraction coupling. These components meet at *junctional triads* where a *T tubule* is flanked by two *terminal cisternae* of the sarcoplasmic reticulum. Triads recur at predictable intervals that mimic the cross striations of the sarcomeres. In mammals, the triads are situated at the junction of the A band and the I band. This periodicity and proximity to the myofibrils signify the intricate role the triads have in control of muscle contraction. They are intimately involved in Ca^{2+} control: sequestration, release, and reuptake.

T tubules are specialized invaginations of the sarcolemma, with which it is continuous at multiple points. T tubules run transverse to the muscle fibers themselves and the sarcolemma and encircle individual muscle fibrils. T tubules form deep invaginations into the sarcolemma. This provides not only more rapid dispersal of muscle membrane depolarization along the muscle fiber, but also allows for propagation along both the surface of the sarcolemma and into the muscle fiber, where it can interact with the deep sarcoplasmic reticulum. T tubules interact directly with components of the sarcoplasmic reticulum, leading to Ca^{2+} release into the sarcoplasm. They also harbor voltage-gated Ca^{2+} channels, the L-type Ca^{2+} channels. These Ca^{2+} channels do not contribute to depolarization or the muscle fiber action potential but instead act as voltage sensors of muscle membrane depolarization. The sarcoplasmic reticulum forms a network of tubules surrounding muscle fibrils inside the sarcolemma.

Junctional sarcoplasmic reticulum (the *terminal cisternae*) stores Ca^{2+} and is the site of Ca^{2+} release in response to a muscle fiber action potential. Junctional sarcoplasmic reticulum contains high amounts of *calsequestrin*, which binds to Ca^{2+} and accounts for the high Ca^{2+} storage of the sarcoplasmic reticulum. The sarcoplasmic reticulum is so efficient in this role that the muscle fiber loses very little Ca^{2+} even after repeated muscle contractions. Junctional sarcoplasmic reticulum is also the site of the Ca^{2+} channel responsible for releasing large stores of calcium into the sarcoplasm, the *ryanodine receptor*, so named for its binding to the plant alkaloid ryanodine.

Sarcoplasmic reticulum voltage-gated Ca^{2+} channels sense the depolarization of the T tubule, interact directly with the ryanodine receptor, and induce it to release Ca^{2+} from the sarcoplasmic reticulum. Free sarcoplasmic reticulum constitutes the remainder of the intrafiber sarcoplasmic reticulum membrane system. It is not associated with the T tubule system and functions in Ca^{2+} reuptake into the sarcoplasmic reticulum. It has a large number of Ca^{2+} adenosine triphosphatase (ATPase) pumps on its surface that function in the energy-dependent reuptake of sarcoplasmic Ca^{2+} and therefore plays a role in muscle relaxation rather than excitation and contraction.

During contraction a motor nerve action potential propagates down the motor nerve axon to the nerve terminal, causing release of acetylcholine (ACh) into

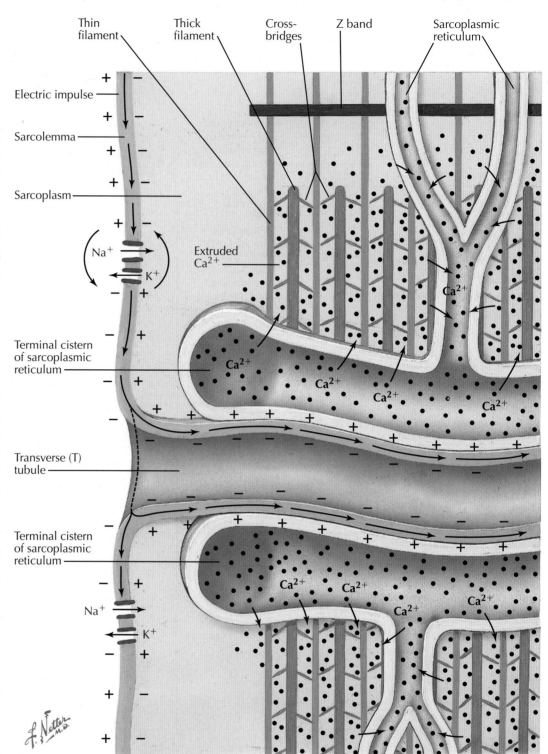

Electric impulse traveling along muscle cell membrane (sarcolemma) from motor endplate (neuromuscular junction) and then along transverse tubules affects sarcoplasmic reticulum, causing extrusion of Ca^{2+} to initiate contraction by "rowing" action of cross-bridges, sliding filaments past one another.

the synaptic cleft of the neuromuscular junction (NMJ). After binding of ACh to the postsynaptic muscle membrane ACh receptor (AChR), there is generation of an *endplate potential*. Suprathreshold endplate potentials generate *muscle fiber action potentials*. These propagate along the sarcolemma, depolarizing the muscle membrane sequentially as they travel along the membrane. The action potential continues down the T tubules. Depolarization of the T-tubule membrane activates the voltage-gated Ca^{2+} channel,

thus activating the ryanodine receptor, releasing large amounts of Ca^{2+} from the sarcoplasmic reticulum into the sarcoplasm. This leads to *cross-bridge formation* between thin and thick filaments, activation of the cross-bridge cycle, *sliding of the thick and thin filaments* past one another, *sarcomere shortening*, and eventually *muscle contraction*. Energy-dependent Ca^{2+} reuptake into the sarcoplasmic reticulum assists in relaxation and replenishes the supply of Ca^{2+} ready for release after the next depolarization.

Plate 12.4

Muscle and Its Disorders

Muscle response to nerve stimulation

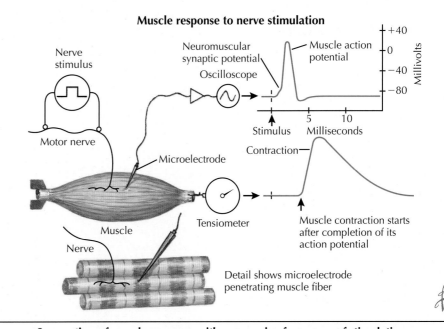

Detail shows microelectrode penetrating muscle fiber

Summation of muscle response with progressive frequency of stimulation

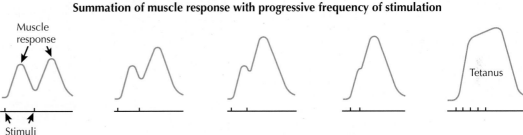

Muscle length–muscle tension relationships

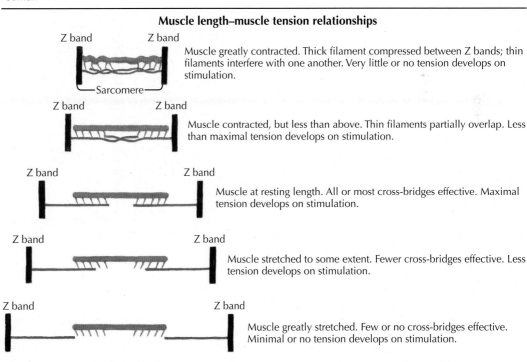

Muscle greatly contracted. Thick filament compressed between Z bands; thin filaments interfere with one another. Very little or no tension develops on stimulation.

Muscle contracted, but less than above. Thin filaments partially overlap. Less than maximal tension develops on stimulation.

Muscle at resting length. All or most cross-bridges effective. Maximal tension develops on stimulation.

Muscle stretched to some extent. Fewer cross-bridges effective. Less tension develops on stimulation.

Muscle greatly stretched. Few or no cross-bridges effective. Minimal or no tension develops on stimulation.

MUSCLE RESPONSE TO NERVE STIMULATION

Stimulation applied to a motor nerve produces a *motor nerve action potential.* This propagates down the motor nerve axon to the nerve terminal. ACh is released from the nerve terminal, binds the AChR on the postsynaptic sarcolemma, and leads to an *endplate potential.* The endplate potential is an *excitatory postsynaptic potential* that, in normal conditions, reaches the threshold to generate a *muscle fiber action potential* that ultimately causes a muscle twitch, or contraction. These potentials are measurable by an intramuscular microelectrode that records the excitatory postsynaptic endplate potential as a small initial deflection immediately preceding the larger muscle fiber action potential. The small delay from the initial stimulus to the initial deflection represents the time it takes to conduct the action potential down the motor nerve axon, release ACh, bind ACh to the postsynaptic membrane receptor, and generate the endplate potential. In addition, the muscle fiber action potential continues along the sarcolemma, down the transverse tubules, leading to massive release of Ca^{2+} from the sarcoplasmic reticulum into the sarcoplasm, initiating the cross-bridge cycle, and eliciting a muscle twitch. This is measurable by a tensiometer during an isometric contraction (with the muscle held at a constant length so it cannot shorten). The time taken for muscle fiber action potential propagation, calcium release, and initiation of the cross-bridge cycle explains the latent period between the muscle fiber action potential and the measurable muscle contraction.

Measurement of the effects of stimulation frequency is possible under similar conditions of isometric contraction. Given that there is all-or-nothing activation and contraction of fibers within a motor unit after stimulation of a single motor neuron, single stimuli produce identical twitch responses with identical tension created. If a second stimulus is given after full relaxation of the muscle, this second twitch intensity will be the same as the first. If, however, the second stimulus is given before full relaxation (i.e., while the muscle is still at least partially contracted) the tension created by the second stimulus will surpass that created by the first. As the frequency of stimulation is increased, this phenomenon, called *summation,* is enhanced. At high enough stimulation frequencies, muscle fibers are unable to relax between stimuli, and they produce a prolonged single-peaked contraction,

known as *tetanus.* This is one mechanism by which muscles generate varying degrees of force.

Isometric contractions also allow for the measurement of the effect of sarcomere length on the development of force generation; that is, the muscle length–tension relationship. Maximal tensile force results when the greatest number of cross-bridges form. This occurs when the muscle is at its resting length and all or most of the cross-bridges are available (i.e., there is maximal overlap of myosin heads with actin), and stimulation will produce

maximum tension. If the sarcomere is shortened, actin filaments begin to overlap or repulse each other and interfere with cross-bridge formation. As a result, fewer cross-bridges form, resulting in less tension. Conversely, when the sarcomere is stretched, actin filaments are pulled laterally, and myosin heads at the middle of the sarcomere no longer overlap with actin. Therefore fewer cross-bridges can form, also resulting in less tension. At the extreme, there is no actin-myosin overlap, and no tension develops after stimulation.

METABOLISM OF MUSCLE CELL

Muscle fiber contraction and relaxation is an energy-dependent process. The source of this energy is ATP. The muscle fiber requires an ongoing supply of ATP to maintain its function. Most ATP is generated in the muscle via utilization of local glycogen stores, free glucose, and free fatty acids.

CARBOHYDRATE METABOLISM

Blood glucose enters the muscle fiber through a specialized muscle-specific glucose transporter. It is then phosphorylated to glucose-6-phosphate and undergoes *glycolysis*. Glucose-6-phosphate is also derived from degradative phosphorylation of muscle glycogen stores. Phosphorylase b kinase activates *myophosphorylase* that initiates *glycogen breakdown*, and a debranching enzyme completes the process by which glucose-1-phosphate is produced. This is also converted to glucose-6-phosphate and enters glycolysis.

The *rate-limiting step* in glycolysis is the conversion of fructose-6-phosphate to fructose-1,6-diphosphate by *phosphofructokinase*. Ultimately, one molecule of glucose is broken down into two molecules of pyruvate, and three molecules of ATP are generated. Under *anaerobic conditions*, pyruvate is converted to lactate. Under *aerobic conditions*, pyruvate is instead converted to acetyl-coenzyme A (acetyl-CoA) and enters the tricarboxylic acid, or Krebs, cycle. Within the mitochondria, this cycle generates carbon dioxide and water, as well as the reduced forms of nicotinamide and flavin adenine dinucleotide (NADH and FADH$_2$, respectively) and guanosine triphosphate (which can transfer phosphate to ADP to produce ATP). NADH and FADH$_2$ then undergo oxidative phosphorylation in the inner mitochondrial membrane, generating additional ATP molecules. Therefore aerobic glycogen and glucose metabolism produces much more ATP than anaerobic glycolysis.

LIPID METABOLISM

Nonesterified fatty acids (NEFAs) enter the muscle fiber from the bloodstream, derived from circulating *very-low-density lipoproteins and triglycerides* stored in adipocytes. *Free fatty acids* are first activated to their acyl-coenzyme A (acyl-CoA) thioesters. *Short- and medium-chain fatty acyl-CoAs* can cross the mitochondrial membranes, where they undergo *beta oxidation*. *Long-chain fatty acyl-CoAs* cannot undergo beta oxidation and require esterification with carnitine by carnitine palmitoyltransferase I (CPT I). The resultant palmitoylcarnitine is then transferred across the inner mitochondrial membrane and converted back into the long-chain fatty acyl-CoA by CPT II. The long-chain fatty acyl-CoA derivative can then enter the beta-oxidation pathway. Beta oxidation occurs via fatty acid chain length–specific enzymes, producing acetyl-CoA that can then enter the Krebs cycle.

Energy utilization in muscle is activity dependent; that is, the specific energy source depends on the level and intensity of activity, type of activity, duration of activity, conditioning, and diet. At rest, the predominant energy source is *fatty acids,* particularly long-chain fatty acids. During low-level, low-intensity exercise, the muscle primarily utilizes glucose and fatty acids. With increasing intensity, glucose utilization is increased, and muscle glycogen becomes a principal energy source. With maximal isometric exercise, anaerobic glycolysis is the primary source. Also, during long-duration

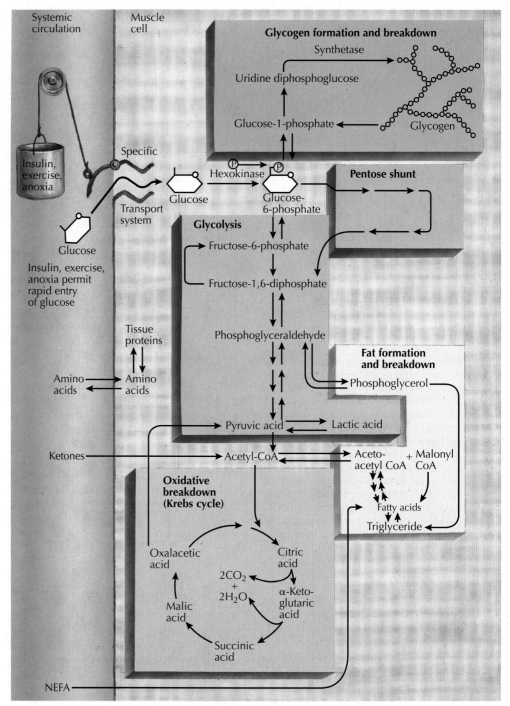

low-level exercise, *lipid metabolism* becomes the main source of energy.

A classic example of a defect of carbohydrate metabolism is *McArdle disease,* or *myophosphorylase deficiency.* Here the deficiency in activity of myophosphorylase leads to the inability to initiate glycogen breakdown. This leads to accumulation of glycogen in the muscle. Because there is no ability to utilize glycogen as an energy source, there is a reduction in the production of pyruvate. As a result, less acetyl-CoA is available to go through the Krebs cycle, and less NADH and FADH$_2$ undergo oxidative phosphorylation. Patients develop exercise intolerance with myalgia, fatigability, exertional weakness, and potentially *rhabdomyolysis.* This is more common with isometric or sustained moderate-intensity exercise.

Patients typically experience a "second wind," whereby a brief rest or reduction in activity leads to improved exercise tolerance. This correlates to increased availability of blood glucose and free fatty acids.

The most common disorder of lipid metabolism is *CPT II deficiency.* CPT II deficiency causes an inability to convert long-chain palmitoylcarnitines back into long-chain fatty acyl-CoAs on the inner mitochondrial membrane. Therefore the long-chain fatty acyl-CoAs cannot enter the beta-oxidation pathway and cannot produce acetyl-CoA to enter the Krebs cycle. Patients develop exercise intolerance and exertional rhabdomyolysis after prolonged exercise, rather than brief, intense exercise, and experience no second-wind phenomenon.

Plate 12.6 Muscle and Its Disorders

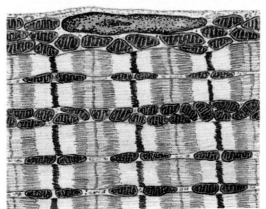

Type I: Dark or red fiber. Large profuse mitochondria beneath sarcolemma and in rows as well as paired in interfibrillar regions. Z lines wider than in type II.

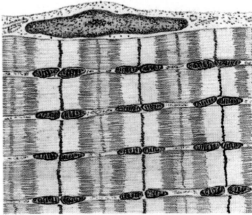

Type II: Light or white skeletal muscle fiber in longitudinal section on electron microscopy. Small, relatively sparse mitochondria, chiefly paired in interfibrillar spaces at Z lines.

MUSCLE FIBER TYPES

Muscle fiber types differ regarding twitch speed, fatigability, and preferential use of glycolytic versus oxidative pathways for energy production. They also differ in muscle color, being white or red. Fiber typing involves differentiating between type I and type II fibers. In addition, type II fibers are further subdivided into type IIa and type IIb fibers.

Type I fibers are adept at utilizing the *aerobic oxidative pathway* for long periods of time. As shown by electron microscopy, they contain large numbers of *mitochondria*, which confer a red color to the muscle itself. They react darkly for oxidative enzymes, such as reduced NADH dehydrogenase, succinate dehydrogenase (SDH), and cytochrome c oxidase. They have low glycolytic activity and react weakly for the glycolytic enzyme myophosphorylase. Accordingly, type I fibers have high lipid but low glycogen content. The myofibrillar ATPase in type I fibers is acid stable and alkaline labile; thus they react darkly for ATPase activity after acid preincubation but do not react for ATPase activity after alkaline preincubation. These are *slow-twitch fibers,* generating low maximum tension. They are, however, fatigue resistant and can maintain activation for longer periods of time. Due to this quality, they are referred to as *slow-twitch, fatigue-resistant fibers.* They are relatively small compared with type II fibers. Type I fibers activate before type II fibers at low levels of muscle contraction, and their motor unit potentials (MUPs) are those that electromyography (EMG) assesses.

Type IIa fibers are fast-twitch fibers with both glycolytic and oxidative metabolic activity. They also contain a large number of mitochondria and react somewhat darkly for oxidative enzymes. Unlike type I fibers, however, they have high glycogen content and stain darkly for glycolytic enzymes. Type IIa myofibrillar ATPase is acid labile and alkaline stable; thus these fibers stain darkly for ATPase activity after alkaline preincubation but not after acid preincubation. As fast-twitch fibers, they are able to generate an intermediate level of maximum tension quickly, but they also fatigue slowly. They are therefore referred to as *fast-twitch, fatigue-resistant* fibers. They are larger than type I fibers and activate later as sustained contractions are required.

Type IIb fibers lie on the opposite end of the spectrum from type I fibers. They harbor few mitochondria and have a white appearance. As a result, they react faintly for oxidative enzymes. They have high glycolytic activity,

Histochemical classification		
Fiber type	**ATPase stain following alkaline preincubation at pH 9.4**	**SDH stain**
1. Fast-twitch, fatigable (IIb) Stain deeply for ATPase following alkaline preincubation but poorly for succinic acid dehydrogenase (SDH), a mitochondrial enzyme active in citric acid cycle. Therefore fibers rapidly release energy from ATP but poorly regenerate it, thus becoming fatigued.		
2. Fast-twitch, fatigue-resistant (IIa) Stain deeply for both ATPase following alkaline preincubation and SDH. Therefore fibers rapidly release energy from ATP and also rapidly regenerate ATP in citric acid cycle, thus resisting fatigue.		
3. Slow-twitch, fatigue-resistant (I) Stain poorly for ATPase following alkaline preincubation but deeply for SDH. Therefore fibers only slowly release energy from ATP but regenerate ATP rapidly, thus resisting fatigue.		

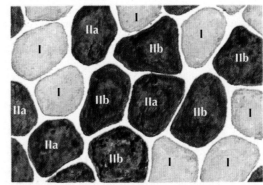

Cross section of skeletal muscle fibers stained for ATPase following alkaline preincubation

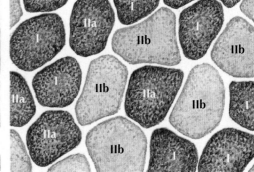

Identical section stained for SDH

however, and react darkly for glycolytic enzymes. They have high glycogen and low lipid content. Their myofibrillar ATPase is acid labile and alkaline stable, similar to type IIa fibers, but they show intermediate reactivity after preincubation at more moderate acidity levels (pH 4.6), unlike type IIa fibers, which have no reactivity under similar conditions. These are fast-twitch fibers but fatigue easily. They are accordingly referred to as *fast-twitch, fatigable fibers.* They reach high maximal force very quickly but only for short periods of time.

Muscle fiber type predominance is reflective of certain types of activity typical for a particular muscle. Short bursts of anaerobic activity (such as sprinting) are especially suited to type IIb fast-twitch, fatigable fibers. Longer aerobic exercise, however, is more suited to type IIa and type I fatigue-resistant fibers. There is evidence that consistent activity mimicking motor nerve activity of neurons that innervate fatigue-resistant fibers can slow contraction and increase fatigue resistance, suggesting that muscle fiber types can change in response to activity type.

OVERVIEW OF MYOPATHIES: CLINICAL APPROACH

In approaching a patient with weakness, the first task of the clinician is lesion localization: to determine by comprehensive clinical evaluation which one of the four organs of the motor unit—motor neuron, peripheral nerve, NMJ, and muscle—is the site of the dysfunction. Once localized to the muscle, a thorough history helps clinicians determine whether the myopathy is inherited or acquired. Characterizing the distribution of muscle weakness provides additional diagnostic clues that help identify specific muscle disorders. Finally, the results of laboratory studies help confirm and refine the diagnosis.

The history provides clinical clues. In most myopathies, weakness is proximal, affecting movements of the hips, thighs, shoulders, and upper arms. Typically, these patients have difficulty climbing stairs, arising from low chairs, and carrying out tasks above their head, such as placing a book on a high shelf or brushing their hair. Less commonly, weakness is distal (affecting movements of the feet/toes and hands/fingers), manifested by tripping over uneven terrain because of footdrop or difficulty opening jars. Much less commonly, weakness affects the cranial muscles producing ocular symptoms (lid drooping, or ptosis), difficulty swallowing (dysphagia), effortful speech (dysarthria), and inability to keep the head straight up, leading to a headdrop.

Associated symptoms of muscle disease include fatigue, exercise intolerance, and muscle atrophy. Myalgias can be associated with toxic or infectious myopathy, certain forms of inflammatory myopathy (those related to a connective tissue disease), and some myotonic myopathies. Cramps suggest metabolic or endocrine myopathies, stiffness or impaired relaxation of muscle points to the possibility of myotonia, episodic tea-colored urine or myoglobinuria is strongly suggestive of a metabolic myopathy, and muscle hypertrophy suggests muscular dystrophy such as a dystrophinopathy.

Determining onset, duration, and evolution of muscle disease enhances the effectiveness of the diagnostic process. For example, weakness presenting at birth suggests some forms of congenital myopathy and infantile myotonic dystrophy; weakness emerging in childhood is typical of most types of muscular dystrophy, congenital myopathy, metabolic and mitochondrial myopathy and, rarely, inflammatory myopathy. Later-onset weakness, coming on in adulthood, is often seen in inflammatory, toxic, and endocrine myopathies and, less commonly, is a first manifestation of muscular dystrophy and metabolic and mitochondrial myopathies.

For most myopathies, weakness is fairly constant over the course of a 24-hour period and uninfluenced by physiologic state (e.g., active or resting, fasting or postprandial). Certain muscle diseases, however, such as periodic paralyses and metabolic myopathies, are characterized by episodic weakness of varying interval and intensity and with or without concomitant metabolic derangements such as myoglobinuria. Disorders of NMJ transmission such as myasthenia gravis have a variation that is worse in the evening and with prolonged activity.

The rate of the progression of weakness over time offers a clue to the character of the myopathy. Acute to subacute progression (i.e., weakness evolving over weeks to several months) is typically seen in inflammatory myopathies (polymyositis [PM]/dermatomyositis [DM]). Chronic progression (with weakness developing over many months to years) is typical of most muscular dystrophies and the inclusion body myositis (IBM) form of inflammatory myopathy. Nonprogressive or mildly progressive weakness over the course of decades is characteristic of most forms of congenital myopathy, which explains why, in some rare instances of mild congenital myopathy, diagnosis is not established until adulthood.

Obtaining a detailed family history in any patient with a suspected myopathy is crucial to unlocking an underlying inherited disorder and identifying its pattern of inheritance. Patients are asked to reflect on certain details of their relatives' medical history, such as overall strength, functional capacity, ability to walk and run, whether there was a need for assistive devices or orthoses to walk, need for a wheelchair or scooter, history of cardiac disease, and whether the patient's (i.e., proband's) symptoms were shared by males and females or were sex specific. Armed with such information, the clinician may have a heightened index of suspicion for an inherited muscle disease. This places the physician in the position to hypothesize the pattern of inheritance (autosomal dominant [AD], autosomal recessive [AR], X-linked, or mitochondrial) and thereby improve the ability to provide genetic counseling.

Clues to the diagnostic process are often found in exploring the patient's medication list, exercise experience, dietary preferences, and motor function in a cool or cold environment. For example, subacute myopathies in adulthood may have a toxic etiology, caused by a cholesterol-lowering agent (statin), colchicine use for gout, or chronic alcohol use. Corticosteroids (CSs) prescribed for a wide spectrum of medical disorders may be responsible for a subacute or chronic myopathy. In susceptible individuals with a glycolytic pathway defect, short bursts of intense activity sometimes lead to muscle cramping, weakness, and myoglobinuria. In contrast, patients with lipid oxidation disorders generally require longer periods of low-intensity exercise to predispose to muscle weakness and myoglobinuria. In individuals with a genetic predisposition to periodic paralysis, a high-carbohydrate meal is sometimes the trigger for an attack of severe muscle weakness. Muscle stiffness worsening with cold exposure is typical of paramyotonia congenita.

The physical examination provides additional clues that help in the diagnostic process. Some muscle disease is part of a multisystem disorder, such as myotonic dystrophy or mitochondrial cytopathy. In myotonic dystrophy, extramuscular involvement may be multiorgan and multisystem, including cataracts, arrhythmia, cognitive impairment, and glucose intolerance. In others, concomitant cardiomyopathy and conduction defects occur as in the dystrophinopathies, Emery-Dreifuss muscular dystrophy (EDMD), and PM/DM. Although the diaphragm is a striated muscle, it is infrequently involved in muscle disease, with notable exceptions including Duchenne muscular dystrophy, myotonic dystrophy type 1, centronuclear myopathy, nemaline myopathy, and acid maltase deficiency.

Muscle bulk can be a clinical feature that points to a dystrophinopathy, limb-girdle muscular dystrophy, or congenital myopathy. *Dysmorphic features* may be seen with congenital myopathies such as nemaline myopathy, in which there is an elongated facies, high-arched palate, and foreshortened toes. *Skin changes,* especially a rash over the face and hands, are typical of DM. *Musculoskeletal contractures* indicate long-standing, usually inherited myopathies such as EDMD and Bethlem myopathy. Myopathy seen in the setting of multiorgan involvement suggests sarcoidosis, amyloidosis, endocrinopathies, connective tissue disorders, infectious disorders, and mitochondrial cytopathies.

Distribution of muscle weakness provides a clue to the diagnostic process. Most myopathies demonstrate a proximal distribution of muscle involvement. *Distal muscle involvement* is characteristic of *myotonic* dystrophy type 1 and dysferlinopathy. *Ocular weakness* is often an early manifestation of mitochondrial myopathy and oculopharyngeal muscular dystrophy (OPMD).

Laboratory tests often provide diagnostic confirmation in the clinical context of a patient with suspected myopathy. These tests include serum creatine kinase (CK) levels, which are elevated in myopathic disorders marked by muscle fiber necrosis and normal in muscle disorders with little injury to the muscle fiber membrane. Electrodiagnostic studies show early recruitment of short-duration, low-amplitude MUPs in weak muscles, irrespective of the cause of the myopathy. However, fibrillation potentials and positive sharp waves primarily occur in aggressive myopathies, including inflammatory, toxic, or dystrophic types. These potentials are less commonly seen in most congenital and endocrine myopathies.

Muscle biopsy analysis by light microscopy can help discriminate inherited and acquired myopathy and can provide diagnostic specificity such as inflammation and necrosis. *Immunohistochemical analysis* of frozen muscle tissue sections identifies specific muscle proteins when muscular dystrophy is suspected. In cases where muscular dystrophy is suspected but cannot be confirmed by immunohistochemical studies, molecular genetic testing by deoxyribonucleic acid (DNA) analysis of leukocytes can sometimes confirm the diagnosis of a muscular dystrophy by identifying a specific known mutation. In selected cases, when metabolic myopathy is suspected, biochemical analysis of frozen muscle tissue for analysis of the glycolytic, oxidative, or mitochondrial metabolic pathways can be performed. Genetic testing is the gold standard diagnostic test for confirmation of any inherited myopathy.

Plate 12.7 continued on next page

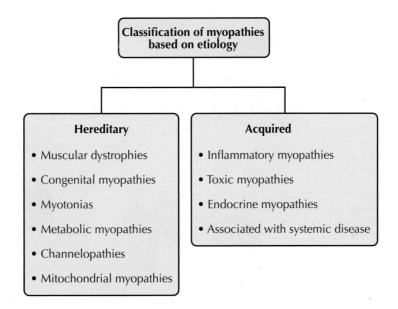

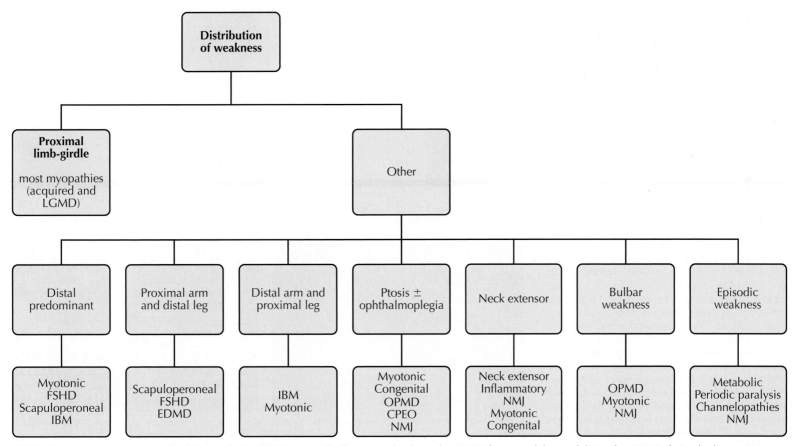

CPEO, Chronic progressive external ophthalmoplegia; EDMD, Emery-Dreifuss muscular dystrophy; FSHD, facioscapulohumeral dystrophy; IBM, inclusion body myositis; LGMD, limb-girdle muscular dystrophy; OPMD, oculopharyngeal muscular dystrophy.

DYSTROPHINOPATHIES

Muscular dystrophies are inherited primary diseases of muscle. Progressive muscle weakness and muscle fiber degeneration are the primary clinical and pathologic characteristics, respectively. A number of distinctive pathologic, clinical, and genetic features provide the means to further classify this diverse group of diseases.

Duchenne muscular dystrophy (DMD) is the most common form of muscular dystrophy (incidence is 1 in 3917 live male births [Norway] to 1 in 4700 [Nova Scotia]). Becker muscular dystrophy (BMD) has a relatively milder clinical course (incidence from about 1 in 18,000 to 1 in 31,000 male births). Both DMD and BMD are inherited as X-linked recessive traits. A third allelic type of dystrophinopathy of intermediate severity is recognized in patients known as "outliers." All three types result from dystrophin deficiency caused by mutations of the *DMD* gene.

Other dystrophinopathies occur at significantly lower incidences. These include carrier females who manifest DMD/BMD, DMD-associated dilated cardiomyopathy (DCM), and muscle cramps with myoglobinuria.

CLINICAL ASPECTS

The clinical features and course of the various dystrophinopathies vary across a wide spectrum. DMD, BMD, and the outliers (intermediate phenotype) have the most severe skeletal muscle involvement, and DCM has the most severe heart muscle involvement. DMD/BMD carrier females may be asymptomatic or manifest mild to severe symptoms. The age of progression to wheelchair use distinguishes DMD and BMD clinically and is usually less than 13 years for DMD in steroid-naive patients, more than 16 years for BMD, and between 13 and 16 years for outliers.

DUCHENNE MUSCULAR DYSTROPHY

The onset of weakness in children with DMD usually occurs between 2 and 3 years of age and nearly always before 5 years. Clinical features include difficulty with running, jumping, going up steps, and other similar activities; an unusual waddling gait; lumbar lordosis; and calf enlargement. Symmetric muscular weakness affects proximal before distal limb muscles and the lower before upper extremities. Affected boys may complain of leg pains and display Gowers sign (using hand support to push themselves from the floor to an upright position). Neck flexor weakness distinguishes boys with DMD from those with milder presentations. Cardiac muscle is also affected. Cognitive function may rarely be average or above average but is usually impaired to a varying degree. Physical examination shows pseudohypertrophy of the calf muscles; possible pseudohypertrophy of quadriceps, gluteal, deltoid, and other muscles; lumbar lordosis; waddling gait; shortening of the Achilles tendons leading to toe walking; and preserved reflexes in the early stage.

Although transient clinical improvement may be seen between 3 and 6 years of age, because normal maturation initially exceeds the early dystrophic process, relentless deterioration gradually follows, leading to wheelchair use. Contractures, scoliosis, and deterioration of pulmonary function follow. Cardiomyopathy affects about one-third of patients by age 14 years, one-half by age 18 years, and all patients after age 18 years. Intestinal hypomotility, also known as intestinal pseudo-obstruction, can be a life-threatening complication in patients with DMD. Cause of death is usually

DUCHENNE MUSCULAR DYSTROPHY: GOWERS MANEUVER

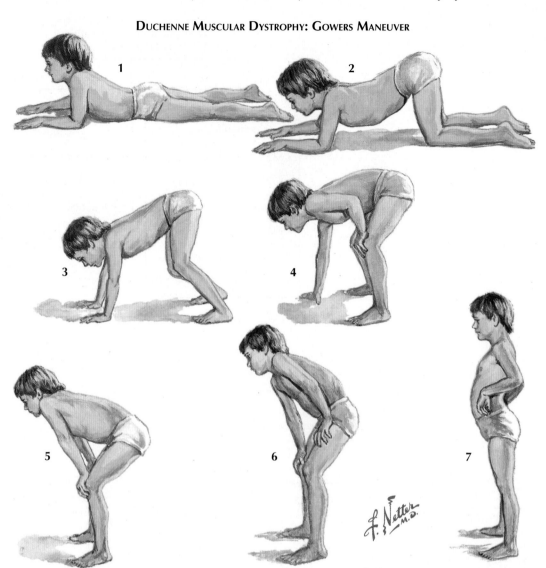

Characteristically, the child arises from prone position by pushing himself up with hands successively on floor, knees, and thighs, as a result of weakness in gluteal and spine muscles. He stands in lordic posture.

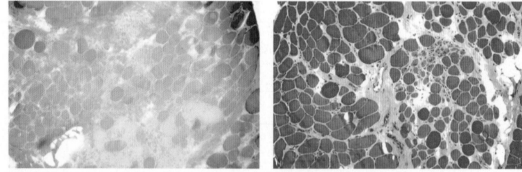

Muscle biopsy specimens showing necrotic muscle fibers being removed by groups of small, round phagocytic cells (*left*, trichrome stain) and replaced by fibrous and fatty tissue (*right*, H&E stain).

respiratory insufficiency or cardiac failure. In the past, most patients with DMD succumbed to disease in their late teens or 20s, but with the advancement of symptomatic and supportive care life expectancy of patients with DMD has increased substantially.

BECKER MUSCULAR DYSTROPHY

Symptoms of BMD usually appear between ages 5 and 15 years but, on occasion, do not appear until the third

or fourth decade or later. The degree of clinical involvement is milder, and cardiac disease and cognitive impairment are not as severe. Gastrointestinal symptoms, contractures, and scoliosis are not as likely to develop in BMD. Neck flexor muscle strength is relatively preserved. Patients with BMD typically remain ambulatory into adult life; they usually survive beyond the age of 30 years. Death occurs from respiratory failure or cardiomyopathy or cor pulmonale between 30 and 60 years of age.

Plate 12.9

Muscle and Its Disorders

DYSTROPHINOPATHIES
(Continued)

MANIFESTING DMD/BMD CARRIER FEMALES

The majority of DMD/BMD carriers, 76% and 81%, respectively, are usually free of symptoms. Mild calf hypertrophy may be seen. However, approximately 8% to 19% of carriers present with mild to moderate and occasionally severe muscle weakness of the limb-girdle type or even with DMD/BMD.

GENETICS

DMD Gene

The *DMD* gene is the largest gene identified in humans, spanning approximately 2.3 megabases on the short arm of the X chromosome at Xp21 including exons 1 to 79. The protein product dystrophin is identified on Western blots of human skeletal muscle proteins using antidystrophin antibodies. The dystrophin-associated protein (DAP) complex also contains many other proteins that are tightly associated. The DAP complex appears to be stabilized and protected from degradation by dystrophin in normal cells; the complex becomes unstable when dystrophin is absent. The muscle tissue of patients with DMD usually shows secondary reduction in the amount of other proteins of the DAP complex.

DMD Gene Mutations. Most *DMD* gene mutations are deletions (about 65%) and duplications (about 10%) of one or more exons with two mutational hot spots concentrated between exons 44 to 53 and exons 3 to 7. The remaining 25% of the mutations are small mutations that include point mutations (nonsense and missense), frameshift mutations, insertion-deletion mutations (indels), and other rare types (small inversions, complex small rearrangements).

No apparent correlation has yet been found between the size of *DMD* gene deletions and the severity and progression of the DMD/BMD phenotype. In most patients, the molecular differentiation of DMD versus BMD appears to be related to the disruption or preservation of the amino acid reading frame by deletion or duplication mutations. The latter either disrupt (DMD) or preserve (BMD) the reading frame in 90% of cases (reading frame hypothesis).

Dystrophin

In greater than 99% of patients with DMD, skeletal muscle biopsy specimens display complete or almost complete absence of dystrophin (0–5% of normal by Western Blot). The intermediate phenotype (mild DMD or severe BMD) appears to develop in patients with dystrophin levels between 5% to 20% of normal, regardless of protein size. Patients with mild to moderate BMD usually have dystrophin levels greater than 20% of either normal or abnormal molecular weight.

DIAGNOSIS

CK values varying between 1000 to 50,000 IU/L are not unusual in DMD/BMD. If serum CK concentration is less 1000 IU/L, the diagnosis should be questioned. From birth through 3 years, serum CK concentration in a child with DMD is always more than 10 times the upper limit of normal (ULN), and in a child with BMD it is usually more than 5 times the ULN. However, CK values do not differentiate reliably between the two types. Serum CK may be mildly increased in asymptomatic carriers and usually much higher in manifest carriers.

DUCHENNE MUSCULAR DYSTROPHY

Sex-linked recessive inheritance

Mother normal, carrier

Father normal

Only males affected, but females may be carriers

2 yr old, affected

5 yr old, normal

8 yr old, affected

10 yr old, normal; may or may not be carrier

15 yr old, affected

2 years — Minimal or no symptoms

8 years

15 years — Severe crippling deformities and contractures

Progression with age { Weakness, especially of pelvic girdle muscles; marked lordosis, enlarged calves

Calf muscles usually but not always enlarged

Lordosis disappears when child sits

Muscle biopsy features include:
- Degeneration and regeneration
- Isolated "opaque" hypertrophic fibers
- Significant replacement of muscle by fat and connective tissue
- Complete or almost complete absence of staining with antidystrophin antibodies in DMD
- Normal or reduced with or without patchy staining of the sarcolemma in BMD. In patients with other neuromuscular diseases, there is homogeneous staining of the plasma membrane.

TREATMENT

Management strategies for DMD have significantly improved, although to date there is no specific treatment. The last 2 decades have seen major breakthroughs in the field of clinical and translational medicine leading to the approval of many treatment strategies for DMD. Despite these advances, DMD remains a relentlessly progressive and ultimately fatal disease. The comprehensive care guidelines for DMD were updated in 2018 and provide a framework for DMD management with

DYSTROPHINOPATHIES
(Continued)

emphasis on a multidisciplinary approach. The neuromuscular physician remains key in the overall care of the patient throughout their lifetime with active participation of several specialists (occupational and physical therapy, rehabilitation, orthopedics, cardiology, pulmonary, gastroenterology and nutrition, endocrine, and psychiatry and psychology).

Oral CSs remain the cornerstone of pharmacologic management in DMD because they have been shown to prolong ambulation, improve upper limb function, preserve cardiorespiratory function, and reduce the need for scoliosis surgery. Current recommendations are to initiate steroids irrespective of the type of mutation at between 3 and 5 years of age. The CS preparations commonly used are prednisone/prednisolone (0.75 mg/kg/day) and deflazacort (0.9 mg/kg/day); the latter was US Food and Drug Administration (FDA) approved in 2017 and is more expensive but causes less weight gain. There are different regimens for steroid dosing: daily, 10 days on/off (0.75 mg/kg/day of prednisone), and high-dose weekend (10 mg/kg of prednisone divided over 2 days over the weekend). There is increasing interest in the development of agents that target the inflammatory cascade similar to CSs but avoid systemic toxicity.

The aim of dystrophin restoration strategies is to realign the reading frame of the *DMD* gene so that partially functioning (BMD-like) dystrophin protein is produced to diminish the severity of the DMD phenotype. Exon skipping therapy in DMD restores the reading frame using synthetic antisense oligonucleotides (ASOs) targeted to the dystrophin pre–messenger RNA, skipping out-of-frame mutations. Eteplirsen is the first ASO (exon 51 skipping) that received accelerated conditional FDA approval in 2016; all ASOs are administered via weekly intravenous infusions. Subsequently there has been approval of golodirsen (exon 53 skipping), viltolarsen (also exon 53 skipping), and casimersen (exon 45 skipping); together they address about 30% of exon skipping–amenable DMD mutations. Ataluren, an oral small molecule effective in promoting read-through of the premature stop codon in nonsense DMD mutations, has received conditional approval in Europe but not yet in the United States. Delandistrogene moxeparvovec-rokl is an adeno-associated virus vector-based gene therapy recently FDA approved for the treatment of ambulatory DMD in boys age 4 to 5 years.

Gene transfer therapy (GTT) utilizes the concept of micro- and mini-dystrophin constructs small enough to be inserted into adeno-associated vectors to drive high levels of targeted tissue transgene expression and produce enough functional dystrophin protein to alter the severity of the DMD phenotype. Three GTT programs utilizing this principle are in early-phase clinical trials through one-time intravenous infusions. A nonrandomized clinical trial using rAAVrh74.MHCK7 micro-dystrophin in patients with DMD showed that it was well tolerated and produced robust expression of micro-dystrophin protein, reduced CK levels, and improved functional scales.

All patients with DMD require cardiac evaluation and noninvasive cardiac imaging after the diagnosis and every 2 years until age 10 years and subsequently every year. Cardiac magnetic resonance imaging (MRI) is the noninvasive imaging modality of choice over echocardiography. It is generally recommended to start prophylactic therapy for cardiomyopathy with angiotensin-converting enzyme inhibitors or angiotensin receptor blockers by age 10 years. Baseline lung function tests should begin by age 5 to

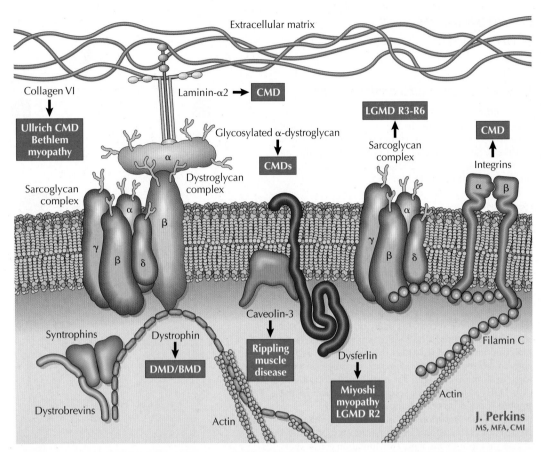

6 years and then as clinically indicated. Cough-assist devices are needed when forced vital capacity (FVC) is less than 50% predicted, and nocturnally assisted noninvasive ventilation should be initiated when there is hypoventilation, sleep-disordered breathing, or FVC less than 50%.

Patients with DMD are at risk of osteoporosis from the combined effect of CS-induced bone toxicity and progressive muscle weakness. Management includes regular screening for vitamin D deficiency, lateral spine

radiographs to detect incidental vertebral fractures, and bone mineral density scans. If there are signs of bone fragility, intravenous bisphosphonate therapy is initiated. The goals of musculoskeletal care in patients with DMD include maintenance of ambulatory status, avoidance of joint contractures, fall and fracture prevention, and preventive care for scoliosis with physical and occupational therapy, rehabilitation, and ongoing neurologic and orthopedic care.

Molecular Genetic Testing Used in the Dystrophinopathies			
Test Method	**Mutations Detected**	**Males with DMD**	**Males with BMD**
Deletion and duplication analysis using MLPA or array CGH	Deletion of one or more exons of *DMD* gene	~50%–65%	~65%–70%
	Duplication of one or more exons of *DMD* gene	~5%–10%	~10%–20%
Mutation scanning and/or sequence analysis	Small insertions/deletions/point mutations/splicing mutations of *DMD* gene	~25%–35%	~10%–20%

BMD, Becker muscular dystrophy; *CGH*, comparative genomic hybridization; *CMD*, congenital muscular dystrophy; *DMD*, Duchenne muscular dystrophy; *LGMD*, limb-girdle muscular dystrophy; *MLPA*, multiplex ligation probe amplification; *PCR*, polymerase chain reaction. (Data from Darras BT, Urion DK, Ghosh PS. Dystrophinopathies. In: Adam MP, Mirzaa GM, Pagon RA, Wallace SE, Bean LJH, Gripp KW, Amemiya A, editors. GeneReviews. University of Washington; 1993–2022. PMID: 20301298.)

Plate 12.11

Muscle and Its Disorders

MYOTONIC DYSTROPHY AND OTHER MYOTONIC DISORDERS

Myotonic dystrophy is a clinically and genetically heterogeneous disorder characterized by myotonia, namely the phenomenon of slowed relaxation after a normal muscle contraction. There are two major forms: type 1 (DM1) and the phenotypically different, milder type 2 (DM2). The prevalence of myotonic dystrophy is 1 in 8000 in the general population, but the relative proportions of DM1 and DM2 are unknown. These AD conditions are among the most common forms of adult-onset muscular dystrophy.

Both DM1 and DM2 are characterized by skeletal muscle weakness and myotonia with additional multisystem involvement. DM1 commonly presents in adolescence and early adult life as well as in a severe congenital form. DM2 typically begins in adulthood. In contrast to DM1, there is no congenital form of DM2. These two genetically determined myotonic disorders occur in relation to expanded repeats in the noncoding regions of the genes *DMPK* (DM1) and *ZNF9*, also known as cellular nucleic acid-binding protein *(CNBP)* DM2 genes.

The onset of DM1 is insidious; patients initially notice distal weakness of the feet and hands, along with myotonia, described by patients as muscle "stiffness," manifested by difficulty in relaxing muscles after strong contractions. Weakness slowly progresses, ultimately involving most muscle groups in a symmetric fashion. The phenotypic appearance of a long face with hanging jaw and hollowing of the temples develops as a result of wasting and weakness of the facial and neck muscles, as well as early-onset cataracts, is very characteristic of DM1. In contrast to many muscle disorders having a stereotyped proximal distribution, DM1 weakness typically has a pronounced distal predominance, resulting in dorsiflexor and finger flexor weakness. Patients have an accompanying cranial musculature weakness characterized by ptosis, dysarthria, nasal voice, and dysphagia. Muscle stretch reflexes are usually reduced or absent. Myotonia is a critical finding; it is elicited by asking the patient to grip the examiner's fingers followed by inability to quickly release. The myotonic response can also be elicited by striking the thenar eminence with a reflex hammer and observing a brisk contraction of the abductor pollicis brevis muscle, followed by a slow relaxation.

DM2 presents with weakness of hip-girdle muscles (difficulty arising from a squat, getting out of a chair, and climbing stairs) and back muscles (resulting in forward flexion or camptocormia when walking); in contrast to DM1, facial and distal weakness is uncommon. In DM2, pain and stiffness are major symptoms, leading patients to their physician in hopes of finding a form of medical therapy. The clinical and EMG features of myotonia are usually less prominent than with DM1.

DM1 is further characterized by the concomitant presence of significant systemic disorders; in contrast, these can be absent or mild in DM2. *Cardiac conduction disturbances* are seen in one-half to two-thirds of patients with DM1 and are less common in DM2; atrial fibrillation and flutter are the most common arrhythmias. *Cataracts* occur in more than 90% of patients with DM1 and DM2; the cataracts are indistinguishable in the two disorders. Changes in cognition and behavior are frequently observed in patients with DM1 but not DM2. Endocrinologic dysfunction is also a prominent issue in DM1 men. They have decreased sperm formation and low testosterone levels; in contrast,

Myotonic Dystrophy

- Frontal balding
- "Hatchet" facies due to atrophy of temporalis muscle
- Cataracts
- Ptosis and drooping mouth due to weakness of facial muscles
- Wasting of sternocleidomastoid muscle
- Gynecomastia

Difficulty in releasing grasp

Myotonia Congenita
(Thomsen disease)

Percussion myotonic reaction. Thumb moves sharply into opposition and adduction on percussion of thenar muscles and returns to initial position slowly.

Electromyogram showing spontaneous myotonic discharge evoked by needle insertion.

Myotonia and muscular overdevelopment. Disease affects both males and females.

menstrual irregularities and infertility occur in women. Early frontal and temporal balding and glucose intolerance and hyperinsulinemia are also common in DM1 but less so in DM2. Respiratory involvement may be seen in DM1, sometimes precipitated by general anesthesia, and excessive daytime somnolence is prevalent. There is an increased risk for malignant hyperthermia (MH) in DM1, so careful planning and precautions must be taken when general anesthesia is required.

Laboratory findings typically demonstrate no to a slight elevation in serum CK in DM1 and a mild hyper-CKemia in DM2. The characteristic EMG finding in both DM1 and DM2 is electrical myotonia, typically consisting of repetitive discharges of muscle fiber

action potentials at 20 to 80 Hz that wax and wane in amplitude and frequency, producing a sound often reminiscent of a dive bomber or a motorcycle engine. Muscle biopsy in DM1 and DM2 is notable for a marked increase in internalized nuclei (arrayed in chains in longitudinal section) and severely atrophic muscle fibers with pyknotic nuclear clumps. Genetic testing confirms the diagnosis for both DM1 and DM2 but may be particularly useful in DM2, especially when EMG myotonia is not prominent.

Congenital DM1 is characterized by profound hypotonia, facial diplegia, poor feeding, arthrogryposis (especially of the legs), and respiratory failure. Affected infants have a characteristic "V" shape of the upper lip

MYOTONIC DYSTROPHY AND OTHER MYOTONIC DISORDERS (Continued)

that results from facial diplegia. With intensive support, most infants survive the neonatal period. In early childhood, there is often a gradual improvement of motor function, but some degree of hypotonia and facial weakness persists. At age 3 to 5 years, foot deformities and learning and behavioral abnormalities present as the main clinical problems. Intellectual disability is a predominant feature of the congenital and childhood forms of DM1. As patients with congenital DM1 age, they develop many of the symptoms and signs of classic, adult-onset DM1.

DM1 results from an expansion of a cytosine-thymine-guanine (CTG) trinucleotide repeat in the 3′-untranslated region of the dystrophica myotonica protein kinase gene *(DMPK)* on chromosome 19q13.3. Wild-type individuals have 5 to 34 CTG repeats at this locus, whereas individuals with DM1 have repeats in the hundreds to thousands. Patients with classic DM1 have repeats in the range of 100 to 1000. When the CTG repeats are elevated to greater than 1000, DM1 may manifest at birth. Inheritance of congenital DM1 is overwhelmingly maternal. The length of the abnormal myotonic dystrophy repeat correlates directly with disease severity and inversely with age of onset. The phenomenon of an earlier age of onset of a more severe clinical phenotype through successive generations is the phenomenon of *anticipation.*

DM2 is caused by an expanded cytosine-cytosine-thymine-guanine (CCTG) tetranucleotide repeat expansion located in intron 1 of the zinc-finger protein 9 gene *(ZNF9)*, also known as the *CNBP* gene, on chromosome 3q21.3. On normal alleles, there are 11 to 26 tetranucleotide repeats; on pathogenic alleles, the number of repeats ranges from 75 to more than 11,000, with a mean of 5000 repeats. There is no correlation between CCTG repeat size and age of onset of weakness or disease severity.

In both DM1 and DM2, the respective disparate gene is transcribed into RNA but is not translated. The mutant RNAs accumulate in the nucleus and alter RNA binding protein activity, which, in turn, results in abnormal function of several genes, including the skeletal muscle chloride channel, the insulin receptor, and cardiac troponin T.

Management of myotonic dystrophy is best carried out in a multidisciplinary neuromuscular clinic. Cardiac follow-up with yearly electrocardiograms (ECGs) is highly recommended because there is a significant risk of sudden death from cardiac dysrhythmias. A trial of medication (mexiletine) may be warranted to ease problematic clinical myotonia. Physical therapy and use of orthoses for the distal leg weakness leading to partial footdrop may be very helpful to optimize motor function.

Other genetic myotonias include *sodium channelopathies (hyperkalemic periodic paralysis)* causing myotonia without weakness until the fifth decade; *paramyotonia congenita,* where myotonia worsens paradoxically with activity (especially in cold environments); and *chloride channelopathy myotonia congenita* (MC).

MC typically becomes symptomatic in infancy or early childhood. The incidence is 2 per 100,000. The most common form is AD (Thomsen disease), characterized by generalized painless myotonia and a complete absence of the extramuscular systemic features characteristic of DM1 and DM2. Affected infants may

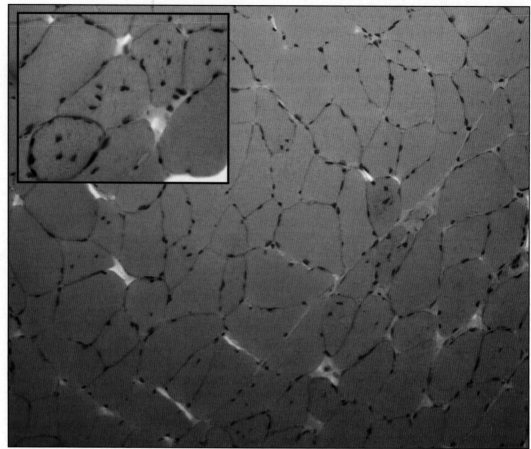

Light microscopy reveals muscle fibers with variation in fiber size and many fibers with internalized nuclei, also appreciated on high power (*inset*). (*Courtesy Declan McGuone, MBBCh, FRCPath.*)

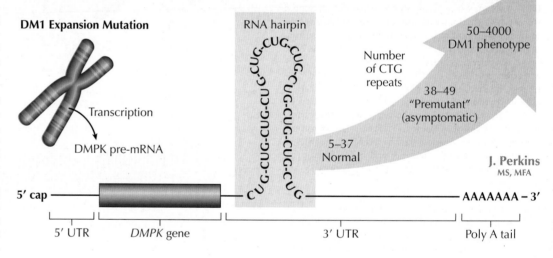

DM1 Expansion Mutation

Transcription

DMPK pre-mRNA

5′ cap

RNA hairpin

CUG-CUG-CUG-CUG-CUG-CUG-CUG-CUG-CUG-CUG-CUG-CUG-CUG-CUG

Number of CTG repeats

50–4000 DM1 phenotype

38–49 "Premutant" (asymptomatic)

5–37 Normal

AAAAAAA – 3′

5′ UTR   *DMPK* gene   3′ UTR   Poly A tail

J. Perkins
MS, MFA

develop eyelid myotonia with crying followed by delayed reopening of the eyes. There is generally little functional impairment with the exception of a tendency to fall when first standing or suddenly trying to run and stiffness symptoms relieved by exercise. There is a warm-up phenomenon: muscles stiff from myotonia are unable to exert normal power but after use are essentially normal in strength. Clinically, muscle size is exaggerated in appearance, leading athletic coaches to mistakenly encourage participation in school sports.

The less common AR form (Becker type) also typically has significant muscle hypertrophy. It may be associated with slowly progressive weakness and greater functional impairment than the more common Thomsen variant. Both have a similar mutation in the muscle chloride channel gene *(CLCN1)* on chromosome 7q25.

Schwartz-Jampel syndrome is not a channelopathy and, strictly speaking, is not a myotonic disorder, but it enters into the differential diagnosis of stiffness in a child. It is a rare AR condition that consists of blepharophimosis, low-set ears, and micrognathia. Affected children have normal intelligence, short stature, multiple joint contractures, and scoliosis. There is continuous muscle stiffness and percussion and grip myotonia. EMG shows complex repetitive discharges but not myotonic discharges.

Plate 12.13

Muscle and Its Disorders

OTHER TYPES OF MUSCULAR DYSTROPHY

Facioscapulohumeral dystrophy (FSHD) is an AD inherited disorder with symptoms of weakness generally appearing before age of 20 years. Weakness and atrophy affect the muscles of facial expression, periscapular muscles (producing prominent scapular winging), biceps, and triceps; the forearm usually remains relatively well preserved. There is early and marked bilateral footdrop. There is modest CK elevation in 50% of patients; the EMG is myopathic, and the muscle biopsy may show prominent inflammatory cells.

FSHD is inherited in an AD fashion with nearly complete penetrance and variable expressivity, with mild and severe cases seen in the same family. It is due to a deletion in the number of D4Z4 repeats in the subtelomeric region of chromosome 4q35. There is a correlation between disease severity and the size of deletion.

Treatment is aimed at encouraging activity with physical therapy, fall prevention, and evaluation for use of assistive devices for mobility. Light foot braces for patients with footdrop are often helpful.

Oculopharyngeal muscular dystrophy (OPMD) is an AD inherited condition with onset in the fifth or sixth decades of life. OPMD is found in individuals of French-Canadian, Spanish-American, and Bukhara-Jewish ancestry. The major clinical features are slowly progressive eyelid ptosis and dysphagia. Ptosis progresses to severe narrowing of the palpebral fissures. Over time, weakness involves the lid, extraocular, facial, neck, and proximal limb muscles in a symmetric fashion. The serum CK is normal or slightly elevated. The EMG shows myopathic features.

OPMD is inherited in an AD fashion, and the mutation is an 11- to 17-trinucleotide expansion of a (guanine-cytosine-guanine [GCG]) 10 repeat encoding for a polyalanine in the (poly A) binding protein nuclear *(PABPN1)* gene, which, when expanded, is thought to cause toxicity to muscle cells by accumulating as intranuclear inclusions. Genetic testing is available to confirm the diagnosis. Dysphagia may be so severe that patients are in danger of aspiration pneumonia, dehydration, and malnutrition; gastrostomy may therefore be necessary.

Limb-girdle muscular dystrophy (LGMD) is an AR or AD inherited disorder and is in a category of muscular dystrophies that is distinct from the more common X-linked DMD and BMD. The onset of weakness ranges from the first to the fourth decade, and the clinical course is one of slowly progressive muscle weakness and wasting with variable disability. The distribution of weakness usually spares the face and predominantly involves proximal and limb-girdle muscle groups. In most patients, the heart and respiratory muscles are spared, but exceptions occur depending on the specific genetic subtype. Serum CK is raised in most subtypes (but not all), EMG reveals fibrillations and myopathic potentials, and muscle biopsy discloses necrosis and regeneration.

Currently, 24 AR and five AD types have been identified. In most of the dominant forms, designated LGMD D, patients have been described in single, large, extended

Classification of Muscular Dystrophies			
Disease	**Inheritance**	**Pattern of weakness**	**Affected protein**
X-linked dystrophies			
Duchenne/Becker	XR	Proximal limb girdle	Dystrophin
Emery-Dreifuss	XR	Proximal arm, distal leg	Emerin
Scapuloperoneal	XR	Proximal arm (scapular winging), distal leg	Four-and-a-half LIM domain protein (FHL1)
Limb-girdle dystrophies			
LGMD1 A-G	AD	Proximal limb girdle	Myotilin, lamin A/C, caveolin-3
LGMD2 A-N	AR	Proximal limb girdle	Calpain 3, dysferlin, sarcoglycans, Fukutin
Other dystrophies			
Facioscapulohumeral	AD	Facial weakness, scapular winging	Unknown
Oculopharyngeal	AD	Ptosis, ophthalmoplegia, pharyngeal weakness	Poly A binding protein 2 (PABP2)
Scapuloperoneal	AD	Scapular and distal leg	Desmin
Myotonic dystrophy 1	AD	Ptosis, distal limbs, myotonia	Dystrophica myotonica protein kinase (DMPK)
Myotonic dystrophy 2	AD	Proximal limbs	Zinc-finger protein 9 (ZNF9)

AD, Autosomal dominant; *AR,* autosomal recessive; *LGMD,* limb-girdle muscular dystrophy; *XR,* X-linked recessive.

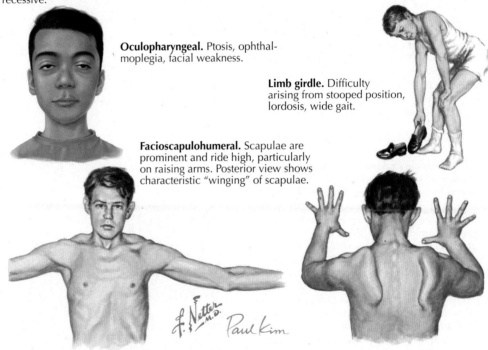

Oculopharyngeal. Ptosis, ophthalmoplegia, facial weakness.

Limb girdle. Difficulty arising from stooped position, lordosis, wide gait.

Facioscapulohumeral. Scapulae are prominent and ride high, particularly on raising arms. Posterior view shows characteristic "winging" of scapulae.

pedigrees and are considered rare. The recessive types, designated LGMD R, are more common, but prevalence is not easily ascertained. The AR subtypes are listed numerically, from LGMD R1 through LGMD R24. Among the 24 subtypes of LGMD R, the most common disorders are associated with mutations in genes coding for calpain (LGMD R1), dysferlin (LGMD R2), Fukutin-related protein (LGMD R9), and anoctamin 5 (LGMD R12). In addition to progressive proximal weakness, each of these disorders has distinctive features. Calpainopathy is characterized by scapular winging, hip adductor weakness, elbow contractures, and tight heel cords. Dysferlinopathy is characterized by atrophy and weakness of calf muscles, and muscle biopsy discloses inflammatory infiltrates. Fukutin-related protein deficiency resembles DMD and BMD, sometimes with cardiomyopathy and diaphragmatic weakness. Anoctamin 5 mutations are

characterized by asymmetric quadriceps weakness and atrophy.

For many LGMD subtypes, genetic testing can be used to identify the specific disease-causing mutation. If unrevealing, a muscle biopsy specimen can be evaluated by immunostaining for candidate proteins for an indirect diagnosis. Patients with LGMD require a comprehensive approach to care best achieved with a multidisciplinary team. Although cardiac and respiratory complications are uncommon, heart assessment by ECG and echocardiogram and lung function evaluation are important to identify and treat proactively for possible underlying complications. Genetic counseling is of importance to families, and prenatal diagnosis is available when the causative mutation has been established. Clinical trials using gene therapy are currently underway for some subtypes of LGMD.

POLYMYOSITIS AND DERMATOMYOSITIS

Inflammatory myopathies are acquired skeletal muscle disorders characterized by muscle weakness, elevated serum CK, and inflammation on muscle biopsy. The major idiopathic inflammatory myopathies that were initially described included polymyositis (PM), dermatomyositis (DM), and inclusion body myositis (IBM). With improved understanding of the pathologic features and presence of myositis antibodies, the category of PM has been further subdivided into subtypes of antisynthetase syndrome and immune-mediated necrotizing myopathy. Connective tissue disorders and underlying malignancy are important associations.

The prevalence of PM/DM is 1 per 100,000 adults, with a female-to-male ratio of 2:1. There is a childhood form of DM. Presenting symptoms include shoulder and pelvic girdle muscle weakness, malaise with fatigue, and occasionally myalgia and muscle tenderness gradually worsening over weeks to months. Patients report difficulty arising from a chair, combing hair, and climbing stairs. A defining symptom of DM is skin rash over the face, hands, neck, and extensor aspects of the extremities.

Clinical examination discloses symmetric proximal muscle weakness of the arms and legs and neck flexor muscles. Distal muscle weakness is usually mild. In DM cutaneous manifestations include Gottron sign (scaly erythematous rash over hand and finger joints and elbow and knee extensor areas), heliotropic rash (violaceous discoloration with upper eyelid edema), V-neck sign (erythematous sign over the anterior neck and chest), shawl sign (erythematous rash over the posterior neck and upper back), erythematous rash over the face (malar region and forehead), periungual telangiectasia (affecting fingernail bed capillaries), "mechanic's hands" (cracking of skin over hands and fingers), and calcinosis cutis (subdermal calcium deposits). In both PM and DM, dysphagia (esophageal weakness), cardiac involvement (heart block or congestive heart failure), and constitutional findings (fever, weight loss, arthritis) may occur.

DM and PM need to be distinguished from other conditions that may cause muscle weakness, including other muscle disorders: muscular dystrophies; toxic (drug-induced), metabolic, and endocrine myopathies; chronic inflammatory demyelinating neuropathy; myasthenia gravis; and, rarely, motor neuron disease.

Diagnosis of DM and PM is based on clinical findings supported by elevated CK (not always present) and an abnormal EMG. Myositis-specific autoantibodies can be present in the blood of many myositis patients and help identify the subtype of myositis. Twenty percent of patients have an antibody to histidyl transfer RNA (tRNA), called anti-Jo1 (the most common myositis antibody), defining a patient subgroup of antisynthetase syndrome with interstitial lung disease and mechanic's hands.

Muscle biopsy of a weak proximal muscle is the definitive study. Histopathologic features of both DM and

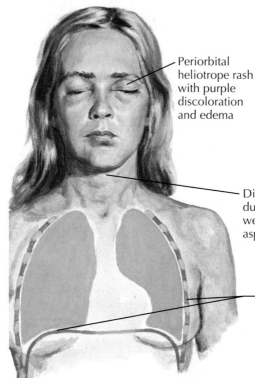

Periorbital heliotrope rash with purple discoloration and edema

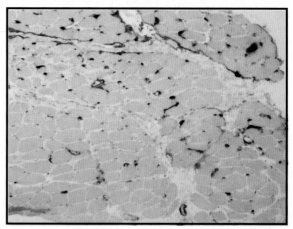

Weakness of central muscle groups evidenced by difficulty in climbing stairs, rising from chairs, and combing hair

Difficulty in swallowing due to pharyngeal muscle weakness may lead to aspiration pneumonia.

Weakness of diaphragm and intercostal muscle causes respiratory insufficiency or failure.

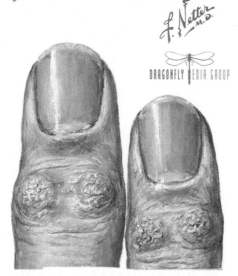

Erythematous or violaceous, scaly papules on dorsum of interphalangeal joints

Deposition of membrane attack complex (MAC) around small blood vessels and capillaries demonstrated by immunoperoxidase stain. (*Courtesy Mathew P. Frosch, MD, PhD, C.S. Kubik Laboratory for Neuropathology, Massachusetts General Hospital and Harvard Medical School.*)

PM include inflammatory cell infiltration and muscle fiber necrosis, with degenerating and regenerating muscle fibers scattered throughout the fascicle. In DM, the inflammatory cell infiltrate, composed mainly of B cells and CD4+ cells, is predominantly perifascicular and perivascular. Muscle atrophy, occurring at the periphery of muscle fascicles, is known as perifascicular atrophy (especially prominent in childhood DM).

Another characteristic finding in DM is deposition of the terminal component of the complement cascade—the membrane attack complex (MAC)—in capillary walls. In contrast, PM is characterized by inflammatory cell infiltration of T cells and macrophages occurring diffusely within the endomysium. Cell-mediated immune mechanisms are important, having increased numbers of cytotoxic CD8+ T cells and increased

Plate 12.15

Muscle and Its Disorders

POLYMYOSITIS AND DERMATOMYOSITIS (Continued)

expression by muscle fibers of major histocompatibility complex (MHC) antigens. Distinct pathologic features of antisynthetase syndrome include necrosis in the perifascicular region, fragmentation of the perimysium, and increased alkaline phosphatase activity in the perimysium. In immune-mediated necrotizing myopathy, the muscle histopathology reveals necrosis and regeneration of muscle fibers with a lack or paucity of lymphocytic infiltrates.

In DM, skin biopsy reveals perivascular lymphoid infiltrate. Immunofluorescence demonstrates deposits of complement, MAC, and immunoglobulin at the dermal-epidermal junction. MRI of muscle is a useful noninvasive adjunct that highlights areas of muscle edema, fatty infiltration, and calcification. MRI can also serve as a guide for muscle biopsy and therapeutic response.

Because malignancy may be associated with PM (up to 10% of patients), and especially with DM (up to 25% of patients older than 40 years), screening for cancer (carcinomas of the breast and ovary in women and lower gastrointestinal tract in men) is important, especially in older adults; routine laboratory studies, mammography, colonoscopy, and computed tomography scanning of the chest and abdomen are performed.

The severity of disease, response to treatment, and prognosis of DM and PM are quite variable and range from mild weakness, which quickly responds to treatment, to progressively worsening weakness, which may be resistant to a number of therapies. Poor prognostic factors are associated with a more than 6-month delay in initiation of therapy from the onset of weakness, dysphagia, interstitial lung disease (Jo1–positive patients), underlying malignancy, presence of collagen vascular disorders, and cardiac involvement. Other clinical features, such as advanced age, severity of weakness, peak CK elevation, and degree of abnormality on muscle biopsy, do not reliably predict the disease course or treatment response.

Treatment with CSs is the initial therapy for both DM and PM. Prednisone dose may vary but can be started at 1 mg/kg/day, with a maximum daily dose of 80 mg. For patients with severe weakness, intravenous glucocorticoid therapy (methylprednisolone 1000 mg/day for 3 days) or intravenous immunoglobulin (2 g/kg divided over 5 days), followed by high-dose oral prednisone, is recommended. Weakness usually improves over weeks. Once muscle strength is significantly improved and stabilized, a slow, gradual taper of prednisone (5–10 mg every 2–3 weeks) is started, aiming for the lowest and yet still effective dose to achieve sustained improvement. This may take up to 1 year. Patients on long-term corticosteroid therapy are treated with calcium, vitamin D, and bisphosphonates (for osteoporosis prevention); antacid or H2 blocker (for gastric mucosa protection); and prophylaxis (usually with Bactrim) for opportunistic infections. In up to 30% of patients,

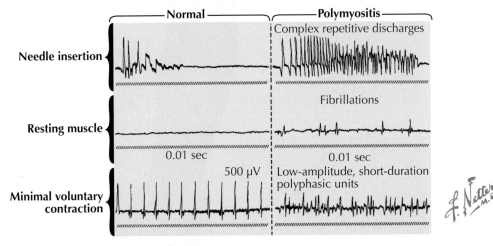

Electromyography

Normal — Polymyositis

Needle insertion — Complex repetitive discharges

Resting muscle — Fibrillations

0.01 sec — 0.01 sec

500 µV — Low-amplitude, short-duration polyphasic units

Minimal voluntary contraction

Muscle biopsy

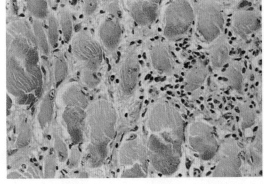
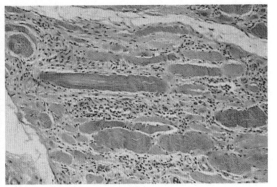

Transverse section ◄——**Muscle biopsy specimens**——► Longitudinal section

Inflammatory reaction: muscle fiber necrosis and regeneration

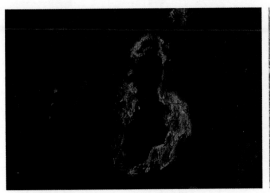
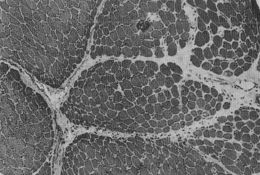

Anti-IgG immunofluorescence of frozen muscle section with positive staining within blood vessel wall, indicating immunologic basis of dermatomyositis

Perifascicular muscle atrophy in child with dermatomyositis

weakness recurs as the dose of prednisone is tapered, and a corticosteroid-sparing immunosuppressive agent is required. Azathioprine, methotrexate, or mycophenolate mofetil have been used in this setting.

Physical therapy and exercise are recommended early in the course of treatment and are tailored to the degree of weakness. Stretching and range-of-motion exercises are helpful in preventing joint contractures

(especially in weak muscles). Appropriate exercise programs, from low levels of isometric and resistive exercises in those with moderate weakness to increasing levels of activity in those with mild weakness, are encouraged throughout the course of disease. Patients with DM may have increased photosensitivity and are advised to avoid prolonged exposure to ultraviolet light.

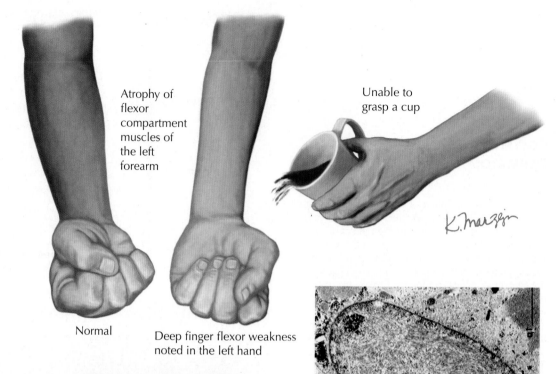

Atrophy of flexor compartment muscles of the left forearm

Unable to grasp a cup

Normal

Deep finger flexor weakness noted in the left hand

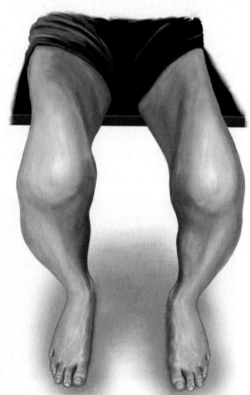

Atrophy and weakness of both quadriceps muscles

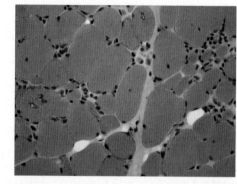

Electron microscopy. 15 to 21-nanometer tubulofilamentous inclusions may be seen in the cytoplasm and nucleus of vacuolated muscle fibers. (From Chad D, Good P, Adelman L, et al: Inclusion body myositis associated with Sjogren's syndrome. Arch Neurol. 1982;39:186-188.)

Light microscopy. Muscle fibers with rimmed vacuoles containing blue amorphous material. Clusters of small atrophied fibers also present (Courtesy Christian J. Davidson, MD.)

INCLUSION BODY MYOSITIS

Inclusion body myositis (IBM) is the most common acquired myopathy over the age of 45 years. Although IBM shares some clinical features and histologic findings with PM and DM, a constellation of distinctive clinical and histopathologic attributes makes IBM unique among the inflammatory myopathies. It has an insidious onset with slow progression over many years. In contrast to PM and DM with symmetric proximal weakness, IBM typically has asymmetric forearm and thigh muscle weakness and atrophy. Weakness and atrophy affecting finger flexors, particularly the flexors pollicis longus and digitorum profundus, quadriceps, and tibialis anterior muscles, are characteristic. Weak pinch as well as hand grip, knee buckling, and sometimes footdrop occur. As the weakness progresses, dysphagia and diaphragmatic weakness resulting in respiratory insufficiency cause increased morbidity.

Serum CK is mildly to moderately elevated ($<$10 times normal). In some patients, the anti-cytosolic 5′-nucleotidase 1A autoantibody is detected. EMG discloses fibrillation potentials and a mixed population of small and large MUPs. MRI of the thigh may reveal a characteristic pattern of fatty infiltration of the vastus lateralis, with sparing of the rectus femoris and posterior compartment.

Muscle biopsy demonstrates distinctive features of inflammatory lymphocytic CD8$^+$ T-cell infiltrates surrounding or invading nonnecrotic myofibers, vacuoles containing basophilic granules (rimmed vacuoles), diffuse MHC class I overexpression, cytochrome c oxidase–negative with SDH-positive fibers suggestive of mitochondrial pathology, and congophilic inclusions. Electron microscopy may help reveal 18-nm filamentous inclusions within muscle nuclei and cytoplasm.

IBM can often be mistaken for PM clinically and by EMG but can be differentiated by muscle biopsy. Toxic (drug-induced) myopathies may show similar vacuoles on muscle biopsy but typically have a subacute course. Hereditary IBMs present similarly with slowly progressive weakness and muscle biopsy demonstrating a vacuolar myopathy with inclusions. However, the family history and sparse inflammation noted in hereditary IBM distinguish it from sporadic IBM. Often, IBM with predominant distal and/or asymmetric weakness is confused with motor neuron disorders and less commonly peripheral neuropathies.

In contrast to other inflammatory myopathies responding robustly to CSs and other immunosuppressive agents, IBM is refractory to immunotherapy. Weakness is gradually progressive; after 10 to 30 years, most patients will require assistance with activities of daily living, a walker for ambulation and, ultimately, a motorized wheelchair. Supportive measures for dysphagia, respiratory insufficiency, and physical therapy help improve quality of life.

Plate 12.17

Muscle and Its Disorders

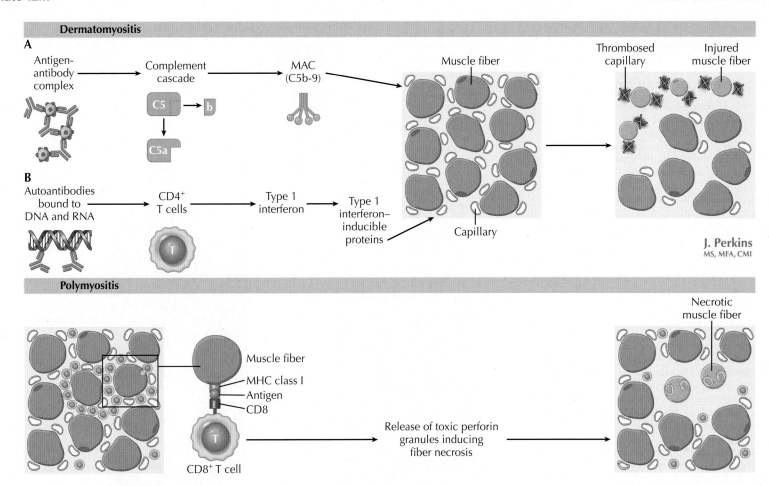

Dermatomyositis

A

Antigen-antibody complex → Complement cascade → MAC (C5b-9) → Muscle fiber

C5 → b
C5 → C5a

Thrombosed capillary   Injured muscle fiber

B

Autoantibodies bound to DNA and RNA → CD4⁺ T cells → Type 1 interferon → Type 1 interferon–inducible proteins → Capillary

J. Perkins
MS, MFA, CMI

Polymyositis

Necrotic muscle fiber

Muscle fiber
MHC class I
Antigen
CD8

CD8⁺ T cell → Release of toxic perforin granules inducing fiber necrosis

IMMUNOPATHOGENESIS OF INFLAMMATORY MYOPATHIES

DM, PM, and IBM share certain pathologic features, including muscle inflammation, fiber necrosis, and regeneration; individual distinctive histopathologic aspects suggest varied pathogenetic mechanisms.

PATHOGENESIS OF DERMATOMYOSITIS

A striking feature observed in muscle biopsies taken from patients with DM is the presence of a diverse collection of cell types: CD4⁺ T lymphocytes, B lymphocytes, plasma cells, macrophages, and dendritic cells located predominantly in a perivascular and perimysial distribution. The role of macrophages and dendritic cells is to present antigen—attached to an MHC class II molecule—to a helper CD4⁺ T cell that, in turn, produces cytokines (such as the interleukins whose targets are principally leukocytes, type 1 interferons [type 1 INF], and chemokines). These molecules amplify the immune response within the muscle microenvironment and have direct deleterious effects on muscle fiber function. The interleukins stimulate B cells to multiply and mature into antibody-producing plasma cells. Additional hallmarks of the DM muscle biopsy are atrophy of muscle fibers occurring specifically on the edges of muscle fascicles, leading to a distinctive pathologic feature known as *perifascicular atrophy,* and presence of MAC with antibodies deposited in capillaries and small blood vessels throughout the endomysium.

One hypothesis proposes that the pathophysiology central to DM is a *microangiopathy* resulting from antibody and MAC-mediated injury of capillaries. MAC is the end product of the complement cascade—consisting of complement components C5b, C6, C7, C8, and polymeric C9—that forms damaging transmembrane channels in the cell membranes of target cells, such as endothelial cells, and causes cell lysis and ultimately cell death. (The specific molecular agents that might trigger the complement cascade in DM have not been identified with certainty; however, antigen-antibody complexes are possible candidates.) The resulting necrosis and thrombosis of capillaries are postulated to result in muscle ischemia subsequently contributing to myofiber damage.

A second pathogenic mechanism underlying muscle injury in DM proposes a central role for INF. Many CD4⁺ cells are plasmacytoid dendritic cells secreting type 1 INF, possibly in response to autoantibodies bound to DNA and RNA located in DM muscle. There is strong evidence that type 1 INF, in turn, induces gene transcription of a host of proteins, some of which have the potential to injure muscle capillaries and muscle fibers and contribute to the pathologic picture of DM, although the precise mechanism of cell injury is not known.

PATHOGENESIS OF POLYMYOSITIS

Examination of muscles biopsies from patients with PM reveals an appearance different from that seen in DM. Inflammatory changes in PM are very similar to IBM (see below), and in biopsies where rimmed vacuoles are not prominently seen it is difficult to distinguish PM from IBM. There is a predominance of CD8⁺ T cells, with a relative smaller percentage of CD4⁺ T lymphocytes; these cells, together with macrophages and dendritic cells, are located within the endomysium. A pathologic signature of PM is the presence of cytotoxic CD8⁺ T cells surrounding and invading nonnecrotic muscle fibers. The CD8⁺ cytotoxic T lymphocytes recognize their targets by binding to antigen associated with MHC class I on muscle fibers and may mediate muscle fiber damage by releasing toxic perforin granules that induce muscle fiber necrosis. The precise character of the antigen or antigens that triggers the immune response and is presented to the T cell by the MHC I protein molecule in PM is not known; it may be an endogenous self-antigen or perhaps an antigen induced by a viral infection. Unlike DM, perifascicular atrophy is not seen, and there is no capillary deposition of complement and immunoglobulin.

PATHOGENESIS OF INCLUSION BODY MYOSITIS

The histopathology of IBM is notable for architectural changes within many fibers: eosinophilic inclusions in muscle fibers as well as rimmed vacuoles are seen, Congo red stains demonstrate amyloid deposits, and electron microscopy discloses tubulofilamentous inclusions in the cytoplasm and nucleus. These findings are perhaps more reminiscent of a neurodegenerative process than one that is immune mediated, and yet a prominent feature is the presence of the invasion of muscle fibers by CD8⁺ cytotoxic cells with MHC class I antigen on the invaded fibers, similar to the cellular reaction in PM. More recent data have suggested that the primary process in IBM may be the inflammatory changes, which then set up a myodegenerative process. The inflammatory cells in IBM are terminally differentiated and have lost the capacity to undergo apoptosis and are thus not responsive to conventional immunotherapy.

ENDOCRINE, TOXIC, AND CRITICAL ILLNESS MYOPATHIES

CORTICOSTEROID MYOPATHIES

Weakness is a common manifestation of both Cushing syndrome and corticosteroid therapy. Muscle weakness begins in the pelvic girdle and proximal legs and, subsequently, shoulder girdle and proximal arms. Predisposing factors include reduced muscular activity, protein malnutrition, and sex (females are more susceptible). CK is typically normal. EMG is often normal but may demonstrate myopathic MUPs with abnormal insertional activity. Muscle biopsy primarily demonstrates fiber diameter diminution, especially histochemical type IIb. Cushing syndrome therapy focuses on identifying and removing the corticosteroid source (i.e., adrenal or pituitary) and dose reduction in patients receiving CSs. Disuse accelerates corticosteroid myopathy, which may be partially prevented by exercise or passive range of motion.

HYPOTHYROID MYOPATHY

Most patients with myxedema (chronic hypothyroidism) report weakness, and 25% have objective proximal muscle weakness. Myoedema, an electrically silent mounding of percussed muscle, occurs in one-third of these patients. The relaxation phase of muscle stretch reflexes is delayed. In childhood, hypothyroid myopathy presents with hypertrophic muscles that slowly contract and relax. In adults, fatigue is associated with muscular spasms and cramps. Serum CK is mildly elevated. EMG may be normal, but in long-standing hypothyroidism increased insertional activity, complex repetitive discharges, and myopathic MUPs are seen. Judicious thyroid replacement restores function.

HYPERTHYROID MYOPATHY

Muscle weakness is common in hyperthyroidism, often affecting the shoulder and pelvic girdle muscles. Rarely, hyperthyroid patients have very brisk muscle stretch reflexes, muscle wasting, and fasciculations mimicking motor neuron disease. CK is normal. Muscle strength and bulk improve as the euthyroid state is restored.

HYPERPARATHYROID MYOPATHY

Weakness and fatigability frequently occur as presenting symptoms of primary hyperparathyroidism. Pelvic girdle and leg muscles are involved before upper extremities. Some patients have unexplained osteomalacia associated with myopathy. Serum parathormone levels are elevated, and serum alkaline phosphatase may be normal or elevated. CK is normal. Patients improve after parathyroidectomy.

HYPOPARATHYROID MYOPATHY

Muscle aches, spasm, twitching, and tremor may occur, but true myopathy in hypoparathyroidism is extremely rare. CK elevations result from muscle damage sustained during prolonged hypocalcemia-induced cramping.

ACROMEGALIC MYOPATHY

Proximal muscle weakness, developing many years after the onset of acromegaly, occurs about 50% of the time. CK and muscle biopsy are normal. The pathogenesis may relate to sustained high levels of growth hormone effects on muscle metabolism. After hypophysectomy,

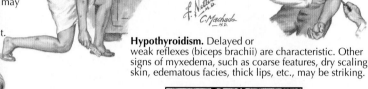

MYOPATHIES SECONDARY TO ENDOCRINE DISORDERS

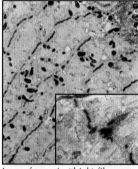

Cushing syndrome. Weakness (difficulty in rising from stooped position) and ecchymoses may be early manifestations. Other stigmata, such as moon face and buffalo hump, may be minimal. Osteoporosis may be present.

Hypothyroidism. Delayed or weak reflexes (biceps brachii) are characteristic. Other signs of myxedema, such as coarse features, dry scaling skin, edematous facies, thick lips, etc., may be striking.

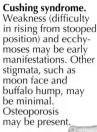

Acromegaly. Weakness in climbing a ladder or stairs and enlargement of jaw and hands may be the first signs.

Loss of myosin (thick) filaments

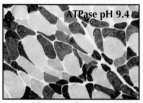

ATPase pH 9.4

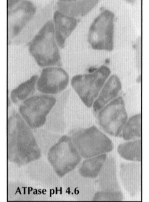

ATPase pH 4.6

Myosin-deficient fibers

Corticosteroid myopathy. Atrophy of type 2 muscle fibers (dark stained), especially the fast-twitch glycolytic type IIb fibers.

Images courtesy T.W. Smith, MD, Pathology Department, University of Massachusetts Medical School.

slow improvement occurs unrelated to postoperative growth hormone level decline.

TOXIC MYOPATHY

Numerous drugs lead to potentially reversible myopathies. Renal insufficiency predisposes because of reduced drug clearance. Cholesterol-lowering agents (e.g., hydroxymethylglutaryl-coenzyme A [HMG-CoA] reductase inhibitors) can cause myopathies characterized by muscle cramping, proximal muscle weakness, and increased serum CK. This is usually a mild myopathy that resolves with drug discontinuation. A more severe complication is the development of an immune necrotizing myopathy associated with autoantibodies to HMG-CoA. Myopathic potentials with myotonia are seen on EMG and muscle fiber necrosis on biopsy. It can be treated successfully with drug cessation and immunotherapy.

Chloroquine causes a vacuolar myopathy with insidious onset of slowly progressive proximal weakness. Electron microscopy discloses autophagic vacuoles containing lamellar or myeloid lipid-containing inclusions and curvilinear bodies. Colchicine induces both an axonal neuropathy and myopathy with vacuolar degeneration, almost always with associated renal insufficiency. Azidothymidine is associated with a myopathy and abnormal mitochondria on muscle biopsy. On rare occasions, penicillamine, cimetidine, and procainamide produce an inflammatory myopathy. Alcohol occasionally leads to chronic myopathies difficult to identify in patients with concomitant neuropathy and malnutrition complications. Acute alcoholic myopathies occur with episodic rhabdomyolysis, acute myalgia, muscle swelling, and weakness.

CRITICAL ILLNESS MYOPATHY

Exposure to intravenous CSs and neuromuscular blocking agents are major critical illness myopathy (CIM) risks; this myopathy also develops with severe systemic illness, multiorgan failure, and sepsis in an intensive care unit setting. Weakness is typically diffuse—flaccid quadriparesis with proximal greater than distal distribution—and sometimes affects the diaphragm, causing failure to wean. Muscle stretch reflexes are depressed or absent. Early in the disease course, serum CK is elevated in 50% of patients. Nerve conduction studies may demonstrate low-amplitude motor responses but preserved sensory responses. EMG reveals fibrillation potentials with myopathic MUPs. Muscle biopsy typically demonstrates selective myosin loss, type II muscle fiber atrophy, and occasional mild fiber necrosis. The pathogenesis is myosin thick filament loss secondary to muscle apoptosis, calpain upregulation, and a transforming growth factor-β/mitogen-activated protein kinase pathway. Inexcitable muscle results from inactivation of sodium channels at the resting membrane potential. Treatment is symptomatic. Intensive insulin therapy (targeting blood glucose concentrations of 80–110 mg/dL) may lower the incidence of CIM. Most patients recover over weeks to months; residual paresis may occur, depending on severity and duration of weakness.

Plate 12.19

Muscle and Its Disorders

Myopathies: Hypokalemia/ Hyperkalemia and Periodic Paralyses Channelopathies

SECONDARY HYPOKALEMIC AND HYPERKALEMIC SYNDROMES

Hypokalemia and hyperkalemia are common electrolyte disturbances associated with muscle weakness. The fall or rise in potassium concentration is often triggered by a medical disorder; the subsequent weakness is considered a secondary effect. Normal range of serum potassium is 3.5 to 5.5 mEq/L, and therefore levels less than 3.5 mEq/L and greater than 5.5 mEq/L define hypokalemia and hyperkalemia, respectively.

Hypokalemia-associated weakness does not usually become problematic until potassium levels fall toward and then below 1.5 mEq/L, with mild weakness, fatigue, and muscle cramping giving way to severe and generalized weakness, myoglobinuria, and cardiac arrhythmias. Common hypokalemia etiologies include excessive renal loss (e.g., diuretic use, primary aldosteronism) and gastrointestinal sources (e.g., vomiting and diarrhea). Mild to moderate hypokalemia is treated safely with oral potassium supplementation, whereas more severe hypokalemia requires intravenous potassium replacement.

Hyperkalemia of moderate to severe degree (>6.5 mEq/L) may be associated with muscle pain and paresthesias and, rarely, muscle weakness. However, cardiac rhythm disturbances with an abnormal ECG (peaked T waves and QRS complex widening) are common, requiring immediate treatment. Common causes include reduced renal excretion secondary to renal failure, drugs inhibiting potassium excretion, metabolic acidosis, and primary adrenocortical insufficiency (Addison disease). Cardiac arrhythmias require treatment with insulin, bicarbonate, and beta-agonists to lower serum potassium rapidly by shifting potassium intracellularly.

PERIODIC PARALYSIS

Weakness associated with hypokalemia and hyperkalemia may be caused by membrane excitability disorders, particularly AD channelopathies. *Hypokalemic periodic paralysis* (HYPOKPP) is caused by a skeletal muscle voltage-sensitive calcium channel gene mutation. *Hyperkalemic periodic paralysis* (HYPERKPP) is secondary to voltage-gated sodium channel *SCN4A* gene mutations. *Andersen-Tawil syndrome* is secondary to potassium channel gene mutations.

HYPOKPP is an AD disorder more frequent and severe in men than women. Episodes of paralysis begin in the second or third decade, often preceded by sensations of muscle tightness and soreness. These vary from quadriplegia to mild weakness in a single limb; muscle stretch reflexes are almost always diminished or absent. Respiratory and cranial nerve–supplied muscles are spared. Attacks average 12 to 24 hours in duration, resolving over 3 to 6 hours, with recovery noted first in muscles initially paralyzed. Provoking factors include rest after exertion, large carbohydrate-rich meals, cold exposure, stress, and alcohol. Attacks often begin during sleep. Between attacks, the examination is usually normal, but in some patients with multiple attacks, prominent limb-girdle weakness develops.

During an attack of total paralysis, serum potassium is usually depressed to 2 to 3 mEq/L, but it may be normal. The paralyzed muscles are electrically inexcitable. Hypokalemia induces cardiographic changes, including bradycardia, U waves, flattened T waves, and lengthened

MYOPATHIES ASSOCIATED WITH DISORDERS OF POTASSIUM METABOLISM

Characteristics of Familial Periodic Paralysis					
Disorder	Inheritance	Chromosome	Gene	Clinical myotonia	Major triggers
Hypokalemic periodic paralysis	AD	1q31–32 (type1)	*CACNA1S* (type 1)	No	Low K⁺, rest after exercise, carbohydrate-rich foods
		17q13.1–13.3 (type 2)	*SCN4A* (type 2)		
Hyperkalemic periodic paralysis	AD	17q13.1–13.3	*SCN4A*	Yes	High K⁺, prolonged rest, fasting
Andersen-Tawil syndrome	AD	17q23.1–24.2	*KCNJ2*	No	Prolonged rest

Hypokalemia

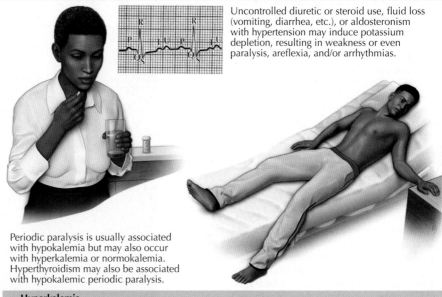

Uncontrolled diuretic or steroid use, fluid loss (vomiting, diarrhea, etc.), or aldosteronism with hypertension may induce potassium depletion, resulting in weakness or even paralysis, areflexia, and/or arrhythmias.

Periodic paralysis is usually associated with hypokalemia but may also occur with hyperkalemia or normokalemia. Hyperthyroidism may also be associated with hypokalemic periodic paralysis.

Hyperkalemia

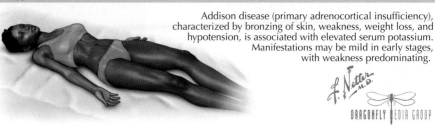

Addison disease (primary adrenocortical insufficiency), characterized by bronzing of skin, weakness, weight loss, and hypotension, is associated with elevated serum potassium. Manifestations may be mild in early stages, with weakness predominating.

P-R and Q-T intervals. CK is elevated during and, less commonly, between attacks.

The acute attack is treated with oral potassium. As prophylaxis, the patient is instructed to avoid high-carbohydrate meals, reduce salt intake, and avoid unaccustomed physical activity. Acetazolamide (125–150 mg/day) prevents most attacks by producing a metabolic acidosis impeding potassium movement into cells.

Thyrotoxic periodic paralysis is a sporadic disorder with an incidence of 2% to 8% of Asian populations with hyperthyroidism, particularly men (80%). Clinical and biochemical features are identical to familial HYPOKPP. Patients with the familial disorder have normal thyroid function, with attacks only when a hyperthyroid state exists. Correction of the hyperthyroid state is the definitive treatment.

HYPERKPP is AD, occurring equally in men and women. Attacks begin earlier than with HYPOKPP, generally before age 10 years. Attacks are usually brief and mild, lasting 0.5 to 4 hours; serum potassium may be slightly elevated but may be normal. Myotonia is prominent clinically and with EMG. Attacks occur

during the day or early in the night. Exercise at the first hint of weakness may delay an attack. Rest after exercise, stress, cold, administration of potassium, and fasting provoke attacks. As in HYPOKPP, permanent proximal limb-girdle muscle weakness may develop with age.

During attacks with elevated serum potassium, there may be electrocardiographic changes, including tall, slender T waves and tachyarrhythmias. CK may be elevated during and between attacks. Between attacks, EMG of weak muscles discloses myotonic discharges. In fully paralyzed muscles, the EMG is silent. Acetazolamide is effective in reducing attack frequency. Mexiletine is the treatment for clinical myotonia.

Andersen-Tawil syndrome is characterized by episodic weakness, dysmorphic features (short stature, hypertelorism, low-set ears, mandibular hypoplasia, clinodactyly), and life-threatening arrhythmias, frequently bigeminy or bidirectional ventricular tachyarrhythmia. Episodic weakness may be associated with hypokalemia, hyperkalemia, or normokalemia. Acetazolamide may reduce attack frequency.

METABOLIC AND MITOCHONDRIAL MYOPATHIES

These disorders are characterized by muscle weakness stemming from three realms of muscle metabolism dysfunction: (1) glycogen breakdown to lactic acid, (2) fatty acids oxidation, and (3) mitochondria ATP production.

McArdle disease, an AR myophosphorylase deficiency leading to glycolytic defects, is the common glycogen storage disease (GSD). Other glycolytic defects—phosphofructokinase, phosphoglycerate mutase, and lactic dehydrogenase deficiencies—produce similar clinical pictures. Children experience easy fatigability and mild weakness. In adolescence, painful muscle cramps develop with more vigorous activity. Muscle necrosis and myoglobinuria occur frequently. Individuals avoid intense activity, preferring less demanding sustained exercise, such as walking. A prominent second-wind phenomenon with renewed strength, attributed to fatty acid mobilization and increased muscle blood flow, occurs after 8 to 10 minutes of exercise when the patient is no longer glycogen dependent. Between attacks, patients are well and lead reasonably typical lives. Mild, permanent weakness occurs in 25%.

Diagnostically, CK is elevated in 90% of resting patients. Venous lactate fails to rise during forearm exercise tests (FETs) because these individuals do not metabolize glycogen. In contrast, peak venous lactate levels normally occur within 3 to 5 minutes after exercise, reaching three to five times preexercise levels. EMG is usually normal between attacks but may show mild myopathic potentials in chronic patients with permanent weakness. Muscle biopsy demonstrates subsarcolemmal glycogen accumulations and completely absent phosphorylase activity. Patients are encouraged to prevent attacks and muscle injury by avoiding high-intensity activity and ingesting glucose before activities.

Pompe disease (PD), or acid maltase (α-1,4-glucosidase) deficiency, is a rapidly fatal infantile AR GSD disorder secondary to an alpha-glucosidase gene mutation. Skeletal muscle glycogen accumulation occurs in the heart and nervous system, leading to severe hypotonia, weakness, and respiratory and heart failure. Milder, later-onset (childhood and adult) forms occur. Symptoms typically begin in the third to fourth decades, with slowly progressive proximal limb, trunk, and respiratory muscle weakness leading to respiratory failure.

Serum CK is elevated. Infantile ECGs are abnormal. EMG discloses myopathic MUPs, fibrillations, complex repetitive potentials, and myotonia. Muscle biopsy reveals a vacuolar myopathy. Electron microscopy demonstrates glycogen granule clusters within cytoplasm and vacuoles. Dried blood spot enzyme analysis provides screening; diagnosis is confirmed by enzyme assay or gene testing. PD is now treatable with intravenous recombinant human alpha-glucosidase.

Carnitine palmitoyl transferase deficiency (CPTd) is an AR, male-predominant lipid metabolism disorder in which muscle cells suffer energy deficits. CPT, an enzyme permitting fatty acid transport into mitochondria, provides muscle cell energy via beta oxidation. Its primary hallmark is recurrent myoglobinuria provoked by prolonged exercise or fasting. Unlike glycolytic disorders, painful cramps do not occur during exercise; thus patients lack warning signals of impending muscle injury. Severe muscle pain, swelling, and tenderness occur during episodes of acute muscle weakness.

CK, normal at rest, rises sharply during attacks. In contrast to McArdle GSD, CPTd venous lactate rises normally during FET. Muscle biopsy is normal except

McArdle Disease

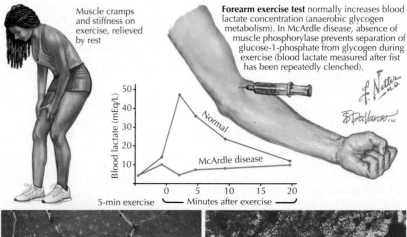

Muscle cramps and stiffness on exercise, relieved by rest

Forearm exercise test normally increases blood lactate concentration (anaerobic glycogen metabolism). In McArdle disease, absence of muscle phosphorylase prevents separation of glucose-1-phosphate from glycogen during exercise (blood lactate measured after fist has been repeatedly clenched).

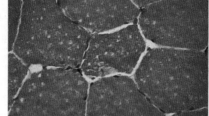

Blood lactate (mEq/L) — Normal — McArdle disease — 5-min exercise — Minutes after exercise

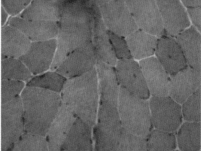

Frozen section of muscle tissue reveals "empty" subsarcolemmal vacuoles (H&E stain).

Frozen section of muscle tissue shows PAS-positive deposits of glycogen (PAS stain).

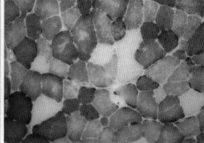

Ragged red fibers result from the accumulation of mitochondria below the sarcolemma of the muscle fibers; best appreciated on modified-Gomori trichrome stain. (*Courtesy Sandra Camelo-Piragua, MD, C.S. Kubik Laboratory for Neuropathology, Massachusetts General Hospital and Harvard Medical School.*)

Scattered muscle fibers show an absence of cytochrome c oxidase (COX) stain. COX stain is directed against one of the subunits encoded by mtDNA. COX negativity in an SDH-positive fiber is suggestive of a mtDNA mutation. (*Courtesy Sandra Camelo-Piragua, MD, C.S. Kubik Laboratory for Neuropathology, Massachusetts General Hospital and Harvard Medical School.*)

with previous myoglobinuric episodes, wherein scattered necrotic and regenerating fibers appear. Prolonged fasting (30–72 hours) leads to significant serum CK increase and delayed or decreased ketone body production. Muscle CPT biochemical assay or genetic testing provides definitive diagnosis.

Frequent meals with a low-fat, carbohydrate-rich diet may improve exercise tolerance. These patients should receive intravenous glucose before and during general anesthesia because prolonged fasting may provoke an attack.

Mitochondrial myopathies are genetically determined metabolic disorders of muscle caused by mitochondrial genome mutations. This circular, double-stranded molecule, consisting of 16,569 base pairs and coding for 22 tRNAs, 2 ribosomal RNAs, and 13 polypeptides contributing to various respiratory chain complexes, is the site of oxidation-reduction reactions generating ATP, the energy currency of the cell. These patients' mitochondria fail to produce sufficient energy for harmonious muscle metabolism function, leading to muscle weakness.

Ocular muscle weakness, notably ptosis and ophthalmoplegia, is a characteristic clinical feature that advances slowly, referred to as *chronic progressive ophthalmoplegia* (CPEO). Cardinal morphologic features include muscle fibers having prominent subsarcolemmal mitochondria accumulations appearing red on modified trichrome stain, designated "ragged red" fibers. *Kearns-Sayre syndrome* is a severe mitochondrial myopathy related to mitochondrial DNA deletion manifesting as a multisystem disorder having retinitis pigmentosa, heart block, elevated cerebrospinal fluid protein (sometimes including ataxia), short stature, endocrinopathy, and cognitive impairment.

Two mitochondrial encephalomyopathies involving muscle and the central nervous system are caused by tRNA mitochondrial mutations. *Myoclonus epilepsy with ragged-red fibers* is characterized by mitochondrial myopathy, myoclonus, ataxia, weakness, and seizures. *Mitochondrial encephalomyopathy* with lactic acidosis has childhood onset, intermittent vomiting, proximal weakness, and recurrent stroke-like episodes.

Plate 12.21

Muscle and Its Disorders

Myoglobinuric Syndromes Including Malignant Hyperthermia

Although virtually all disorders of muscle eventually require the attention and expertise of the medical community for diagnosis and management, myoglobinuria is distinctive because it is a medical emergency that demands immediate attention. This disorder often signifies a life-threatening and usually reversible systemic medical illness that must be rapidly treated; left untreated it may result in irreversible kidney damage.

Myoglobinuria—the presence in urine of a 17.8-kDa red pigment, iron-protein compound called *myoglobin*—results from rhabdomyolysis, which is the acute breakdown or necrosis of skeletal muscle fibers whose contents (among them myoglobin) subsequently leak into the circulation. Rhabdomyolysis reflects a fundamental problem involving disturbed muscle metabolism. The disorder is not uncommon; a recent study reported 26,000 cases per year annually from patient discharge databases. There tends to be a male predominance with a male-to-female ratio of 2:1.

The most common cause of rhabdomyolysis, amounting to 46% of cases, is exposure to exogenous myotoxic agents, such as illicit drugs, alcohol, and prescribed medications, including antipsychotics (the most common), statins, colchicine (in the setting of renal insufficiency), selective serotonin reuptake inhibitors, and lithium. Statins are commonly associated with myalgia and sometimes modest increases in CK but uncommonly with frank rhabdomyolysis. Synthetic statins such as atorvastatin are more likely to produce myoglobinuria than first-generation agents such as pravastatin.

Recurrent rhabdomyolysis occurs in 10% of patients with metabolic myopathies due to impaired glycogen metabolism or fatty acid oxidation, usually triggered by prolonged fasting or strenuous exertion. Defects in the mitochondrial respiratory chain, where ATP is produced, also need consideration. These are ultimately caused by mutations or microdeletions in the cytochrome b oxidase gene or in genes encoding cytochrome oxidase subunits. Rarely, recurrent myoglobinuria may be caused by mitochondrial tRNA mutations.

The clinical manifestations of rhabdomyolysis are muscle weakness, pain, tenderness and swelling, severely elevated serum levels of CK, and tea- or cola-colored urine caused by the presence of myoglobin. This pigment is grossly visible as tea-colored when serum concentration surpasses 100 mg/dL. Weakness may be profound and generalized, but respiratory and bulbar muscles are not affected. Between attacks, strength is typically normal, but in the case of alcohol-induced rhabdomyolysis, a chronic myopathy may emerge after repeated attacks. Patients often have a low-grade fever and leukocytosis. Myoglobin is detected in the urine by dipstick and ultrafiltration and is probably found in only 20% of cases.

Acute renal failure complicates almost 15% to 30% of cases of rhabdomyolysis, and among patients with rhabdomyolysis, there is a fatality rate of 3%. However,

Severe muscle cramps and collapse on exertion (as in soldier on long march)

Paroxysmal rhabdomyolysis

Malignant hyperthermia

Extreme temperature elevation in anesthetized patient

108°F (42°C)

Urine brown, scanty (myoglobinuria)

Renal shutdown

Serum CK elevated

Creatinine elevated

most patients respond to hydration, sodium bicarbonate and mannitol, or furosemide diuresis.

MH is an AD disorder caused by a ryanodine receptor gene defect on the long arm of chromosome 19. Occasionally, patients with MH have mild subclinical weakness, CK elevation, and nonspecific muscle biopsy changes. MH is associated with several well-characterized myopathies, including DMD, central core disease, myotonic dystrophy, and idiopathic hyper-CKemia. The pathophysiology involves an abnormality in the sarcoplasmic reticulum's ability to regulate intracellular calcium.

Succinylcholine or inhalational anesthetics lead to a rapid rise in intracellular calcium. Within minutes, an alarming clinical syndrome of increased muscle metabolism unfolds, characterized by rigidity secondary to muscle contracture, hyperthermia (temperature may soar, rising at a rate of 1 degree every 5 minutes, to as high as 43°C), metabolic acidosis, cardiovascular

instability, and myoglobinuria. Urgent treatment consists of immediately stopping anesthesia, uncoupling excitation and contraction with dantrolene, reducing body temperature, providing intravenous fluids and diuresis, and correcting metabolic acidosis with bicarbonate. Certain anesthetics, including nitrous oxide, opiates, barbiturates, and droperidol, are considered safe to use in patients at risk of MH.

MH bears some resemblance to neuroleptic malignant syndrome (NMS) because both share features of hyperthermia, rigidity, and myoglobinuria. NMS is triggered by a variety of neuroleptic agents, including phenothiazines and haloperidol, or by the withdrawal of dopaminergic drugs. It has additional clinical characteristics, including extrapyramidal and autonomic dysregulation. The primary pathophysiology is inhibition of central dopaminergic receptors so that heat generation is increased and heat dissipation is attenuated. Treatment requires dantrolene and dopamine agonists.

Section 1 Cranial Nerve and Neuro-ophthalmologic Disorders

Baehr M, Frotscher M. *Duus' Topical Diagnosis in Neurology: Anatomy, Physiology, Signs, Symptoms*. 4th ed. Thieme; 2005.

Biousse V, Newman NJ. *Neuro-Ophthalmology Illustrated*. Thieme; 2009.

Brazis PW, Masdeu JC, Biller J. *Localization in Clinical Neurology*. 5th ed. Lippincott, Williams & Wilkins; 2007.

Doty RL. The olfactory system and its disorders. *Semin Neurol*. 2009;29:74-81.

Gilchrist JM. Seventh cranial neuropathy. *Semin Neurol*. 2009;29:5-13.

Gonella MC, Fischbein NJ, So YT. Disorders of the trigeminal system. *Semin Neurol*. 2009;2:36-44.

Kim SY, Naqvi IA. *Neuroanatomy, Cranial Nerve 12 (Hypoglossal)*. StatPearls; 2022.

Landau MD, Barner KC. Vestibulocochlear nerve. *Semin Neurol*. 2009;29:66-73.

Lin HC, Barkhaus PE. Cranial nerve XII: the hypoglossal nerve. *Semin Neurol*. 2009;29:45-52.

Miller NR, Newman NJ, Biousse V, Kerrison JB, eds. *Walsh and Hoyt's Clinical Neuro-Ophthalmology*. 6th ed. Lippincott, Williams & Wilkins; 2005.

Ong CK, Chong V. The glossopharyngeal, vagus and spinal accessory nerves. *Eur J Radiol*. 2010;74:359-367.

Roper SD, Chaudhari N. Taste buds: cells, signals and synapses. *Nat Rev Neurosci*. 2017;18(8):485-497.

Wilson-Pauwels L, Akesson EJ, Stewart PA, Spacey SD. *Cranial Nerves in Health and Disease*. 2nd ed. BC Decker; 2002.

Section 2 Spinal Cord: Anatomy and Myelopathies

Avila MJ, Hurlbert RJ. Central cord syndrome redefined. *Neurosurg Clin North Am*. 2021;32:353-363.

Bosscher HA, Grozdanov PN, Warraich II, MacDonald CC, Day MR. The anatomy of the peridural membrane of the human spine. *Anat Rec (Hoboken)*. 2021;304:677-691.

Brinjikji W, Colombo E, Cloft HJ, Lanzino G. Clinical and imaging characteristics of spinal dural arteriovenous fistulas and spinal epidural arteriovenous fistulas. *Neurosurgery*. 2021;88:666-673.

Diehn FE, Krecke KN. Neuroimaging of spinal cord and cauda equina disorders. *Continuum (Minneap Minn)*. 2021;27:225-263.

DiGiorgio AM, Virk MS, Mummaneni PV. Spinal meningiomas. *Handb Clin Neurol*. 2020;170:251-256.

Eli I, Lerner DP, Ghogawala Z. Acute traumatic spinal cord injury. *Neurol Clin*. 2021;39:471-488.

Flint G. Syringomyelia: diagnosis and management. *Pract Neurol*. 2021;21:403-411.

Gailloud P. Spinal vascular anatomy. *Neuroimaging Clin North Am*. 2019;29:615-633.

Ghogawala Z, Terrin N, Dunbar MR, et al. Effect of ventral vs dorsal spinal surgery on patient-reported physical functioning in patients with cervical spondylotic myelopathy: a randomized clinical trial. *JAMA*. 2021;325:942-951.

Goyal A, Cesare J, Lu VM, et al. Outcomes following surgical versus endovascular treatment of spinal dural arteriovenous fistula: a systematic review and meta-analysis. *J Neurol Neurosurg Psychiatry*. 2019;90:1139-1146.

Gregg L, Gailloud P. Neurovascular anatomy: spine. *Handb Clin Neurol*. 2021;176:33-47.

Hussain I, Parker WE, Barzilai O, Bilsky MH. Surgical management of intramedullary spinal cord tumors. *Neurosurg Clin North Am*. 2020;31:237-249.

Lallemant-Dudek P, Durr A. Clinical and genetic update of hereditary spastic paraparesis. *Rev Neurol (Paris)*. 2021;177:550-556.

Lannon M, Kachur E. Degenerative cervical myelopathy: clinical presentation, assessment, and natural history. *J Clin Med*. 2021;10:3626.

Lawton AJ, Lee KA, Cheville AL, et al. Assessment and management of patients with metastatic spinal cord compression: a multidisciplinary review. *J Clin Oncol*. 2019;37:61-71.

Lemon R. The cortical "upper motoneuron" in health and disease. *Brain Sci*. 2021;11:619.

Mirian A, Korngut L. The utility of the laboratory work up at the time of diagnosis of amyotrophic lateral sclerosis. *J Neuromuscul Dis*. 2018;5:35-38.

Moon N, Aryan M, Westerveld D, Nathoo S, Glover S, Kamel AY. Clinical manifestations of copper deficiency: a case report and review of the literature. *Nutr Clin Pract*. 2021;36:1080-1085.

Ong B, Wilson JR, Henzel MK. Management of the patient with chronic spinal cord injury. *Med Clin North Am*. 2020;104:263-278.

Onofrei LV, Henrie AM. Cervical and thoracic spondylotic myelopathies. *Semin Neurol*. 2021;41:239-246.

Otten M, McCormick P. Natural history of spinal cavernous malformations. *Handb Clin Neurol*. 2017;143:233-239.

Parks NE. Metabolic and toxic myelopathies. *Continuum (Minneap Minn)*. 2021;27:143-162.

Pittock SJ, Zekeridou A, Weinshenker BG. Hope for patients with neuromyelitis optica spectrum disorders—from mechanisms to trials. *Nat Rev Neurol*. 2021;17:759-773.

Sciubba DM, Pennington Z, Colman MW, et al. Spinal metastases 2021: a review of the current state of the art and future directions. *Spine J*. 2021;21:1414-1429.

Taga M, Charalambous CC, Raju S, et al. Corticoreticulospinal tract neurophysiology in an arm and hand muscle in healthy and stroke subjects. *J Physiol*. 2021;599:3955-3971.

Section 3 Spinal Trauma

Karsy M, Hawryluk G. Modern medical management of spinal cord injury. *Curr Neurol Neurosci Rep*. 2019;19(9):65.

Liu Z, Yang Y, He L, et al. High-dose methylprednisolone for acute traumatic spinal cord injury: a meta-analysis. *Neurology*. 2019;93(9):e841-e850.

Steinmetz MP, Benzel EC. *Benzel's Spine Surgery: Techniques, Complication Avoidance and Management*. 4th ed. Elsevier; 2016.

Section 4 Nerve Roots and Plexus Disorders

Cervical Disk Herniation

Wong JJ, Côté P, Quesnele JJ, Stern PJ, Mior SA. The course and prognostic factors of symptomatic cervical disc herniation with radiculopathy: a systematic review of the literature. *Spine J*. 2014;14(8):1781-1789.

Back Pain and Lumbar Disk Disease

Fritz JM, Magel JS, McFadden M, et al. Early physical therapy vs usual care in patients with recent-onset low back pain: a randomized clinical trial. *JAMA*. 2015;314(14):1459-1467.

Tavee J, Levin KH. Low back pain. *Continuum (Minneap, Minn)*. 2017;23:467-486.

Lumbosacral Spinal Stenosis

Lurie J, Tomkins-Lane C. Management of lumbar spinal stenosis. *BMJ*. 2016;352:h6234.

Zaina F, Tomkins-Lane C, Carragee E, Negrini S. Surgical versus non-surgical treatment for lumbar spinal stenosis. *Cochrane Database Syst Rev*. 2016;(1):CD010264.

Diabetic Lumbosacral Radiculoplexus Neuropathy

Dyck PJ, Thaisetthawatkul P. Lumbosacral plexopathy. *Continuum (Minneap Minn)*. 2014;20:1343-1358.

Brachial Plexopathy

Rubin DI. Brachial and lumbosacral plexopathies: a review. *Clin Neurophysiol Pract*. 2020;5:173-193.

Brachial Plexus and Cervical Nerve Root Injuries at Birth

Chauhan SP, Blackwell SB, Ananth CV. Neonatal brachial plexus palsy: incidence, prevalence, and temporal trends. *Semin Perinatol*. 2014;38(4):210-218.

Frade F, Gómez-Salgado J, Jacobsohn L, Florindo-Silva F. Rehabilitation of neonatal brachial plexus palsy: integrative literature review. *J Clin Med*. 2019;8(7):980.

Socolovsky M, Costales JR, Paez MD, Nizzo G, Valbuena S, Varone E. Obstetric brachial plexus palsy: reviewing the literature comparing the results of primary versus secondary surgery. *Childs Nerv Syst*. 2016;32(3):415-425.

Section 5 Mononeuropathies

Aminoff M. *Electrodiagnosis in Clinical Neurology*. 5th ed. Elsevier; 2005.

Beltran LS, Bencardino J, Ghazikhanian V, Beltran J. Entrapment neuropathies III: lower limb. *Semin Musculoskelet Radiol*. 2010;14:501-511.

Bird TD. Hereditary neuropathy with liability to pressure palsies. In: Pagon RA, Bird TD, Dolan CR, Stephens K, eds. *Gene-Reviews*. University of Washington; 1993-1998.

Caliandro P, La Torre G, Padua R, Giannini F, Padua L. Elbow. *Cochrane Database Syst Rev*. 2011;(2):CD006839.

Cartwright MS, Yoon JS, Lee KH, Deal N, Walker FO. Diagnostic ultrasound for traumatic radial neuropathy. *Am J Phys Med Rehabil*. 2011;90:342-343.

Dang AC, Rodner CM. Unusual compression neuropathies of the forearm, part I: radial nerve. *J Hand Surg Am*. 2009;34:1906-1914.

Dang AC, Rodner CM. Unusual compression neuropathies of the forearm, part II: median nerve. *J Hand Surg Am*. 2009;34:1915-1920.

Daube J, Rubin D. *Clinical Neurophysiology*. 3rd ed. Oxford University Press; 2009.

Deymeer F, Jones HR. Pediatric median mononeuropathies: a clinical and electromyographic study. *Muscle Nerve*. 1994;17:755-762.

Escolar D, Jones HR. Pediatric radial mononeuropathies: a clinical and electromyographic study of 16 children with review of the literature. *Muscle Nerve*. 1996;19:876-883.

Faridian-Aragh N, Chalian M, Soldatos T, et al. High-resolution 3T MR neurography of radial neuropathy. *J Neuroradiol*. 2011;38:265-274.

Felice KJ, Jones HR. Pediatric ulnar mononeuropathy, report of 21 electromyography-documented cases and review of the literature. *J Child Neurol*. 1996;11:116-120.

Felice KJ, Jones HR. Focal neuropathies is children. In: Holmes G, Moshé S, Jones HR, eds. *Clinical Neurophysiology of Infancy, Childhood, and Adolescence*. Elsevier; 2005:615-644.

Greenberg SA. Pearls: neuromuscular disorders. *Semin Neurol*. 2010;30:28-34.

Gross PT, Jones HR. Proximal median neuropathies: electromyographic and clinical correlation. *Muscle Nerve*. 1992;15:390-395.

Holmes G, Moshé, S, Jones HR. *Clinical Neurophysiology of Infancy, Childhood, and Adolescence*. Elsevier; 2005.

Hunderfund AN, Boon AJ, Mandrekar JN, Sorenson EJ. Sonography in carpal tunnel syndrome. *Muscle Nerve*. 2011;44:485-491.

Jones HR, De Vivo D, Darras BT. *Neuromuscular Disorders of Infancy, Childhood, and Adolescence*. Elsevier; 2003.

Jones HR, Felice KJ, Gross PT. Pediatric peroneal mononeuropathy: clinical and electromyographic aspects. *Muscle Nerve*. 1993;16:1167-1173.

Keen NN, Chin CT, Engstrom JW, Saloner D, Steinbach LS. Diagnosing ulnar neuropathy at the elbow using magnetic resonance neurography. *Skeletal Radiol*. 2011;4:401-407.

Larner AJ. Pitfalls in the diagnosis of ulnar neuropathy: remember the deep palmar branch. *Br J Hosp Med (Lond)*. 2010;71:654-655.

Levin K, Luders H. *Comprehensive Clinical Neurophysiology*. WB Saunders; 2000.

Malipeddi A, Reddy VR, Kallarackal G. Posterior interosseous nerve palsy: an unusual complication of rheumatoid arthritis: case report and review of the literature. *Semin Arthritis Rheum*. 2011;40:576-579.

Srinivasan J, Ryan MM, Escolar DM, Darras BT, Jones HR. Sciatic pediatric neuropathies a 30-year prospective study. *Neurology*. 2011;76:976-980.

Stewart J. *Focal Peripheral Neuropathies*. 4th ed. JBJ Publishing; 2010.

van den Ende KI, Steinmann SP. Radial tunnel syndrome. *J Hand Surg Am*. 2010;35:1004-106.

Venna N, Bielawski M, Spatz EM. Sciatic nerve entrapment in a child: case report. *J Neurosurg*. 1991;75:652-654.

Visser LH, Ngo Q, Groeneweg SJ, Brekelmans G. Long-term effect of local corticosteroid injection for carpal tunnel syndrome: a relation with electrodiagnostic severity. *Clin Neurophysiol*. 2012;123:838-841.

Werner RA, Andary M. Electrodiagnostic evaluation of carpal tunnel syndrome. *Muscle Nerve*. 2011;44:597-607.

Section 6 Peripheral Neuropathies

Barohn RJ, Amato AA. Pattern-recognition approach to neuropathy and neuronopathy. *Neurol Clin*. 2013;31(2):343-361.

Burns JM, Mauermann ML, Burns TM. An easy approach to evaluating peripheral neuropathy. *J Fam Pract*. 2006;55:853-861.

Burns TM. Guillain-Barré syndrome. *Semin Neurol*. 2008;28:152-167.

Burns TM, Schaublin GA, Dyck PJ. Vasculitic neuropathies. *Neurol Clin*. 2007;25:89-113.

Collins MP, Dyck PJ, Gronseth GS, et al. Peripheral Nerve Society guideline on the classification, diagnosis, investigation, and immunosuppressive therapy of non-systemic vasculitic neuropathy: executive summary. *J Peripher Nerv Syst*. 2010;15(3):176-184.

Dispenzieri A. POEMS syndrome: update on diagnosis, risk-stratification, and management. *Am J Hematol*. 2015;90(10):951-962.

Katz JS, Saperstein DS, Gronseth G, Amato AA, Barohn RJ. Distal acquired demyelinating symmetric neuropathy. *Neurology*. 2000;54:615-620.

Klein CJ. Charcot-Marie-Tooth disease and other hereditary neuropathies. *Continuum (Minneap Minn)*. 2020;26(5):1224-1256.

Klein CJ, Moon JS, Mauermann ML, et al. The neuropathies of Waldenström's macroglobulinemia (WM) and IgM-MGUS. *Can J Neurol Sci*. 2011;38(2):289-295.

Lamb CJ, James P, Dyck B. Chronic inflammatory demyelinating polyneuropathy. *Pract Neurol*. Jul/Aug 2021.

Latov N, Gorson KC, Brannagan TH III, et al. Diagnosis and treatment of chronic immune-mediated neuropathies. *J Clin Neuromuscul Dis*. 2006;7:141-157.

Mauermann ML, Burns TM. The evaluation of chronic axonal polyneuropathies. *Semin Neurol*. 2008;28:133-151.

Naddaf E, Mauermann ML. Peripheral neuropathies associated with monoclonal gammopathies. *Continuum (Minneap Minn)*. 2020;26(5):1369-1383.

Saperstein DS, Katz JS, Amato AA, Barohn RJ. Clinical spectrum of chronic acquired demyelinating polyneuropathies. *Muscle Nerve*. 2001;24:311-324.

Saporta AS, Sottile SL, Miller LJ, Feely SM, Siskind CE, Shy ME. Charcot-Marie-Tooth disease subtypes and genetic testing strategies. *Ann Neurol*. 2011;69:22-33.

Shelly S, Shouman K, Paul P, et al. Expanding the spectrum of chronic immune sensory polyradiculopathy: CISP-plus. *Neurology.* 2021;96(16):e2078-e2089.

Siskind CE, Shy ME. Genetics of neuropathies. *Semin Neurol.* 2011;31:494-505.

Tesfaye S, Boulton AJ, Dyck PJ, et al. Diabetic neuropathies: update on definitions, diagnostic criteria, estimation of severity, and treatments. *Diabetes Care.* 2010;33:2285-2293.

Tracy JA, Dyck PJ. Investigations and treatment of chronic inflammatory demyelinating polyradiculoneuropathy and other inflammatory demyelinating polyneuropathies. *Curr Opin Neurol.* 2010;23:242-248.

Section 7 Autonomic Nervous System and Its Disorders

Blom H, Andersson C, Olofsson BO, Bjerle P, Wiklund U, Lithner F. Assessment of autonomic nerve function in acute intermittent porphyria; a study based on spectral analysis of heart rate variability. *J Intern Med.* 1996;240:73-79.

Darnell RB, Posner JB. Paraneoplastic syndromes involving the nervous system. *N Engl J Med.* 2003;349:1543-1554.

Gilman S, Wenning GK, Low PA, et al. Second consensus statement on the diagnosis of multiple system atrophy. *Neurology.* 2008;71:670-676.

Low PA, Benarroch EE, eds. *Clinical Autonomic Disorders.* 3rd ed. Lippincott, Williams & Wilkins; 2008.

Low PA, Walsh JC, Huang CY, McLeod JG. The sympathetic nervous system in diabetic neuropathy. *Brain.* 1975;98:341-356.

Mathias CJ, Bannister R. *Autonomic Failure: A Textbook of Clinical Disorders of the Autonomic Nervous System.* 5th ed. Oxford University Press; 2012.

Robertson D, Biaggioni I, Burnstock G, Low PA, Paton JFR. *Primer on the Autonomic Nervous System.* 3rd ed. Academic Press; 2012.

Suhr OB, Wiklund U, Ando Y, Ando E, Olofsson BO. Impact of liver transplantation on autonomic neuropathy in familial amyloidotic polyneuropathy: an evaluation by spectral analysis of heart rate variability. *J Intern Med.* 1997;242:225-229.

Tuck RR, McLeod JG. Autonomic dysfunction in Guillain-Barré syndrome. *J Neurol Neurosurg Psychiatry.* 1981;44:983-990.

Vernino S, Low PA, Fealey RD, Stewart JD, Farrugia G, Lennon VA. Autoantibodies to ganglionic acetylcholine receptors in autoimmune autonomic neuropathies. *N Engl J Med.* 2000;343:847-855.

Section 8 Pain

Basbaum AI, Bautista DM, Scherrer G, Julius D. Cellular and molecular mechanisms of pain. *Cell.* 2009;139:267-284.

Benarroch EE. Descending monoaminergic pain modulation: bidirectional control and clinical relevance. *Neurology.* 2008;7:217-221.

Bennett GJ, Watson CP. Herpes zoster and postherpetic neuralgia: past, present and future. *Pain Res Manag.* 2009;14:275-282.

Bogduk N. On the definitions and physiology of back pain, referred pain, and radicular pain. *Pain.* 2009;147:17-19.

Bril V, England J, Franklin GM, et al. Evidence-based guideline: treatment of painful diabetic neuropathy: report of the American Academy of Neurology, the American Association of Neuromuscular and Electrodiagnostic Medicine, and the American Academy of Physical Medicine and Rehabilitation. *Neurology.* 2011;76:1758-1765.

Brown MD, Gomez-Marin O, Brookfield KF, Li PS. Differential diagnosis of hip disease versus spine disease. *Clin Orthop Relat Res.* 2004;419:280-284.

Bruehl S. An update on the pathophysiology of complex regional pain syndrome. *Anesthesiology.* 2010;113:713-725.

Chou R, Qaseem A, Snow V, Casey D, Cross Jr JT, Shekelle P, et al. Diagnosis and treatment of low back pain: a joint clinical practice guideline from the American College of Physicians and the American Pain Society. *Ann Intern Med.* 2007;147:478-491.

Costigan M, Scholz J, Woolf CJ. Neuropathic pain: a maladaptive response of the nervous system to damage. *Annu Rev Neurosci.* 2009;32:1-32.

Craig AD. Pain mechanisms: labeled lines versus convergence in central processing. *Annu Rev Neurosci.* 2003;26:1-30.

Cummins TR, Sheets PL, Waxman SG. The roles of sodium channels in nociception: implications for mechanisms of pain. *Pain.* 2007;131:243-257.

Dejerine J, Roussy G. Le syndrome thalamique. *Rev Neurol.* 1906;12:521-532.

Derry S, Lloyd R, Moore RA, McQuay HJ. Topical capsaicin for chronic neuropathic pain in adults. *Cochrane Database Syst Rev.* 2009;(4):CD007393.

De Santi L, Monti L, Menci E, Bellini M, Annunziata P. Clinical-radiologic heterogeneity of occipital neuralgiform pain as multiple sclerosis relapse. *Headache.* 2009;49:304-307.

Devigili G, Tugnoli V, Penza P, et al. The diagnostic criteria for small fibre neuropathy: from symptoms to neuropathology. *Brain.* 2008;131(Pt 7):1912-1925.

Dickinson BD, Head CA, Gitlow S, Osbahr AJ III. Maldynia: pathophysiology and management of neuropathic and maladaptive pain—a report of the AMA Council on Science and Public Health. *Pain Med.* 2010;11:1635-1653.

Dieleman JP, Kerklaan J, Huygen FJ, Bouma PA, Sturkenboom MC. Incidence rates and treatment of neuropathic pain conditions in the general population. *Pain.* 2008;137:681-688.

Duffy RL. Low back pain: an approach to diagnosis and management. *Prim Care.* 2010;37:729-741.

Dyck P. The stoop-test in lumbar entrapment radiculopathy. *Spine (Phila Pa 1976).* 1979;4:89-92.

Garza I. Craniocervical junction schwannoma mimicking occipital neuralgia. *Headache.* 2007;47:1204-1205.

Hashiguchi A, Mimata C, Ichimura H, Kuratsu J. Occipital neuralgia as a presenting symptom of cervicomedullary dural arteriovenous fistula. *Headache.* 2007;47:1095-1097.

Heinricher MM, Tavares I, Leith JL, Lumb BM. Descending control of nociception: specificity, recruitment and plasticity. *Brain Res Rev.* 2009;60:214-225.

Kalichman L, Hunter DJ. Lumbar facet joint osteoarthritis: a review. *Semin Arthritis Rheum.* 2007;37:69-80.

Maihofner C, Seifert F, Markovic K. Complex regional pain syndromes: new pathophysiological concepts and therapies. *Eur J Neurol.* 2010;17:649-660.

Markman JD, Gaud KG. Lumbar spinal stenosis in older adults: current understanding and future directions. *Clin Geriatr Med.* 2008;24:369-388.

Melzack R. Evolution of the neuromatrix theory of pain. The Prithvi Raj lecture: presented at the Third World Congress of World Institute of Pain, Barcelona 2004. *Pain Pract.* 2005;5:85-94.

Millan MJ. The induction of pain: an integrative review. *Prog Neurobiol.* 1999;57:1-16.

Mueller NH, Gilden DH, Cohrs RJ, Mahalingam R, Nagel MA. Varicella zoster virus infection: clinical features, molecular pathogenesis of disease, and latency. *Neurol Clin.* 2008;26:675-697, viii.

Pavan-Langston D. Herpes zoster antivirals and pain management. *Ophthalmology.* 2008;115:S13-S20.

Rinkus KM, Knaub MA. Clinical and diagnostic evaluation of low back pain. *Semin Spine Surg.* 2008;20:93-101.

Saab CY, Waxman SG, Hains BC. Alarm or curse? The pain of neuroinflammation. *Brain Res Rev.* 2008;58:226-235.

Schaible H, Grubb BD. Afferent and spinal mechanisms of joint pain. *Pain.* 1993;55:5-54.

Sharma RR, Parekh HC, Prabhu S, Gurusinghe NT, Bertolis G. Compression of the C-2 root by a rare anomalous ectatic vertebral artery. case report. *J Neurosurg.* 1993;78:669-672.

Tanenberg RJ, Irving GA, Risser RC, et al. Duloxetine, pregabalin, and duloxetine plus gabapentin for diabetic peripheral neuropathic pain management in patients with inadequate pain response to gabapentin: an open-label, randomized, noninferiority comparison. *Mayo Clin Proc.* 2011;86:615-626.

Todd A, Koerber H. Neuroanatomical substrates of spinal nociception. In: McMahon S, Koltzenburg M, eds. *Wall and Melzack's Textbook of Pain.* 5th ed. Elsevier; 2006:73.

Tough EA, White AR, Cummings TM, Richards SH, Campbell JL. Acupuncture and dry needling in the management of myofascial trigger point pain: a systematic review and meta-analysis of randomised controlled trials. *Eur J Pain.* 2009;13:3-10.

Tracey I, Mantyh PW. The cerebral signature for pain perception and its modulation. *Neuron.* 2007;55:377-391.

van der Windt DA, Simons E, Riphagen II, et al. Physical examination for lumbar radiculopathy due to disc herniation in patients with low-back pain. *Cochrane Database Syst Rev.* 2010;(2):CD007431.

Vanelderen P, Lataste A, Levy R. Occipital neuralgia. *Pain Pract.* 2010;102:137-144.

Varlotta GP, Lefkowitz TR, Schweitzer M, et al. The lumbar facet joint: a review of current knowledge: part II: diagnosis and management. *Skeletal Radiol.* 2011;40:149-157.

Vinik A. The approach to the management of the patient with neuropathic pain. *J Clin Endocrinol Metab.* 2010;95:4802-4811.

Wiech K, Farias M, Kahane G, Shackel N, Tiede W, Tracey I. An fMRI study measuring analgesia enhanced by religion as a belief system. *Pain.* 2008;139:467-476.

Willis Jr WD. Pain pathways in the primate. *Prog Clin Biol Res.* 1985;176:117-133.

Willis WD, Westlund KN. Neuroanatomy of the pain system and of the pathways that modulate pain. *J Clin Neurophysiol.* 1997;14:2-31.

Section 9 Floppy Infant

Darras BT, Jones Jr HR, Ryan MM, De Vivo DC, eds. *Neuromuscular Disorders of Infancy, Childhood, and Adolescence: A Clinician's Approach.* 2nd ed. Academic Press; 2014.

McMillan HJ, Kang PB. *Pediatric Electromyography: Concepts and Clinical Applications.* Springer; 2017.

Mercuri E, Pera MC, Brogna C. Neonatal hypotonia and neuromuscular conditions. *Handb Clin Neurol.* 2019;162:435-448.

Mercuri E, Pera MC, Scoto M, et al. Spinal muscular atrophy—insights and challenges in the treatment era. *Nat Rev Neurol.* 2020;16:706-715.

Prasad AN, Prasad C. Genetic evaluation of the floppy infant. *Semin Fetal Neonatal Med.* 2011;16:99-108.

Volpe JJ. Neonatal hypotonia. In: Darras BT, Jones HR, Ryan MM, De Vivo DC, eds. *Neuromuscular Disorders of Infancy, Childhood, and Adolescence: A Clinician's Approach.* 2nd ed. Academic Press; 2015:85-95.

Volpe JJ, Inder TE, Darras BT, de Vries LS, du Plessis AJ, Neil JJ, Perlman JM, eds. *Volpe's Neurology of the Newborn.* 6th ed. Elsevier; 2017.

Section 10 Motor Neuron and Its Disorders

Bento-Abreu A, Van Damme P, Van Den Bosch L, Robberrecht W. The neurobiology of amyotrophic lateral sclerosis. *Eur J Neurosci.* 2010;31:2247-2265.

Brugman F, Veldink JH, Franssen H, et al. Differentiation of hereditary spastic paraparesis from primary lateral sclerosis in sporadic adult-onset upper motor neuron syndromes. *Arch Neurol.* 2009;66:509-514.

Kiernan MC, Vucic S, Cheah BC, et al. Amyotrophic lateral sclerosis. *Lancet.* 2011;377:942-955.

Singer MA, Statland JF, Wofe GI, Barohn RJ. Primary lateral sclerosis. *Muscle Nerve.* 2007;35:291-302.

Strong MJ, Gordon PH. Primary lateral sclerosis, hereditary spastic paraplegia and amyotrophic lateral sclerosis: discrete entities or spectrum? *Amyotroph Lateral Scler Other Motor Neuron Disord.* 2005;6:8-16.

Tartaglia MC, Rowe A, Findlater K, Orange JB, Grace C, Strong MJ. Differentiation between primary lateral sclerosis and amyotrophic lateral sclerosis: examination of symptoms and signs at disease onset and during follow up. *Arch Neurol.* 2007;64:232-236.

Wijesekera LC, Leigh PN. Amyotrophic lateral sclerosis. *Orphanet J Rare Dis.* 2009:4:3.

Zinman L, Cudowicz M. Emerging target and treatments in amyotrophic lateral sclerosis. *Lancet Neurol.* 2011;10:481-490.

Section 11 Neuromuscular Junction and Its Disorders

Beeson D, Higuchi O, Palace J, et al. Dok-7 mutations underlie a neuromuscular junction synaptopathy. *Science.* 2006;313:1975-1978.

Ben Ammar, Petit AF, Alexandri N, et al. Phenotype genotype analysis in 15 patients presenting a congenital myasthenic syndrome due to mutations in DOK7. *J Neurol.* 2010;257:754-766.

Burke G, Cossins J, Maxwell S, et al. Rapsyn mutations in hereditary myasthenia: distinct early- and late-onset phenotypes. *Neurology.* 2003;61:826-828.

Burns TM, Russell JA, Lachance DH, Jones HR. Oculobulbar involvement is typical with Lambert-Eaton myasthenic syndrome. *Ann Neurol.* 2003;53:270-273.

Chevessier F, Faraut B, Ravel-Chapuis A, et al. MUSK, a new target for mutations causing congenital myasthenic syndrome. *Hum Mol Genet.* 2004;13:3229-3240.

Deymeer F, Serdaroglu P, Poda M, Gulsen-Parman Y, Ozcelik T, Ozdemir C. Clinical characteristics of a group of Turkish patients having a benign phenotype with ptosis and marked ophthalmoparesis and mutations in the acetylcholine receptor epsilon subunit gene. *Acta Myol.* 2000;19:29-32.

Donger C, Krejci E, Serradell AP, et al. Mutation in the human acetylcholinesterase-associated collagen gene, COLQ, is responsible for congenital myasthenic syndrome with end-plate acetylcholinesterase deficiency (Type Ic). *Am J Hum Genet.* 1998;63:967-975.

Drachman DB. Myasthenia gravis. *N Engl J Med.* 1994;330:1797-1810.

Engel AG, Ohno K, Bouzat C, Sine SM, Griggs RC. End-plate acetylcholine receptor deficiency due to nonsense mutations in the epsilon subunit. *Ann Neurol.* 1996;40:810-817.

Engel AG, Ohno K, Sine SM. Congenital myasthenic syndromes. In: Engel A, Franzini-Armstrong C, eds. *Myology.* McGraw-Hill; 2004:1755-1790.

Engel AG, Shen XM, Selcen D, Sine SM. What have we learned from the congenital myasthenic syndromes. *J Mol Neurosci.* 2010;40:143-153.

Gottstein B, Pozio E, Nöckler K. Epidemiology, diagnosis, treatment, and control of trichinellosis. *Clin Microbiol Rev.* 2009;22:127-145.

Gronseth GS, Barohn RJ. Practice parameter: thymectomy for autoimmune myasthenia gravis (an evidence-based review): report of the Quality Standards Subcommittee of the American Academy of Neurology. *Neurology.* 2000;55:7-15.

Gutmann L, Phillips LH, Gutmann L. Trends in the association of Lambert-Eaton myasthenic syndrome with carcinoma. *Neurology.* 1992;42:848-850.

Huze C, Bauche S, Richard P, et al. Identification of an agrin mutation that causes congenital myasthenia and affects synapse function. *Am J Hum Genet.* 2009;85:155-167.

Keesey JC. Clinical evaluation and management of myasthenia gravis. *Muscle Nerve.* 2004;29:484-505.

Lambert EH, Eaton LM, Rooke ED. Defect of neuromuscular conduction associated with malignant neoplasms. *Am J Physiol.* 1956;187:612-613.

Lashley D, Palace J, Jayawant S, Robb S, Beeson D. Ephedrine treatment in congenital myasthenic syndrome due to mutations in DOK7. *Neurology.* 2010;74:1517-1523.

Meriggioli MN, Sanders DB. Myasthenia gravis: diagnosis. *Semin Neurol.* 2004;24:31-39.

Mihaylova V, Müller JS, Vilchez JJ, et al. Clinical and molecular genetic findings in COLQ-mutant congenital myasthenic syndromes. *Brain.* 2008;131(Pt 3):747-759.

Mihaylova V, Salih MA, Mukhtar MM, et al. Refinement of the clinical phenotype in musk-related congenital myasthenic syndromes. *Neurology.* 2009;73:1926-1928.

Milone M, Shen XM, Selcen D, et al. Myasthenic syndrome due to defects in rapsyn: clinical and molecular findings in 39 patients. *Neurology.* 2009;73:228-235.

Muller JS, Herczegfalvi A, Vilchez JJ, et al. Phenotypical spectrum of DOK7 mutations in congenital myasthenic syndromes. *Brain.* 2007;130(Pt 6):1497-1506.

Muller JS, Mildner G, Müller-Felber W, et al. Rapsyn N88K is a frequent cause of congenital myasthenic syndromes in European patients. *Neurology.* 2003;60:1805-1810.

Ohno K, Brengman J, Tsujino A, Engel AG. Human endplate acetylcholinesterase deficiency caused by mutations in the collagen-like tail subunit (ColQ) of the asymmetric enzyme. *Proc Natl Acad Sci U S A.* 1998;95:9654-9659.

Ohno K, Engel AG, Shen XM, et al. Rapsyn mutations in humans cause endplate acetylcholine-receptor deficiency and myasthenic syndrome. *Am J Hum Genet.* 2002;70:875-885.

Ohno K, Hutchinson DO, Milone M, et al. Congenital myasthenic syndrome caused by prolonged acetylcholine receptor channel openings due to a mutation in the M2 domain of the epsilon subunit. *Proc Natl Acad Sci U S A.* 1995;92:758-762.

Ohno K, Tsujino A, Brengman JM, et al. Choline acetyltransferase mutations cause myasthenic syndrome associated with episodic apnea in humans. *Proc Natl Acad Sci U S A.* 2001;98: 2017-2022.

Ohno K, Wang HL, Milone M, et al. Congenital myasthenic syndrome caused by decreased agonist binding affinity due to a mutation in the acetylcholine receptor epsilon subunit. *Neuron.* 1996;17: 157-170.

O'Neil JH, Murray NMF, Newsom-Davis J. The Lambert-Eaton myasthenic syndrome: a review of 50 cases. *Brain.* 1988;111: 577-596.

Palace J, Lashley D, Newsom-Davis J, et al. Clinical features of the DOK7 neuromuscular junction synaptopathy. *Brain.* 2007;130 (Pt 6):1507-1515.

Phillips LH. The epidemiology of myasthenia gravis. *Semin Neurol.* 2004;24:17-20.

Sanders DB, El-Salem K, Massey JM, McConville J, Vincent A. Clinical aspects of MuSK antibody positive seronegative MG. *Neurology.* 2003;60:1978-1980.

Schara U, Christen HJ, Durmus H, et al. Long-term follow-up in patients with congenital myasthenic syndrome due to CHAT mutations. *Eur J Paediatr Neurol.* 2010;14:326-333.

Schara U, Lochmüller H. Therapeutic strategies in congenital myasthenic syndromes. *Neurotherapeutics.* 2008;5:542-547.

Selcen D, Milone M, Shen XM, et al. Dok-7 myasthenia: phenotypic and molecular genetic studies in 16 patients. *Ann Neurol.* 2008;64:71-87.

Sine SM, Ohno K, Bouzat C, et al. Mutation of the acetylcholine receptor alpha subunit causes a slow-channel myasthenic syndrome by enhancing agonist binding affinity. *Neuron.* 1995;15:229-239.

Skeie GO, Apostolski S, Evoli A, et al. Guidelines for treatment of autoimmune neuromuscular transmission disorders. *Eur J Neurol.* 2010;17:893-902.

Sobel J. Diagnosis and treatment of botulism: a century later, clinical suspicion remains the cornerstone. *Clin Infect Dis.* 2009;48: 1674-1675.

Sobel J, Painter J. Illnesses caused by marine toxins. *Clin Infect Dis.* 2005;41:1290-1296.

Titulaer MJ, Maddison P, Sont JK, et al. Clinical Dutch-English Lambert-Eaton Myasthenic syndrome (LEMS) tumor association prediction score accurately predicts small-cell lung cancer in the LEMS. *J Clin Oncol.* 2011;29:902-908.

Tseng-Ong L, Mitchell WG. Infant botulism: 20 years' experience at a single institution. *J Child Neurol.* 2007;22:1333-1337.

Tsujino A, Maertens C, Ohno K, et al. Myasthenic syndrome caused by mutation of the SCN4A sodium channel. *Proc Natl Acad Sci U S A.* 2003;100:7377-7382.

Vincent A, McConville J, Farrugia ME, et al. Antibodies in myasthenia gravis and related disorders. *Ann N Y Acad Sci.* 2003;998:324-335.

Section 12 Muscle and Its Disorders

Ahmed ST, Craven L, Russell OM, Turnbull DM, Vincent AE. Diagnosis and treatment of mitochondrial myopathies. *Neurotherapeutics.* 2018;15:943-953.

Barohn RJ, Dimachkie MM, Jackson CE. A pattern recognition approach to patients with a suspected myopathy. *Neurol Clin.* 2014;32(3):569-593.

Bockhorst J, Wicklund M. Limb girdle muscular dystrophies. *Neurol Clin.* 2020;38(3):493-504.

Cabral BMI, Edding SN, Portocarrero JP, Lerma EV. Rhabdomyolysis. *Dis Mon.* 2020;66:101015.

Darras BT, Urion D, Ghosh PS. *Dystrophinopathies.* University of Washington; 2018.

De Visser M. Late-onset myopathies: clinical features and diagnosis. *Acta Myol.* 2020;39(4):235-244.

Domingos J, Sarkozy A, Scoto M, Muntoni F. Dystrophinopathies and limb-girdle muscular dystrophies. *Neuropediatrics.* 2017;48(4): 262-272.

Doughty CT, Amato AA. Toxic myopathies. *Continuum (Minneap Minn).* 2019;25:1712-1731.

Findlay AR, Goyal NA, Mozaffar T. An overview of polymyositis and dermatomyositis. *Muscle Nerve.* 2015;51(5):638-656.

Goyal NA. Immune-mediated myopathies. *Continuum (Minneap Minn).* 2019;25(6):1564-1585.

Greenberg SA. Inclusion body myositis: clinical features and pathogenesis. *Nat Rev Rheumatol.* 2019;15(5):257-272.

Hamel J, Tawil R. Facioscapulohumeral muscular dystrophy: update on pathogenesis and future treatments. *Neurotherapeutics.* 2018;15(4):863-871.

Johnson NE. Myotonic muscular dystrophies. *Continuum (Minneap Minn).* 2019;25(6):1682-1695.

Katzberg HD, Kassardjian CD. Toxic and endocrine myopathies. *Continuum (Minneap Minn).* 2016;22:1815-1828.

Kaya Y, Sarikcioglu L. Sir William Richard Gowers (1845-1915) and his eponym. Yasemin Kaya & Levent Sarikcioglu. *Childs Nerv Syst.* 2015;31:633-635.

Kress JP, Hall JB. ICU-acquired weakness and recovery from critical illness. *N Engl J Med.* 2014;370:1626-1635.

Lawal TA, Todd JJ, Witherspoon JW, et al. Ryanodine receptor 1-related disorders: an historical perspective and proposal for a unified nomenclature. *Skelet Muscle.* 2020;10:32.

Lilleker JB, Keh YS, Roncaroli F, Sharma R, Roberts M. Metabolic myopathies: a practical approach. *Pract Neurol.* 2018;18(1):14-26.

Meola G. Myotonic dystrophy type 2: the 2020 update. *Acta Myol.* 2020;39(4):222-234.

Mohassel P, Mammen AL. Anti-HMGCR myopathy. *J Neuromuscul Dis.* 2018;5(1):11-20.

Riazi S, Kraeva N, Hopkins PM. Malignant hyperthermia in the post-genomics era: new perspectives on an old concept. *Anesthesiology.* 2018;128:168-180.

Selva-O'Callaghan A, Pinal-Fernandez I, Trallero-Araguás E, Milisenda JC, Grau-Junyent JM, Mammen AL. Classification and management of adult inflammatory myopathies. *Lancet Neurol.* 2018;17(9):816-828.

Statland JM, Fontaine B, Hanna MG, et al. Review of the diagnosis and treatment of periodic paralysis. *Muscle Nerve.* 2018;57:522-530.

Stunnenberg BC, LoRusso S, Arnold WD, et al. Guidelines on clinical presentation and management of nondystrophic myotonias. *Muscle Nerve.* 2020;62(4):430-444.

Tanboon J, Nishino I. Classification of idiopathic inflammatory myopathies: pathology perspectives. *Curr Opin Neurol.* 2019;32(5):704-714.

Tarnopolsky MA. Myopathies related to glycogen metabolism disorders. *Neurotherapeutics.* 2018;15:915-927.

Uruha A, Goebel HH, Stenzel W. Updates on the immunopathology in idiopathic inflammatory myopathies. *Curr Rheumatol Rep.* 2021;23(7):56.

Wang LH, Tawil R. Current therapeutic approaches in FSHD. *J Neuromuscul Dis.* 2021;8(3):441-451.

Weihl CC. Sporadic inclusion body myositis and other rimmed vacuolar myopathies. *Continuum (Minneap Minn).* 2019;25(6): 1586-1598.

Yamashita S. Recent progress in oculopharyngeal muscular dystrophy. *J Clin Med.* 2021;10(7):1375.

Z'Graggen WJ, Tankisi H. Critical illness myopathy. *J Clin Neurophysiol.* 2020;37:200-204.